Handbook of Motivation and Cognition
VOLUME 2

HANDBOOK OF
MOTIVATION AND COGNITION
Foundations of Social Behavior
VOLUME 2

Edited by

E. Tory Higgins
Columbia University

Richard M. Sorrentino
University of Western Ontario

THE GUILFORD PRESS
New York • London

© 1990 The Guilford Press
A Division of Guilford Publications, Inc.
72 Spring Street, New York, NY 10012

Printed in the United States of America

This book is printed on acid-free paper.

Last digit is print number: 9 8 7 6 5 4 3 2 1

Library of Congress Cataloging-in-Publication Data

(Revised for volume 2)

Handbook of motivation and cognition.

Includes bibliographies and indexes.
1. Motivation (Psychology) 2. Cognition. 3. Inter-
personal relations. I. Sorrentino, Richard M.
II. Higgins, E. Tory (Edward Tory), 1946–
BF503.H36 1986 153.8 85-24916
ISBN 0-89862-667-6 (v. 1)

ISBN 0-89862-432-0 (v. 2)

Contributors

John A. Bargh, PhD, Department of Psychology, New York University, New York, New York

Charles S. Carver, PhD, Department of Psychology, University of Miami, Coral Gables, Florida

Robert B. Cialdini, PhD, Department of Psychology, Arizona State University, Tempe, Arizona

Norman T. Feather, PhD, Department of Psychology, The Flinders University of South Australia, Adelaide, South Australia, Australia

Peter M. Gollwitzer, PhD, Max-Planck-Institut für psychologische Forschung, Münich, Federal Republic of Germany

E. Tory Higgins, PhD, Department of Psychology, Columbia University, New York, New York

Larry L. Jacoby, PhD, Department of Psychology, McMaster University, Hamilton, Ontario, Canada

Marcia K. Johnson, PhD, Department of Psychology, Princeton University, Princeton, New Jersey

Colleen M. Kelley, PhD, Department of Psychology, Williams College, Williamstown, Massachusetts

Arie W. Kruglanski, PhD, Department of Psychology, University of Maryland–College Park, College Park, Maryland

Richard R. Lau, PhD, Department of Political Sciences, Rutgers University, New Brunswick, New Jersey

David C. McClelland, PhD, Center for Applied Social Science, Boston University, Boston, Massachusetts

Leonard S. Newman, PhD, Department of Psychology, New York University, New York, New York

Janet Polivy, PhD, Department of Psychology, University of Toronto, Erindale Campus, Mississauga, Ontario, Canada

Joel O. Raynor, PhD, Department of Psychology, State University of New York at Buffalo, Amherst, New York

William S. Rholes, PhD, Department of Psychology, Texas A&M University, College Station, Texas

Diane N. Ruble, PhD, Department of Psychology, New York University, New York, New York

Mark Schaller, PhD, Department of Psychology, University of Texas at Arlington, Arlington, Texas

v

Michael F. Scheier, PhD, Department of Psychology, Carnegie Mellon University, Pittsburgh, Pennsylvania

Norbert Schwarz, Dr. phil. habil., Zentrum für Umfragen, Methoden und Analysen, ZUMA, Mannheim, and Department of Psychology, University of Heidelberg, Federal Republic of Germany

Steven J. Sherman, PhD, Department of Psychology, Indiana University, Bloomington, Indiana

Judith-Ann C. Short, PhD, Children's Psychiatric Unit, Victoria Hospital, London, Ontario, Canada

Richard M. Sorrentino, PhD, Department of Psychology, University of Western Ontario, London, Ontario, Canada

William B. Swann, Jr., PhD, Department of Psychology, University of Texas-Austin, Austin, Texas

Yaacov Trope, PhD, Department of Psychology, Hebrew University, Jerusalem, Israel

Joel Weinberger, PhD, Derner Institute of Advanced Psychological Studies, Adelphi University, Garden City, New York

Jo Marie Zubek, BA, Department of Psychology, State University of New York at Buffalo, Amherst, New York

Preface

This is the second volume of the *Handbook of Motivation and Cognition: Foundations of Social Behavior*. The general purpose of both volumes has been to elicit original chapters specifically for the *Handbook* that present theory and research on the interface of motivation and cognition. Obtaining such chapters was somewhat more difficult in the first volume because at that time there was less explicit consideration of motivation–cognition interrelations. Since then, synergistic approaches to motivation and cognition, the "Warm Look," have become rather hot in psychology. Thus, this time the problem has been more how to select chapters for the second volume. Indeed, a series of volumes on the motivation–cognition interface is probably necessary at this stage to cover the full extent of this exciting new area. Nevertheless, the chapters in this volume, together with those in the first volume, cover many of the most influential and exciting research programs and theories in this area.

This second volume of the *Handbook* continues to emphasize theory and research on the motivation–cognition interface, but it expands the range of approaches considered by including contributions reflecting clinical, developmental, political, and cognitive psychological perspectives in addition to social and personality perspectives. While expanding the range of approaches considered, this volume also addresses specific issues at a greater level of detail than the previous volume, including such key issues as the nature of self-regulation and self-control, the role of affect, value, and inference in social action, and motivation–cognition relations in social understanding.

CHAPTER SUMMARIES

In order to provide the reader (and re-reader) with a brief description of the issues, proposals, and perspectives found in each chapter, we have written a brief summary of each chapter. These summaries emphasize the authors' proposals and perspectives rather than research findings because we believe that new ideas are especially likely to inspire new research on the motivation–cognition interface.

Part I addresses issues concerning *self-regulation and self-control*. Carver and Scheier propose that human behavior is a continual process of moving toward various kinds of represented goals and that this movement occurs by a process of feedback control. They suggest that a system of self-regulation, an internal guidance system, underlies human behavior. Stored knowledge is used both for understanding in information processing and for use as a prescriptive guide for action. There is a weaving together of interpretive knowledge and behavioral knowledge into patterns of association, which in different situations can evoke different behavior options. People are motivated to reduce any sensed discrepancy between existing conditions and some reference value. Self-focused attention promotes monitoring of such discrepancies. Feedback systems can be interconnected and ordered hierarchically. Disengagement of the self-regulatory process can occur when expectations of successful discrepancy reduction are low. Emotion is both a determinant and a consequence of self-regulation. A key determinant of people's emotions is their sense of progress in reducing their discrepancies—their sensed rate of progress as well as changes in the rate of progress.

Gollwitzer asks the question, "How do people choose, plan, enact, and evaluate actions?" His chapter first reviews the previous literature that has addressed this question. Choice motivation is distinguished from control motivation. Four distinct phases in the course of action are described. The predecisional action phase involves wishing and deliberating. The decision-making and preactional phase involves transforming wishes into goal intentions and goal planning. The action initiation phase involves commitment to implementing the goal and volitional strength. The goal achievement and postactional phase involves evaluating outcomes of the action. Gollwitzer suggests that the concept of "mind-set" can be used to specify the distinct tasks or demands to be solved at each of the four phases; what phase-typical cognitive orientation promotes completion of each task? A deliberative mind-set, for example, should promote relatively accurate, open, and impartial processing in regard to the desirability and feasibility of alternative goals. In contrast, an implemental mind-set should promote relatively biased, closed, and partial processing that is optimistic with respect to a chosen goal's desirability and feasibility. Evidence supporting the distinction between a deliberative versus an implemental mind-set is then presented.

Bargh raises the issue of how much control a person exercises over his or her own thought and behavior in social situations. What other agents of control exist and what is the extent of their influence? Bargh argues that while responses may be strongly influenced by the environment and preconscious processes, an intervening intention is required to make the response itself. Intentional, goal-directed responding can overcome automatic tendencies in information processing and action. Bargh suggests that the key question then becomes, "Where do goals come from?" He proposes that instead of being under "executive" control, much goal-setting activity may be initiated by patterns of environmental features. It may be the environment itself that activates the goal or intent. More specifically, chronic representations of goals (or intents) and those environmental features with which they are frequently and consistently associated (e.g., because these are the situations in which the goals are typically pursued) may become interconnected in memory. Thus, goals or intentions would be automatically activated whenever relevant situational features were present in the environment. And these goals and intentions can guide thought and behavior outside of awareness in the service of the individual and not simply to satisfy the desires or demands of the social environment.

Polivy describes a model that integrates feelings that arise from or are accompanied by sensations inside the body (including emotions, hunger, thirst, sexual arousal, drug cravings) with cognitions and behaviors. She suggests that internal sensations are cues for behavior. They may be interpreted cognitively and then acted upon either appropriately (i.e., in accordance with the internal feeling) or inappropriately. Inappropriate action includes inhibiting the appropriate behavior or attempting to substitute an alternative. Polivy focuses on the effects of suppressing internally cued behavior. She proposes that ignoring internal signals for behavior or inhibiting appropriate behavioral responses produces distress and maladaptive behavior. And this is true for almost any internal drive or activity of "feeling." Various costs of inhibiting behaviors are then described, including how repressive coping styles, inhibiting trauma experiences, and inhibiting or suppressing internally cued behaviors (e.g., eating, smoking, alcohol drinking) all lead to or promote health problems and behavioral excess. The difficulty of inhibiting stimulated behavior and the role of society in pressing for inhibition are then discussed. Polivy then considers the functions of emotions as a behavior cue, how emotions both guide action for the individual and communicate appropriate reactions to observers. Catharsis is beneficial when it involves responding appropriately to one's feelings. To ignore one's feelings has negative consequences. Cognition can cause problems if it causes one to respond inappropriately to emotional cues.

Part II considers *the role of affect, value, and inference as sources of action.* Feather provides a review and update of expectancy–value theory. This theory relates people's actions to their perception of the attractiveness or aversiveness of expected outcomes. It is used to investigate relations between the values that people hold and their actions in defined situations. Expectations include beliefs about whether a particular action can be performed to some required standard that defines a successful outcome and beliefs about the various positive and negative consequences that might follow the outcome. Values induce valences on events and objects within the psychological environment. There are developmental trends in the emergence of value priorities. Values play a key role in the choices that individuals make, in the plans that guide their behavior, and in the way they justify their decisions. Values express both motivational concerns and societal demands. They have a normative quality and also function as criteria or frameworks for testing expectations. Values are more readily activated in a situation if they are strongly held and there are cues in the situation that trigger them off. Expectations and values can affect one another.

Sorrentino, Raynor, Zubek, and Short propose that a combination of Raynor's theory of personality functioning and change and Sorrentino's research and theory on uncertainty orientation can provide the basis for an integration of the two major camps in developmental psychology: the organismic–structuralists and the mechanistic–functionalists. Uncertainty orientation is proposed as a fundamental organismic variable that governs development in the cognitive, moral, and ego-identity areas. The authors' purpose is to specify more precisely the conditions under which motivational and environmental forces will enhance or inhibit development in each of these areas. They propose that as a consequence of past experience, people will emerge from childhood with markedly different expectations about themselves and the world around them. And, most important, people will move toward or away from later developmental stages depending upon the informational and affective value they perceive in situations related to these stages. The theory of personality functioning assumes that maximization of positive value (both informational and affective) and minimization of negative value are the basic functions of personality. In regard to the self-system, affective value involves self-esteem from evaluation (feelings about me) and informational value involves clarity or confusion about self-attributes (knowledge about who I am). Uncertainty orientation reflects individual differences in information value and strategies for possessing clarity. It is hypothesized that uncertainty-oriented individuals are more likely than certainty-oriented individuals to reach the final stages described by developmental stage theorists, to prefer principled moral reasoning, and to reach the highest levels of ego-identity development.

Higgins and Trope propose a new model, "activity engagement theory," to address the issue of what determines people's motivational responses when they are engaging an input. They first consider this issue by reviewing the previous literature distinguishing intrinsic from extrinsic motivation. Activity engagement theory is then presented as an alternative perspective on people's affective and inferential responses to engaging an input. Activity engagement theory proposes that there are many possible activity identifications for any input, including both primary and secondary identifications. The primary activity identification determines the relevance and significance of the different input properties. The relation between the primary and secondary activity identifications influences people's affective and inferential responses to the input. These responses, in turn, influence subsequent engagement with the input depending upon how the input is subsequently identified. Higgins and Trope then propose to define intrinsic and extrinsic motivation in terms of whether it is properties inherent to or extraneous from the input, respectively, that the primary identification has made relevant. Previous and prospective research on intrinsic and extrinsic motivation is then considered in terms of this proposal.

Schaller and Cialdini begin by pointing out that although there has been no shortage of possible explanations for the effects of mood on helping, the focus of each has been on a constrained set of moderators or mediators of particular theoretical interest. An intergrative reconciliation of alternative accounts has not been provided. Schaller and Cialdini suggest that what needs to be considered is how attentional and cognitive processes interact with motivational processes in directing effects of mood on helping. They then offer a model to fulfill this aim, with the effects on helping of happiness and sadness as temporary mood states receiving specific emphasis. The model contains a variety of proposals. For example, it is proposed that sad individuals will withdraw attention from the environment and focus upon the self, whereas happy individuals will be more likely to focus upon the environment. The helping responses of sad individuals will be more dependent upon careful consideration of factors related to hedonic consequences. Sadness leads to an enhanced drive to restore a disrupted mood state to its prior level, whereas happiness leads to a less focused motive toward greater personal attainment. Sadness is more likely to lead to a reduced level of arousal and activity. And sadness and happiness differ in whether negative versus positive thoughts, respectively, are relatively more accessible. These and other proposed differences between sadness and happiness are then used to account for a wide variety of findings in the literature on helping behavior.

Lau's chapter focuses on individuals' political actions and begins with the premise that the study of individual political behavior must be based, at least implicitly, on some underlying psychological theory of human motivation and behavior. Lau reviews the changes in the dominant theories of individual political behavior from the 1950s to the '80s. In the '50s, "psychodynamic" models were influential, with emphasis on unconscious motivations, displacement of intrapsychic needs, such as power needs, and so on. As for psychology in general, motivational theories of political action dominated in the '60s—in particular, motivation for cognitive consistency, such as perceiving and acting consistent with party identifications and beliefs. As psychology became more "cognitive" in the '70s, so too did models of individual political behavior. Economic, rational-choice models predominated, in which it was assumed that people were motivated to calculate self-interest rationally in relation to financial and material goals. Following this review, Lau describes two major challenges to the "economic" model. First, the "symbolic politics" model argues that individuals possess important motives other than self-interest and financial or material gain, such as symbolic attitudes of collective significance (e.g., nationalism, racism). Second, "information-processing" models argue that individuals' calculations are often not as "rational" as the economic model assumes because of people's cognitive limitations. Evidence of constraints on processing is then presented.

Part III considers *the role of motivation and cognition in understanding self and others*. Kruglanski begins by asking, "Are motivational and informational factors parameters of the same process whereby all attributions are made?" He then raises the issue of whether any motive is potentially relevant to the attribution process. His position is that any judgment, attributional or otherwise, is at once motivated and informationally based. Kruglanski supports this position by discussing the relation between lay epistemic motivations and attributional processes. The lay epistemic process involves a two-phase sequence: hypothesis generation and hypothesis validation. Two sources of cessation of each phase are capability (availability and accessibility) and the epistemic motivations of closure seeking (seek–avoid) and specificity (specific–nonspecific). All epistemic motivations are assumed to arise from the individual's perceived costs/benefits analysis of given epistemic end states, which can vary by situation or by person. The system is "unfrozen" (set in motion) when there is a perceived discrepancy between the actual versus desired epistemic end state. Kruglanski reviews various studies demonstrating the effects of the different kinds of epistemic motivations on judgment and behavior. He then describes how motivation is an inseparable part of judgmental activities in general, and how lay epistemic motivations function together with "informational" attribution principles in particular.

Rholes, Newman, and Ruble describe how developmental changes in children's understanding of dispositions impact on their motivational processes. They argue that during early and middle childhood, as a function of both cognitive changes and social-life-phase changes, children gradually come to understand dispositions to be invariant structures, that is, abiding, constant aspects of persons that exert a consistent influence on behaviors across situations and time. Because of this development, some social experiences and information acquire new meanings and importance for children. And this, in turn, can transform their motivational processes, including their achievement motivation, self-evaluation, interpersonal interactions, and internalization of prosocial values. Rholes et al. point out significant parallels between the determinants and consequences of dispositional knowledge and the determinants and consequences of gender constancy, which is another form of knowledge about personal invariance. They also distinguish among various expectancy-formation processes for predicting behavior, such as matching situation to situation, behavioral valence to behavioral valence, behavioral labeling to behavioral labeling, and inferred behavioral source to inferred behavioral source. Finally, they outline a set of principles concerning the relation between social-cognitive developmental changes and changes in motivation and behavior, including cognitive consistency needs, the meaning of events, and interest in acquiring trait-relevant information.

Swann considers the interplay of self-enhancement and self-verification. He asks, "What do people want to believe about themselves?" He argues that both self-enhancement and self-verification processes are sufficiently robust that neither can be ruled out. It is true both that people like to be liked and that people are motivated to maintain an idea about themselves. And these motivations can work together (e.g., high-self-esteem persons) or be in conflict (e.g., low-self-esteem persons). With respect to social feedback in particular, people are motivated both to receive positive feedback about themselves (because of their need for praise and love) and to receive feedback that is consistent with their self-beliefs (because of their need to believe that the social world is predictable and controllable). Swann proposes that the process of self-enhancement requires only that the feedback be identified as favorable or unfavorable. In contrast, the process of self-verification requires identification of the self-attribute contained in the feedback, accessing stored beliefs about one's self-attributes, and comparing these self-attributes. Swann suggests that this difference means that self-verification has more complex conditional rules for approaching and avoiding feedback than does self-evaluation, which, in turn, means that self-verification requires additional mental work. He then describes a variety of motivational implications of this difference in mental effort, such as the effects of depriving people of cognitive resources or manipulating the accessibility or certainty of people's self-beliefs.

Part IV considers *various forms of motivation–cognition interrelations*. Jacoby and Kelley present the thesis that behavior is often guided by unconscious influences of memory for prior episodes, and that the presence of such unconscious influences places limits on conscious, intentional control of behavior. They suggest that the unconscious influences originate from a myriad of mundane experiences rather than from traumatic experiences or unresolved conflicts. Their concern is with the effects of prior experience independent of conscious memory for the relevant prior experience. They propose that a consideration of unconscious influences of memory for prior episodes has advantages over the traditional emphasis on influences of abstract knowledge representations, such as schemas. They argue that behavior is locally controlled by the specific configuration of a situation that elicits the retrieval of similar prior events, and that the effects of motivational variables are more controlled by local circumstances than would be expected if an abstract knowledge representation were responsible for directing behavior. As for episodic memory in general, factors that affect encoding and retrieval should both be important for motivation. They dispute the classic notion of drive plus habit producing behavior, and suggest instead that often the source of the energy for a behavior is not separate from the control of the behavior by prior experiences. Jacoby and Kelley also distinguish between "memory as tool" and "memory as object." With regard to the latter, they present evidence suggesting that the subjective experience of remembering an episode depends on attributional processes and thus is vulnerable to errors of source attribution and heuristic biases (e.g., a "fluency heuristic").

Johnson and Sherman ask the question, "To what extent are our memories of the past and anticipations of the future veridical?" They propose that the past, present, and future fold backward and forward like Japanese origami. Both the past and the future are constructed and reconstructed in the present, and the past and future construct the present. This origami quality of time derives from many psychological factors, including preconceptions, confusions about sources of information, mood, focus of attention, considerations of possible alternatives, and strategies for seeking and evaluating information. In origami time, cognition and motivation often have a mutually metamorphic relation that makes it difficult to separate cognitive and motivational sources of bias. Motivation and cognition interact both at a given moment in time and across time. Johnson and Sherman review evidence of various psychological factors involved in the construction and reconstruction of the past and future. In discussing the past, they raise the issue of veridicality—how do people distinguish reality from fantasy? Reality monitoring and reality constraints are described. Constraints on thinking about the future are also considered, as well as how prediction, biased imaginings, and other thoughts about the future can help to create the future.

Schwarz examines the informative functions of affective states and proposes that affective states inform people about the nature of the situation in which the affective states are experienced. He argues that the impact of affective states on evaluative judgments are not mediated by the effects of affective states on selective recall. Rather, the affective state is a piece of information that may bear on the judgment task according to a "how do I feel about it?" heuristic. He also suggests that in decision making or problem solving affective states may influence the choice of processing strategies. Negative affect informs the person that its current situation is problematic, which motivates changing and carefully assessing the current situation and fosters the use of effortful, detail-oriented analytical processing. In contrast, positive affect informs the person that the personal world is nonproblematic and there is little need to engage in effortful cognitive activity, which fosters the use of less effortful heuristic strategies. Schwarz also raises the question, "When are judgments based on one's affective state rather than on other kinds of information?" He suggests that judgments may be based on one's affective state when the judgment at hand is affective in nature and/or is too complex or cumbersome to make on the basis of a piecemeal information-processing strategy. He also suggests the need to distinguish between different types of negative and positive affective states and to consider the cognitive asymmetry between approach and avoidance situations.

Weinberger and McClelland are concerned with contrasting and reconciling two major approaches to motivation: traditional motivation theories that see motivation as primarily affective and theories that treat motivation as a cognitive phenomenon. As an exemplar of the former approach, McClelland's most recent and complete model of motivation is described. Then, various informational cognitive conceptions of motivation are reviewed. These two types of approaches are then critically compared. Although these two approaches are apparently irreconcilable, Weinberger and McClelland propose a resolution in terms of there being two distinct kinds of motivation—one affectively based and one cognitively based. They suggest that these two kinds of motivation reflect different kinds of phenomena, predict different classes of behavior, and follow qualitatively different rules (although they can function in parallel). Affectively based motives, or "implicit motives," are based on a limited number of biologically based needs that exist in everyone. Individual differences in these needs are innate or are the result of prelinguistic learning. They are best measured in free-response situations. Cognitively based motives, or "self-attributed motives," are tied to self-conceptions learned after language acquisition and are activated by making the self-system relevant. They are unique to humans. There are an unlimited number of potential motives and there are large individual differences. They are best assessed by self-report measures.

It is evident from the foregoing chapter summaries that an extensive array of perspectives on the motivation–cognition interface is covered in the present volume. Synergistic approaches are presented that include the cognitive underpinnings of motivational processes and action (e.g., Bargh; Carver & Scheier; Gollwitzer; Higgins & Trope; Jacoby & Kelley; Rholes, Newman, & Ruble), the motivational underpinnings of cognitive processes and action (e.g., Feather; Kruglanski; Johnson and Sherman; Polivy; Schwarz), and distinctions between different kinds of motivation-cognition relations underlying action (e.g., Lau; Schaller & Cialdini; Sorrentino, Raynor, Zubek, & Short; Swann; Weinberger & McClelland). Within this range of approaches, many of the most important and fascinating questions concerning the motivation–cognition interface are addressed in this book.

ACKNOWLEDGMENTS

We wish first to express our sincere appreciation to the contributors to this volume who are, in fact, the coauthors of this book. Once again, it is evident from their chapters that issues concerning the motivation–cognition interface and the "Warm Look" excite them as much as they excite us. Like the eventual reader, we have learned a tremendous amount from reading (and re-reading) the chapters in this volume. The Guilford Press, and particularly Seymour Weingarten, has again given us the kind of support and encouragement that makes this enterprise both worthwhile and enjoyable. As the roots of our deepest thoughts and feelings, we give our warmest thanks to our wives and children—Robin, Judy, Kayla, and Eric!

Contents

PART I   *Self-Regulation and Self-Control*

CHAPTER 1   **Principles of Self-Regulation: Action and**   3
Emotion   *Charles S. Carver* and
Michael F. Scheier

CHAPTER 2   **Action Phases and Mind-Sets**   53
Peter M. Gollwitzer

CHAPTER 3   **Auto-Motives: Preconscious Determinants of**   93
Social Interaction   *John A. Bargh*

CHAPTER 4   **Inhibition of Internally Cued Behavior**   131
Janet Polivy

PART II   *Affect, Value, and Inference as Sources of Action*

CHAPTER 5   **Bridging the Gap between Values and Actions:**   151
Recent Applications of the Expectancy–Value
Model   *Norman T. Feather*

CHAPTER 6   **Personality Functioning and Change:**   193
Informational and Affective Influences on
Cognitive, Moral, and Social Development
Richard M. Sorrentino, Joel O. Raynor,
Jo Marie Zubek, and *Judith-Ann C. Short*

CHAPTER 7   **Activity Engagement Theory: Implications of**   229
Multiply Identifiable Input for Intrinsic
Motivation   *E. Tory Higgins* and *Yaacov Trope*

CHAPTER 8   **Happiness, Sadness, and Helping: A Motivational**   265
Integration   *Mark Schaller* and *Robert B. Cialdini*

CHAPTER 9   **Political Motivation and Political**   297
                   Cognition   *Richard R. Lau*

    PART III   *Motivation and Cognition in Understanding Self*
               and Others

CHAPTER 10   **Motivations for Judging and Knowing:**   333
                   Implications for Causal Attribution
                   Arie W. Kruglanski

CHAPTER 11   **Understanding Self and Other: Developmental**   369
                   and Motivational Aspects of Perceiving Persons in
                   Terms of Invariant Dispositions   *William S. Rholes,*
                   Leonard S. Newman, and *Diane N. Ruble*

CHAPTER 12   **To Be Adored or to Be Known?: The Interplay of**   408
                   Self-Enhancement and Self-Verification
                   William B. Swann, Jr.

    PART IV   *Theories Relating Motivation and Cognition*

CHAPTER 13   **An Episodic View of Motivation: Unconscious**   451
                   Influences of Memory   *Larry L. Jacoby* and
                   Colleen M. Kelley

CHAPTER 14   **Constructing and Reconstructing the Past and the**   482
                   Future in the Present   *Marcia K. Johnson* and
                   Steven J. Sherman

CHAPTER 15   **Feelings as Information: Informational and**   527
                   Motivational Functions of Affective
                   States   *Norbert Schwarz*

CHAPTER 16   **Cognitive versus Traditional Motivational Models:**   562
                   Irreconcilable or Complementary?
                   Joel Weinberger and *David C. McClelland*

    Author Index   598
    Subject Index   613

PART I

Self-Regulation and Self-Control

CHAPTER 1

Principles of Self-Regulation

Action and Emotion

CHARLES S. CARVER
University of Miami

MICHAEL F. SCHEIER
Carnegie Mellon University

What is the nature of the basic processes that underlie overt human behavior? The concept of motivation, which is prominent in the title of this handbook, was developed as part of the attempt to answer this question. People act in particular ways because they are "motivated" to do so. To say this is a start, but hardly more than that. To say that motives result in behavior says nothing about the nature of the processes referenced by (or following from) the term "motive"; it says only that such processes exist, somewhere within the organism.

What is the nature of these processes? Various theorists have given varied answers over the decades. The answers have been so diverse that one sometimes wonders whether the theorists were even portraying the same organism. Human behavior has sometimes been seen as reflecting the dynamics of internal energy systems competing for ascendence (Freud, 1940/1949; see also Hull, 1943). Another view holds that behavior simply emerges directly from a system of competing needs (Murray, 1938). To others, human behavior is a set of patterns coded into our genes over eons of evolution (e.g., Wilson, 1975). It has also been argued, of course, that the concept of motive is irrelevant and misleading—that human behavior is the product of a history of external events coming together to form a pattern of reinforcement contingencies (Skinner, 1938).

In this chapter, we argue for the usefulness of yet another view. The position we take here is that human behavior is a continual process of moving toward various kinds of mental goal representations, and that this movement occurs by a process of feedback control. This view treats behavior as being the consequence of an internal guidance system that is inherent in the way humans are organized. For this reason, we tend to refer to the mechanism underlying human behavior as a system of "self-regulation." In what follows we describe this viewpoint, which has been central in our thinking about human behavior for over a decade (Carver, 1979; Carver & Scheier, 1981a, 1983). Our goal in this chapter is to create a sense of how such a model of behavior can be fit to the human experience.

We have also made a special effort to consider the relationship between the ideas we are presenting here and ideas that are being used by other people. Resemblances among theories exist more often than most people realize, and we have paused periodically to point out some that strike us as interesting. The chapter is divided into sections, each dealing with one aspect of the conceptual analysis under discussion. The final portion of each section consists of a brief glance at the landscape of contemporary psychological thought, with an eye toward similarities among theories.

We should point out before we begin that what we are going to be describing here would not be regarded by most motivational theorists as a complete picture of motivation or self-regulation (cf. Kuhl, 1984; see Ford, 1987, for an even broader perspective). Our aim is not so much to paint a complete picture as it is to create a sense of the importance of certain kinds of constructs (e.g., goal values and feedback processes) in analyzing human functioning.

GOALS AND FEEDBACK CONTROL

We begin by briefly sketching out a few minimal assumptions about the mental organization of the organism whose self-regulation we are trying to describe. We tacitly take the view that is prevalent in contemporary discussions of cognition and social cognition. That is, we assume that people impose order on their experiences, based on regularities that they encounter across time and events. This "order" presumably takes the form of schematic organization in memory. Once schemas have been developed, they are used to recognize, understand, and interpret newly encountered objects and events, and to make predictions regarding future events (for reviews of the burgeoning literature, see, e.g., Cantor & Kihlstrom, 1987; Sherman, Judd, & Park, 1989; Showers & Cantor, 1985; Srull & Wyer, 1989; Wyer & Srull, 1984).

Construing Situations and Specifying Goals

Cognitive structures can be used for at least two purposes. Some of the knowledge stored in memory is used for perceiving, construing, and interpreting things. Some knowledge, in contrast, is stored for use as a prescription for action.[1] Though these types of knowledge can be distinguished from each other in principle, in practice they are often closely associated or interconnected in memory. For example, Schank and Abelson (1977) noted that mental representations of social scripts are used both to understand the actions of others and to guide one's own actions. These two functions of the script require two distinguishable but closely related kinds of information. Presumably, use of the interpretive part of the script begins to call up the associated knowledge of actions that fit the script (cf. Prinz, 1987). Activating interpretive schemas in memory thus should cause the predictable emergence of particular qualities in the person's behavior.

The linkage between interpretive knowledge and related qualities of action has been demonstrated in a number of studies, two examples of which we note briefly here (see also Fazio, 1986). Wilson and Capitman (1982) had male undergraduates read a boy-meets-girl story (under a ruse), thereby activating a particular category of interpretive knowledge in memory. When an attractive girl entered the room moments later, these subjects displayed more of the behavioral qualities linked to that category than did control subjects. Similarly, Carver, Ganellen, Froming, and Chambers (1983) activated an aggressive schema in some subjects via a sentence construction task, and found that those subjects were more aggressive later in an unrelated context. In both cases, alterations in behavior apparently were induced by activating interpretive mental structures to which the behavioral qualities were linked.

The weaving together of interpretive knowledge and behavioral knowledge in memory provides one way to think about how various goals emerge as salient to people from minute to minute. As people perceive or construe or think about the situations they are in, the behavioral qualities associated with the categories that come to mind also become activated (cf. Trzebinski, McGlynn, Gray, & Tubbs, 1985). As situations change, different behavioral qualities are evoked. Indeed, as one's thoughts about a single situation shift and change, the evolving thoughts also cue associations that sometimes evoke different behavioral options. This fluid and continuous activation of patterns of association in memory would seem to represent one mechanism by which behavioral qualities are brought forward for potential execution in behavior. It seems likely that in the course of day-to-day affairs a great many actions involve this sort of spur-of-the-moment mediation, being evoked by the simple process of activation of schemas in memory, through construal of situations and persons.

Clearly, however, this is not the only way for a behavioral quality to be evoked. For example, Ajzen and Fishbein (e.g., Ajzen, 1985; Ajzen & Fishbein, 1980) have spent considerable effort analyzing the process by which people formulate behavioral intentions. This process involves systematic use of several aspects of knowledge, which are weighed and integrated into an intention to take some specific sort of action. The formation of an intention presumably induces the activation of behavioral knowledge relevant to actions that logically follow from the intent. The conscious development of intentions thus is a second way by which behavioral qualities can become active.

We said at the outset that we regard human action as being fundamentally goal-directed. In the preceding paragraphs, we have written not so much about goals as about behavioral knowledge in memory. These two concepts may not be identical, but they surely are closely related. Saying that someone has taken up a behavioral goal is in some sense equivalent to saying that the person wants to manifest in his or her actions a particular quality that is represented in a knowledge structure in his or her memory. Accordingly, we assume throughout this discussion that the behavioral goals underlying human action are specified in memory as elements of behavioral knowledge.

We should point out that goals (and action knowledge) can exist at several levels of abstraction. The attributes of behavioral schemas can be extremely concrete (e.g., levels of muscle tension), or they can be abstract (e.g., the quality of grace or dignity in a person's bearing or in a person's handling of a situation). Goals can be restricted in scope and quickly attained (e.g., to pick up a pencil), or they can be elaborate and attained slowly (e.g., to acquire a good reputation in one's work). Since both types of goals imply the need for physical movements, there presumably is a translation process by which abstract aspects of schemas are translated into concrete act qualities. Very concrete aspects of behavioral schemas are of particular interest to contributors to the literature of motor control (e.g., Adams, 1976; Kelso, 1982; Rosenbaum, 1987; Salmoni, Schmidt, & Walter, 1984; Schmidt, 1976, 1987), but in this chapter we focus primarily on goals that are of higher levels of abstraction.

The idea that human behavior—indeed, human personality—is best analyzed in terms of the goals that people adopt is one that has been prominent in the writings of many theorists in recent years. Here are a few examples (see Pervin, 1989, for detailed discussion of a range of views). Elliott and Dweck (1988) have emphasized the importance of knowing the nature of people's "goals" in their achievement efforts. Klinger (1975, 1977) has used the phrase "current concern" to describe the goals with which a person is presently engaged. Cantor and Kihlstrom (1987) have written about the "life tasks" that occupy people at various periods of their lives. Markus and Nurius (1986) have described "possible selves," defined as representations of desired and undesired qualities of the self, goals to be attained and to be avoided. Emmons (1986) has argued that personality can be described in terms of the patterns of "personal strivings" that characterize the individual. Palys and Little (1983) discuss "personal projects." The notion that goals are intrinsic to human action is also implicit in Higgins's (1987) concept of "self-guide" and Vallacher and Wegner's (1985) concept of "action identification."

Though distinctions can be drawn among these various concepts, what we wish to emphasize here is not their differences but rather their similarities. In each case, the central theme is that human action is defined in terms of the individual's goals. High-level goals are translated in some manner into lower-level prescriptions for action, into more concrete knowledge that specifies overt movements. The knowledge needed for this translation is drawn from memory, if it is available there. If not, it is sought out elsewhere. In each of the theoretical notions just listed, there is an emphasis on the idea that understanding the person means understanding the person's goals.

From Goals to Behavior

Although the activation of goals (or action knowledge) sets the stage for behavior to occur, the mere activation of this knowledge in memory does not necessarily mean that those behavioral qualities will be reflected in action. How do people get from a state of having information in working memory to displaying the comparable quality in overt action? Before addressing this question, we must distinguish between two classes of actions: those that are intentional, effortful, and consciously mediated versus those that are highly automatic. Because our focus in this chapter is on conscious, effortful action, we consider this case first.

It seems to us that conscious, effortful action is easily construed in terms of the principles of feedback control (for more general statements on this perspective, see, e.g., MacKay, 1963, 1966; Miller, Galanter, & Pribram, 1960; Powers, 1973). In a feedback loop (see Figure 1.1), some existing condition is compared against a reference value (through a device generically termed a "comparator"). If a discrepancy between the two is noticed, an output function is engaged. The output creates an adjustment of some sort in the existing state of affairs, which is aimed at diminishing the discrepancy. If the adjustment is effective, subsequent perceptions will be more closely aligned with the reference value. The overall function of this arrangement is to negate or minimize sensed deviations from a comparison value.

These functions seem to be implicit in consciously mediated human behavior. When behavioral information has become active in memory, it is put in place as a "guide," a "reference point," or a "standard of comparison" (we use these terms interchangeably throughout the chapter). People periodically check on their present activities, states, or personal qualities (input function) and compare these perceptions against the reference values active in memory. If the perception or construal of behavior is discrepant with what the person intends to be doing, the result is a change in behavior, aimed at diminishing or removing the discrepancy (see also Norman, 1981). This feedback mechanism provides a way by which procedural knowledge is manifest in overt action.

In the logic of the feedback loop, behavior is inherently purposive (even if the purposes underlying certain acts are relatively trivial), undertaken in the

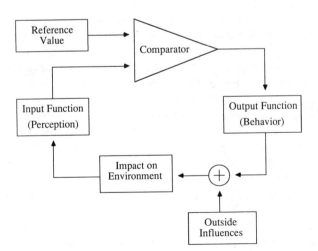

FIGURE 1.1 Schematic diagram of a discrepancy reducing feedback loop, showing the basic processes presumed to underlie self-corrective behavioral self-regulation.

service of creating perceptions of conformity to some reference value. Human life is viewed as a continual process of establishing goals and intentions, and adjusting current patterns of behavior so as to match these values more closely, using informational feedback as a guide to progress (cf. Locke, Shaw, Saari, & Latham, 1981, especially pp. 135–136).

Self-Attention and Engagement of the Comparator

Some time ago, we suggested that some of the empirical consequences of self-focused attention could be best understood in terms of these feedback processes (Carver, 1979; Carver & Scheier, 1981a).[2] More specifically, we argued that when a person is in a situation in which a reference value has been evoked in memory, self-directed attention causes the engagement of the comparator of a feedback loop guiding action. Indeed, making this argument was what first caused us to think seriously about the usefulness of principles of feedback control as a model of human behavior.

The argument that self-focus engages the comparator of a feedback system has two implications. The first and more straightforward of the two is that self-focus should cause an increase in the frequency or probability of making comparisons between the present state and the standard of comparison. Though this argument is logically straightforward, the effect is a difficult one to demonstrate, and the evidence is necessarily somewhat indirect. The assumption is that when people make this sort of mental comparison, it is occurring at an abstract level. Yet, being able to make the abstract comparison often requires certain kinds of concrete information. Accordingly, we tried to establish situations in which we could observe subjects as they sought to gain access to concrete information that would assist in making the abstract comparison we expected them to be making (Scheier & Carver, 1983).

Subjects in this research were trying to perform well at an experimental task, and we expected them to check periodically on the adequacy of their performance in comparison to some reference point. The concrete information that was made available to them varied from study to study. In two studies, seeking information was operationalized as the frequency with which subjects re-examined patterns that they were trying to copy accurately. In two other studies, seeking information was operationalized as the extent to which subjects chose to obtain performance norms for a test. In each case, subjects with high levels of self-focus were more likely than those with less self-focus to seek out this concrete information. Our inference is that the self-attentive subjects (more than the less self-attentive subjects) were engaging in an abstract mental comparison between behavior and standard.

If self-focus engages the comparison process, a second consequence should also follow: Behavior should be adjusted so that it conforms more closely to the reference value being used by the person. Does self-focus promote better self-regulation? Yes. There is abundant evidence that increased self-focus does promote a closer correspondence between ongoing behavior and salient behavioral standards (see Carver & Scheier, 1981a, for a review). The evidence comes from studies with widely varying subject populations, widely varying behavioral standards, and widely varying operationalizations of self-focus. The basic effect has been replicated so often that there can be little doubt of its reality.

There is also evidence that reductions in self-awareness can cause behavior to become more poorly self-regulated, with the person becoming more impulsive and responsive to cues of the moment. This sort of effect has been obtained in several studies in which self-awareness was reduced through deindividuation (e.g., Diener, 1979; Prentice-Dunn & Rogers, 1982); similar behavioral effects often follow from the consumption of alcohol, which Hull (1981) has argued reduces self-awareness.

Feedforward and Automatization

We view the feedback principle as very important in human behavior. Our emphasis on the role of feedback sometimes inclines us to disregard two other matters, to which we now point briefly. Both relate to the fact that a good deal of human behavior consists of relatively smooth performances of well-known acts. There often is little or no evidence of any discrepancy at all between ongoing behavior and desired behavior. Rather, the action flows easily and in close conformity to the act intended.

There are two points to be made about this. First, this continuous close conformity between behavior and reference value suggests the existence of what is sometimes termed a feed*forward* process in self-regulation, as well as a feedback process. (There is controversy, however, regarding the feedforward principle and its applicability to psychological phenomena; see, e.g., Gardner & Gardner, 1988, and the succeeding commentaries.)

The easiest way to grasp the concept of feedforward is to imagine that the operation of a feedback loop begins with a reference value in place and an output function that begins to act before an input is sensed. It would make little sense for the initial output of such a system to be random. It would be far more functional for the initial output to be a relatively good approximation of the act that would yield conformity to the reference value. Feedforward, in essence, is a first-approximation output, occurring before input is sensed and compared. If it is a good *enough* approximation, the input function will correspond well to the reference value. If it is a poorer approximation, a discrepancy will be noted and adjusted via subsequent output. This line of argument fits the fact that initial behavioral output in a given act is often such that little discrepancy ever arises between actual and desired conditions.

Note that feedforward does not inherently displace the feedback process. That is, a well-regulated system must ensure that the action produced does indeed create conformity to the reference value. Very good first approximations can sometimes create a false impression that the feedback function (i.e., the input and comparison) is not taking place when it actually is. On the other hand, it is reasonable to ask whether there are circumstances in which feedforward is relied on to the point that feedback is discontinued altogether.

It is sometimes assumed that this is what happens when an action is repeated often enough that it ceases to be consciously controlled and becomes instead fully automatic (cf. Shiffrin & Schneider, 1977). Increased automaticity means that recognition of the behavioral context evokes an act quality from memory and that the act quality is executed without monitoring (see Stelmach & Larish, 1980). This is sometimes referred to as "open-loop" control, because of the absence of a return cycle of feedback and comparison.

Does automaticity mean the complete removal of feedback processing? There are at least two reasons for hesitating to accept that conclusion too readily (see also Schmidt, 1987, for a broader discussion of issues). First, the effortful–automatic dichotomy may not really be a dichotomy but a continuum (Cohen, Dunbar, & McClelland, 1988). Repeating acts makes them *more* automatic, but how often does an act become *completely* automatic? Unless it has attained that status, can it really be said to have escaped entirely from the use of feedback? Perhaps it is more appropriate to assume that use of feedback *diminishes* as the action becomes more automatic, rather than ending altogether. Indeed, it is not entirely clear that the use of feedback is equivalent to the use of attentional resources, and it is the latter that constitutes the usual metric for discussing automaticity (cf. Schmidt, 1987).

A second reason for not assuming too readily that automatic actions no longer depend upon feedback is that even highly automated acts do not always produce the consequences to which they are directed. Human beings clearly have a mechanism for error recognition in such cases (Norman, 1981), and this error recognition implies the use of feedback.

Taking a Look Around

Let us stop for a moment, and consider how the principles we have outlined thus far relate to several theoretical statements made by others. Four comparisons are noteworthy. The first one concerns the self-regulatory role we ascribed to self-focused attention in this section of the chapter and the effects of self-focus in Duval and Wicklund's (1972) self-awareness theory. In a sense, the effects ascribed by the two views are absolutely identical. Duval and Wicklund (1972) held that self-directed attention induces a comparison between present self and salient standards of comparison, and that this comparison in turn can cause behavior to shift into closer conformity with the standard. Indeed, our own first empirical examinations of the effects of self-awareness took place within the framework of their theory. Only later did it occur to us to think about the issues around which the first part of this chapter is organized.

What makes our viewpoint on these matters fundamentally different from that articulated by Duval and Wicklund (1972) is a difference in *why* we think these effects take place. Why does self-directed attention lead to a comparison between present behavior and standard? Why does the comparison lead to adjustments in behavior? In the view we have just presented, these events take place because voluntary behavior is self-regulated through a process of adjustment through feedback, and feedback control intrinsically entails such a comparison. In Duval and Wicklund's view, by contrast, the comparison process takes place because human beings are inherently self-critical and naturally drift to comparisons with standards to which they are inferior. Discrepancy reduction takes place (within their theoretical framework) as a way of diminishing an aversive drive state caused by awareness of the discrepancy.

Although the empirical predictions made by these two views are in many cases the same, the underlying dynamics assumed by the two viewpoints seem very different phenomenologically. There are places where the two approaches do make different predictions, but it is rare that the divergence of prediction bears on the point now under discussion (though see Carver & Scheier, 1981b). As is often true of disagreements that depend more on metatheoretical than on theoretical matters, which portrayal of the underlying dynamics is preferable depends partly on which of the underlying world views one finds more congenial. If nothing else, this comparison illustrates the ease with which alternative construals can be imposed on the phenomena of empirical reality.

Other comparisons make a very different point, illustrating the fact that the logic of feedback control (if not the label per se) has begun to permeate thinking in contemporary personality and social psychology. Consider Bandura's views on personality and behavior. Bandura began his major theoretical efforts at a time when learning theories were coming into their own as a model of human behavior. His social learning theory (e.g., Bandura, 1969) became widely known as a major variant within that tradition. As time has gone by, however, his ideas have moved farther and farther away from learning principles, focusing more and more on self-regulatory cognitive activities. Indeed, the word "learning" has even disappeared from the term by which he refers to his theory, which currently consists wholly of modifiers (Bandura, 1986).

The themes that Bandura has recently emphasized include the ideas that people symbolically represent their goals, that people engage in self-reflective monitoring of their behavior; that people's actions have an impact on the settings in which the action takes place, as well as vice versa (reciprocal determinism); and that both goal setting and knowledge of performance are needed for optimal self-regulation of behavior (Bandura, 1982, 1986). These themes all map easily onto the elements of the feedback loop shown in Figure 1.1. In short, in practice (if not in vocabulary), Bandura seems to have adopted the principle of feedback control as a tool for analyzing behavior.

Although Bandura has been reluctant to adopt the vocabulary of feedback principles, this is less true of other theorists whose position is otherwise similar to Bandura's. A good example is a discussion by Kanfer and Busemeyer (1982) of the nature of therapy. They argue that the therapy process is best viewed as a dynamic feedback system consisting of several stages. The client uses feedback both from the therapy session and from actions taken outside therapy to guide movement through a longer-term plan of behavior change. Indeed, Kanfer and Busemeyer argue that the same feedback is also used to re-evaluate both the appropriateness of the short-term goals of therapy as means to attain longer-term goals, and also the nature of the longer-term goals themselves. Kanfer and Busemeyer's (1982) discussion represents a good illustration of the way in which feedback concepts can be applied meaningfully to very important kinds of situations in human action.

A final useful comparison goes beyond the points made thus far in the chapter, by considering how the principles of feedback apply in the context of dyadic interaction. Thus far we have limited ourselves to considering one person at a time. We have characterized that person as having goals and intentions in mind, and as trying to act in ways that will confirm that the goals were being attained. When two people interact with each other, they do so as feedback systems interacting with each other, each with its own goals and its own perceptions. In the past few years, several theorists have discussed social interchange from this perspective, though without using the feedback concept explicitly.

For example, Darley and Fazio (1980) described a set of processes by which people's expectancies about others cause them to orient and act toward those others in ways that confirm the initial expectancy. One of the main points in that discussion is that both parties in the interaction play two roles: Both are perceivers and both are targets of the other's actions and perceptions. In a similar vein, Swann (1987) has emphasized that the nature of social reality is not typically dictated by one person in an interaction, but rather is negotiated by the two people in the interaction, each of whom is acting both as a perceiver and as a target. The themes of both of these discussions are very much in accord with a feedback-based view of human behavior.

HIERARCHICAL ORGANIZATION

The feedback loop may be an important construct, but by itself it is inadequate to account for the elaboration and flexibility of human behavior. Complexity is added, however, by considering the fact that feedback systems can be interconnected. Of primary interest at present is the idea that feedback systems can be ordered in a hierarchy. Powers (1973) has argued that this sort of organization underlies the self-regulation of behavior in living organisms, and arguments of a similar form have also been made by other theorists focusing on very different aspects of behavior (e.g., Broadbent, 1977; Dawkins, 1976; Gallistel, 1980; Vallacher & Wegner, 1987; for models of brain function compatible with this line of thought, see, e.g., Baron, 1987; Stuss & Benson, 1986). We have found aspects of this argument interesting, and accordingly have adopted this position as a conceptual heuristic.[3]

In a hierarchical organization of feedback systems, there are relatively superordinate feedback loops and relatively subordinate loops. The output function of the superordinate system consists of the resetting of reference values at the next lower level of abstraction (see Figure 1.2). To put it somewhat differently, higher-order or superordinate systems "behave" by providing reference values to the systems just subordinate to them in the hierarchy. Presumably, the selection of a

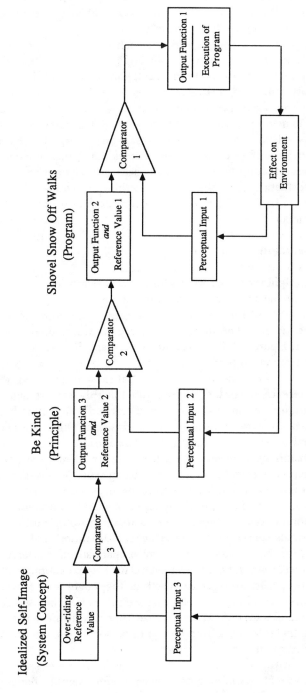

FIGURE 1.2 Schematic diagram of a three-tiered hierarchy of feedback systems, illustrating the "cascade" of control that flows from higher to lower levels, as superordinate loops set the reference values for the loops that are directly subordinate. The levels of control illustrated here are those at the top of the hierarchy proposed by Powers (1973). In this case, the example depicts a cross-section of the behavior of a woman who is actively attempting to match her self-perceptions to her idealized self by following the principle of conscientiousness, which is being manifested in terms of the programmatic activity of shoveling snow from the walks of an elderly neighbor.

13

particular reference value depends at least in part on associations that have developed between classes of perceptions and classes of actions that have proven to be discrepancy-reducing in similar situations in the past.

The reference values that are being specified as behavioral outputs become more concrete and restricted as one moves from higher to lower levels of a hierarchy. Control at each lower level reflects regulation of some quality that contributes to the quality controlled at the next higher level, though not actually defining it. Each level within the hierarchy monitors input at a level of abstraction that is appropriate to its own functioning, and each level adjusts output so as to minimize discrepancies at that level. Powers (1973) argued that this identity between output at one level and resetting of reference values at the next lower level is maintained from whatever level is presently acting as superordinate, on downward through the hierarchy, to the level of setting reference values for muscle tensions. Thus the hierarchy creates the physical execution of whatever action is taking place.

Upper Levels of Abstraction

We have focused on the implications of Powers's hierarchy at relatively high levels of abstraction, which are the levels of our own greatest interest (though see Marken, 1986, and Rosenbaum, 1987, for evidence regarding the usefulness of similar notions at lower levels). The illustration of the nature of hierarchical organization provided in Figure 1.2 also illustrates the several highest levels of abstraction in the organization proposed by Powers. At the highest level shown (labeled "system concepts") are such values as the global sense of idealized self. Self is not the only reference value that might be used at this level, though it probably is the most intuitive example of the type of standard that occurs here and may be the most frequently used reference value at this level. Other possibilities include the idealized sense of a relationship or of a society.

Reference values at this level are very abstract. As one considers the attempt to self-regulate with respect to such values, a reasonable question to ask is what behavioral outputs are even relevant to the attempt. How does a person act so as to minimize discrepancies between these highly abstract values and his or her behavior? What behavioral outputs will create the desired correspondence?

As we indicated just above, the answer that Powers (1973) suggested is that the behavioral output of this highest-order system consists of providing reference values to the next lower level, which he termed the level of "principle control." To put it more concretely, people act to "be" who they think they ought to be or want to be by using any of several guiding principles that are implied by the idealized self to which they aspire. The makeup of the idealized self to which the person aspires will obviously differ somewhat from person to person. Thus, the principles that will be specified as output will also vary.

Principles begin to provide some form for behavior. Principles are aspects of behavior for which we have names in everyday language—for example, honesty, responsibility, thrift, and expedience. The form that principles provide for behavior is still fairly abstract, however. Principles are not specifications of acts so much as they are specifications of qualities that can be manifest in acts of many types (see also Schank & Abelson's [1977] discussion of the concept of "metascript"). People do not just go out and "do" honesty, or responsibility, or thrift, or expedience. Rather, people can manifest any one (or more) of these qualities in their behavior by doing any number of specific activities.[4]

These specific activities, in which behavior finally becomes recognizable as behavior, are termed "programs." A program is similar to what Schank and Abelson (1977) termed a "script." A program specifies a course of action, but with many of the details left blank. The details are left unspecified because what is done at any particular point in the script depends upon the nature of the circumstances that are encountered at that point. Clearly, much of what people do in their day-to-day lives appears program- or script-like in character. Going to the grocery store, cooking dinner, writing a report, taking a walk—all these are programs.

Principles provide reference values for program-level control in two ways. The first is by suggesting certain kinds of programs as potential reference values. For example, the principle of thrift or frugality would provide as one output a program involving dinner at home rather than a dining-out program. The second way in which principles provide reference values pertains to choices that are made within programs. A person already committed to the dining-out program might be influenced by the thrift principle to choose an inexpensive restaurant rather than a pricier alternative, or to choose the least expensive dish on the menu and avoid drinks, appetizers, and dessert.

Programs are the sort of activities that most people take for granted as "behavior." Although programs often are undertaken in order to attain relatively abstract goals, the programs themselves are sufficiently concrete and overt that they are easily recognizable as actions. It is very easy to describe the actions in a program. Executing them, however, is more complex a process than is naming them. In the model proposed by Powers (1973), programs act by specifying yet more restricted qualities as reference values to lower-level control structures.

More concretely, one enacts a program (in part) by enacting sequences of movement. One difference between programs and sequences is that programs involve choice points where decisions must be made (ranging from trivial to important), whereas the constituents of a sequence are executed "all of a piece." When an action becomes sufficiently well learned that its enactment (once begun) is automatic rather than effortful, it can be thought of as having become a sequence rather than a program. Sequences, in turn, are composed of even more restricted qualities (which we ignore here).

This process of specifying high-order, abstract qualities in terms of lower-order, more concrete qualities of action brings to mind the notion of means–end analysis (e.g., Newell & Simon, 1972). The "end" in this phase is a high-level goal; the "means" is a set of lower-level action qualities that can be used to attain it. This phrase was coined in the context of problem solving, to refer to an active process of analyzing a behavioral problem into component steps that will resolve it, working from the higher level toward very concrete acts. One might think of a means–end analysis as creating a new program of action, as opposed to using a program that is already familiar.

In general, when the term "means–end analysis" is used, it is assumed that the analysis taking place is conscious and effortful. In the hierarchy now under discussion, by contrast, this assumption is not made. In the functioning of this hierarchy, something akin to the outcome of a means–end analysis is being evoked from memory, as standards are specified downward through the hierarchy. The process is often implicit and relatively automatic, however, rather than conscious and effortful. On the other hand, some degree of conscious means–end analysis often occurs as a result of such circumstances as the need to choose from among several potential action strategies within a broad program of behavior.

As we noted earlier, many theorists believe that highly automatic actions use no feedback in their execution. This is not, however, the position taken by Powers (1973). Powers believes that the use of feedback is inherent throughout the hierarchy he has proposed (which includes five additional levels below control of sequences). Loops at each level of the hierarchy presumably monitor qualities that are appropriate to that level of control. It does seem clear from other research that motor programs embody hierarchical organization (e.g., Rosenbaum, 1987), but there is no unanimity on the role of feedback in their execution when they have become well learned (cf. Schmidt, 1987). At a minimum, feedback information would seem to be necessary in order to be able to modify or refine lower-level outputs; on the other hand, if an action is completely automatic, presumably no modification or refinement is currently taking place.

Hierarchical Organization: Additional Points

There are several more points that should be made about the theme of hierarchical organization in behavior, and we make them here in no particular order of importance.

First, as should be apparent from the foregoing discussion, this view holds that control of behavior occurs simultaneously at all levels below whatever level is functionally superordinate. That is, a person does not engage in a high-order action, and then stop and wait for lower-level activities to catch up. Nor does a person engage in low-level act qualities as preparation for the attainment of high-level acts. Rather, the process of carrying out a high-level act *consists of* the carrying out of low-level acts (see also Vallacher & Wegner, 1985, 1987). Thus, if you are matching your behavior to the principle of kindness by doing a favor for a neighbor, the matching is being enhanced throughout the doing of the favor, not just when the favor has been completed. In this view, exceedingly restricted and concrete behavioral acts (e.g., changes in level of muscle tension, changes in postural orientation) are intrinsically embedded in the creation of very abstract behavioral qualities (e.g., conveying a certain mood in a piece of art, being gracious to others, delivering a speech with style). To put it differently, whenever a high level of control is engaged, so are all levels below it.

On the other hand, it is *not* necessarily the case that all upper levels of the hierarchy are engaged at all times. There are many circumstances in which behavioral self-regulation appears not to be guided by the superordinate sense of self, but rather by reference values at the level of program control. To put it differently, levels of control below that of system concepts are functionally superordinate whenever the person's current concern is at a lower level (cf. Klinger, 1975; Shallice, 1978; Vallacher & Wegner, 1985, 1987).

This would appear to be the case, for example, when people engage in the "maintenance" activities of which life seems so full—for instance, shopping for groceries, washing dishes, driving to work. During such actions people may lose sight of higher-order goals, as they focus on the concrete realities of the situations confronting them (cf. Norman, 1981). Indeed, we have argued elsewhere (Carver & Scheier, 1981a) that it is common for program control to be functionally superordinate in people's behavior because of the frequent need for decision making that occurs at the program level. Though most behavior probably involves at least the level of program control, it is arguable that states such as deindividuation and alcohol intoxication diminish even program control, rendering sequence control functionally superordinate. This view would be consistent with the impulsive, spontaneous character of actions that occur in those states.

We have tended to assume that self-regulation at any level higher than the level that is functionally superordinate is suspended until attention is refocused on reference values at the higher level. This does not mean that actions taken while under low-level control have no implications for higher-level discrepancies. When behavior is being controlled at lower levels, discrepancies at higher levels can remain unchanged, can be decreased, and can even be increased, depending on the consequences of the lower-level activity in which the person is engaging. Effects on high-level discrepancies presumably would not be noted, however, until and unless attention were redirected to the higher level. We should acknowledge that this argument is speculative. It might well be that high-level values always influence behavior, with the influence simply being slighter and more subtle when these values are not focal in one's attention.

Thus far we have addressed behavior as having a single purpose at a time. We should note, however, that people often attempt to move toward a number of goals simultaneously. We mean to convey more here than the idea that lower-order values are always being matched in the service of higher-order values in any hierarchical system. Rather, we mean that multiple goals are often operative even within a given level of the hierarchy. In some cases the reference values are entirely compatible with each other (e.g., being frugal while also being austere). In other cases the values are more mutually exclusive (e.g., being frugal while also being a patron of the arts; losing weight quickly while maintaining good health). Reducing discrepancies with respect to one of these values means enlarging discrepancies with respect to the other value, resulting in conflict. Indeed, this sort of conflict is a major source of dissatisfaction in life (Emmons, 1986; Van Hook & Higgins, 1988).

Although the hierarchy we are discussing is in some ways very simple, it has implications for several basic problems in thinking about human behavior. For one thing, it is implicit in this approach that goals at any given level can often be achieved by a variety of means at lower levels. This flexibility in goal attainment is particularly apparent as one examines the upper levels of the hierarchy, where the goals are more abstract. As we noted earlier, a particular principle can usually be realized in many programs of action in many different behavioral domains. This flexibility in goal attainment permits the hierarchical approach to address in a meaningful way the fact that people sometimes shift radically the manner in which they attain a goal when the goal itself has not changed appreciably (cf. Wicklund & Gollwitzer, 1982).

Just as a given goal can be obtained via multiple pathways, so can a specific behavioral act be performed in the service of diverse goals. For example, you could buy someone a gift in order to make that person feel good, to repay a kindness, to put the other person in your debt, or to satisfy part of your perceived holiday season role. Indeed, a given act can be aimed at meeting goals at different levels of abstraction. For example, walking through a door and closing it behind you may be a mindless *sequence* of action; it may be part of a *program* of choices (reflecting a decision to go somewhere other than the room you are in); or it may be a manifestation of a *principle* (choosing to leave a room where someone is behaving dishonorably).

Thus, a given physical act can have strikingly different meanings, depending on the purpose that it is intended to serve. This is an important subtheme of the viewpoint on behavior under discussion here: Behavior can be understood only by identifying the goals to which the behavior is addressed. The fact that this is not always easy to do does not make it any less critical.

A final implication of the notion of hierarchical organization concerns the fact that goals in behavior are not equivalent in their importance. The higher one goes into the organization, the more fundamental to the overriding sense of self (or whatever value is in place at the superordinate level) are the qualities that are encountered. A related point is that the "importance" of reference values at low levels is at least partly a product of the degree to which their attainment contributes to success in the attempt to reduce discrepancies at higher levels.

Taking a Look Around

As was true earlier in the chapter, the ideas that we have outlined in this section share conceptual ground with ideas that are discussed elsewhere in contemporary psychology, three of which we would like to note briefly.

As we noted earlier in this section, we have adopted the hierarchical analysis from Powers (1973) as a conceptual heuristic. We find many of its implications interesting, and have more to say about some of those implications later on in the chapter. We have not, however, directly examined the hierarchical model in any of our own empirical work. On the other hand, others have used related concepts in ways that seem very consistent with the reasoning just outlined.

Of greatest relevance is a body of recent work by Vallacher and Wegner

(1985, 1987). This work appears to argue strongly for the viability of the notion of hierarchical organization, as that notion applies to relatively high levels of control. Vallacher and Wegner are interested in how people identify or construe their actions. They have pointed out that people can identify any given act in a variety of ways, some of which are concrete and some more abstract. Futhermore, the level of abstraction at which people identify their actions can have predictable influences on behavior.

Vallacher and Wegner make two assumptions about variations in level of action identification. The first is that people tend to construe (and presumably to regulate) their activities in as abstract a fashion as they can manage without difficulty. For example, students are in general more likely to construe their behavior as "attending classes," or "listening to a lecture," or even "obtaining an education," than they are to construe the same acts as "walking into a building, sitting down, and listening to another person." The second assumption is that when people have difficulties in carrying out an action, they tend to move to a lower-level identification of the same activity. To put it in slightly different terms, difficulties in self-regulating at a high level of abstraction typically cause a lower level to become functionally superordinate.

Some of the research that Vallacher and Wegner have conducted to support their theory has used techniques that induce a high-level act identification in some subjects and a lower-level identification in other subjects. The research then examines the susceptibility of the two groups of subjects to cues implying a particular high-level identity for the ongoing behavior. The typical result (e.g., Wegner, Vallacher, Kiersted, & Dizadji, 1986) is that subjects led to have higher-order understanding of their behavior early on are unlikely to reconstrue their actions on the basis of these later cues. Subjects with lower-order orientations early on are more likely to reconstrue their actions, and to behave subsequently in a manner consistent with this reconstrual.

Research stemming from Vallacher and Wegner's theory is interesting in its own right, and has potentially important implications with regard to self-regulatory processes. The point we wish to make about their work at present, however, is that it seems to bear out the usefulness of a hierarchical view of behavior. Furthermore, most of the behavioral qualities by which Vallacher and Wegner illustrate variations in act identification are easily assimilated to three levels of control in the hierarchy proposed by Powers (1973): principle control, program control, and sequence control. We suggest that Vallacher and Wegner's research constitutes prima facie evidence of the reasonableness of these levels of the Powers hierarchy, and of the more general argument that behavior is hierarchically organized. We also infer that these three levels of control are represented especially easily in verbal descriptions. Perhaps this is because they are fundamental qualities in self-regulation.

A second similarity between these ideas and other models in contemporary social and personality psychology is somewhat broader and more diffuse. A number of theories incorporate the idea that people choose their actions and their orientations toward their experience so as to maintain a positive self-evaluation or a positive self-image. For example, a wide range of evidence supports the idea that people make self-serving attributions for good and bad outcomes that they experience (e.g., Weary, 1980; see also Taylor & Brown, 1988). There is also evidence that people will go out of their way to create esteem-protective explanations for potential bad outcomes before they occur, even to the extent of handicapping their own performance by doing so (e.g., Snyder, Higgins, & Stucky, 1983). In the same vein, Tesser (1980, 1986; Tesser & Campbell, 1983) has analyzed the circumstances under which people take personal pride in the accomplishments of others who are close to them, versus avoiding similar information when it results in unflattering comparisons with their own accomplishments.

Each of these literatures appears to reflect people's attempts to prevent discrepancies from arising between a desired sense of self and present perceptions of self. In each case, people are trying to protect a quality that is important and central to them, by taking concrete and overt steps of one sort or another. Although the parallelism is somewhat fuzzy, the principle demonstrated by each of these literatures appears to be compatible with the logic of hierarchical organization. That is, people attempt to minimize discrepancies at the highest level by the concrete expedient of taking steps to create certain perceived realities at lower levels.

It is also interesting and relevant to the point we are making that theories of this sort often incorporate a provision to the effect that self-evaluation or self-esteem maintenance is a concern for people only under certain circumstances. This seems very similar to the idea that people sometimes operate in such a manner that lower levels of control are functionally superordinate. Only when attention is directed to higher-order reference values does the potential for creating discrepancies at that level become obvious.

The notion of hierarchical organization as outlined here also bears some resemblance to ideas from the phenomenological perspective on personality. Several theorists represented in that literature have argued that the highest-order motive underlying human behavior is self-actualization (Maslow, 1970; Rogers, 1961). Self-actualization is a concept that is hard to define easily, but it typically is described as a tendency to realize one's own potential in one's behavior, a tendency to become everything that one is capable of being. There is considerable superficial similarity between the concept of self-actualization and the notion of self-regulation with respect to system concept values. That is, self-regulation at this highest level promotes the sense of personal wholeness and integration that self-actualization is believed to bring. Effective regulation at the level of system concepts means living up to one's potential. Maslow (1970) argued that self-actualization stands at the top of a hierarchy of motivational qualities. At the lower levels of his hierarchy stand basic biological needs and motives to attain physical safety and security. In the middle are motives that pertain to social interaction, and at the top is self-actualization. Self-actualization exerts a subtle influence on behavior, in Maslow's view, because of the fact that lower-order needs are more demanding than higher-order needs. Maslow argued that people are not free to engage in self-actualization unless lower-level needs are satisfied.

The behavioral contents of Maslow's hierarchy are quite different from the behavioral qualities in the hierarchy we have been discussing. Indeed, the nature of the hierarchical organization is also quite different. In the hierarchy we have been discussing, lower-level actions contribute to the attainment of higher-level values; in Maslow's hierarchy, lower-level needs do not serve this function. Nevertheless, there is one interesting functional similarity between the two views. Inherent in both is the idea that action aimed at higher-order concerns is disrupted if difficulties are encountered at lower levels. Indeed, this idea is also a cornerstone of Vallacher and Wegner's (1985, 1987) theory (the idea that people adopt lower-level identifications of their actions when they encounter problems carrying them out). Thus, one cannot self-regulate with respect to one's idealized self (i.e., cannot self-actualize) if one is unable to enact a needed principle or program. When this happens, attention typically is drawn downward, disrupting control at higher levels (cf. Kimble & Perlmuter, 1970).

A final point we would like to make concerns a superficial similarity between our description of hierarchical organization and Freud's (1923/1962) structural model of personality. Freud held that personality has three elements: id, which is impulsive and unresponsive either to practice reality or to ideals; ego, which is planful and practical and acts to restrain id impulses according to the needs of the situation; and superego, which embodies pressure toward ideals, particularly moralistic ideals. Freud viewed these aspects of personality as competitors for influence, rather than as hierarchically organized. Yet there is an interesting similiarity between the actions that stem from these elements of personality and actions as they are produced at various levels of the control hierarchy under discussion.

When all higher-level control is removed temporarily and sequence control is given free rein, people appear more impulsive in their behavior. They are more responsive to passing cues of the moment (both internal and external) that touch off sequences of action. It is as though lower-level sequences, once begun, run off by themselves unless overruled by control at a higher level. This impulsive character of action at low levels of abstraction is reminiscent of characteristics of id functioning in the psychoanalytic model.

Though we would hesitate to press the similarity between sequence control and id functioning too far, there is a relatively strong resemblance between the notion of program control in the hierarchy under discussion and descriptions of ego functioning. Program control involves planning, decision making, and an attempt to behave in a pragmatic manner (in the absence of higher-level control), as opposed to behaving in either an impulsive or an idealistic manner. These characteristics are also seen in the functioning of the ego.

The levels of control higher than program control also resemble in some ways the functioning of the superego. Engaging the level of principle control causes an attempt to conform to principles, some of which are moralistic. We have characterized control at the highest (system concept) level as an attempt to conform to idealized representations of the self (or other comparable qualities). The efforts represented by these two levels of control are similar in some respects to the attempt to conform to the ego ideal. The fit is far from perfect, at least partly because not all principles in the hierarchy under discussion are moralistic. Yet it seems reasonable to ask whether Freud's emphasis on morality to the exclusion of other ideals might not have been a reflection of the times in which he developed his ideas. The similarities otherwise seem sufficiently intriguing to warrant additional scrutiny.

INTERRUPTION AND DISENGAGEMENT

The processes outlined thus far in the chapter bear on self-regulation of behavior in situations where the attempt to act proceeds unimpeded. People are not always successful or effective, however, in what they try to do. People often encounter obstacles in their attempts to execute plans, realize intentions, or attain goals. Attempts to minimize and eliminate discrepancies do not always work out. Thus, any approach to analyzing human action that is to be even minimally effective must address the question of what happens when people confront such obstacles.

We believe that self-regulatory efforts are interrupted when obstacles to goal attainment are encountered (cf. Simon, 1967). The interruptions can be either momentary or prolonged. They can occur prior to the initial action attempt (if the difficulties are anticipated) or during the attempt itself (if unforeseen problems arise along the way). The interruption may occur only once, or may occur repeatedly through the course of acting. In each case, we presume that interruption leads the person to evaluate the situation that he or she is in, and derive an outcome expectancy—the subjective likelihood of successful discrepancy reduction, given continued effort (Figure 1.3). Expectancy assessment (about which we say more later) presumably involves the integration of information from a number of different sources, including an analysis of the physical and social constraints impinging on one's actions, and a consideration of the depth and breadth of one's resources.

We think of the consequences of this expectancy assessment as forming a rough dichotomy, which forms around a behavioral "watershed," or discontinuity. If expectancies for success are sufficiently favorable, the person returns to efforts at goal attainment, returning thereby to the self-regulatory feedback process that had been engaged before the interruption. If expectancies are sufficiently unfavorable, the person begins to disengage from the attempt at goal attainment (cf. Klinger, 1975; Kukla, 1972), thereby diminishing the engagement of the feedback process with respect to that goal and attempting to avoid the behavior–goal comparison (Carver, Antoni, & Scheier, 1985). We have assumed that both the return to effort (which is no different in principle from any discrepancy reduction attempt) and the disengagement tendency are enhanced by further self-focus. Thus, in early studies intended to test this aspect of our thinking, the prediction

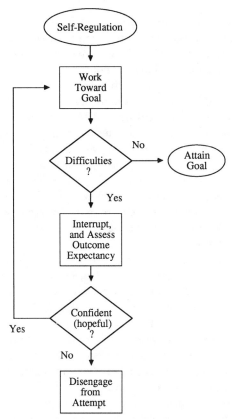

FIGURE 1.3 Flow chart depiction of self-regulatory possibilities, indicating that action sometimes continues unimpeded; that obstacles to goal attainment induce a sequence of evaluation and decision making; and that if expectancies are sufficiently unfavorable the person may disengage from further effort. Adapted from Carver and Scheier (1981a).

was for a spreading interaction, such that the effects of favorable and unfavorable expectancies would both be exaggerated by higher levels of self-attention.

Although virtually all behavioral responses to impediments can be construed in this dichotomous fashion, we should note another issue in passing. Specifically, the level of subjective probability at which continued efforts give way to disengagement (i.e., the behavioral watershed) presumably varies with the importance of the behavioral dimension in question. That is, in general people presumably will continue to pursue goals that are very important to them even when expectancies are relatively negative, whereas goals that are less important may be abandoned when expectancies are less negative.[5] This is a theoretical point that we have not pursued empirically, but it is a point that should be borne in mind.

The sequence of interruption and expectancy assessment can be prompted by several antecedent conditions. The simplest circumstance leading to this sequence is frustration—the existence of an obstacle to goal attainment, either external (impediments or constraints) or internal (deficits of skill, knowledge, or effort). Another class of potential interruptors is rising anxiety. Anxiety occurs when contemplating or engaging in the activity is threatening for some reason. In both of these cases, the logic outlined above should apply.

This analysis has received research support with respect to both of these categories of situations. In one study, the model was applied to persistence in the face of failure (Carver, Blaney, & Scheier, 1979b). Subjects were given a failure pretreatment on what was described as a test of intelligence. Later they worked on a second task, which consisted in reality of one unsolvable puzzle. Some subjects were led to be optimistic concerning their performance on the second task, and others were led to be pessimistic. Those induced to hold negative expectancies for the second task persisted on that task less when self-focus was high than when it was lower. Those whose expectancies were more favorable persisted longer when self-attention was higher than when it was lower (a pattern that was conceptually replicated by Scheier & Carver, 1982).

Another project conducted at about the same time examined responses to fear (Carver, Blaney, & Scheier, 1979a). Subjects were selected as having uniformly moderate fear of nonpoisonous snakes. They varied, however, in self-reported expectancies of being able to pick up and hold a snake if asked to do so. Self-attention during a behavioral approach task led to self-reports of heightened anxiety among all subjects, and presumably to interruption and outcome assessment at an earlier stage of the task (see also Scheier, Carver, & Gibbons, 1981). The effect of self-attention on overt behavior, however, depended on subjects' preassessed levels of confidence. Doubtful subjects stopped the approach task earlier in the approach sequence when self-focus was high than when it was lower, whereas confident subjects tended to persist longer under conditions of heightened self-focus.[6]

When Disengagement Is More Difficult

Though a disengagement impetus occurs when people are sufficiently discouraged or doubtful, it is not always easy to disengage overtly from the goals one has taken up, no matter how unfavorable one's expectancies (see Figure 1.4). In some cases the social context does not sanction withdrawal (and in some cases the physical environment does not permit it). We have assumed that when there are such constraints on overt disengagement, the result is often a psychological or mental disengagement from the behavioral dimension in question (cf. Heckhausen, 1967; Lewin, 1935). This may be reflected in task-irrelevant thinking, daydreaming, and the like (cf. Brunson & Matthews, 1981; Diener & Dweck, 1978), as well as the tendency to avoid information that would indicate how poorly one is doing (cf. Carver et al., 1985). This mental disengagement may in some circumstances be useful—for example, by permitting debilitating anxiety to diminish. However, if the situation is such that mental disengagement has implications for performance (e.g., if there is time pressure), the result is likely be a performance deficit (Carver, Peterson, Follansbee, & Scheier, 1983; Carver & Scheier, 1982).

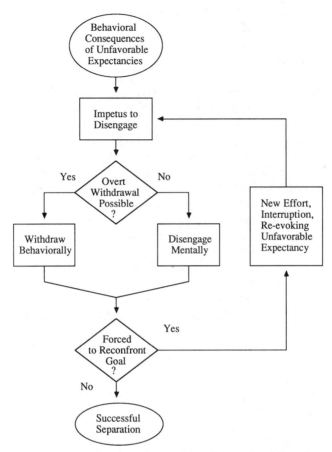

FIGURE 1.4 Elaborated depiction of behavioral possibilities that follow from unfavorable expectancies, including both overt and covert disengagement, either of which can be overridden by circumstances that force the person to reconfront the behavioral goal from which he or she is attempting to disengage.

Though mental disengagement may provide a temporary channel for expressing the impulse to withdraw, even this expression cannot always be sustained (Figure 1.4). There are many reference values from which complete disengagement is simply not feasible, even if doubts about discrepancy reduction are intense. Many high-order goals fit this description, goals such as doing well in one's chosen profession or having a good and fulfilling relationship with another person. Other goals that are less central to the sense of self, such as getting along with the people with whom one must interact repeatedly, may also be in this category. When a person perceives that matching such a value is unlikely, an attempt at disengagement may result. This temporary disengagement will sooner or later be followed by a renewed confrontation with the reference value, however, given life's circumstances. The result is a repeated cycle of sporadic effort, doubt, and disengagement.

Expectancies and Affect

Thus far we have limited ourselves to a consideration of the effects of interruption and expectancy assessment on action. We believe that these events also have an influence on affect. That is, deciding that goal attainment is or is not feasible should also have an impact on how one feels. The perception that goal attainment is unlikely should lead to negative affect—feelings of upset, frustration, and depression. A favorable expectancy, even if the situation is a difficult one, should lead to positive affect—feelings of excitement, happiness, and hope (cf. Stotland, 1969). Presumably, the intensity of this affect is proportional to the subjective importance of the behavioral dimension in question.

We have assumed that outcome expectancies set the general tone of the person's affective response—that is, influence whether the affect will be positive or negative. The more precise quality of the affect is determined by other considerations, primarily the perceived bases for the expectancy. That is, if the outcome expectancy is favorable and if the basis for the expectancy is the person's abilities or efforts, the feeling is experienced as heightened self-esteem or pride. If the expectancy arises instead because of aspects of one's environment (e.g., powerful and helpful others, or a benign situation), the positive feeling is experienced instead as gratitude.

Similarly, the exact qualities of the negative affect associated with doubt depends on attributional considerations. If the negative expectancy is seen as a product of one's own inadequacies or shortcomings, the result is lowered self-esteem or shame. If the expectancy depends instead upon external influences (e.g., powerful and hostile others, or a situation with insuperable obstacles), the feelings experienced are more likely to have overtones of anger and resentment. This line of reasoning was supported in a study of task performance in which good or bad expected outcomes were attributed to oneself or to a partner (Carver & Scheier, 1982).

Disengagement: When Is It Appropriate and When Is It Not?

In addressing the disengagement process in the preceding sections, we have emphasized the idea that confidence produces persistence, whereas doubt leads to giving up. It is important to point out that we do not mean to say thereby that the disengagement function is inherently maladaptive. Though disengagement always implies giving up, in many contexts it is quite sensible to give up or defer goals that presently are difficult or impossible to attain (cf. Janoff-Bulman & Brickman, 1982). It makes little sense, for example, to continue to shop for groceries once you discover that you have left your wallet—and thus all your money—at home. In this case, it is fully reasonable to defer the shopping.

There are other contexts, of course, in which disengagement is less adaptive. These are cases in which abandonment of the goal is premature, or in which the goal is one that should not (or cannot) be abandoned so easily. In such situations, the withdrawal of effort appears to be an ineffective way of coping with the ordinary difficulties of life. In line with this assertion, the line of reasoning presented in this section of the chapter has been used to analyze a variety of problems that seem to involve giving up on goals prematurely—problems including low self-esteem (Brockner, 1979) and both test anxiety and social anxiety (Burgio, Merluzzi, & Pryor, 1986; Carver, Peterson, et al., 1983; Carver, Scheier, & Klahr, 1987; Rich & Woolever, 1988; Schlenker & Leary, 1982). Though a full treatment of those literatures is beyond the scope of this chapter, more focused discussions have been presented elsewhere (Carver & Scheier, 1984, 1986a).

Taking a Look Around

It is very easy to point to commonalities between the ideas presented in this section and ideas appearing elsewhere. The expectancy construct has had a long history in psychology, dating back at least to Tolman (1932, 1938). It forms an essential part of expectancy–value approaches to achievement behavior (e.g., Atkinson & Feather, 1966; Atkinson & Raynor, 1974); it provides the cornerstone of learned helplessness theory (e.g., Abramson, Seligman, & Teasdale, 1978; Miller & Norman, 1979; Roth, 1980; Seligman, 1975; Weiner & Litman-Adizes, 1980); and it is incorporated into a number of other theories as well (e.g., Bandura, 1977, 1986; Feather, Chapter 5, this volume; Kanfer & Hagerman, 1981, 1985; Klinger, Barta, & Maxeiner, 1981; Mischel, 1973; Rotter, 1954; Wortman & Brehm, 1975). The convergence among such a wide range of theories attests to the explanatory power of the expectancy concept.

On the other hand, we should note that although the construct has been very widely used, it has been used (with various modifiers) in rather diverse ways. The diverging connotations of variations on this concept can be confusing. Four expectancy concepts are perhaps most common in analyses of behavioral self-regulation. One of them is the expectation that a particular action will lead to a given outcome (which Bandura, 1977, 1986, terms "outcome expectancy"). In most applications, though not all, this construct is used primarily as a foil for other expectancies.[7] That is, knowing that a given behavior will produce a given outcome is useful only to the extent that people also feel themselves capable of executing the behavior (a perception that Bandura terms "efficacy expectancy"). The expectancy of being able to execute the needed behavior is similar to another commonly used construct: the "expectancy of control" over the outcome.

Both efficacy and control expectancies focus on personal agency as a causal force. We are less convinced, however, of the need to assume that personal agency is the only important cause of people's efforts and their consequent outcomes (see also Wong & Sproule, 1984). Accordingly, we use an expectancy construct that is more ambiguous in that respect. We use the term "outcome expectancy" to refer to the subjective likelihood that a desired outcome will occur, given that one continues to exert efforts toward its attainment.

We de-emphasize personal agency in this construct in recognition of the fact that there are many circumstances in which people see outcomes as being subject to important influences besides their own skills or efforts. We believe that people often take these various influences into account simultaneously, arriving at an overall sense of whether or not the desired outcome is likely to occur. Thus, our outcome expectancy construct intrinsically incorporates a niche for such perceived influences on anticipated outcomes as a benign or hostile environment, religious faith, or belief in the effectiveness (or ineffectiveness) of a placebo (cf. Chambliss & Murray, 1979). Bandura's theory, in which self-efficacy is the final pathway to behavior, appears to force the position that personal efficacy is the only causal process that people consider with respect to their expectancies for success or failure.[8]

Our position regarding the role of personal efficacy is sometimes seen as an argument that personal control over outcomes is never important. This is a misperception. There are many circumstances (particularly in Western society) in which the goal underlying a person's behavior is to do something oneself, with no assistance from anyone else, and indeed with no aid from chance or the fates. We do not, however, believe that this depiction accurately characterizes all of human goal-directed behavior (see also Burger, 1989). Many outcomes are desirable in themselves (e.g., meeting enjoyable people, having a relaxing vacation, owning a Porsche, having one's tax returns consistently overlooked by Internal Revenue Service auditors), and precisely what causes those outcomes to occur is less important than the perception that they *will* occur.

To put it more formally, let us think of good outcomes as a broad category of experience, with outcomes produced by personal agency being a subset of that category. When the goal being pursued does not include the requirement of personal agency, people will have favorable expectancies for goal attainment any time a positive outcome is anticipated, regardless of whether personal agency is perceived to underlie the outcome. If the goal being pursued has the additional requirement of personal causality, however, the person will have a favorable expectancy only when a positive outcome is anticipated *and* it is perceived that personal agency is the basis for that outcome.

A similar principle is embedded in our thinking about the nature of the affect that surrounds favorable and unfavorable expectancies. That is, we assume that the valence of the expectancy creates an overall affective tone, which is modulated by the person's perceptions of the causes of the expectancy. This position, which we adopted on an intuitive basis, turns out to be very similiar to the position that Weiner (e.g., 1979, 1982, 1986a, 1986b) has taken for more systematic theoretical reasons. Weiner and his colleagues have also developed considerable empirical support for his theory. Certain affects (happiness, depression, frustration, and upset) are typically associated with outcome, independent of the attribution for the outcome. Other affects are associated with specific attributions. For example, ability attributions are associated with feelings of greater or lesser competence and pride. Attributions involving other persons are associated with feelings of gratitude or anger.

EMOTION

The preceding section of the chapter has described how expectancies influence the manner in which people deal with adversity, either encountered or anticipated. The general outlines of that analysis seem sensible to us, and it has been supported by a fair amount of research. That description has something of an ad hoc flavor to it, however, in the sense that it incorporates none of the language of feedback processes. We think we have a way of reconciling the ideas just outlined and the feedback concepts that we emphasized in an earlier section, but to do so we must take up in greater detail another aspect of the puzzle of self-regulation. The concept that must be considered more fully is emotion.

Although the preceding section includes some mention of the existence of feelings (in parallel to expectancies), we have not addressed directly the question of how good and bad feelings come to arise. Where exactly do feelings come from? There currently is a good deal of discussion of the circumstances under which various feeling qualities seem to occur and the psychological meaning of those feeling qualities (e.g., Hoffman, 1986; Ortony, Clore, & Collins, 1988; Srull & Wyer, 1986; Weiner, 1986a, 1986b). But there remains a sense in which these theories fail to address the question of the mechanism by which the underlying positive and negative affective tone comes to exist. Most theories include a statement to the effect that positive feelings arise from goal attainment and negative feelings arise from failure. This statement, we think, says both too much (because it is not always correct) and too little (because it fails to speak to cases in which feelings exist when neither success nor failure has occurred).

We have recently suggested a way of approaching this question (Carver & Scheier, 1990), in a way that makes use of the logic of feedback control. The ideas are, at this point, untested speculation. We think they are provocative, however, and they do appear to provide a way to round out the picture of self-regulation we have been trying to develop in this chapter. In this section we describe these ideas.[9] We do so by reconsidering, in somewhat different terms, some of the events described earlier.

We began this chapter by characterizing people's conscious self-regulation as a process of monitoring present actions and comparing the qualities perceived therein to the reference values that presently are salient, making adjustments as necessary to render discrepancies minimal. In this section, we use the term "monitoring" as a shorthand way of referring to this feedback process. As indicated earlier, we see this monitoring loop as fundamental to the control of intentional behavior.

Consider now the possibility that there is also a second feedback process that (in a sense) builds on this one, but does so in a fashion that is orthogonal to the hierarchical organization discussed earlier. This second loop operates simultaneously with the monitoring loop and in parallel to it. The second feedback system serves what we will term a "metamonitoring" function.

Discrepancy Reduction and the Pace of Discrepancy Reduction

The most intuitive way to describe what this metamonitoring function is doing is to say that the meta loop is checking on how well the action loop is doing at reducing the behavioral discrepancies that the action loop is itself monitoring. More concretely, the perceptual input for the metamonitoring loop is a representation of the *rate of discrepancy reduction in the behavioral (monitoring) system over time*. What is important to the meta loop is not merely *whether* the action loop is reducing sensed discrepancies, but *how rapidly* it is doing so. If discrepancies are being reduced rapidly, the action loop's rate of progress (which is the meta loop's perceptual input) is a high value. If discrepancies are not being reduced at all, the action loop's progress (the meta loop's perceptual input) is zero. Any time discrepancies are enlarging at the level of action monitoring, of course, the action loop's progress is inverse. (In the remainder of this section, we will treat phrases such as "progress of the action loop" as shorthand for "rate of discrepancy reduction in the action loop.")

We find an analogy useful in describing the functioning of these two systems. Because action implies change between states, let us consider action to be analogous to distance (treating distance as a vector, because perception of one's action incorporates both the difference between successive states and also the direction of the difference). If the monitoring loop deals with distance, and if the meta loop assesses the rate of progress of the monitoring loop, then the meta loop is dealing with the psychological equivalent of velocity (also directional). In mathematical terms, velocity is the first derivative of distance over time. To the extent that the physical analogy is meaningful, the input to the meta loop would be the first derivative over time of the same input information as is used by the action loop.

If metamonitoring functions as a feedback loop, there must be more going on than mere sensing of the rate of discrepancy reduction in the action loop. Sensing this quality provides an input, but no more. If the meta loop is a feedback system, this input must be compared against a reference value (cf. Frijda, 1986, 1988). In the case of the meta loop, the reference value is some acceptable or desired rate of change with respect to behavioral discrepancy reduction. As in any feedback system, the comparison yields an assessment of discrepancy or deviation from the standard.

We think that the outcome of this meta-level comparison is manifest phenomenologically in two forms. The first is a hazy and nonverbal sense of outcome expectancy. The second is affect, a feeling quality, a sense of positiveness or negativeness.

When sensed progress in the action loop conforms to the desired rate of progress, the metamonitoring system registers no discrepancy (see Table 1.1, example 1). Given an absence of any discrepancy at the meta level, affect is neutral. When the action loop is making continuous, steady progress toward

TABLE 1.1   Three Conditions of Behavior over Time, How They Would Be Construed at the Level of the Action Loop, How They Would Be Construed at the Level of the Metamonitoring Loop, and the Affect That Theoretically Would Be Experienced

Depiction of behavior	Action loop construal	Meta loop construal	Affect
1. Progress toward goal, at a rate equal to the standard	Discrepancy reduction	No discrepancy	None
2. Progress toward goal, at a rate lower than the standard	Discrepancy reduction	Discrepancy	Negative
3. Progress toward goal, at a rate higher than the standard	Discrepancy reduction	Positive discrepancy	Positive

Note. From "Origins and Functions of Positive and Negative Affect: A Control-Process View" by C. S. Carver and M. F. Scheier, 1990, *Psychological Review*, 97, 19–35. Copyright 1990 by the American Psychological Association. Reprinted by permission.

reducing its own discrepancy but its rate of discrepancy reduction is slower than the metamonitoring system's reference value, a discrepancy exists for the meta loop (Table 1.1, example 2). The result in this case should be a degree of doubt and negative affect, proportional to the size of this meta-level discrepancy. When the rate of discrepancy reduction in the action loop is higher than the meta loop's reference value (Table 1.1, example 3), there is a positive discrepancy at the meta loop—an overshoot of the reference value that is reflected in confidence and in positive feelings.

It is clear that the two systems under discussion (monitoring and metamonitoring) are related to each other (they use some of the same information, but modified in different ways). It is our view, however, that only one of them has direct implications for affect. In all of the cases shown in Table 1.1, the action loop is successfully reducing discrepancies. Affect, however, differs from case to case. Affect may be neutral, it may be positive, or it may even be negative, depending on the adequacy of the *rate* of discrepancy reduction. Assessing the adequacy of the rate of progress of the first system implies the existence of a second system.

It is also important to note that in this view the size of the discrepancy confronted by the action loop at any given point does not play an important role in the perceptual input to the meta loop. A large discrepancy—even a *very* large discrepancy—perceived at the level of the action loop can be associated with perceptions of either abundant progress or insufficient progress. This same discrepancy thus can be associated with either favorable or unfavorable expectancies and with either positive or negative affect. The only thing that matters with respect to the metamonitoring system is whether or not the perceived *rate of progress* in the action system is adequate.

Indeed, the same point can also be made of cases in which the behavioral discrepancy is relatively small. If the metamonitoring system senses that there is an abundant rate of change toward complete discrepancy reduction, there should be positive affect and a feeling of confidence. If it senses an inadequate rate of change, there should be negative affect and doubt.

Thus, ironically, it should be possible for a person who has a large discrepancy at the action loop to feel more positively than a person who has a small discrepancy at the action loop, if the first person is perceiving a more acceptable rate of progress than the second person. In terms of the physical analogy, the first person is more distant from the goal, but is moving toward it with a higher velocity.

Just as the monitoring of action apparently can take any of several levels in a hierarchy of behavioral control as superordinate, so should the meta system be able to function at any of several levels. It seems likely, however, that discrepancies noted by the meta system have greater emotional impact when they concern a central element of self than when they bear only on a more peripheral goal (a program or a sequence of action). Sometimes a task failure has a big impact on one's feelings, sometimes not (cf. Dweck & Elliott, 1983; Dweck & Leggett, 1988; Elliott & Dweck, 1988; Hyland, 1987; Srull & Wyer, 1986). The difference between these cases would seem to be the level of abstraction at which the person is focusing. The consequences of metamonitoring are more intense, or have a greater impact, at higher levels than at lower levels of the hierarchy (see also Frijda, 1988).

The view that affect derives from a feedback process has a further implication that is in some respects highly counterintuitive, though in other respects it fits well with intuition. The implication is this: If the meta loop is really a bidirectional feedback system, it follows that overshooting the reference value (the condition creating positive affect) should lead to a self-corrective attempt to return to the reference value. This reasoning fits with intuition in suggesting that people who have exceeded their desired rate of progress are likely to slow their subsequent efforts and coast for a while. What is counterintuitive is the suggestion that something about the way the human organism is organized naturally works against the continued existence of good feelings (as well as bad feelings).

The existence of such a natural tendency seems, at first glance, highly unlikely. A plausible basis for such a tendency can be seen, however, in the idea that human behavior is hierarchically organized and involves multiple current concerns. That is, people typically are working toward several goals more or less simultaneously, and many lower-level efforts contribute to minimizing discrepancies at high levels. To the extent that movement toward goal attainment is more rapid than expected in one domain, it permits the person to shift attention and effort toward goal strivings in another domain, at no cost. To continue the unnecessarily rapid pace in the first domain may increase positive affect regarding that activity, but by thus diverting effort from other goals, that action creates the potential for negative affect in other domains.

Rate and Changes in Rate

What we have said thus far concerns various rates of progress toward action goals (above, below, and equal to the reference value). It should be obvious that the rate of discrepancy reduction at the action loop can *change over time*. Changes in rate at the action loop are subjectively manifested not as affect, but as change of affect. The subjective experience will in some respects depend on the initial and final rates. An increase in rate from below to above the criterion value will be experienced as a change from negative affect to positive affect. An increase in rate from well below the criterion value to a point equal to that value will be experienced as a change from negative affect to no affect.

These shifts in rate can be gradual, or they can be more abrupt. The more abrupt an increase in the action loop's progress, the more the subjective experience incorporates a rush of exhilaration, reflecting the contrast between the more negative feelings and more positive feelings (cf. Frijda's [1988, p. 350] description of "sentimentality"). The more abrupt the slowing of the action loop's progress, the more the subjective experience should incorporate the well-known "sinking feeling" (de-exhilaration?) that reflects the contrast when feelings suddenly shift in a negative direction. Indeed, it may be that a shift toward more negative feelings is often precisely what causes the person to interrupt ongoing action, as we described earlier, and consciously evaluate the probability of eventual success.

We earlier suggested a physical analogy, such that sensed progress of the action loop is analogous to the physical quality of velocity. To take this analogy one step further, changes in rate of progress are analogous to the physical quality of acceleration. Returning to this analogy allows us to make one more point. In the same way that physical distance and velocity are independent of each other, both of these qualities are independent of acceleration. (An object moving 20 feet per second can be accelerating or decelerating, or its velocity can be constant; the same is true of an object moving at 80 feet per second.)

We suggest that the same independence also exists on the other side of the analogy. That is, we argued earlier that the affect a person experiences is independent of the degree of discrepancy at the action level (see Table 1.1). In the same fashion, the exhilaration associated with acceleration of progress is distinct from both the size of the discrepancy at the action level and the rate of discrepancy reduction at the action level. In other words, the affect and the exhilaration are separate qualities.

To use an example, a person with a large discrepancy at the action level will have positive affect if the rate of discrepancy reduction is greater than needed. This positive affect will be relatively free of exhilaration if the rate of discrepancy reduction is constant. If the rate has suddenly shifted upward (to the same ending value), the positive feelings should be accompanied by a greater sense of exhilaration. Similar reasoning can be applied to negative affect and the experience of de-exhilaration.

Further Processing and Differences between Immediate and Subsequent Expectancies

In describing the postulated metamonitoring function, we suggested that one manifestation of its operation is a hazy sense of expectancy. Obviously, however, people's expectancies for an outcome do not rest entirely on their currently sensed rate of progress toward the outcome. Indeed, as we outlined in a previous section of the chapter, our own research has consistently emphasized the fact that temporary frustration or anxiety is less important than are other sources of information in leading to the coping expectancies that determine subsequent behavior (Carver et al., 1979a, 1979b; Carver, Peterson, et al., 1983). Thus, although metamonitoring during a period of threat and difficulty yields a sense of doubt, this transient doubt is often modified in the light of additional thought. This additional thought means stepping away from the meta loop temporarily (though not necessarily too far away).

In judging outcome probability more deliberatively, people depend to a large extent on memories of their prior outcomes in similar situations. They also reflect on additional resources they might bring to bear on the problem (cf. Lazarus, 1966), on the possibility of alternative approaches to the problem, and on social comparison information (e.g., Wills, 1981; Wood, Taylor, & Lichtman, 1985). In sum, the more conscious and verbalizable expectancies that people generate when they interrupt their efforts and think about the likely outcomes of those efforts are influenced by additional processing, potentially involving a fairly wide range of information.

In many instances, this additional processing is very simple. It may involve nothing more than retrieving a summary memory regarding prior outcomes in this class of situations (e.g., "I always do poorly at standardized tests"; "People never like me") or engaging in self-exhortation ("You can do it—try harder"). Other instances, however, involve a more wide-ranging search of diverse memories, or a more extensive analysis of possibilities with respect to the present situation. This more complex search might involve thinking about such questions as whether additional information about the situation is obtainable, whether other people might be able and willing to provide assistance, or whether important aspects of the situation are likely to change soon enough to make any difference.

How do these various thoughts influence subsequent expectancies and affect? In the first set of cases noted, the mechanism is probably very simple. When people retrieve chronic expectancies from memory in summary form, the information is already coded in the form of expectancies. Presumably, these memories represent summaries or consolidations of the products of earlier instances of metamonitoring during behavior. When evoked from memory, this information presumably contributes directly to a subsequent sense of confidence or doubt. Memories of expectancies may also be linked to memories of the corresponding affective qualities, thus directly influencing subsequent affective tone.

In the second set of cases noted above, a more complex mechanism may apply—a mechanism that is tied to the theory we are outlining. When people stop and analyze the situation they are in, they typically bring to mind a series of possible ways of approaching the situation or ways in which the situation might change. In order for these possibilities to influence subsequent expectancies, their likely consequences must be evaluated. How are they evaluated? One plausible argument is that they are briefly played through mentally as behavioral scenarios. Playing through the scenarios should lead to conclusions that influence the person's outcome expectancy for the actual situation ("If I approach it this way instead of that way, it should work better"; This is the only thing I can see to do, and it will just make the situation worse").

It seems reasonable to suggest that this evaluation process engages the same mental apparatus as handles metamonitoring during overt behavior. When one's progress is currently stalled, playing through a scenario that is confident and optimistic will indicate a higher rate of behavioral progress than is currently being experienced. The meta loop thus will yield a more optimistic outcome assessment than is currently being derived from overt action. If the scenario is negative and hopeless, reflecting further diminished progress, the meta loop will yield an assessment of greater doubt. Thus, expectancy-related rumination can either reduce or exacerbate a person's initial hesitancy and doubt, depending on the scenario that comes to mind. We suggest, however, that the influence on subsequent expectancies (and affect, as well) may involve the same processing mechanism as that producing more momentary effects on expectancies during the actual flow of behavior.

Illustrations

Thus far in this section, our discussion has been quite abstract. We believe, however, that the implications of the principles we have described are more accessible intuitively than may be apparent thus far. Let us apply the principles to a couple of common experiences, to try to make this clearer. These examples also will illustrate two ways in which our arguments differ from those typically made about the source of affect.

We have argued that positive feelings arise from a high rate of discrepancy reduction in the action loop, even if a large discrepancy remains to be reduced. In thinking about this, consider the experience of being stuck on a problem in your work. Sometimes the realization occurs that you know a different way to approach the problem (sometimes even know that this approach will eventually lead to a solution). This event constitutes both a high rate of progress and an acceleration in progress. Such a realization often produces a flash of elation—even if the behavioral goal itself (i.e., the problem's actual solution) is very distant. Thus, affect does not depend on attaining a success. Affect can arise at any stage of the process of goal-directed action.

Success usually produces positive feelings; this has led many to use success as the defining condition for positive affect. Paradoxically, however, success sometimes has the opposite effect. At first glance, a crowning success might seem to be the ultimate in progress. But a great deal depends on the context in which the success is embedded. If the goal attained leads to a dead end, rather than opening up the possibility of other goals to move toward, the success leads in some sense to a halt in progress. The former goal may remain active because it was highly valued, or simply because it has been in place so long, but there is no longer any progress toward it. In such a case, the success may be followed (or even accompanied) by a sense of dysphoria, rather than elation. Success is most likely to lead to sustained positive feelings when the attainment of one goal slides smoothly into a sense of progress toward attaining other goals.

These examples both concern overt actions in which movement toward behavioral goals is progressing at either an adequate or inadequate rate. It is not necessary, however, that a person be engaged in overt action for emotion to be generated. As we suggested earlier, we suspect that the metamonitoring processes we have outlined here are often engaged as a person plays out a scenario mentally, as well as when a physical action is taking place. Thus, a person can feel either hope or despair over the anticipated progress of an event that has not yet begun (cf. Markus & Nurius, 1986). Similarly, a person can renew feelings (as opposed to simply recalling them) by mentally reliving an event that has already happened. The more vivid the reliving, the stronger the affect experienced (see also Frijda, 1988). In such a case, the affect would not simply be retrieved from memory; it would be regenerated.

Reference Values Used for Metamonitoring

What reference value is used by the metamonitoring system? We assume that this system is capable of monitoring with respect to varying definitions of adequate progress for the action loop (just as the action loop is capable of monitoring with respect to varying actions). Sometimes the reference value is imposed from outside (as in a tenure review decision), and sometimes it is self-imposed (as in someone with a personal timetable for career development). Sometimes the reference value is very demanding; sometimes it is less so.

As an example in which the meta standard is both stringent and externally imposed, consider the requirements of degree programs in medical or law school. In such cases, even continuous progress in an absolute sense (i.e., successful mastery of required material) is adequate only if it occurs at or above the rate required by the degree program. Thus, as the person attempts to attain the action goal of becoming a physician or lawyer, the reference value for metamonitoring will be a relatively stringent one.

How stringent a standard is being used at the meta level has straightforward implications for the person's emotional life. If the pace of progress used as a reference point is too high, the person's rate of behavioral discrepancy reduction will rarely live up to it, even if (objectively) the person's rate of progress is extraordinarily high. In such a case, the person will experience negative affect often and positive affect rarely. If the pace of progress used as a reference point is very low, the person's rate of behavioral discrepancy reduction will more frequently exceed it. In this case, the person will experience positive affect more often and negative affect more rarely.[10]

What variables influence the stringency of the meta-level standard being used? One important determinant is the extent to which there is time pressure on the activity being regulated. This, of course, varies greatly from one activity to another. Some actions are clearly time-dependent ("That report must be turned in by 5:00"); others are more vaguely so ("It's about the time of year to fertilize the lawn"), and the time dependency is even hazier for others ("I want to go to China some day"; "I'd like to have a boat before I get to be too old to enjoy it"). When an activity has demanding time constraints, the meta-level reference value used necessarily is stringent. When there is a relative lack of time pressure, a lax standard is more likely to be used.

Although time dependence is clearest in situations that require a rapid pace, there also seems to be a second sort of time dependence. This occurs in behavioral activities that people wish to have completed but have no desire to do (a common view of chores). Such goals are highly time-dependent, in the sense that people wish their attainment to be instantaneous. Given this, the meta-level reference value is at a very high level. Because the rate of progress therefore cannot meet the standard, positive affect is nearly impossible and aversiveness is almost inevitable when the activity is being engaged in. (On the other hand, the intensity of this affect is proportional to the importance of the activity, which is often relatively low.) This set of relations would seem to define the experience of drudgery.

Mixed Feelings, and the Independence of Positive and Negative Affect

Our discussion thus far has focused on the existence of one feeling at a time. Affect associated with goal-directed effort need not be purely positive or purely negative, however. It is entirely possible for a single event to produce both of these feelings, depending on how it is viewed in metamonitoring.

Sometimes more than one view may be taken on an event, even when the event is considered with respect to a single goal (cf. Ortony et al., 1988, pp. 51–52). For example, sometimes the experience of a failure yields the realization of how to attain future success. The failure is displeasing, but the insight is elating. Feelings generated by the event thus are mixed. Focusing more on the present failure to attain the goal (inadequate progress) will yield a greater sense of negative affect. Focusing more on the insight (progress toward future success) will yield a greater sense of positive affect. Both feelings, however, are produced by different aspects of the same outcome, and both can be felt at once (or as alternating time-shared experiences).

It is perhaps more common that an action or an outcome has implications for two distinct goals. The goals making up the hierarchy of a person's self-definition are not always perfectly compatible with each other, and occasionally two conflicting goals become salient at the same time (see also Emmons, 1986;

Van Hook & Higgins, 1988). For example, the goal of career advancement and the goal of spending a lot of time with one's young children may both be desirable, but the 24-hour day imposes limitations on the time available for trying to attain them. Sometimes the actions that permit progress toward one goal (working extra hours at the office) simultaneously interfere with progress toward the other goal (spending time with one's children). To the extent that both goals remain salient, the result is mixed feelings. In this case, however, the two feeling qualities stem from metamonitoring with respect to each of two distinct goals.

This general line of thought also suggests a perspective on the assertion, made frequently in recent years, that positive and negative affective experiences are not inversely associated but rather are independent (e.g., Diener & Emmons, 1984; Diener & Iran-Nejad, 1986; Warr, Barter, & Brownbridge, 1983; Watson & Tellegen, 1985; Zevon & Tellegen, 1982). This argument, which usually focuses on the experience of moods rather than on the nature of affect, means in part that people's moods can incorporate mixed feelings. A mood can be partly good and partly bad, though only rarely are both of these feelings intense at the same time (Diener & Iran-Nejad, 1986).

This argument also means that knowing a person is not depressed does not make it reasonable to infer that the person is happy. Knowing a person is not happy does not make it reasonable to infer that the person feels bad. Sometimes people are affectively neutral. The relative independence of these qualities thus has important methodological implications. To know about both positive and negative qualities in people's overall feelings, one must assess both (cf. Wortman & Silver, 1989).

Although these two qualities of mood have been observed to vary relatively independently, there has been very little discussion of why this is so. Diener and Iran-Nejad (1986) noted that their subjects sometimes reported moderate amounts of both positive and negative affect, but they did not speculate on why. Watson and Tellegen (1985) noted the possibility that different parts of the brain might be involved in the two affect qualities, but did not address the question of why people might ever experience mixed feelings.

The preceding discussion suggests a very simple explanation for these findings. People often have many goals at once. A person who is making rapid progress on some of his or her current concerns and poor progress on others should experience positive feelings with respect to the former and negative feelings with respect to the latter. The experience of mixed outcomes must be common, even in the course of a single day. The diversity of these "progress reports" from the metamonitoring system should disrupt any inverse correlation between reports of having experienced positive affect and reports of having experienced negative affect in a given time span, particularly if that span is relatively long. As the time span narrows to a given "emotional" event, one would expect the independence of the two affects to diminish, because the person is more likely to be dealing with only one goal (and only one perspective on it) than would otherwise be the case. This is precisely what seems to happen (Diener & Iran-Nejad, 1986).

Negative Affect and Disengagement: Additional Issues

This section has focused on the attempt to conceptualize feeling qualities and expectancies within a framework resting on feedback principles. There are, however, several issues that arise when one considers this approach to emotion in conjunction with one aspect of the model of self-regulation outlined earlier. In particular, an important aspect of that model is the idea that if a person's expectancies of goal attainment are sufficiently unfavorable, the person may disengage from pursuit of the goal (see also Klinger, 1975; Kukla, 1972; Wortman & Brehm, 1975). Considering this disengagement response, and the emotions that often surround it, raises a variety of questions.

One issue stems from the idea that behavior is hierarchically organized, and that goals are increasingly important as one moves upward through the hierarchy. We assume that it rarely is difficult to disengage from values low in the hierarchy of control. Indeed, the nature of programs is such that disengagement from efforts at subgoals is quite common, even while the person continues to pursue the overall goal of the program (e.g., if you go to buy something and the store is closed for inventory, you often head for another store that stocks the item rather than give up altogether).

Sometimes, however, disengaging from a lower-order goal has serious implications for discrepancy reduction or enlargement at a higher level. Sometimes the standards or reference values from which one is attempting to disengage have implications for higher-order goals that are important, even central to one's life. One cannot withdraw from these values permanently without substantially reorganizing one's value system (Carver & Scheier, 1986b; Kelly, 1955; Millar, Tesser, & Millar, 1988). Disengagement from certain goals, then, is quite difficult.

Now recall the affective consequences of being in this situation. The desire to disengage was prompted in the first place by unfavorable expectancies for discrepancy reduction. These expectancies are paralleled by negative affect. In this situation, then, the person is experiencing strong negative feelings (because of an inability to make adequate progress toward behavioral discrepancy reduction) and is unable to do anything about those feelings (because of an inability to give up the behavioral reference value). The person in this situation simply stews in the feelings that arise from irreconcilable discrepancies (see also Martin & Tesser, 1989). In our view, this bind—being unable to let go of something that is unattainable—often lies at the heart of exogenous depression (cf. Hyland, 1987; Klinger, 1975; Pyszczynski & Greenberg, 1987). It seems important to recognize that the existence of this bind often stems in part from the hierarchical quality of people's goal systems.

A second issue is also raised by the idea that effort gives way to disengagement as expectancies become more negative. Though we believe this does occur, there is a conceptual discontinuity between this idea and the feedback ideas we presented in this section of the chapter. In the conceptual model of negative affect presented earlier in this section, where is there a mechanism to produce disengagement? We portrayed metamonitoring as a feedback system in which discrepancies (inadequate progress) produce doubt and negative affect. Why should this system (and the corresponding monitoring system) not just continue endlessly to attempt to reduce discrepancies, however ineffectively? Why should the negative affect not simply persist or intensify? What permits the person ever to disengage?

The answer has to be that in normal self-regulation there is an override mechanism of some sort that is capable of taking precedence over this feedback system and causes disengagement from the reference value currently being used to guide action. In the jargon of the computer metaphor, there must be a "break" function, which permits ongoing action to be suspended or abandoned altogether. In circumstances where disengagement is adaptive, it is adaptive precisely because it frees the system to take up other reference values; it enables the person to turn to the pursuit of substitute or alternate goals. Such an override function is a critically important element in human self-regulation, inasmuch as there are any number of goals from which people simply must disengage, either temporarily or permanently (see Klinger, 1975, for a broader discussion of commitment to and disengagement from incentives).

Although it seems necessary to assume an override function in adaptive self-regulation, it should also be re-emphasized that disengagement does not always take place, even when the desire to disengage is there. As we have just noted, when the goal toward which the person is unable to make progress is central to that person's implicit definition of self, the person for that reason often cannot disengage from it. Disengagement from such a goal means disengagement from oneself. Such a circumstance, we suggested, yields substantial distress.

Indeed, there is evidence that the inability (or unwillingness) to disengage is a correlate of depression. Depression has been linked to behavioral indicators of failing to disengage mentally from experimentally created failures (Kuhl, 1984, 1985; Pyszczynski & Greenberg, 1985, 1987). Depression has also been linked to concurrent self-reports of a tendency to perseverate mentally on failure (Carver, La Voie, Kuhl, & Ganellen, 1988) and to ruminate on personally valued activities during forced suspension of those activities (Millar et al., 1988). Mental perseveration among depressed people is not limited to major life goals, but can occur even for transient and relatively trivial intentions (Kuhl & Helle, 1986). Thus, there is evidence suggesting that depression is bound up with a general failure to override and disengage. It is not clear why this should be so, but in some sense this failure seems to be at the core of the dynamics of depression (see also Klinger, 1975).

Discussion of this issue also raises a more general question. People clearly vary in how easily they put previously valued goals behind them and move on to new ones. This is true whether the goal has been removed permanently by some external event—for example, the death of a loved one (cf. Wortman & Silver, 1989)—or whether the person has simply decided to abandon the previously sought-after goal, as happens when people break off close relationships or give up desired careers. Some people disengage quickly and move on, experiencing relatively little distress; others take longer to disengage, and consequently experience more negative affect. What makes people differ from each other in this way seems an important question.

Taking a Look Around

The ideas proposed in this section of the chapter share certain elements with several other current approaches to emotion. For example, frequent citations to Frijda (1988) in the course of our description reflect the fact that our ideas have commonalities with the tone of his far more extensive theory of emotion (Frijda, 1986). Somewhat more straightforward and easier to discuss is the relationship between our ideas and two other theories of emotion. One of them has recently been proposed by Higgins (1987). His model makes considerable use of the concept of discrepancy, as does ours, though it does so in somewhat different ways.

Higgins (1987) proposed that certain emotions occur as the consequences of discrepancies between pairs of psychological entities. For the sake of simplicity, we deal here with only two kinds of discrepancy. The first is between one's perceived actual self and one's "ideal" self (actual–ideal discrepancies). The second is between one's perceived actual self and one's "ought" self (actual–ought discrepancies). (We also disregard the fact that ideals and oughts can be one's own, or can also be imposed on one by significant others.)

An ideal self is a desired self, a self to which one aspires. This mental entity is reward-based. Living up to the ideal means attaining something desired, acquiring reward. An ought self, in contrast, is a duty or obligation, a self that one feels compelled to be, rather than desires to be. This entity is punishment-based. Living up to an ought means doing something so as to avoid a punishment. Each person has ideals, and each person has oughts (which may be either interrelated or distinct); the perceived actual self may be compared to each of these reference points.

According to Higgins, large discrepancies between ideal and actual yield depressed affect. Pure depression thus represents a failure to attain rewards. In contrast, large discrepancies between ought and actual are said to yield anxiety. Pure anxiety thus represents an impending failure to avoid punishment. This separation of reference values for the self into ideal versus ought is reminiscent of Gray's (1981, 1982) discussion of behavioral approach and behavioral avoidance systems in behavior, which he believes are mediated by distinct physiological structures.

Three differences between this theory and our approach deserve comment. First, Higgins (1987) proposed that depressed affect is a consequence of a discrepancy between an actual and an ideal representation of the self. As described in this section of the chapter, we think that the discrepancy that matters is a discrepancy in sensed rate of *progress* toward that representation. Thus, from our point of view, a person who is discrepant from the ideal but perceives rapid enough movement toward it should experience positive rather than negative affect.

A second difference between theories is also implicit in this last statement. The model we outlined here deals explicitly with both positive and negative affect. The theory proposed by Higgins, in contrast, focuses almost exclusively on negative affect. Although Higgins did mention positive affect in passing (1987, p. 336), this mention seems to us to have raised more questions about the meaning of positive affect within his framework than it answered. In particular, Higgins appears to have taken the position that positive affect consists of the absence of negative affect—a position we are not at all sure is tenable. Although a complete discussion of the issue is beyond the scope of this chapter, this seems an important issue to resolve.

The third comparison between theories concerns the distinction between ideals and oughts. This is the most novel aspect of the Higgins analysis, providing him a conceptual basis for differentiating anxiety from depression. We, in contrast, have never attempted to make this differentiation between negative affects. On the other hand, this aspect of the Higgins model can be translated into feedback terms with relatively little difficulty. Higgins framed the distinction between ideals and oughts in terms of reward and punishment contingencies. There is a rough correspondence between these contingencies and two kinds of feedback systems. A negative feedback loop, to which our discussion has been limited thus far, is a discrepancy-*reducing* or -negating loop (thus the label "negative"). This system has a positive reference value, a desired goal. This sort of system would be construed by some people as reinforcement-based.

A positive feedback loop, in contrast, is a discrepancy-*amplifying* loop (Carver & Scheier, 1981a, Ch. 2; Ford, 1987, Ch. 3; Maruyama, 1963; see DeAngelis, Post, & Travis, 1986, for applications). The reference value of this system is an undesired quality. Discrepancy-amplifying loops attempt to move the currently perceived value as far away as possible from the reference value. This sort of system would be construed by some as punishment-based. Deviation-amplifying loops are believed to be less common in naturally occurring systems than discrepancy-reducing systems, because they are unstable. Nevertheless, whenever the motive behind an act is the desire to prevent a condition from existing, the behavior would seem to reflect a positive feedback loop (for examples, see Carver & Scheier, 1981a, pp. 157–165; Ogilvie, 1987).

Presumably, metamonitoring can occur with respect to both types of loops, providing (in terms of our ideas) a basis for affect in either case. If the distinction made by Higgins is valid, then, we would say that depressed affect occurs when there is insufficient progress in a negative feedback system (an approach system) and that anxiety occurs when there is insufficient progress in a positive feedback system (an avoidance system). Thus, there is a way to reconcile this aspect of Higgins's theory with the metatheoretical orientation we are promoting.

Our ideas also have an interesting relation to another emotion theory. Mandler (1984; Mandler & Watson, 1966) has proposed that interruption of an organized sequence of action causes autonomic arousal, which creates the potential for emotion (*à la* Schachter & Singer, 1962). He sees anxiety as the emotion most likely to occur after interruption, because interruptors often leave people without alternate ways to reach desired goals; this (to Mandler) is what induces the label "anxiety" (cf. Millar et al., 1988).

Though Mandler sees anxiety as the most likely emotional consequence of interruption, sometimes interruption leads to other emotions, even positive ones. Berscheid (1983), in applying Mandler's theory to interpersonal attraction, has developed this idea more completely. She argued for two cases in which interruptions *facilitate* completion of action sequences, thus producing positive emotion. In the first case, an interruption is removed or shown to have less of an impact than it first appeared to have. In the second case, the interruption is an event that produces attainment of a desired goal sooner than anticipated. In either of these cases, interruption can result in positive feelings.

There are obvious similarities between this view and ours. One is the idea that obstructions to goal attainment can cause emotional reactions. We agree with Mandler and Berscheid that a person who feels helpless and disorganized after an interruption will experience negative affect. In our view, however, impeding or disrupting efforts at goal attainment yields negative affect intrinsically, rather than merely creating a condition of affect-free arousal that must be assigned affective meaning (cf. Chwalisz, Diener, & Gallagher, 1988).

The two situations said by Berscheid (1983) to produce positive affect seem to us to reduce to a single phenomenon: In each case, there occurs a shift toward higher levels of progress toward goal attainment. When an interrupting condition is removed, a loss of progress (the interruption) is followed by *enhanced* progress. When goal attainment occurs unexpectedly quickly, the increase in progress is immediate (i.e., without an initial slowing). Both cases satisfy our condition for positive affect, in that both suggest progress at a rate that exceeds the likely reference point.

We would hold, however, that the position taken by Berscheid on positive affect minimizes two important points. In the case of removal of an interrupting condition, we would argue that there is negative affect during the period between onset and removal of that initial interruption. Only when the removal occurs (or is anticipated) does affect shift, because only then does progress return to a high level. Second, we would argue that it is not *completion* of act sequences that is pleasing (as both Mandler and Berscheid hold), but movement toward completion at a rate higher than needed.

CLOSING COMMENT

In this chapter, we have tried to indicate some of the ways in which feedback principles can be of use in approaching an understanding of the human experience. The feedback-based view of behavior is one in which people's goals and values are inherently of central importance. Of similar importance are the skills that serve as means by which these ends are to be attained. From this view, it is important to understand the structure of people's representations of their goals and subgoals, and the processes by which they develop better understandings of how higher-order goals are attained through lower-order actions. In this view, self-regulation is a cycle of creating representations of outcomes that one wants to have come to pass, and then trying to make reality match those representations. Finally, it is important to understand that emotion plays an important role in self-regulation—a role that is not necessarily as mysterious as it might once have seemed.

Although the easiest illustrations of the principles outlined in this chapter probably come from domains of achievement and instrumental activity, we do not mean to suggest that these ideas apply only to achievement goals. We believe that this approach to behavior applies to all goal-directed action, and we see the category of goal-directed action as very broad indeed. Human goals such as developing and maintaining a sound relationship, being a good mother or father, dealing honorably and pleasantly with acquaintances, seeing someone you care about be happy and fulfilled, having a full and rich life, and becoming immersed in the fictional lives portrayed in a novel are fully amenable to analysis in these terms.

Finally, it should be clearly understood that we do not regard this theoretical statement as an endpoint, but rather as a way station. There are many places in the preceding sections where important issues remain to be resolved, where speculation stands in the place of understanding. We hope, however, that these ideas are intriguing enough to represent a useful starting place for others in the exploration of how human motivation translates into action.

Notes

1. This distinction is related to that made between declarative and procedural knowledge (e.g., Cantor & Kihlstrom, 1987; Smith, 1984), though it is not the same. The phrase "procedural knowledge" is used to denote responses that are coded in memory as productions rather than as propositions (for detail see Smith, 1984). Some of these responses are acts, but others are purely mental events. What we refer to here as "act-specifying information" may be a subtype of procedural knowledge.

2. Our use of terms such as "self-awareness" and "self-focus" does not imply a searching or in-depth examination of the self. As used here, they merely denote momentary shifts of one's attention to that aspect of self pertinent to what one is doing and what one is intending to do.

3. The Powers (1973) model is one example of a broader class of possibilities (cf. Bower, 1978; Kelso & Kay, 1987; Newell, 1973). The details of these approaches are at present less important to us than are commonalities of the models as a class. We focus on Powers's hierarchy because it seems to capture the qualities of human action that we find most interesting.

4. We note in passing that some goals in behavior are private, in the sense that they stand apart from the needs or wishes of other people; other goals are public, social, or self-presentational in nature, with the desires and perceptions of others playing a significant role. There is considerable evidence that focusing on private aspects of the self causes behavior to shift toward the former goals, and that focusing on public aspects of the self causes behavior to shift toward the latter goals. Though a full treatment of that literature is beyond the scope of this chapter, our view is that the level of principle control is where the private–public distinction is most important, as the person adopts either a personal or a social orientation to behavior (for an expanded discussion, see Carver & Scheier, 1985).

5. Some may question the universality of this principle. Consider people whose primary interest is in avoiding failure on the behavioral dimension, rather than in attaining success. To them, an important goal is more threatening than a trivial one (cf. Atkinson & Feather, 1966). They therefore will tend to avoid entering important situations, choosing (when possible) less important ones. The critical question, however, is whether they will abandon an important goal (once an attempt has been begun) more quickly than a less important one. Because giving up means failure, withdrawal from the situation should be just as threatening as doing poorly in it. Although we are not experts in

the achievement literature and have not searched that literature exhaustively, we are not aware of data that address this question.

6. Although our emphasis in this discussion is on situational or domain-specific expectancies, we should note that we have undertaken a program of work investigating the effects of generalized expectancies—optimism versus pessimism. The logic underlying predictions in that research is the same as is outlined here, and results to date strongly support the applicability of that logic to the effects of generalized expectancies (see Scheier & Carver, 1987, 1988, for reviews).

7. There are other literatures, however, in which the anticipation or belief of contingency is a critical issue. In alcohol research, for example, an important question is what consequences people expect drinking to produce. Beliefs that drinking enhances social or sexual capabilities (which take the same logical form as this expectancy) constitute an important reason why some people drink (e.g., Goldman, Brown, & Christiansen, 1987).

8. We might note that this divergence of emphasis appears to be a natural consequence of differences in the origins of the approaches. A major impetus to Bandura's self-efficacy theory was the desire to understand therapeutic behavior change. The observation that people often know exactly what to do but lack confidence in their ability to do it led him to the two expectancy constructs that he uses. Lack of self-confidence certainly is an important and central problem in therapy. However, given the way Bandura's theory is structured, it has no room to address additional causal forces. This is problematic once the theory is taken outside the therapy context.

9. The ideas presented in this section of the chapter raise many questions and issues that go beyond the scope of our discussion here. Readers interested in examining a broader range of issues are referred to the more complete presentation elsewhere (Carver & Scheier, 1990).

10. Reference values for the meta loop presumably can shift as a result of time and experience (see also Lord & Hanges, 1987). As people acquire more experience in a given domain, adjustments (either upward or downward) often occur in the pacing that they expect and demand of their goal-directed efforts. Though this point is quite important, discussion of it goes beyond the scope of this chapter (see Carver & Scheier, 1990).

References

Abramson, L. Y., Seligman, M. E. P., & Teasdale, J. D. (1978). Learned helplessness in humans: Critique and reformulation. *Journal of Abnormal Psychology, 87*, 49-74.

Adams, J. A. (1976). Issues for a closed-loop theory of motor learning. In G. E. Stelmach (Ed.), *Motor control: Issues and trends* (pp. 87-107). New York: Academic Press.

Ajzen, I. (1985). From intentions to actions: A theory of planned behavior. In J. Kuhl & J. Be_mann (Eds.), *Action control: From cognition to behavior* (pp. 11-39). New York: Springer-Verlag.

Ajzen, I., & Fishbein, M. (1980). *Understanding attitudes and predicting social behavior.* Englewood Cliffs, NJ: Prentice-Hall.

Atkinson, J. W., & Feather, N. T. (Eds.). (1966). *A theory of achievement motivation.* New York: Wiley.

Atkinson, J. W., & Raynor, J. O. (Eds.). (1974). *Motivation and achievement.* Washington, DC: V. H. Winston.

Bandura, A. (1969). *Aggression: A social learning analysis.* Englewood Cliffs, NJ: Prentice-Hall.

Bandura, A. (1977). Self-efficacy: Toward a unifying theory of behavior change. *Psychological Review, 84*, 191-215.

Bandura, A. (1982). Self-efficacy mechanism in human agency. *American Psychologist, 37*, 122-147.

Bandura, A. (1986). *Social foundations of thought and action: A social cognitive theory.* Englewood Cliffs, NJ: Prentice-Hall.

Baron, R. J. (1987). *The cerebral computer: An introduction to the computational structure of the human brain.* Hillsdale, NJ: Erlbaum.

Berscheid, E. (1983). Emotion. In H. H. Kelley, E. Berscheid, A. Christiansen, J. H. Harvey, T. L. Huston, G. Levinger, E. McClintock, L. A. Peplau, & D. R. Peterson (Eds.), *Close relationships* (pp. 110-168). San Francisco: W. H. Freeman.

Bower, G. H. (1978). Contacts of cognitive psychology with social learning theory. *Cognitive Therapy and Research, 2*, 123-146.

Bower, G. H., & Cohen, P. R. (1982). Emotional influences in memory and thinking: Data and theory. In M. S. Clark & S. T. Fiske (Eds.), *Affect and cognition: The seventeenth annual Carnegie Symposium on Cognition* (pp. 291-331). Hillsdale, NJ: Erlbaum.

Broadbent, D. E. (1977). Levels, hierarchies, and the locus of control. *Quarterly Journal of Experimental Psychology, 29*, 181-201.

Brockner, J. (1979). The effects of self-esteem, success-failure, and self-consciousness on task performance. *Journal of Personality and Social Psychology, 37*, 1732-1741.

Brunson, B. I., & Matthews, K. A. (1981). The Type A coronary-prone behavior pattern and reactions to uncontrollable stress: An analysis of performance strategies, affect, and attributions during failure. *Journal of Personality and Social Psychology, 40*, 906-918.

Burger, J. M. (1989). Negative reactions to increases in perceived personal control. *Journal of Personality and Social Psychology, 56*, 246-256.

Burgio, K. L., Merluzzi, T. V., & Pryor, J. B. (1986). Effects of performance expectancy and self-focused attention on social interaction. *Journal of Personality and Social Psychology, 50*, 1216-1221.

Cantor, N., & Kihlstrom, J. F. (1987). *Personality and social intelligence.* Englewood Cliffs, NJ: Prentice-Hall.

Carver, C. S. (1979). A cybernetic model of self-attention processes. *Journal of Personality and Social Psychology, 37*, 1251-1281.

Carver, C. S., Antoni, M., & Scheier, M. F. (1985). Self-consciousness and self-assessment. *Journal of Personality and Social Psychology, 48*, 117-124.

Carver, C. S., Blaney, P. H., & Scheier, M. F. (1979a). Focus of attention, chronic expectancy, and responses to a feared stimulus. *Journal of Personality and Social Psychology, 37*, 1186-1195.

Carver, C. S., Blaney, P. H., & Scheier, M. F. (1979b). Reassertion and giving up: The interactive role of self-directed attention and outcome expectancy. *Journal of Personality and Social Psychology, 37*, 1859-1870.

Carver, C. S., Ganellen, R. J., Froming, W. J., & Chambers, W. (1983). Modeling: An analysis in terms of category accessibility. *Journal of Experimental Social Psychology, 19*, 403-421.

Carver, C. S., La Voie, L., Kuhl, J., & Ganellen, R. J. (1988). Cognitive concomitants of depression: A further examination of the roles of generalization, high standards, and self-criticism. *Journal of Social and Clinical Psychology, 7*, 350-365.

Carver, C. S., Peterson, L. M., Follansbee, D. J., & Scheier, M. F. (1983). Effects of self-directed attention on performance and persistence among persons high and low in test anxiety. *Cognitive Therapy and Research, 7*, 333-354.

Carver, C. S., & Scheier, M. F. (1981a). *Attention and self-regulation: A control-theory approach to human behavior.* New York: Springer-Verlag.

Carver, C. S., & Scheier, M. F. (1981b). The self-attention-induced feedback loop and social facilitation. *Journal of Experimental Social Psychology, 17*, 545-568.

Carver, C. S., & Scheier, M. F. (1982). Outcome expectancy, locus of attribution for expectancy, and self-directed attention as determinants of evaluations and performance. *Journal of Experimental Social Psychology, 18*, 184-200.

Carver, C. S., & Scheier, M. F. (1983). A control-theory model of normal behavior, and implications for problems in self-management. In P. C. Kendall (Ed.), *Advances in cognitive-behavioral research and therapy* (Vol. 2, pp. 127-194). New York: Academic Press.

Carver, C. S., & Scheier, M. F. (1984). Self-focused attention in test anxiety: A general theory applied to a specific phenomenon. In H. van der Ploeg, R. Schwarzer, & C. D. Spielberger (Eds.), *Advances in test anxiety research* (Vol. 3, pp. 3-20). Hillsdale, NJ: Erlbaum.

Carver, C. S., & Scheier, M. F. (1985). Aspects of self, and the control of behavior. In B. R. Schlenker (Ed.), *The self and social life* (pp. 146-174). New York: McGraw-Hill.

Carver, C. S., & Scheier, M. F. (1986a). Analyzing shyness: A specific application of broader self-regulatory principles. In W. H. Jones, J. M. Cheek, & S. R. Briggs (Eds.), *Shyness: Perspectives on research and treatment* (pp. 173-185). New York: Plenum.

Carver, C. S., & Scheier, M. F. (1986b). Self and the control of behavior. In L. M. Hartman & K. R. Blankstein (Eds.), *Perception of self in emotional disorder and psychotherapy* (pp. 5-35). New York: Plenum.

Carver, C. S., & Scheier, M. F. (1990). Origins and functions of positive and negative affect: A control-process view. *Psychological Review, 97,* 19-35.

Carver, C. S., Scheier, M. F., & Klahr, D. (1987). Further explorations of a control-process model of test anxiety. In H. van der Ploeg, R. Schwarzer, & C. D. Spielberger (Eds.), *Advances in test anxiety research* (Vol. 5, pp. 15-22). Lisse, The Netherlands: Swets & Zeitlinger.

Chambliss, C. A., & Murray, E. J. (1979). Efficacy attribution, locus of control, and weight loss. *Cognitive Therapy and Research, 4,* 349-353.

Chwalisz, K., Diener, E., & Gallagher, D. (1988). Autonomic arousal feedback and emotional experience: Evidence from the spinal cord injured. *Journal of Personality and Social Psychology, 54,* 820-828.

Cohen, J. D., Dunbar, K., & McClelland, J. L. (1988). *On the control of automatic processes: A parallel distributed processing model of the Stroop effect* (Technical Report No. AIP-40). Pittsburgh: Carnegie Mellon University, Department of Psychology.

Darley, J. M., & Fazio, R. H. (1980). Expectancy confirmation processes arising in the social interaction sequence. *American Psychologist, 35,* 867-881.

Dawkins, R. (1976). Hierarchical organization: A candidate principle for ethology. In P. P. G. Bateson & R. A. Hinde (Eds.), *Growing points in ethology* (pp. 7-54). Cambridge, England: Cambridge University Press.

DeAngelis, D. L., Post, W. M., & Travis, C. C. (1986). *Biomathematics: Vol. 15. Positive feedback in natural systems.* Berlin: Springer-Verlag.

Diener, C. I., & Dweck, C. S. (1978). An analysis of learned helplessness: Continuous changes in performance strategy and achievement cognitions following failure. *Journal of Personality and Social Psychology, 36,* 451-462.

Diener, E. (1979). Deindividuation, self-awareness, and disinhibition. *Journal of Personality and Social Psychology, 37,* 1160-1171.

Diener, E., & Emmons, R. A. (1984). The independence of positive and negative affect. *Journal of Personality and Social Psychology, 47,* 1105-1117.

Diener, E., & Iran-Nejad, A. (1986). The relationship in experience between various types of affect. *Journal of Personality and Social Psychology, 50,* 1031-1038.

Duval, S., & Wicklund, R. A. (1972). *A theory of objective self-awareness.* New York: Academic Press.

Dweck, C. S., & Elliott, E. S. (1983). Achievement motivation. In E. M. Hetherington (Vol. Ed.), *Handbook of child psychology* (4th ed): *Vol. 4. Socialization, personality, and social development* (pp. 643-691). New York: Wiley.

Dweck, C. S., & Leggett, E. L. (1988). A social-cognitive approach to motivation and personality. *Psychological Review, 95,* 256-273.

Elliott, E. S., & Dweck, C. S. (1988). Goals: An approach to motivation and achievement. *Journal of Personality and Social Psychology, 54,* 5-12.

Emmons, R. A. (1986). Personal strivings: An approach to personality and subjective well being. *Journal of Personality and Social Psychology, 51,* 1058-1068.

Fazio, R. (1986). How do attitudes guide behavior? In R. M. Sorrentino & E. T. Higgins (Eds.), *Handbook of motivation and cognition: Foundations of social behavior* (Vol. 1, pp. 204-243). New York: Guilford Press.

Ford, D. H. (1987). *Humans as self-constructing living systems: A developmental perspective on behavior and personality.* Hillsdale, NJ: Erlbaum.

Freud, S. (1962). *The ego and the id.* New York: Norton. (Original work published 1923)

Freud, S. (1949). *An outline of psychoanalysis.* New York: Norton. (Original work published 1940)

Frijda, N. H. (1986). *The emotions.* Cambridge, England: Cambridge University Press.

Frijda, N. H. (1988). The laws of emotion. *American Psychologist, 43,* 349-358.

Gallistel, C. R. (1980). *The organization of action: A new synthesis.* Hillsdale, NJ: Erlbaum.

Gardner, R. A., & Gardner, B. T. (1988). Feedforward versus feedbackward: An ethological alternative to the law of effect. *Behavioral and Brain Sciences, 11,* 429-447.

Goldman, M. S., Brown, S. A., & Christiansen, B. A. (1987). Expectancy theory: Thinking about drinking. In H. T. Blane & K. E. Leonard (Eds.), *Psychological theories of drinking and alcoholism* (pp. 181–226). New York: Guilford Press.

Gray, J. A. (1981). A critique of Eysenck's theory of personality. In H. J. Eysenck (Ed.), *A model for personality* (pp. 246–276). Berlin: Springer-Verlag.

Gray, J. A. (1982). *The neuropsychology of anxiety: An enquiry into the functions of the septo-hippocampal system.* New York: Oxford University Press.

Heckhausen, H. (1967). *The anatomy of achievement motivation.* New York: Academic Press.

Higgins, E. T. (1987). Self-discrepancy: A theory relating self and affect. *Psychological Review, 94,* 319–340.

Hoffman, M. L. (1986). Affect, cognition, and motivation. In R. M. Sorrentino & E. T. Higgins (Eds.), *Handbook of motivation and cognition: Foundations of social behavior* (Vol. 1, pp. 244–280). New York: Guilford Press.

Hull, C. L. (1943). *Principles of behavior.* New York: Appleton-Century-Crofts.

Hull, J. G. (1981). A self-awareness model of the causes and effects of alcohol consumption. *Journal of Abnormal Psychology, 90,* 586–600.

Hyland, M. (1987). Control theory interpretation of psychological mechanisms of depression: Comparison and integration of several theories. *Psychological Bulletin, 102,* 109–121.

Janoff-Bulman, R., & Brickman, P. (1982). Expectations and what people learn from failure. In N. T. Feather (Ed.), *Expectations and actions: Expectancy-value models in psychology* (pp. 207–237). Hillsdale, NJ: Erlbaum.

Kanfer, F. H., & Busemeyer, J. R. (1982). The use of problem-solving and decision-making in behavior therapy. *Clinical Psychology Review, 2,* 239–266.

Kanfer, F. H., & Hagerman, S. (1981). The role of self-regulation. In L. P. Rehm (Ed.), *Behavior therapy for depression: Present status and future directions* (pp. 143–179). New York: Academic Press.

Kanfer, F. H., & Hagerman, S. (1985). Behavior therapy and the information processing paradigm. In S. Reiss & R. R. Bootsin (Eds.), *Theoretical issues in behavior therapy* (pp. 3–33). New York: Academic Press.

Kelly, G. A. (1955). *The psychology of personal constructs.* New York: Norton.

Kelso, J. A. S. (Ed.). (1982). *Human motor behavior: An introduction.* Hillsdale, NJ: Erlbaum.

Kelso, J. A. S., & Kay, B. A. (1987). Information and control: A macroscopic analysis of perception-action coupling. In H. Heuer & A. F. Sanders (Eds.), *Perspectives on perception and action* (pp. 3–32). Hillsdale, NJ: Erlbaum.

Kimble, G. A., & Perlmuter, L. C. (1970). The problem of volition. *Psychological Review, 77,* 361–384.

Klinger, E. (1975). Consequences of commitment to and disengagement from incentives. *Psychological Review, 82,* 1–25.

Klinger, E. (1977). *Meaning and void: Inner experience and the incentives in people's lives.* Minneapolis: University of Minnesota Press.

Klinger, E., Barta, S. G., & Maxeiner, M. E. (1981). Current concerns: Assessing therapeutically relevant motivation. In P. C. Kendall & S. D. Hollon (Eds.), *Assessment and strategies for cognitive-behavioral interventions* (pp. 161–196). New York: Academic Press.

Kuhl, J. (1984). Volitional aspects of achievement motivation and learned helplessness: Toward a comprehensive theory of action control. In B. A. Maher (Ed.), *Progress in experimental personality research* (Vol. 13, pp. 99–170). New York: Academic Press.

Kuhl, J. (1985). Volitional mediators of cognition–behavior consistency: Self-regulatory processes and action versus state orientation. In J. Kuhl & J. Beckmann (Eds.), *Action control: From cognition to behavior* (pp. 101–128). New York: Springer-Verlag.

Kuhl, J. & Helle, P. (1986). Motivational and volitional determinants of depression. The degenerated-intention hypothesis. *Journal of Abnormal Psychology, 95,* 247–251.

Kukla, A. (1972). Foundations of an attributional theory of performance. *Psychological Review, 79,* 454–470.

Lazarus, R. S. (1966). *Psychological stress and the coping process.* New York: McGraw-Hill.

Lewin, K. (1935). *A dynamic theory of personality*. New York: McGraw-Hill.

Locke, E. A., Shaw, K. N., Saari, L. M., & Latham, G. P. (1981). Goal setting and task performance: 1969-1980. *Psychological Bulletin, 90*, 125-152.

Lord, R. G., & Hanges, P. J. (1987). A control system model of organizational motivation: Theoretical development and applied implications. *Behavioral Science, 32*, 161-178.

MacKay, D. M. (1963). Mindlike behavior in artefacts. In K. M. Sayre & F. J. Crosson (Eds.), *The modeling of mind: Computers and intelligence* (pp. 225-241). Notre Dame, IN: University of Notre Dame Press.

MacKay, D. M. (1966). Cerebral organization and the conscious control of action. In J. C. Eccles (Ed.), *Brain and conscious experience* (pp. 422-445). Berlin: Springer-Verlag.

Mandler, G. (1984). *Mind and body: Psychology of emotion and stress*. New York: Norton.

Mandler, G., & Watson, D. L. (1966). Anxiety and the interruption of behavior. In C. D. Spielberger (Ed.), *Anxiety and behavior* (pp. 263-288). New York: Academic Press.

Marken, R. S. (1986). Perceptual organization of behavior: A hierarchical control model of coordinated action. *Journal of Experimental Psychology: Human Perception and Performance, 12*, 267-276.

Markus, H., & Nurius, P. (1986). Possible selves. *American Psychologist, 41*, 954-969.

Martin, L., & Tesser, A. (1989). Toward a model of ruminative thought. In J. S. Uleman & J. A. Bargh (Eds.), *Unintended thought: The limits of awareness, intention, and control* (pp. 306-326). New York: Guilford Press.

Maruyama, M. (1963). The second cybernetics: Deviation-amplifying mutual causal processes. *American Scientist, 51*, 164-179.

Maslow, A. H. (1970). *Motivation and personality*. New York: Harper & Row.

Millar, K. U., Tesser, A., & Millar, M. G. (1988). The effects of a threatening life event on behavior sequences and intrusive thought: A self-disruption explanation. *Cognitive Therapy and Research, 12*, 441-458.

Miller, G. A., Galanter, E., & Pribram, K. H. (1960). *Plans and the structure of behavior*. New York: Holt, Rinehart & Winston.

Miller, I. H., & Norman, W. H. (1979). Learned helplessness in humans: A review and attribution theory model. *Psychological Bulletin, 86*, 93-118.

Mischel, W. (1973). Toward a cognitive social learning reconceptualization of personality. *Psychological Review, 80*, 252-283.

Murray, H. A. (1938). *Explorations in personality*. New York: Oxford University Press.

Newell, A. (1973). Production systems: Models of control structures. In W. G. Chase (Ed.), *Visual information processing* (pp. 463-526). New York: Academic Press.

Newell, A., & Simon, H. A. (1972). *Human problem solving*. Englewood Cliffs, NJ: Prentice-Hall.

Norman, D. A. (1981). Categorization of action slips. *Psychological Review, 88*, 1-15.

Ogilvie, D. M. (1987). The undesired self: A neglected variable in personality research. *Journal of Personality and Social Psychology, 52*, 379-385.

Ortony, A., Clore, G. L., & Collins, A. (1988). *The cognitive structure of emotions*. Cambridge, England: Cambridge University Press.

Palys, T. S., & Little, B. R. (1983). Perceived life satisfaction and the organization of personal project systems. *Journal of Personality and Social Psychology, 44*, 1221-1230.

Pervin, L. (Ed.). (1989). *Goal concepts in personality and social psychology*. Hillsdale, NJ: Erlbaum.

Powers, W. T. (1973). *Behavior: The control of perception*. Chicago: Aldine.

Prentice-Dunn, S., & Rogers, R. W. (1982). Effects of public and private self-awareness on deindividuation and aggression. *Journal of Personality and Social Psychology, 43*, 503-513.

Prinz, W. (1987). Ideo-motor action. In H. Heuer & A. F. Sanders (Eds.), *Perspectives on perception and action* (pp. 47-76). Hillsdale, NJ: Erlbaum.

Pyszczynski, T., & Greenberg, J. (1985). Depression and preference for self-focusing stimuli after success and failure. *Journal of Personality and Social Psychology, 49*, 1066-1075.

Pyszczynski, T., & Greenberg, J. (1987). Self-regulatory perseveration and the depressive self-focusing style: A self-awareness theory of reactive depression. *Psychological Bulletin, 102*, 122-138.

Rich, A. R., & Woolever, D. K. (1988). Expectancy and self-focused attention: Experimental support for the self-regulation model of test anxiety. *Journal of Social and Clinical Psychology, 7,* 246–259.

Rogers, C. R. (1961). *On becoming a person.* Boston: Houghton Mifflin.

Rosenbaum, D. A. (1987). Hierarchical organization of motor programs. In S. Wise (Ed.), *Neural and behavioral approaches to higher brain function* (pp. 45–66). New York: Wiley.

Roth, S. (1980). A revised model of learned helplessness in humans. *Journal of Personality, 48,* 103–133.

Rotter, J. B. (1954). *Social learning and clinical psychology.* New York: Prentice-Hall.

Salmoni, A. W., Schmidt, R. A., & Walter, C. B. (1984). Knowledge of results and motor learning: A review and critical reappraisal. *Psychological Bulletin, 95,* 355–386.

Schachter, S., & Singer, J. E. (1962). Cognitive, social, and physiological determinants of emotional state. *Psychological Review, 69,* 379–399.

Schank, R. C., & Abelson, R. P. (1977). *Scripts, plans, goals, and understanding.* Hillsdale, NJ: Erlbaum.

Scheier, M. F., & Carver, C. S. (1982). Self-consciousness, outcome expectancy, and persistence. *Journal of Research in Personality, 16,* 409–418.

Scheier, M. F., & Carver, C. S. (1983). Self-directed attention and the comparison of self with standards. *Journal of Experimental Social Psychology, 19,* 205–222.

Scheier, M. F., & Carver, C. S. (1987). Dispositional optimism and physical well-being: The influence of generalized outcome expectancies on health. *Journal of Personality, 55,* 169–210.

Scheier, M. F., & Carver, C. S. (1988). A model of behavioral self-regulation: Translating intention into action. In L. Berkowitz (Ed.), *Advances in experimental social psychology* (Vol. 21, pp. 303–346). New York: Academic Press.

Scheier, M. F., Carver, C. S., & Gibbons, F. X. (1981). Self-focused attention and reactions to fear. *Journal of Research in Personality, 15,* 1–15.

Schlenker, B. R., & Leary, M. R. (1982). Social anxiety and self-presentation: A conceptualization and model. *Psychological Bulletin, 92,* 641–669.

Schmidt, R. A. (1976). The schema as a solution to some persistent problems in motor learning theory. In G. E. Stelmach (Ed.), *Motor control: Issues and trends* (pp. 41–65). New York: Academic Press.

Schmidt, R. A. (1987). The acquisition of skill: Some modifications to the perception–action relationship through practice. In H. Heuer & A. F. Sanders (Eds.), *Perspectives on perception and action* (pp. 77–103). Hillsdale, NJ: Erlbaum.

Seligman, M. E. P. (1975). *Helplessness: On depression, development, and death.* San Francisco: W. H. Freeman.

Shallice, T. (1978). The dominant action system: An information-processing approach to consciousness. In K. S. Pope & J. L. Singer (Eds.), *The stream of consciousness: Scientific investigations into the flow of human experience* (pp. 117–157). New York: Wiley.

Sherman, S. J., Judd, C. M., & Park, B. (1989). Social cognition. *Annual Review of Psychology, 40,* 281–326.

Shiffrin, R. M., & Schneider, W. (1977). Controlled and automatic human information processing: II. Perceptual learning, automatic attending, and a general theory. *Psychological Review, 84,* 127–190.

Showers, C., & Cantor, N. (1985). Social cognition: A look at motivated strategies. *Annual Review of Psychology, 36,* 275–305.

Simon, H. A. (1967). Motivational and emotional controls of cognition. *Psychology Review, 74,* 29–39.

Skinner, B. F. (1938). *The behavior of organisms.* New York: Appleton-Century-Crofts.

Smith, E. R. (1984). Model of social inference processes. *Psychological Review, 91,* 392–413.

Snyder, C. R., Higgins, R. L., & Stucky, R. J. (1983). *Excuses: Masquerades in search of grace.* New York: Wiley.

Srull, T. K., & Wyer, R. S., Jr. (1986). The role of chronic and temporary goals in social information processing. In R. M. Sorrentino & E. T. Higgins (Eds.), *Handbook of motivation and cognition: Foundations of social behavior* (Vol. 1, pp. 503–549). New York: Guilford Press.

Srull, T. K., & Wyer, R. S., Jr. (1989). Person memory and judgment. *Psychological Review, 96*, 58-83.

Stelmach, G. E., & Larish, D. D. (1980). A new perspective on motor skill automation. *Research Quarterly for Exercise and Sport, 51*, 141-157.

Stotland, E. (1969). *The psychology of hope.* San Francisco: Jossey-Bass.

Stuss, D. T., & Benson, D. F. (1986). *The frontal lobes.* New York: Raven Press.

Swann, W. B., Jr. (1987). Identity negotiations: Where two roads meet. *Journal of Personality and Social Psychology, 53*, 1038-1051.

Taylor, S. E., & Brown, J. D. (1988). Illusion and well-being: A social psychological perspective on mental health. *Psychological Bulletin, 103*, 193-210.

Tesser, A. (1980). Self-esteem maintenance in family dynamics. *Journal of Personality and Social Psychology, 39*, 77-91.

Tesser, A. (1986). Some effects of self-evaluation maintenance on cognition and action. In R. M. Sorrentino & E. T. Higgins (Eds.), *Handbook of motivation and cognition: Foundations of social behavior* (Vol. 1, pp. 435-464). New York: Guilford Press.

Tesser, A., & Campbell, J. (1983). Self-definition and self-evaluation maintenance. In J. Suls & A. G. Greenwald (Eds.), *Psychological perspectives on the self* (Vol. 2, pp. 1-31). Hillsdale, NJ: Erlbaum.

Tolman, E. C. (1932). *Purposive behavior in animals and men.* New York: Appleton-Century-Crofts.

Tolman, E. C. (1938). The determiners of behavior at a choice point. *Psychological Review, 45*, 1-41.

Trzebinski, J., McGlynn, R. P., Gray, G., & Tubbs, D. (1985). The role of categories of an actor's goals in organizing inferences about a person. *Journal of Personality and Social Psychology, 48*, 1387-1397.

Vallacher, R. R., & Wegner, D. M. (1985). *A theory of action identification.* Hillsdale, NJ: Erlbaum.

Vallacher, R. R., & Wegner, D. M. (1987). What do people think they're doing? Action identification and human behavior. *Psychological Review, 94*, 3-15.

Van Hook, E., & Higgins, E. T. (1988). Self-related problems beyond the self-concept: Motivational consequences of discrepant self-guides. *Journal of Personality and Social Psychology, 55*, 625-633.

Warr, P., Barter, J., & Brownbridge, G. (1983). On the independence of positive and negative affect. *Journal of Personality and Social Psychology, 44*, 644-651.

Watson, D., & Tellegen, A. (1985). Toward a consensual structure of mood. *Psychological Bulletin, 98*, 219-235.

Weary, G. (1980). An examination of affect and egotism as mediators of bias in causal attributions. *Journal of Personality and Social Psychology, 38*, 348-357.

Wegner, D. M., Vallacher, R. R., Kiersted, G., & Dizadji, D. (1986). Action identification in the emergence of social behavior. *Social Cognition, 4*, 18-38.

Weiner, B. (1979). A theory of motivation for some classroom experiences. *Journal of Educational Psychology, 71*, 3-25.

Weiner, B. (1982). The emotional consequences of casual ascriptions. In M. S. Clark & S. T. Fiske (Eds.), *Affect and cognition: The 17th annual Carnegie Symposium on Cognition* (pp. 185-209). Hillsdale, NJ: Erlbaum.

Weiner, B. (1986a). *An attributional theory of motivation and emotion.* New York: Springer-Verlag.

Weiner, B. (1986b). Attribution, emotion, and action. In R. M. Sorrentino & E. T. Higgins (Eds.), *Handbook of motivation and cognition: Foundations of social behavior* (Vol. 1, pp. 281-312). New York: Guilford Press.

Weiner, B., & Litman-Adizes, T. (1980). An attributional, expectancy–value analysis of learned helplessness and depression. In J. Garber & M. E. P. Seligman (Eds.), *Human helplessness: Theory and applications* (pp. 35-57). New York: Academic Press.

Wicklund, R. A., & Gollwitzer, P. M. (1982). *Symbolic self-completion.* Hillsdale, NJ: Erlbaum.

Wills, T. A. (1981). Downward comparison principles in social psychology. *Psychological Bulletin, 90*, 245-271.

Wilson, E. O. (1975). *Sociobiology: The new synthesis.* Cambridge, MA: Harvard University Press.

Wilson, T. D., & Capitman, J. A. (1982). The effects of script availability on social behavior. *Personality and Social Psychology Bulletin, 8*, 11-19.

Wood, J. V., Taylor, S. E., & Lichtman, R. R. (1985). Social comparison in adjustment to breast cancer. *Journal of Personality and Social Psychology, 49,* 1169-1183.

Wong, P. T. P., & Sproule, C. F. (1984). An attribution analysis of the locus of control construct and the Trent Attribution Profile. In H. M. Lefcourt (Ed.), *Research with the locus of control construct: Vol. 3. Extensions and limitations* (pp. 310-360). New York: Academic Press.

Wortman, C. B., & Brehm, J. W. (1975). Responses to uncontrollable outcomes: An integration of reactance theory and the learned helplessness model. In L. Berkowitz (Ed.), *Advances in experimental social psychology* (Vol. 8, pp. 277-336). New York: Academic Press.

Wortman, C. B., & Silver, R. C. (1989). The myths of coping with loss. *Journal of Consulting and Clinical Psychology, 57,* 349-357.

Wyer, R. S., Jr., & Srull, T. K. (Eds.). (1984). *Handbook of social cognition* (3 vols.), Hillsdale, NJ: Erlbaum.

Zevon, M. A., & Tellegen, A. (1982). The structure of mood change: An idiographic/nomothetic analysis. *Journal of Personality and Social Psychology, 43,* 111-122.

CHAPTER 2

Action Phases and Mind-Sets

PETER M. GOLLWITZER
Max-Planck-Institut für psychologische Forschung

The focus of this chapter is on the course of action, which is understood to be a temporal, horizontal path starting with a person's desires and ending with the evaluation of the achieved action outcome. The phenomena of choosing an action goal, initiating the appropriate actions, and executing these actions are assumed to be situated in between. This comprehensive perspective conceives of the course of action as a number of consecutive, distinct segments or phases. It raises questions concerning how people *choose* action goals, *plan* and *enact* their execution, and *evaluate* their efforts. The concept of "mind-set" is employed to find answers to these questions in terms of the cognitive processes or orientations that allow for easy completion of the different action phases.

A PHASE MODEL OF ACTION

Goal Setting and Goal Striving

"Being motivated" implies a number of different phenomena. But how many distinct aspects of being motivated to pursue a desired goal are there? Kurt Lewin (Lewin, Dembo, Festinger, & Sears, 1944) made a major distinction between goal striving and goal setting. "Goal striving" is behavior directed toward existing goals, and thus addresses questions of moving toward the chosen goal. "Goal setting," on the other hand, addresses the question of what goals a person will choose, and thus considers the expected value of the available choice options. Noticing the unique nature of both of these problems, Lewin adopted a distinct theoretical perspective for each of them. He referred to an expectancy × value model when goal setting was at issue—for instance, when he and his colleagues were attempting to explain people's changes in aspiration level (Lewin et al., 1944). Issues of goal striving, however, were explained in terms of his theory of tension systems (Lewin, 1926), through which he tried to discover the forces that move a person toward a chosen goal. Lewin considered the strength of these forces to be related not only to the valence of the chosen goal, but also to the individual's perceived distance from the goal. By introducing the variable of potency, Lewin (1936) tried to explain which of the many goals people entertain at a given time actually guide their behavior in specific situations.

German researchers studying goal-oriented behavior before Lewin devoted themselves solely to the issue of goal striving by studying the initiation and execution of actions serving chosen goals or instructions given by others. This research tradition has become known as the German "will psychology"; its most prominent figure was Narziss Ach (1905, 1910, 1935). Researchers in this tradition fiercely disagreed on the key questions of will psychology, such as whether intentions specifying an appropriate opportunity to act favor smooth action initiation, regardless of the importance of the respective superordinate goal (Ach, 1935; Selz, 1910). Nevertheless, they unanimously considered goal striving to be different from goal setting, which they referred to as the "battle of motives." For German will psychologists, it was clear that people's goal setting depends primarily on their desires, needs, and interests, whereas a host of additional variables determines whether and how people act on their chosen goals. It was the latter that they tried to identify and that they explored in their theories.

Researchers studying goal-oriented behavior after Lewin shifted their attention from goal striving to goal setting. Stimulated by Lewin's as well as Festinger's work on shifts in the level of aspiration (Festinger, 1942; Lewin et al., 1944), Atkinson (1957) presented a formal model of risk taking that made it possible to compute the motivational tendency to choose tasks representing various difficulty levels. Like Lewin, Atkinson considered goal setting and goal striving to be the two major problems requiring solution in any psychology of motivation:

> The first problem is to account for an individual's selection of one path of action among a set of possible alternatives. The second problem is to account for the amplitude of the action tendency once it is initiated, and for its tendency to persist for a time in a given situation. (1957, p. 359)

However, Atkinson hoped that the two distinct problems could be reduced to one and thereby could be accounted for by a single theoretical model. In his view, the theory best suited to accomplish this purpose was the risk-taking model (Atkinson, 1957) or a modified version of it (Atkinson & Reitman, 1956). This model implies that the motivational tendency that makes a person choose a certain task will also account for the effort the person exerts when working on the chosen task and for the quality of the achieved performance.

Empirical studies investigating this implication sometimes observed the predicted performance-enhancing effects of motivation, but more often failed to do so (see Atkinson, 1974, for a review). Atkinson attributed the "now you see it, now you don't" character of this effect to what he called "overmotivation" (and its opposite, "undermotivation"). Referring to the Yerkes–Dodson law (Yerkes & Dodson, 1908), he postulated that there should be an ideal motivational tendency for each individual task. Tasks differ with respect to the amount of motivation that leads to most efficient performance: Low levels of motivation are more appropriate for some tasks, whereas medium or high levels are more appropriate for others. Since which tasks belong to which category was unknown, Atkinson suggested establishing this classification empirically. Once it was known what level of motivation is ideal for a given task, researchers would finally be able to develop valid predictions of task performance, based solely on their knowledge of the individual's motivation.

As compared to this empirical Sisyphus-like work, a more theoretical solution to the troublesome motivation–performance issue certainly exists. That is, one can re-establish the old distinction between goal setting and goal striving. Eric Klinger (1977) recognized this possibility when he introduced his concept of "current concerns." He pointed out (1977, pp. 22–24, 329–330) that expectancy × value theories have been only very modestly successful in predicting vital aspects of goal striving, such as work effort and quality of performance. Consequently, his theory of current concerns focuses solely on issues of goal striving. This theory has no difficulties in accounting for the commonly observed invigoration of activity in the face of obstacles en route to a chosen goal—a phenomenon that cannot be explained by expectancy–value theories, because the setback must be assumed to reduce the expectancy of achieving the goal and thus the individual's motivation to work for it.

Kuhl (1983) also re-established the classic distinction by introducing the concepts of "choice motivation" and "control motivation." In his opinion, models of choice motivation relate to goal setting, and he saw Atkinson's risk-taking model and its many reformulations and extensions (e.g., Feather, 1967; Heckhausen, 1977; Raynor, 1969; Weiner, 1974) as more or less valid examples of such models. Kuhl noted a lack of theories on goal striving and offered his own model, which he labeled "control theory" (Kuhl, 1984). Stimulated by Atkinson and Birch's (1970) assumption that a person is always affected by numerous motivational tendencies, all in constant flux, Kuhl saw effective goal striving as dependent on people's efforts to shield it from competing action tendencies. Accordingly, whether people make progress with respect to a chosen goal is no longer seen as dependent only on the motivation that originally made them choose this goal. Rather, it is also a question of how successfully people shield (control) the actions that lead to goal achievement.

The Rubicon Model of Action Phases

The "Rubicon model" of action phases (Heckhausen, 1987b; Heckhausen & Gollwitzer, 1986, 1987) goes beyond the useful conceptual distinction between goal setting and goal striving. Although the model keeps these two problems of goal-oriented behavior separate, it encompasses both within a single theoretical model, thus permitting them to be analyzed in relation to each other. Furthermore, it provides a temporal perspective that begins with the awakening of a person's wishes prior to goal setting and continues through the evaluative thoughts entertained after goal striving has ended.

Separating the sequence of events occurring within this comprehensive time frame into discrete phenomena, the model posits four distinct phases: first, the predecisional phase; second, the postdecisional but still preactional phase; third, the actional phase; and last, the postactional phase. These phases are separated by three clear boundaries or transition points: the making of a decision, the initiation of respective actions, and the conclusion of these actions. But what distinct phenomena are associated with each phase?

Predecisional Action Phase

The first phase is characterized by wishing and deliberating. People's motives (McClelland, 1980) produce certain wishes: For instance, a person with a strong power motive and a weak affiliation motive is expected to experience more wishes related to power than to affiliation. However, people cannot act on all of their wishes but must choose among them, because some wishes may contradict each other, others are too difficult to implement, and life is simply too short to follow all of one's wishes. People have to deliberate over which of their many wishes they prefer to pursue.

How can people establish such preferences? They may employ the criteria of feasibility and desirability. With respect to feasibility, people may contemplate whether they can obtain the outcome implied by a given wish through their own activity and whether the situational context they face is facilitating or impeding. Accordingly, they should also become concerned with questions such as whether they will find enough time to strive for the desired outcomes and whether the necessary means or opportunities will be available.

The desirability of the wanted outcome is determined by reflecting on its expected value. The expected value is derived by estimating the pleasantness–unpleasantness of potential short-term and long-term consequences and by assessing the probability that achieving the desired outcome will lead to these consequences. Such consequences include the following: a positive or negative self-evaluation, a positive or negative evaluation by significant others, progress toward some important life goal, or some pleasant or unpleasant side effects unrelated to the specific wish that initially started the person's striving (Heckhausen, 1977). In addition, incentives associated with the process of achieving the desired outcome (e.g., joy experienced while trying to establish the desired outcome) should also be relevant when the desirability of a given wish is deliberated.

Proper assessment of the feasibility and desirability of a given wish, however, requires that this wish be seen in relation to other wishes. A wish associated with many attractive consequences may suddenly appear less desirable when scrutinized in the light of a superordinate wish (e.g., the wish to dine in fine restaurants becomes less desirable when it conflicts with the wish to buy a house). Or it might become more feasible when contemplated in connection with the realization of other wishes (e.g., a busy person's wish to learn to play tennis may appear more feasible when it is contemplated together with the wish to take an extended vacation).

Making a Decision and the Preactional Phase

Even when a wish is accorded high desirability and feasibility and thus is given highest preference, the model of action phases assumes that wish fulfillment further demands transforming the wish into an intention. Phenomenologically, this transformation is characterized as a resolution resulting in a feeling of determination to fulfill the wish (or at least a feeling of assurance that one will act on the wish at hand; Michotte & Prüm, 1910). The goal state or desired outcome specified by the wish thus becomes an end state that the individual feels committed to achieve. The model describes this sense of obligation in stating that the individual has acquired a "goal intention." To catch the flavor of this transition from the fluid state of deliberation to a firm sense of commitment, Heckhausen (1987b) employed the metaphor of "crossing the Rubicon."

After forming a goal intention, people move to the preactional phase. The phenomenon associated with this action phase is planning. Planning is often necessary because newly formed goal intentions cannot be implemented immediately if the individual is engaged in alternative activities that first need to be completed or if relevant opportunities to act are not yet available. In addition, most goal intentions specify goal states (e.g., to graduate from college) that cannot be achieved in a single step. Consequently, the individual is interrupted (or must pause) repeatedly and is forced to await future opportunities to work towards this goal.

The model of action phases assumes that people do *not* use these time breaks or pauses to weigh the positive or negative consequences of goal achievement; rather, the feeling of obligation associated with the goal intention makes people concerned with the issue of how to promote achieving the chosen goal. Accordingly, they should address questions of *when* and *where* to start acting, *how* to act, and *how long* to act. Whenever people anticipate difficulties with respect to any of these implementational issues, they should commit themselves to one of the many possible ways of initiating, executing, and terminating a relevant course of action.

Committing oneself to a particular implementational course constitutes forming behavioral intentions. These behavioral intentions (i.e., initiation intentions, execution intentions, and termination intentions) focus on a person's behavior in pursuing the chosen goal. The model distinguishes behavioral intentions from goal intentions, since the latter focus on desired goal states. In line with the ideas of German will psychology (Ach, 1935), it is assumed that behavioral intentions promote the smooth initiation, execution, and termination of activities in pursuing a person's goal intentions.

Action Initiation and the Actional Phase

When does a goal intention lead to initiating relevant actions? It primarily depends on the goal intention's volitional strength—that is, how strongly a person is committed to implementing the chosen goal. The genuine amount of volitional strength is considered to be a positive function of the goal's desirability and feasibility as perceived prior to choosing this goal. However, this volitional strength may vary, depending on a person's experiences with attempting to initiate relevant actions. If a person repeatedly ignores good opportunities to initiate relevant actions, volitional strength may decrease over time. On the other hand, volitional strength may spontaneously and momentarily increase when the individual encounters obstacles.

More importantly, goal intentions and their effects on the initiation of relevant actions cannot be discussed without considering that many different goal intentions may compete for implementation at any given point in time. One would expect that under these circumstances the intention with the comparatively highest volitional strength would prevail. However, the situation at hand may not be equally conducive to implementing all of these competing intentions; it may favor implementing some of these intentions more than others. In addition, for some intentions the situation at hand may be better suited for smooth implementation than any future situation for which the individual hopes. Consequently, the individual may be very eager to take the opportunity at hand and to postpone the implementation of competing intentions, even if these intentions are associated with comparatively higher volitional strength.

To summarize: Whether a given goal intention leads to the initiation of relevant actions depends on its volitional strength (as compared with that of other competing goal intentions) *and* on how favorable the situation is for readily initiating the particular goal intention (as compared with initiating competing goal intentions *and* as compared with relevant future opportunities one hopes to encounter). Finally, a goal intention that has been furnished with initiation intentions during the postdecisional (preactional) phase should have an additional advantage over competing goal intentions, given that the opportunity specified by the initiation intention is present. In this case, the opportunity to act should be more easily recognized and, once recognized, should elicit a special impulse to start acting on it.

Action initiation is the demarcation line signaling the transition to the actional phase. The phenomenon characteristic of this phase is acting toward goal achievement. A person's efforts to pursue a goal intention are again assumed to be related to the goal intention's volitional strength. The amount of volitional strength serves as a kind of threshold value for the individual's effort exertion. This threshold, however, may be spontaneously moved upward if hindrances are encountered, thus allowing for a reactive, momentary increase in volitional strength. Spontaneous nonconscious increases in effort exertion were originally reported by German will psychologists (Ach, 1935; Hillgruber, 1912), who interpreted these reactive responses of the individual as attempts to hold on to one's goal commitment. These ideas should *not* be confused with considerations expressed by models of effort calculation. For example, Brehm, Wright, Solomon, Silka, and Greenberg (1983), Kukla (1972), and Meyer (1973) specified how the reflective appraisal of perceived ability, perceived difficulty, and subjective value of goal attainment determine a person's effort exertion.

Heckhausen (1987a) assumed that the course of action is directed by the mental representation of the goal, and that determination to achieve a goal originates from the mental goal representation even when the goal itself is outside of conscious awareness. The goal may be defined at various levels of abstraction (i.e., at the lowest level to the intricacies of the actions to be executed, at an intermediate level to the intended outcome, and at the highest level to the consequences that this outcome is expected to mediate), depending on the difficulties the person encounters when acting on it. In line with Vallacher and Wegner's (1987) action identification theory, goals are assumed to be defined on low levels of abstraction (i.e., necessary implementational steps as compared to the intended outcome and its desired consequences) when smooth goal pursuit is thwarted.

Goal Achievement and the Postactional Phase

The phenomenon associated with the final action phase is evaluating the question of whether one's goal striving has succeeded. What criteria govern this evaluation? Two successive evaluative questions must be answered by the individual. First is the question of whether the intended outcome has been achieved, so that the individual may stop acting and await the desired consequences. This question is easily answered whenever the outcome is a discrete performance (e.g., to send a birthday gift to a friend). It becomes a problem difficult to solve and full of uncertainty whenever the intended outcome can be continuously improved or extended (e.g., to prepare well for a mathematics test). In the latter case, the individual may resort to termination intentions (e.g., "I will work through the practice examples twice" or "I will stop when I succeed in solving every other practice problem"), thus defining clear standards regarding when the intended outcome is achieved.

Second, the individual must address the question of whether the actual value of the goal striving matches its expected value. This implies that the individual must wait for the desired consequences of the achieved outcome before this question can be answered. Only then will the individual be in a position to compare the actual value with the desired value, regardless of whether the desired consequences are a positive self-evaluation, positive evaluation by others, progress toward some superordinate goal, or some pleasant side effects. In reality, the actual value may not measure up to the expected value as assessed during predecisional deliberation. The desirability of the goal may have been overestimated because certain negative consequences were neglected or underestimated, whereas positive consequences were overestimated. Future predecisional deliberation should benefit from such evaluations; that is, the estimation of expected values should become more accurate. In this sense, postactional individuals look not only back into the past, but also to the future.

Postactional evaluation may not only benefit future deliberation, but may also help a person's future planning. Whenever the individual recognizes that the achieved outcome does not meet the intended standards or that the achieved outcome is not good enough to lead to the desired consequences, the individual may furnish the goal intention with new initiation and execution intentions, thus improving the chances of successful implementation. Or the person may lower the standards related to the quality of the outcome or the attractiveness of its consequences. If such measures are not taken or if all of these efforts fail, the goal intention may linger on without successful implementation. Whenever a situation is encountered that could be perceived as conducive to implementing the goal intention, it still should become activated, although chances to implement it are rather slim. Since this activation occupies cognitive capacity, it may even hinder the implementation of competing goal intentions, thus turning the individual into a procrastinator who keeps failing to act on his or her intentions.

Summary and Discussion

The Rubicon model of action phases takes a comprehensive temporal (horizontal) perspective on the course of action, and thus differs from most current models of action. The latter are of a strict vertical, hierarchical nature (e.g., Carver & Scheier, 1981; Gallistel, 1980, 1985; Hacker, 1985; Semmer & Frese, 1985); they assume that the individual, when executing a course of action, advances from a concern with abstract, superordinate, higher-level goals to concrete, subordinate, lower-level goals. The temporal dimension of action is addressed solely with respect to the organization of single acts or action units within the course of action (von Cranach, 1982).

The horizontal perspective as suggested by the model of action phases has so far not been very popular in psychology. The German philosopher and psychologist Christoph Sigwart (1889) introduced this perspective prior to the heyday of will psychology. Although his work did not stimulate any systematic research, it at least prevented German will psychologists from confounding problems of goal setting (which they referred to as problems of motivation) with goal striving (which they referred to as problems of willing or volition). Recently, Heckhausen and Kuhl (1985) employed a horizontal perspective when they reflected on the long way from a person's wishes to the execution of relevant actions. Although their primary focus was on the mental examinations that wishes must pass before winning access to a person's behavior, they made a strong distinction between pre- and postintentional processes, which they also referred to as motivational and volitional processes, respectively.

The Rubicon model of action phases incorporates this distinction; however, instead of focusing on a person's mental efforts (or blocks) in turning a wish into relevant action, it attempts to delineate distinct phenomena of goal-oriented behavior whose functioning obeys distinct principles. In temporal order, these phenomena are deliberating, planning, acting, and evaluating. The Rubicon model may lead to a number of misconceptions if taken too literally. These misconceptions are as follows:

1. The model does *not* imply that every single initiation of action is directly preceded by deliberation of the desirability and feasibility of the underlying goal and the forming of a goal intention. Many initiations of action are simply resumptions of activities that were started some time before; forming the underlying goal intention anew is therefore unnecessary. The same is true for action initiations postponed because of a lack of opportunities to act. Finally, people

entertain goal intentions that imply superordinate, identity-related goals, such as becoming a psychologist. These identity intentions (Gollwitzer, 1987) lead to initiating relevant actions without prior reflection on the desirability and feasibility of the underlying goal; the individual needs only to check whether a given opportunity is conducive to pursuing this goal.

2. The model does *not* imply that forming a goal intention is necessarily followed by intense planning concerning where, when, how, and how long to implement the chosen goal. It is rather assumed that such concerns originate *only* when smooth implementation of the goal intention is threatened. Initiation may be cumbersome (a) whenever special circumstances or means are required that still need to be developed or created; (b) whenever the critical opportunity may be missed because it is difficult to recognize, happens infrequently, or presents itself only for a short moment; and (c) when competing goal intentions continue to block implementing the critical goal intention. Execution is hampered when the course of action runs into difficulties because the individual does not possess the necessary competencies or fails to focus attention on the goal pursuit when conscious control of the activity is needed. Finally, termination of the implementational activities becomes problematic whenever it is unclear exactly what suffices as the intended outcome. In all of these cases pertaining to the initiation, execution, and termination of implementational actions, planning that results in the formation of the respective behavioral intentions is to be expected.

3. The model of action phases does *not* exclude the possibility of overlap between action phases. In the predecisional phase, deliberation of wishes concerning a goal can easily be interrupted so that actions in the service of other already chosen goals may be planned, initiated, completed, or evaluated. Also, in the postdecisional (preactional) phase, the individual may deliberate various wishes and evaluate some completed goal pursuit while waiting for the opportunity to act on a chosen goal; the individual may even act on some other goal when these actions do not demand much cognitive capacity (i.e., when they are automatized). Similarly, during the execution of goal-related actions, individuals may deliberate wishes, ready themselves for implementing other goals, or evaluate some terminated goal pursuit as long as executing the critical actions is largely automatized.

4. The model of action phases does *not* ignore the fact that goal striving is hierarchically organized. This is most evident in the model's distinction between goal intentions and behavioral intentions. Behavioral intentions are supplements to goal intentions and serve to promote the implementation of goal intentions. Accordingly, the formation of a goal intention precedes the formation of behavioral intentions, and the latter are justified by the former. But not all of the intentions formed subordinately to some goal intention must be behavioral intentions. People frequently form goal intentions in the service of other (superordinate) goal intentions (e.g., when a person who has decided to become a psychologist makes up his or her mind to go to school abroad). In this case, the formation of the subordinate goal (i.e., going to school abroad) should be preceded by a concern not only for the feasibility of this goal, but also for its desirability.

5. The model uses the metaphor of crossing the Rubicon to describe forming a goal intention. The allusion is not so much to having gone beyond a point of no return as it is to putting incessant deliberation to a rest. The model assumes that making a goal decision stops the "babble of competing inner voices" (Jones & Gerard, 1967, p. 181). After the decision has been made, but prior to the initiation of actions, no deliberation of the pros and cons relative to the chosen goal is expected to occur; rather, the individual is assumed to explore efficient implementation of the chosen goal (Beckmann & Gollwitzer, 1987).

Still, the model assumes that making a goal decision creates a rather durable commitment to pursue this goal, so that hindrances to one's goal pursuit do not lead to immediate retreat. Rather, the individual is expected to attempt to conquer hindrances by spontaneously increasing effort, employing different means, taking more time to overcome these hindrances, or trying to get around them by taking alternative routes to goal achievement (Gollwitzer & Wicklund, 1985). Obviously, the concept of commitment employed by the Rubicon model of action phases is dissimilar to commitment notions that link commitment to the execution of action, as conceived by dissonance researchers (Brehm & Cohen, 1962; Wicklund & Brehm, 1976), and also by Brockner and Rubin (1985), Farrell and Rusbult (1981), Kiesler (1971), and Salancik (1977). Since behavior is less revocable than thoughts (Jones & Gerard, 1967), the latter conceptualization furnishes commitment with a point-of-no-return quality. Contrary to this approach, the action phases model conceptualizes commitment in terms of an obligation to a goal, as portrayed in research on maintaining relationships (Kanter, 1972; Kelley, 1983; Lund, 1985; Rosenblatt, 1977), on identification with an organization (Buchanan, 1974; Mowday, Porter, & Steers, 1982; O'Reilly & Chatman, 1986), and on self-defining goals (Wicklund & Gollwitzer, 1982) or personal strivings (Emmons, 1989).

At the core of the Rubicon model of action phases is the assumption that the realm of goal-oriented behavior comprises various phenomena (deliberating, planning, acting, evaluating) that are ruled by different principles. But how is it possible to specify these principles so that one may test postulated differences? In the next section, I show that employing the concept of mind-set provides an interesting solution to this problem.

THE CONCEPT OF MIND-SET

If we assume that the phenomena associated with each phase of the Rubicon model are efforts at solving distinct tasks, we may try to specify the tasks to be solved at each of the four phases of the model. In the predecisional phase, the person's task is to make the best possible choice between potential action goals, whereas in the postdecisional (preactional) phase the task is to promote the initiation of actions that imply moving toward the chosen goal. In the actional phase the person faces the task of efficiently executing such actions, whereas the task in the postactional phase may best be described as trying to determine whether the intended outcome and its desired consequences actually accrued. We may further assume that involvement in these tasks creates a congruent "mind-set"—that is, a phase-typical cognitive orientation that promotes task completion (Gollwitzer, 1990). This implies that analyzing the task demands of each action phase should lead to hypotheses about the unique qualities of the respective mind-set. Before this analysis is attempted, however, a historical review of the concept of mind-set is presented.

Historical Background

In 1904 Oskar Külpe, the founder of the Würzburg school (see Boring, 1950, pp. 401–406; Gibson, 1941; Humphrey, 1951, pp. 30–131), reported his experiments on what he called "abstraction." Subjects viewed pictures of four nonsense syllables, each written in a different color. The letters composing the syllables, the positioning of the colors, and syllables themselves were varied over trials. Most importantly, Külpe also varied instructions prior to each picture presentation. Subjects had to attend to a particular aspect of the stimulus display (e.g., the frequency of a certain letter, the positioning of the colors, the figure represented by the positioning of the syllables, or the kind of letters composing the syllables). Immediately after each stimulus presentation, lasting 0.125 second, he requested the subjects to report the solutions to the tasks; in addition, he asked them to recall the other aspects of the stimulus display, of which they had not been instructed to take notice. The results showed drastic effects of instruction: Whenever the experimenter's questions were related to the instructions prior to viewing the display (e.g., subjects were asked to attend to the positioning of the colors and then asked to recall it), subjects were highly accurate in their answers; however, whenever there was a mismatch (e.g., subjects were asked to attend to the positioning of the colors but had to report on the different letters composing the four different syllables), subjects were extremely inaccurate.

In a very similar experiment, Chapman (1932) observed comparatively more accurate reports when the instructions given prior to stimulus presentation matched the inquiry posed after stimulus presentation. Watt (1905), another representative of the Würzburg school of thought, used particular words to talk about such effects, speaking of the instructions prior to stimulus presentation as constituting an *Aufgabe* (task), which creates in the individual who accepts it a corresponding *Einstellung* (mind-set). This mind-set in turn should "prepare" the individual so that the stimulus material presented should be analyzed efficiently, resulting in proper task completion.

Mind-Sets Related to Action Phases

In earlier papers stimulated by the Rubicon model of action phases, two distinct mind-sets or states of mind were postulated (Gollwitzer, 1987; Heckhausen, 1987b; Heckhausen & Gollwitzer, 1986, 1987). The predecisional and postactional phases were seen as being similar, because in both phases the desirability and feasibility of a goal are at issue. Because this issue is the master theme of the modern psychology of motivation (Atkinson, 1964), we referred to these action phases and the associated mind-sets as "motivational." Likewise, the postdecisional (preactional) phase and the actional phase were seen as being similar, since in both phases implementing the chosen goal is at issue. Because this was the master theme of will psychology, these action phases and the associated mindsets were referred to as "volitional." Moreover, the motivational mind-set was said to be characterized by a so-called "reality orientation"—that is, an orientation toward processing available information in a nonselective, unbiased manner. On the other hand, the volitional mind-set was said to be characterized by a so-called "realization orientation"—that is, an orientation toward processing available information in a selective manner biased in favor of attaining the chosen goal.

This original conceptualization, however, created confusion. For instance, it can be argued (Kornadt, 1988) that not only predecisional but also postactional individuals try to achieve (realize) something—namely, to make proper decisions or to develop correct evaluations, respectively. Therefore, realization orientation should also be present in the latter action phases. Similarly, people in the process of planning or executing an intricate course of action have to scrutinize available situational information rather realistically, and thus should also evidence a strong reality orientation.

This original conceptualization also failed to exploit the theoretical power of the concept of mind-set. Applying the mind-set concept to the action phases, first of all, requires critically analyzing the tasks individuals set for themselves in the various action phases. Second, having discovered the characteristic task demands, one is finally in a position to form hypotheses about the unique cognitive orientation of the respective mind-sets. Our original conceptualization discouraged this approach because it lumped the predecisional and the postactional phases together, banning the idea that different tasks are solved in these action phases. The same was done with the postdecisional (preactional) phase and the actional phase. Moreover, the characterization of the cognitive characteristics of the delineated mind-sets was either extremely general (reality orientation) or did not even relate to a cognitive orientation, but rather to the task expected to elicit the mind-set (realization orientation). In the following discussion, our original conceptualization is abandoned. Instead, an analysis of the tasks to be solved at each action phase is presented. As a result, four distinct mind-sets (i.e., the deliberative, implemental, actional, and evaluative mind-sets) are postulated, and their distinctive cognitive orientations are spelled out.

Deliberative Mind-Sets

When reflecting on the task to be solved in the predecisional phase, one has to keep in mind that predecisional individuals deliberate in order to determine which of their wishes are not only most desirable but also feasible. Solving this task requires that an individual be primarily concerned with information relevant to the positivity–negativity of the expected consequences of a given wish's outcome in order to estimate its desirability. In addition, information that allows the individual to assess the chances of achieving this outcome seems crucial in determining its feasibility. Reliable estimates should be favored when *all* of the relevant information for assessing desirability and feasibility is discovered and processed. Since it is unclear at the outset which pieces of information or knowledge may be relevant to assessing desirability and feasibility, a general open-mindedness toward processing incoming or stored information seems beneficial. Finally, being concerned with information that addresses (or potentially addresses) the desirability of the wish under scrutiny will not do much good if deliberation is not conducted in an impartial manner. Ignoring negative consequences or overemphasizing positive consequences may make the deliberated wish appear more desirable than is actually justified. Similarly, if information pertaining to the feasibility of the wish under scrutiny is not analyzed in a manner that favors accurate assessments, the individual may overestimate his or her capabilities to implement the desired wish, and thus may judge its feasibility to be higher than it actually is.

Accordingly, the mind-set that clearly facilitates the task of the predecisional phase (i.e., to choose the most desirable wish that is also feasible) should evidence the following characteristics: First, there should be cognitive tuning toward information relevant to the issues of feasibility and desirability. Second, there should be an orientation toward accurate and impartial processing of such information. And finally, there should be an open-mindedness or heightened receptivity to information in general. This deliberative mind-set should originate whenever people become intensely involved with deliberating their wishes.

Implemental Mind-Sets

The task to be solved by the postdecisional (preactional) individual is planning when, where, and how to act in order to promote action initiation. Solving this task effectively requires the individual to be primarily concerned with information related to these questions. Moreover, task solution is facilitated whenever the individual commits himself or herself to a certain favorable opportunity to act—that is, forms an initiation intention. In this way attention is focused on a specified opportunity to act, and the probability that the individual will forego this opportunity is reduced. However, all of these concerns will fail to benefit action initiation if the individual starts to question the desirability or feasibility of the chosen goal. Accordingly, any such doubts should be countered by the individual's boosting the desirability and feasibility of the chosen goal, thus maintaining persistence in initiating actions to reach the chosen goal.

Therefore, the mind-set that facilitates solving the task of the postdecisional (preactional) phase should evidence the following characteristics: First, there should be cognitive tuning toward information relevant to when, where, and how to act. Second, there should be closed-mindedness in the sense of concentrating on information that helps to promote the chosen goal. And finally, there should be a partial and optimistic analysis of information related to the chosen goal's desirability and feasibility, respectively. This implemental mind-set should originate whenever people become intensely involved with planning the implementation of their goal intentions.

Actional Mind-Sets

The task of the actional phase may be described as acting toward the goal so that goal achievement is promoted. Solving this task requires one to avoid disruptions, because any halting of the flow of action postpones goal achievement. The mind-set that facilitates this should therefore evidence characteristics of what Csikszentmihalyi (1975) called "flow experience" and Wicklund (1986) labeled "dynamic orientation." The individual no longer reflects on the qualities of the goal to be achieved, on his or her capacities to achieve the goal, or on alternative strategies on goal achievement; nor does the individual form behavioral intentions regarding when, where, and how to act. Rather, the individual is completely caught up in the actions currently being executed. Accordingly, only those aspects of the self and the environment that sustain the course of action are attended to, whereas any potentially disruptive aspects (e.g., self-reflective thoughts, competing goal intentions, distractive environmental stimuli) are ignored. Therefore, the mind-set that facilitates the promotion of goal achievement is one of closed-mindedness to information that could trigger a re-evaluation of the goal that is pursued, a re-evaluation of the chosen route toward goal attainment, or any self-evaluation (e.g., "Can I be proud of my performance? Am I suited for this activity?"). Rather, the actional mind-set should evidence cognitive tuning toward internal and external cues that guide the course of action toward goal attainment. It should originate whenever people move effectively toward goal attainment.

Evaluative Mind-Sets

The task to be solved in the postactional phase is evaluating outcomes and consequences of goal striving in order to discover whether the intended outcome has been reached and its desired consequences have been obtained. Solving this task, therefore, requires the individual to be primarily concerned with the quality of the outcome (standards) and the actual desirability of its consequences. Task solution should be facilitated when the individual simply compares what is achieved (outcomes) and obtained (consequences) with what was intended and desired when the goal intention was formed. This comparison should benefit from a correct assessment of the quality of the outcome and an objective, impartial view of the desirability of its consequences.

Accordingly, the mind-set that facilitates the task of evaluation in the postactional phase should evidence the following characteristics: First, there should be cognitive tuning toward information relevant to assessing the quality of the achieved outcome and the desirability of its consequences. Second, there should be an orientation toward accurate and impartial processing of this information. And finally, there should be a comparative orientation; that is, the intended outcome and the desired consequences should be compared with the actual outcome and its consequences. This evaluative mind-set should originate whenever people become intensely involved with evaluating outcomes and consequences of goal striving.

Summary

The various action phases of the Rubicon model differentiate four distinct phenomena of goal-oriented behavior: deliberating, planning, acting, and evaluating. Since each of these phenomena implies solving a distinct task, it is inferred that different mind-sets evolve whenever one is involved in these particular tasks. For each of these distinct mind-sets (i.e., deliberative, implemental, actional, evaluative), the associated cognitive orientation is specified by analyzing concrete task demands.

MIND-SETS AND COGNITIVE FUNCTIONING: RECENT FINDINGS

So far, we have concentrated our empirical efforts on testing the cognitive orientations postulated for the deliberative and implemental mind-sets. Our experiments have focused on three key issues: (1) the postulated cognitive-tuning effects; (2) the distinct way of processing information related to feasibility and desirability; and (3) the postulated differences in open-mindedness.

Mind-Sets and Cognitive Tuning

We hypothesized that both the deliberative and the implemental mind-sets achieve cognitive tuning toward task-congruous information. The deliberative mind-set should lead to cognitive tuning toward information related to the feasibility of the intended outcome (action–outcome expectancy) and to the desirability of the expected consequences (expected value), whereas the implemental mind-set should evoke cognitive tuning toward information related to action initiation (when, where, and how to get started). How does one test these hypotheses? In principle, there are two possible approaches. The first approach focuses on the subjects' thoughts while they are in a deliberative or implemental mind-set; it is expected that congruous thoughts will be experienced more frequently than incongruous thoughts. The second approach focuses on the subjects' readiness to encode or retrieve task-congruous information; here it is expected that congruous information will be encoded and retrieved comparatively more effectively.

Thought Sampling

The first approach led us to conduct three different but related experiments. In the first experiment (Heckhausen & Gollwitzer, 1987, Study 1), experimental subjects chose between two different sets of test material designed to measure creativity, one set consisting of black-and-white pictures and the other set consisting of color pictures. Subjects were told that they would later write a creative story about whichever set of pictures they chose. The reason given for offering a choice was that some people more easily reach their full creative potential when working with color pictures, whereas others perform better with black-and-white pictures. Subjects were encouraged to avoid snap choices between test materials, but to engage instead in full-fledged deliberation. For this purpose, we had subjects view a series of sample pictures (six black-and-white and six color pictures).

We interrupted one group of subjects 90 seconds after they had viewed the sample pictures (the predecisional group), while still undecided as to which set of test material they wanted to choose. In a thought-sampling task, they were requested to report their thoughts experienced during the 90-second time period, starting with the last sample picture up to the point of interruption. To increase the validity of this self-report, we proceeded as follows: Subjects first were to write down their most recent thought, and then the second most recent thought. Next, the first thought was to be reported, and then everything they had thought of in between. According to Ericsson and Simon (1980), this procedure should produce valid self-reports because subjects can retrieve the most recent thought from short-term memory. Writing down the most recent thought should then facilitate recall of the thoughts experienced immediately before, since these should be connected through episodic associations in long-term memory.

Another group of subjects was not interrupted until a decision had been made and subjects had spent 90 seconds waiting for the test material they had chosen (the postdecisional group). These postdecisional subjects reported their thoughts experienced during the 90-second time period starting with having made a decision up to the point of interruption.

Finally, we employed two groups of control subjects. Both groups were simply assigned a set of test material (yoked with the pre- and postdecisional subjects' choices). One of these groups was interrupted before this assignment (the preassignment group) and the other group afterwards (the postassignment group). The time periods on which control subjects had to focus when reporting their thoughts were closely matched to those of the respective experimental subjects.

Content analysis of subjects' reported thoughts revealed that thoughts related to expected values (e.g., "Being a creative person is important") and thoughts related to action–outcome expectancies (e.g., "I would do better with the color material") were much more frequent in predecisional subjects than in any of the other three groups of subjects. The frequency of implementation-related thoughts (i.e., considerations and expressed intentions about what kind of story would be told and how this should be done) was elevated in both the postdecisional and postassignment groups. However, hardly any implemental thoughts were reported by predecisional and preassignment subjects.

If it is assumed that predecisional subjects engaged in intensive deliberation and thus developed a deliberative mind-set, the observed predominance of task-congruous thoughts in predecisional subjects supports our cognitive-tuning hypothesis. Similarly, because both postdecisional and postassignment subjects were planning to write a creative story on the test material, both of these groups of subjects should have developed an implemental mind-set. Observing comparatively more implemental thoughts in these two groups again supports our hypothesis of task-congruous cognitive tuning.

Distance from Making a Change Decision

One could argue that the findings described above are rather trivial, because subjects simply entertained those thoughts that they were told to entertain. One has to remember, however, that we did not tell predecisional subjects to think of issues related to action–outcome expectancies and expected values; nor did we tell postdecisional subjects to stop thinking about such issues and to turn their attention to implementational issues instead. A still more convincing test of the cognitive-tuning hypothesis may be performed if the independent and dependent variables are exchanged—that is, if one asks people who harbor a personal, unresolved problem pending a change decision to engage in exactly those mental activities hypothesized to be associated with a deliberative mind-set. If our hypothesis of mind-set-congruous cognitive tuning is correct, one should expect these subjects to become lost in deliberation and therefore to feel predecisional—that is, far from making a change decision. But if such people are asked to engage in mental activities that we believe to be associated with an implemental mind-set, they should become intensely involved in the postdecisional task of planning the implementation of the change decision not yet made. Consequently, they should feel postdecisional and thus closer to making a change decision.

To test these ideas, the following experiment was conducted (Gollwitzer, Heckhausen, & Ratajczak, 1990). Subjects first named an unresolved personal problem that was pending a change decision. They named problems such as "Should I move away from home?" "Should I switch my major?" or "Should I break up with my boyfriend?" In order to measure subjects' perceived distance from making a change decision, we asked subjects at the outset of the experiment how determined they felt at that very moment, how much resolution it would still take them to arrive at a change decision, and how far away they felt from the act of making a change decision. Next, one group of subjects (the deliberation group) was asked to estimate the expected value of making the change decision. They listed the potential immediate consequences and the delayed positive and negative consequences, and they estimated the probability of these consequences' occurring. In addition, they assessed the chances of achieving the respective outcomes. Another group of subjects (the implementation group) was asked to plan the implementation of the not-yet-made change decision by listing a number of different activities that could serve the purpose of implementing it. Subjects then had to decide on a course of action and to imagine themselves executing this plan.

When subjects were asked again about their perceived distance from a change decision (employing the three items listed above), deliberation subjects continued to describe themselves as undetermined and irresolute—that is, far from making a change decision. Implementation subjects, however, indicated an increase in determination and resolution—that is, perceived themselves as closer to making a change decision. An analysis of the potential mediators of this effect ruled out an increase in desirability or feasibility, but instead pointed to having committed oneself to a certain implementational plan as the critical variable. In other words, forming behavioral intentions most strongly contributed to approaching the change decision.

In summarizing the two studies reported thus far, I would like to point out the following: Predecisional subjects showed comparatively more thoughts related to action–outcome expectancies and expected values, and when (undecided) people were made to entertain such thoughts, they felt strongly predecisional. Postdecisional subjects, on the other hand, showed comparatively more implemental thoughts, and when (undecided) people were made to entertain such thoughts they felt less predecisional—that is, closer to the act of decision. These findings suggest that a deliberative mind-set produces cognitive tuning toward thoughts related to action–outcome expectancies and expected values, whereas the implemental mind-set tunes one toward issues of how to achieve a chosen goal.

Writing Fairy Tales

The most convincing demonstration that deliberative and implemental mind-sets entail congruous thought production is provided by the findings of the following experiment (Gollwitzer, Heckhausen, & Steller, 1989, Study 1). First, subjects were placed either into a deliberative or an implemental mind-set by being asked to deliberate an unresolved personal problem pending a change decision or to plan a personal project pending realization, respectively. Again, subjects were allowed to work on personal problems or projects of their choice; career-related, lifestyle-related, and interpersonal issues were named with approximately equal frequency. The deliberative mind-set group received the same instructions as described above in the distance-from-a-change-decision experiment. Subjects in the implemental mind-set group were instructed to list five implementational steps required to complete the intended project they had named. For each of these steps, subjects had to commit themselves as to when, where, and how they planned to execute it. The control group did not receive any mind-set manipulation.

In the second part of the experiment, subjects were presented with the beginnings of three different fairy tales and were asked to continue these tales with three sentences each. All of these tales ended at a point where the main character of the story faced a goal decision. In the first story, for example, a widowed king faced the choice of going to war or staying at home to protect his beloved daughter. The sentences were scored on the basis of whether deliberative or implementational efforts were imputed to the king: Any verbs relating to the king were classified according to whether the king was engaged in the predecisional task of choosing between goals or the postdecisional task of implementing a chosen goal. The phrase "The king racked his brain wondering what to do," for instance, was scored as imputing a deliberative effort to the king, whereas the phrase "The king ordered a trusted officer to stay at home at the castle and protect his daughter" was scored as imputing an implementational effort.

As expected, subjects' mind-sets affected their flow of creative thought when completing their fairy tales. Deliberative mind-set subjects imputed more deliberative efforts to the king than implemental mind-set subjects, with control subjects' imputations falling between those of the other two groups. An analogous congruency effect was observed with imputing implementational efforts. The implemental mind-set group scored higher than the deliberative mind-set group, and the control group again scored in between these two groups.

Telling fairy tales follows a certain story grammar (Rabkin 1979; Rumelhart, 1975, 1977): Only when a solution is found to the problem introduced at the beginning may the story come to an end. Since these solutions come about more easily if the main character takes action, ascribing implementational efforts to the king should have been the more common response. This was actually the case in the control group: Subjects imputed about 10 times as many implementational efforts as deliberative efforts to the king. However, although telling a fairy tale strongly favors producing implementational thoughts, the deliberative mind-set weakened this preorientation and the implemental mind-set strengthened it. It seems important to note that these mind-sets had been elicited when subjects meditated on quite different issues (i.e., unresolved personal problems or intended projects related to career, lifestyle, or interpersonal issues), and that some minutes had passed before subjects proceeded with the fairy tales.

Cued Recall of Mind-Set-Congruous Information

Deliberative and implemental mind-sets not only should make congruous thoughts more readily available, but also should allow for more effective processing of congruous information. That is, people operating within a deliberative mind-set should be particularly effective in processing information related to outcome expectancy and expected value, whereas people operating within an implemental mind-set should be more adept at processing information related to when, where, and how to act on a chosen goal. Demonstrating potent mind-sets implies, in addition, that this prediction should hold true not only for information relevant to the meditated unresolved problem that has led to the deliberative mind-set, or for information relevant to the planned project that has led to the implemental mind-set. Rather, these mind-sets' cognitive-tuning effects should transfer to unrelated deliberative or implementational information.

To explore this supposition, we asked subjects to view a series of slides (Gollwitzer et al., 1989, Study 2). Each of the eight slides depicted a different person said to be experiencing a personal conflict of the following kind: Should I do X or not? The accompanying slide specified this conflict (e.g., "Should I sell my apartment or not?") and presented thoughts presumably entertained by the person depicted. Two of these thoughts were related to the expected values of the change decision ("It would be good because . . ."; "It would be bad because . . ."), and two were related to the question of how to initiate relevant actions, given that the change decision had been made. One of these latter two was related to the timing of relevant actions ("If I should decide to do it, then I won't . . . before

. . ."), and the other to the sequencing of relevant actions ("If I should decide to do it, then I will first . . . and then . . .").

We created deliberative and implemental mind-sets by employing the choice paradigm introduced above (i.e., the first study reported). The choice offered was between materials for a creativity test that required constructing collages from material cut out of newspapers. Two sets of collage segments were said to be available, one set consisting of black-and-white elements and the other of color elements. Subjects were told that people could reach their full creative potential only if they chose the type of material (black-and-white or color) they found personally most appealing.

One group of subjects viewed the slides and had to recall the information depicted on the sides prior to making a decision. Another group received and recalled the information after a decision had been made. If mind-set-congruous information is processed more effectively, predecisional subjects should have recalled information related to expected values better than implemental information, whereas the reverse should have been true for postdecisional subjects. Finally, we employed a group of control subjects who received and recalled the same information without either expecting to make a decision or having made one.

Control subjects' cued-recall performance (the beginnings of the sentences as listed above were provided as recall cues) was the same for expected-value-related information (positive and negative consequences) and the implementation-related information (timing and sequencing of relevant actions). Predecisional subjects, however, did better with expected-value-related information than with implementation-related information, whereas the reverse was true for postdecisional subjects. This pattern of recall performance strongly suggests that mind-set-congruous information is processed more effectively than incongruous information. The present study should not be confused with experiments designed to explore whether there is differential recall of information that is consistent with or contradictory to the decision made (Dellarosa & Bourne, 1984). In the present study, the information provided was not even relevant to the choice to be made, neither supporting nor undermining subjects' decisions.

What kind of memory processes account for the present finding that mind-set-congruous information is recalled comparatively more effectively? If we assume that subjects' retrieval attempts necessitate constructing descriptions of what they are trying to retrieve (Bobrow & Norman, 1975; Norman & Bobrow, 1976, 1979), it seems possible that mind-sets provide perspectives (Bobrow & Winograd, 1977) that allow for the easy construction of specific descriptions. The deliberative mind-set, for instance, should favor descriptions phrased as pros and cons, benefits and costs, hopes and fears, all tied to the specific conflicts of the depicted characters given as retrieval cues. In other words, the deliberative mind-set makes for the ready construction of descriptions that specify expected-value-related information, whereas the implemental mind-set helps constructing descriptions that specify implementation-related information. As Norman and Bobrow (1979) point out, quick construction of specific descriptions at the time of retrieval further successful retrieval. Norman and Bobrow also assume that whenever the description of the information sought matches the elaboration of this information at the time of encoding, recall performance is particularly enhanced. It seems possible, then, that deliberative and implemental mind-sets favor congruous recall via congruous elaboration at the time of encoding and via the ready construction of congruous descriptions at the time of retrieval.

Summary

The results of the four experiments reported show that deliberative and implemental mind-sets tune people's cognitive functioning so that congruous thoughts become readily accessible and congruous information is processed effectively. Most interestingly, both mind-sets possess some stability over time and generalize across situations (the third and fourth studies reported).

Mind-Sets and Biased Inferences

The studies presented above primarily address the questions of what types of thoughts or information are congruous with the deliberative and implemental mind-sets, whether congruous thoughts are more pervasive, and whether congruous information is processed more effectively. However, both mind-sets can also be assumed to differentially affect the way in which congruous or incongruous information is handled. We hypothesized that information related to feasibility and to desirability are analyzed in a distinct manner. Whereas in a deliberative mind-set information related to desirability is assessed impartially, assessment partial to the chosen goal is expected in an implemental mind-set. Also, feasibility is expected to be assessed rather accurately in a deliberative mind-set, whereas optimistic assessments that overestimate the actual feasibility of the intended outcome are expected in an implemental mind-set. We conducted two studies on each of these issues. The first two studies were thought-sampling studies related to predecisional individuals' assessment of desirability. The second two studies used the illusion-of-control paradigm (Alloy & Abramson, 1982) and related to assessing feasibility when a deliberative or implemental mind-set has been created experimentally.

The Counterplea Heuristic

Is there an impartial analysis of expected value in individuals with a deliberative mind-set? To answer this question, we (Gollwitzer & Heckhausen, 1987, Study 2) asked female university students to name an unresolved personal problem for which they wished resolution but that for some reason they had not resolved yet (e.g., "Should I move from home?" "Should I switch my major?" "Should I study abroad?"). Then we asked subjects to achieve clarity with respect to whether they wanted to make a change decision; we expected this instruction to trigger intensive deliberation and to create a deliberative mind-set. We also asked subjects to report back to the experimenter when they felt that further mentation would not achieve greater clarity.

Subjects were then given the thought-sampling questionnaire (described above), because subjects' answers to this questionnaire allowed us to study the temporal order of the flow of conscious thought. We scored subjects' thoughts according to a coding scheme that differentiated between positive and negative consequences of having achieved the desired outcome as implied by a change decision. First, we noticed that positive and negative consequences were pondered with equal frequency. More interestingly, when we put the thoughts reported into the correct temporal order, we discovered that deliberation followed a certain pattern. Deliberation started with reflection on the positive incentives of wish fulfillment (e.g., having moved from home). However, subjects did not indulge in these positive consequences, but immediately turned toward reflecting on negative incentives. It seemed that these deliberating people played their own devil's advocate: Their initial enthusiasm about the positive aspects was tempered with a counterplea pointing to negative consequences.

We tried to replicate this observed pattern of meditating on positive and negative consequences with a different sample of subjects—that is, male students at a military academy (Gollwitzer & Heckhausen, 1987, Study 2). Although these students named rather different unresolved problems (e.g., "Should I acquire a flying license?" "Should I buy new skiing equipment?" "Should I learn how to hang-glide?"), the same temporal pattern of thinking about the positive and negative consequences emerged. Obviously, people who become intensely involved with deliberating an unresolved personal problem attempt an impartial analysis of potential consequences. Even though the positive consequences are most salient at the beginning, negative prospects are quickly compiled in order to contrast the desired positive consequences with potential negative consequences. Thus, desired consequences are pitted against those that are feared; therefore, there is no partial analysis focusing exclusively or primarily on desired consequences.

The issue of impartial information processing prior to making a decision is not new. Festinger (1964) reported a number of studies that addressed the cognitive functioning of predecisional subjects. All of these studies assumed that an impartial analysis would not affect the initial divergence of attractiveness between choice alternatives (Davidson & Kiesler, 1964; Jecker, 1964; Walster & Festinger, 1964). Other studies defined impartiality as an equal amount of attention paid to each of the choice alternatives, as measured by looking time (Gerard, 1967), listening time (Brock & Balloun, 1967), or more recently in terms of recall performance (Beckmann & Gollwitzer, 1987).

However, these different approaches to predecisional impartiality do not capture the individual's analysis of decision-relevant information. An impartial analysis does not necessarily leave the divergence of attractiveness between choice alternatives untouched, and a partial analysis may be conducted even when the attention paid to choice alternatives (as measured in terms of encoding time or recall performance) is about equal. Not surprisingly, then, conflicting findings have been reported by studies that adhere to these operationalizations of impartiality (e.g., Janis & Mann, 1968; Mann, Janis, & Chaplin, 1969). Therefore, the somewhat old-fashioned thought-sampling technique we employed may actually provide the most valid data on the question of whether predecisional deliberation is impartial, because it captures subjects' actual thought processes.

We have not yet used our thought-sampling technique to test the hypothesis that the implemental mind-set leads to a partial analysis of expected-value-related information. But rather unambiguous support for such partial information processing after a decision is available elsewhere (Wicklund & Brehm, 1976). Researchers in the tradition of dissonance theory observed that postdecisional subjects increased the attractiveness of the chosen alternative and decreased the attractiveness of the nonchosen alternative (Brehm, 1956). In addition, postdecisional individuals were found to selectively seek information that potentially supported their choice and to actively avoid nonsupportive information (Frey, 1986). These findings have been interpreted either in terms of justifying one's decision in order to fulfill a need for consistency (Insko, Worchel, Folger, & Kutkus, 1975) or in terms of justifying one's decision for the purpose of arriving at an "unequivocal action orientation" that precludes further deliberation of the choice alternatives (Jones & Gerard, 1967; Wicklund & Frey, 1981).

This latter interpretation of postdecisional partiality is similar to our perspective that an implemental mind-set yields a partial analysis of expected-value-related information in order to promote immediate and persistent implementation of the chosen goal. The minor difference between the two perspectives may be the following: The mind-set perspective suggests that doubts about the actual desirability of the chosen goal are first of all avoided by concentrating on the implementation of the chosen goal. Only when this fails are postdecisional individuals assumed to resort to justifying their choices by increasing their expected desirability.

Illusion of Control

How do the deliberative and implemental mind-sets affect the analysis of information related to the issue of feasibility? Our hypothesis was that the deliberative mind-set should spawn an accurate assessment of the probability of achieving a certain outcome, whereas the implemental mind-set should lead to inaccurate, optimistic assessments. We tested these hypotheses in two experiments employing an illusion-of-control paradigm (Gollwitzer & Kinney, 1989).

In the contingency learning task designed by Alloy and Abramson (1979), subjects perform numerous trials on a single-stimulus apparatus. In this task, subjects are asked to determine to what degree they can influence the onset of a target light (outcome) by choosing to press or not to press a button (alternative actions). By observing whether or not the target light turns on, subjects estimate how much influence or control they have over the target light onset. The experimenter can vary the actual degree of control by manipulating the frequency of light onset associated with each of the two action alternatives (pressing or not pressing). The smaller the difference between these two frequencies, the less objective control subjects have over target light onset.

An extensive body of research (for a comprehensive review, see Alloy & Abramson, 1988) has revealed that nondepressed individuals claim to possess control over desired outcomes that are noncontingent on subjects' actions, whenever these outcomes occur frequently (e.g., in a 75-75 problem, where the target light comes on in 75% of pressing and 75% of nonpressing responses) as compared to infrequently (e.g., in a 25-25 problem). We hypothesized that the inaccurate, optimistic judgments of control (action–outcome expectancy) found with noncontingent but frequent outcome problems should be attenuated in deliberative mind-set subjects, and that they should be aggravated in implemental mind-set subjects.

In our first study (Gollwitzer & Kinney, 1989, Study 1), we modified the Alloy and Abramson (1979) paradigm by adding a second apparatus and by asking subjects to work on five sets of 20 trials. To create a deliberative mind-set, we told subjects that their objective in the first part of the experiment was to decide (after completing the five sets) on which of the two available apparatuses they wanted to work during the second part of the experiment. To allow for an informed decision, subjects were encouraged to alternate between the two apparatuses. We attempted to create an implemental mind-set by asking subjects to decide on the sequence of alternation between apparatuses with respect to all five sets of trials *before* starting the first set, and then to try to produce as many light onsets as possible.

Two problem conditions were established, a 75-75 problem and a 25-25 problem. Accordingly, both apparatuses presented either noncontingent frequent or noncontingent infrequent onset of the target light. When target light onset was frequent (the 75-75 problem), implemental mind-set subjects reported inaccurately high, illusionary judgments of control, whereas deliberative mind-set subjects showed modest control judgments. Apparently, the deliberative mind-set prevents people from being lured into illusionary optimism; that is, they recognize that high frequency of a desired outcome is not necessarily a valid indicator of one's degree of influence over the outcome. With respect to the 25-25 problem, both mind-set groups showed modest control judgments. This indicates that implemental mind-set subjects do adapt to the constraints of reality. They do not blindly perpetuate an impression of control over target outcomes, but rather accept that they have little control when too many failures are encountered.

This experiment may be criticized on two different grounds. First, one could argue that the implemental mind-set subjects may have been reluctant to tell the experimenter that they made a bad choice of alternation between apparatuses; consequently, they may have inflated their control judgments simply to keep up a good impression. Second, Barry Schwartz (1988) recently reported an illusion-of-control experiment where he pretrained subjects on a button-pushing task that offered only two buttons. In the pretraining task, he either established a rule discovery orientation (subjects had to determine which sequences of button pressing led to reinforcement in three different sequence problems) or a reward orientation (subjects were reinforced for four pushes, in any order, on each of the two buttons). Rule discovery subjects showed less illusion of control than reward subjects in a subsequent Alloy and Abramson type of contingency learning task. One could argue that our deliberative mind-set manipulation was actually a rule discovery manipulation, since subjects were instructed to determine on which of the two apparatuses they would do better, whereas the implemental mind-set manipulation was a reward orientation manipulation, since subjects were instructed to produce as many target light onsets as possible.

Both problems can easily be avoided, however, when a mind-set manipulation is employed, as described in the fairy tale experiment above. Accordingly, we ran a second study (Gollwitzer & Kinney, 1989, Study 2) where one-third of the subjects meditated on an unresolved personal problem requiring a change decision by carefully deliberating the expected value of making a change decision (deliberative mind-set). Another third made specific plans for implementing an intended project by delineating exactly when, where, and how they wanted to initiate relevant actions (implemental mind-set). Once both groups of subjects had finished these mentations, they were asked to work on a contingency problem that presented frequent noncontingent target outcomes (a 75–75 problem). The instructions for completing this task were identical for both groups of subjects; that is, they had to discover *how* to produce target light onset. A set of 40 trials was offered. We also added a control group (the last third of the subjects) that did not receive any mind-set manipulation, but worked only on the contingency problem.

Deliberative mind-set subjects again showed the most accurate judgments of control; that is, their control judgments were lower than those of control and implemental subjects. Implemental mind-set subjects evidenced control judgments that were even (albeit not significantly) more illusionary than those of control subjects. Supporting our mind-set interpretation of these findings, deliberative mind-set subjects' judgments of control correlated negatively with the reported "personal importance" of the problem pondered during the predecisional mentation. Apparently, the more involved subjects' deliberation was, the more realistic their subsequent judgments of control were. A parallel finding was observed for implemental subjects. Here, judgments of control were positively related to subjects' anticipated frustration if the project should (for whatever reason) fail to be implemented.

The present findings not only support our hypothesis that a deliberative mind-set spawns accurate control judgments whereas the implemental mind-set favors illusionary optimism, but also offer a new perspective on the phenomenon of illusion of control. It seems possible that illusion of control is generally based on an implemental mind-set. That is, whenever subjects commit themselves to achieving a desired outcome, they are likely to experience illusion of control. Data from Martin, Abramson, and Alloy (1984) and Vazquez (1987) support this line of thought: Whenever it was made difficult for subjects to commit themselves to achieving the target outcome, subjects failed to evidence illusion of control. Also, when Langer (1975) introduced the concept of illusion of control, she discovered that various factors making a luck task (i.e., random outcomes) appear to be a skill task manage to produce illusion of control. Viewed in the context of our theoretical framework, the presence of skill-related aspects in a task may induce subjects to commit themselves to the goal of achieving the desired outcome, even though its appearance is solely determined by chance. In other words, a goal commitment emerges that allows for the development of an implemental mind-set.

Finally, our mind-set conceptualization also provides a new framework from which to view "depressive realism" (i.e., the observation that depressed people do not experience illusion of control when noncontingent outcomes appear frequently). Conceivably, depressives find it particularly difficult to set for themselves the goal at hand (e.g., to maximize target light onset) because of pervasive negative beliefs about themselves—that is, their abilities, past performances, intelligence, and strengths (Beck, 1967, 1976). Such beliefs should generate doubts concerning the attainability of the given goal and thus should hinder goal commitment. Consequently, no implemental mind-set may evolve, and depressed people thereby remain insusceptible to feelings of illusionary optimism.

Summary

The findings of the last four experiments reported suggest strongly that deliberative mind-set subjects do analyze the positive and negative consequences of a prospective goal impartially. In addition, they make rather accurate estimates of action–outcome probabilities. The latter is definitely not true of implemental mind-set subjects: They overestimate these probabilities, thus showing illusionary optimism.

One wonders whether the deliberative mind-set favors accurate probability judgments in general, and not only when action–outcome expectancies are at stake. When wishes are deliberated, the probability (certainty) that the desired outcome may be reached is an important concern. Clearly, part of the answer to this question is related to action–outcome expectancy (i.e., how certain people are that they can control the desired outcome). However, there are other possible answers. The more general answer relates to people's beliefs that they possess relevant action potentials (i.e., their self-concepts of relevant competencies); the more specific answer relates to beliefs associated with specific courses of action (i.e., how cerain is it that doing X will lead to the desired outcome). Certainty is of relevance again when an individual ponders the probability that the achieved outcome will lead to a desired consequence. To answer this question, the individual must estimate the probability that certain events will occur. As we know from decision research (Baron, 1988; Slovic, Lichtenstein, & Fischhoff, 1988), people have difficulty with deriving accurate estimates. They employ numerous heuristics to ease this task (Nisbett & Ross, 1980; Tversky & Kahneman, 1973, 1974), but more often than not go astray (e.g., the gambler's fallacy, the conjunction fallacy). In particular, they are overconfident when estimating the probability of desired events (Hoch, 1985) or frequent events (Fischhoff, Slovic, & Lichtenstein, 1977). In addition, they cling to an initial estimate even when evidence accrues that urges correction; in other words, people generally fail to apply Bayes's theorem (Birnbaum & Mellers, 1983).

Should deliberative mind-set subjects do better in all of these probability judgments? Or do improvements in probability judgments generally require instruction in statistics (Nisbett, Fong, Lehman, & Cheng, 1987)? For some of the above-reported failures in assessing the probability of certain events correctly, intensive instruction in statistics seems necessary to achieve noticeable improvements (e.g., when the application of the Bayesian theorem is called for); however, for other failures, such as the overconfidence phenomenon, benefit may result from a deliberative mind-set. With respect to probability judgments related to the feasibility of the desired outcome, however, one would expect that all relevant judgments should become more accurate in a deliberative mind-set.

Moreover, one wonders whether the deliberative mind-set may also reduce shortcomings people evidence when analyzing the desirability of a choice. As decision researchers have repeatedly observed (Baron, 1988; Slovic et al., 1988), people ignore minor differences between options; they employ simplified strategies (e.g., elimination by aspects); they avoid tradeoffs between equally important consequences; they weight negative consequences differently from positive consequences, thus falling prey to framing effects; and they overweight consequences that are absolutely certain (the certainty effect). Moreover, many potential consequences are not even considered, and relevant values, attitudes, and goals that allow one to estimate the attractiveness of consequences are ignored (in particular, those that are contradictory). Again, one may raise the question of whether people need explicit training to avoid these shortcomings. So far, no research has been conducted to explore whether a deliberative mind-set reduces these shortcomings.

Research conducted in the realm of person memory suggests that this may be possible. During impression formation, people give greater attention and processing to relatively infrequent behaviors that do not match the overall picture of the target person (i.e., are inconsistent or contradictory). However, once an impression has been formed, it is the consistent information that is preferentially encoded and better remembered (for reviews, see Higgins & Bargh, 1987; Ruble & Stangor, 1986). Apparently, as soon as one is ready to act on an impression formed (implemental mind-set), the thorough analysis of the information at hand (associated with the deliberative mind-set during impression formation) vanishes.

Mind-Sets and Open-Mindedness

We hypothesized that the deliberative mind-set increases a person's receptiveness to a broad range of incoming information, whereas the implemental mind-set decreases such receptiveness. We thought that two different structural qualities of a person's information processing might account for this. First, the more heeded information (i.e., information to which individuals are attending) people can encode into short-term memory, the higher their receptivity should be. Second, people should show higher receptivity if their allocation of attention is very mobile and flexible, because that should allow them to pick up peripheral information. Accordingly, we conducted experiments that measured amount of heeded information encoded and allocation of attention in deliberative and implemental mind-sets.

Noun Span

As pointed out by Dempster (1985) and others (Case, Kurland, & Goldberg, 1982; Chi, 1976), the width of a person's noun span is a good indicator of the amount of heeded information a person successfully encodes into short-term memory. In a typical noun span experiment, subjects are read a list of words presented less than 1 second apart. When the experimenter has pronounced the last word of the list, subjects are requested to immediately repeat all of the words in the order presented.

For our experiment, we (Heckhausen & Gollwitzer, 1987, Study 2) prepared a whole set of word lists, including lists consisting of five, six, and seven one-syllable nouns. We read a first block of word lists to subjects to obtain baseline scores of their noun span. Then subjects were given the cover story of the first experiment reported above, which offered subjects a choice between test materials for a creativity test (Heckhausen & Gollwitzer, 1987, Study 1). The subjects were interrupted either prior to making a choice of test material (the deliberative mind-set group) or shortly thereafter (the implemental mind-set group). Immediately after the interruption, another block of word lists was read to the subjects. The words on the lists for the baseline measure and the critical second test were irrelevant to making a choice between test materials. We also employed a control group that was never offered a choice between test materials, but still took the baseline and critical noun span test.

When computing the noun spans via a classic procedure described by Woodworth and Schlosberg (1954, p. 696), we found that deliberative mind-set subjects showed a broader span in the second, critical assessment, as compared to their baseline scores. Their noun span increased after they had moved from the ordinary test situation (testing session for baseline data) into a deliberative mind-set associated with contemplating the choice of test material. This increased noun span was also significantly elevated as compared to both the first and second assessments of the control group. For the implemental mind-set group, no significant decrease in noun span was observed between the first and second assessments; possibly, the task of planning one's performance on the chosen creativity test was just not complex and involving enough to create a pronounced implemental mind-set.

It might be suggested that the superior performance of the deliberative mind-set subjects on the noun span test may have been rooted in an increase in nonspecific activation caused by disrupting deliberation. However, the results of a further study (Heckhausen & Gollwitzer, 1986, Study 3) do not support this explanation. This study employed exactly the same paradigm as the noun span experiment, except that subjects worked on simple arithmetic tasks instead of recalling lists of nouns. We thought that performing highly routinized and nearly informationless mental tasks such as these should profit from an increased level of activation. Accordingly, if performance on such tasks was not facilitated when these tasks were solved within a deliberative mind-set, nonspecific activation was unlikely to have produced the increase in noun span. As it turned out, no differences in performance were observed between the groups.

Mobile Allocation of Attention

The last study to be presented here suggests that a deliberative mind-set involves a greater receptivity to incoming information, because comparatively more heeded information is encoded. But there should be a second source of greater receptivity—that is, an increased readiness to encode peripheral, incidental information. Flexible, mobile allocation of attention should enhance the individual's chances of encoding such information, whereas allocating attention solely to information that is already heeded should reduce them.

We conducted the following experiment (Gollwitzer & Heckhausen, 1987, Study 1) to explore whether the deliberative mind-set increases flexible allocation of attention and the implemental mind-set reduces it. The idea underlying this study drew on research done by developmental psychologists interested in the development of attentional processes in children (Hagen & Hale, 1973). Much of this research (e.g., Miller & Weiss, 1981) has involved the so-called "central-incidental learning task," in which children are asked to remember the location of certain objects designated as central while other objects designated as incidental serve as potential distractors. At the end of this task, children are unexpectedly asked to recall the incidental objects in addition to the central objects; this determines whether attention was also allocated to the incidental information.

We modified this task so that adults would also find it involving. In our task, the central information was a short story consisting of factual statements about a small university in northern Germany. This story was presented sentence by sentence, and subjects were told to memorize it for later recall. The incidental information took the form of single, unrelated two-syllable nouns placed next to each sentence. These nouns also were irrelevant to the decisional problem that was used to create deliberative and implemental mind-sets (see below). After presentation of the stimulus material, a recognition test for the incidental information was applied. Recognition of the incidental material seemed a more appropriate measure than recall, because recall speaks to the accessibility of information in memory, whereas the availability of the incidental information was at issue here. The latter is more sensitively captured by a recognition procedure (see Bargh & Thein, 1985; Srull, 1981, 1984).

Subjects viewed the information and had to recall it either prior to making a decision (deliberative mind-set group) or shortly thereafter (implemental mind-set group). In the control group, subjects worked on the central–incidental task, neither having made nor expecting to make a decision. The decision that subjects had to make was embedded in the following cover story: Subjects were to play the part of a personnel manager. The problem at hand was to hire one of two applicants for the position of a product manager.

Deliberative mind-set subjects recognized the incidental information significantly better than implemental mind-set subjects, with control subjects showing a recognition performance that tended to be better than that of the implemental mind-set subjects and worse than that of the deliberative mind-set subjects. In addition, there was no difference among these three groups with respect to how certain they felt about the correctness of their judgments. Accordingly, the hypothesis that the motivational mind-set is characterized by more mobile allocation of attention than the implemental mind-set finds support in this pattern of data.

Summary

The last two experiments presented suggest that deliberative mind-set subjects are more receptive to available information than are implemental mind-set subjects. This is because deliberative mind-set subjects (1) encode comparatively more heeded information into short-term memory, and (2) show more mobile allocation of attention. The conducted experiments suggest that the deliberative mind-set enhances receptivity via encoding of heeded information and that it tends to do so via mobile allocation. With respect to the implemental mind-set's postulated reduction in receptivity, our findings are much weaker. There is no reduction in terms of encoding, and only a tendency with respect to allocation of attention. Possibly we failed to create strong implemental mind-sets in both experiments reported. Subjects may not have experienced a full-blown implemental mind-set, and this may have been the reason why we did not observe any significant reductions in receptivity.

MIND-SET EFFECTS: THEIR CORRELATES AND MECHANISMS

Not all mind-sets influence cognitive processing to an equal degree; some are more potent than others. What are the correlates (variables) that accompany these differences? These variables should be different for each of the action-related mind-sets outlined at the beginning of this chapter (the deliberative, implemental, actional, or evaluative mind-set). But all of these variables are related to the individual's involvement with trying to solve the task associated with the respective action phase (the predecisional, preactional, actional, or postactional phase).

For instance, in the predecisional phase the task is to determine which of one's wishes is most desirable but still feasible. Whether intensive task involvement (i.e., intense deliberation) will actually occur depends on the wish that is scrutinized, the surrounding environment, and various personal attributes. Intense deliberation should be hindered when the individual's freedom of choice is restricted by others (e.g., superiors who make the final decision); when habit or need intervenes (i.e., there is no question which wish will be chosen); or when already chosen superordinate goals determine which subordinate wish will be implemented (i.e., goal-closed decisions; Toda, 1976). It should be stimulated whenever conflict exists between wishes that appear equally desirable or between feasibility and desirability of a given wish. Other variables that should stimulate intense deliberation are the accountability and irreversibility of the individual's choice and the amount of information available. A number of potentially relevant personal attributes, such as certainty orientation (Sorrentino & Short, 1986), state orientation (Kuhl, 1984), sensitization coping style (Olson & Zanna, 1979), failure threat and depression (Pietromonaco & Rook, 1987), and the state of private self-awareness (Wicklund & Ickes, 1972), may all favor intense deliberation. Finally, it also seems possible to intensify deliberation through self-instructions and through instructions given by the experimenter (see Mischel's [1983] work on self-regulation).

All of these variables determine how involved a person may become with deliberating wishes, and thus have to be considered as potential correlates with the potency of the deliberative mind-set. Similarly, becoming intensely involved with the task of promoting the initiation of actions (implemental mind-set), the effective execution of goal-directed activities (actional mind-set), and the proper evaluation of the effects of one's goal striving (evaluative mind-set) should all depend on the specific qualities of the problem at hand, the situational context, and various personality attributes. I have tried to specify these variables elsewhere (Gollwitzer, 1990); as it turns out, there are different correlates with the potency of each of these mind-sets. I do not repeat this analysis here, but instead raise the question of what types of mechanisms produce mind-set effects.

The classic definition of mind-set (*Einstellung*) advanced by the Würzburg school suggests that the mechanisms mediating mind-set effects are located in the cognitive processes advancing the solution of the task that stimulated the mind-set. In the presented research on deliberative and implemental mind-sets, we observed that mind-sets affected subjects' thought production, the recall of congruous information, the analysis of desirability-related information, the inferences made on the basis of feasibility-related information, and finally the attentional processes when irrelevant information had to be encoded. It appears, then, that deliberative and implemental mind-sets make any knowledge that helps to solve the respective task more accessible. Part of this knowledge is categorical or episodic and relates to the specific problem at hand (i.e., the decision to be made or the project to be planned). The other part is procedural and relates to how wishes are deliberated (deliberative mind-set) or how projects are planned (implemental mind-set) in general. It is this latter part that we found to transfer to subsequent, unrelated tasks.

In this sense, the observed mind-set effects are most similar to the cognitive-tuning effects originally analyzed by Zajonc (1960) and extended by Brock and Fromkin (1968), Cohen (1961), Leventhal (1962), and most recently by Higgins, McCann, and Fondacaro (1982). This research employs a paradigm in which subjects are assigned different tasks. Half of the subjects are told to transmit their impression of a target person to others, whereas the other half are told to receive others' impressions of the target person. Subsequently, how subjects organize information on the target person and what kind of information is suppressed are analyzed. Clearly, these studies also demonstrate that different task assignments may act as steering mechanisms for organizing presented information. The research reported here expands on this idea by stating that the tasks people face at the various action phases create distinct mind-sets that tune people's cognitive functioning.

The observed mind-set effects should not be confused with research findings reported under the heading of the "New Look" in perception (Bruner, 1957; Bruner & Goodman, 1947). This research introduced the notion of "category accessibility." It is assumed that the ease with which a given stimulus input is coded in terms of a given category depends not only on the match between the features of the stimulus and of the category; other factors, such as expectancy and need states, can also increase the likelihood that a particular category rather than an alternative will be applied to the input. More recently, it has been demonstrated that simply activating (priming) a concept in one task is capable of increasing the accessibility of that construct in an unrelated subsequent task where subjects are asked to categorize a target person's behavior (Higgins, Rholes, & Jones, 1977; Srull & Wyer, 1979). In general, this research focuses on how a certain category is made more accessible so that it influences the interpretation of available information in its own terms. Our mind-set research, on the other hand, explores the effects that becoming intensely involved with the task of deliberating or planning has on the accessibility of appropriate cognitive procedures. In this sense, our research is more similar to recent attempts to delineate effects of goals or roles on the elaboration and organization of available information, as reported by Srull and Wyer (1986) and Zukier (1986), respectively.

Also, there is the question of whether mind-set effects are based on active, conscious processes involving deliberate strategies and control, or on passive, unconscious processes that occur automatically and are uncontrolled (Higgins & King, 1981; Posner & Warren, 1972). As Bargh (1989) pointed out, these aspects of being an intentional (active) process characterized by awareness and control may not always come in the two configurations described (i.e., all three are present or all three are absent), as seems to be the case with our subjects. First, our subjects were *not* aware of the mind-set effects we observed in the illusion-of-control study or in the mobile-allocation-of-attention study (i.e., subjects' certainty ratings were high and did not differ between groups). Second, however, if we had made subjects aware of them (and this is also true for the fairy tale study), subjects could have easily halted (controlled) them. Finally, deliberative and implemental mind-set effects would not occur in the absence of an explicit intention to deliberate an unresolved problem or to plan a chosen project, respectively. So it appears that mind-sets carry more of the qualities of active sets than of passive sets (Higgins & King, 1981).

Finally, how do we account for the observed transfer of the cognitive processes stimulated by deliberating or planning to subsequent unrelated tasks? This effect reminds of Luchins's (1942) problem-solving experiments, in which he demonstrated that when subjects repeatedly solved a given type of arithmetic problem suggesting a certain strategy, they then applied this strategy to subsequent arithmetic problems even when other ways of solving the problem were possible or necessary. Obviously, practiced mental operations may transfer from the training context to subsequent contexts to which they do not immediately apply. The questions of what features of the subsequent context enhance this effect, how much time may pass before such effects vanish, and what exactly happens to mental procedures during practice remain open. Recent research by J. R. Anderson on the acquisition of cognitive skill has begun addressing these issues (Anderson, 1982, 1987; in the realm of social cognition, see Smith, Branscombe, & Borman, 1988; Smith & Lerner, 1986).

GENERAL SUMMARY AND CONCLUSION

The starting point of this chapter is the question of whether the course of events associated with goal-oriented behavior is homogeneous. Although early researchers (e.g., Narziss Ach, Kurt Lewin) studying goal-oriented behavior vehemently argued against such a view by suggesting that goal setting and goal striving are ruled by different principles, this insight was widely ignored in later research on motivation (e.g., in research stimulated by Atkinson's risk-taking model). We introduced a model of action phases in a renewed attempt to delineate the various distinctive phenomena of goal-oriented behavior. These phenomena are considered to be deliberating wishes (potential goals), planning the implementation of chosen goals, acting on these goals, and evaluating one's goal striving (i.e., the outcome and its consequences).

Under the assumption that these phenomena present themselves to individuals engaged in goal-oriented endeavors as tasks that need to be solved in succession, the concept of mind-set has been introduced. It has been argued that being involved with these tasks leads to characteristic cognitive orientations (mind-sets) that are beneficial for solving these tasks efficiently. The cognitive orientations related to each of these tasks (or phenomena) have been spelled out. Finally, a number of experiments have been reported that empirically tested the cognitive orientations postulated for the deliberative and implemental mind-sets. This research has shown that the deliberative mind-set is characterized by cognitive tuning toward outcome expectancy and expected-value-related thoughts and information, by an accurate analysis of outcome-expectancy-related information and an impartial analysis of expected-value-related information, and by a heightened general receptivity to available information. The implemental mind-set, on the other hand, is characterized by cognitive tuning toward the implementational thoughts and information, and by an optimistic analysis of expectancy-related information.

These findings strongly suggest that researchers of motivation should question the still-common view that goal-oriented behavior is a homogeneous phenomenon. It seems more appropriate to conceive of goal-oriented behavior as a succession of distinctive phenomena that are ruled by their own principles. The very recent revival of interest in goal concepts (Pervin, 1989) and in the issue of commitment (Brickman, 1987) seems based on this view.

But the presented findings are also important in their own right. They suggest that the individual's cognitive apparatus readily adjusts to the various demands of goal-oriented behavior, and they thus stimulate a new perspective on common topics in the psychology of motivation (e.g., illusion of control), clinical psychology (e.g., depressive realism), decision making (e.g., certainty judgments), and social cognition (e.g., impression testing vs. impression formation). Finally, they imply interesting answers to the question of how people can more effectively turn their wishes into action.

Acknowledgments

This chapter is dedicated to the memory of Heinz Heckhausen. I am grateful to John Bargh, Tory Higgins, Christine Liu, Richard Sorrentino, and Robert Wicklund for their comments on an earlier draft.

References

Ach, N. (1905). *Über die Willenstätigkeit und das Denken* [Willing and thinking]. Göttingen: Vandenhoeck & Rupprecht.

Ach, N. (1910). *Über den Willensakt und das Temperament* [Temperament and the act of willing]. Leipzig: Quelle & Meyer.

Ach, N. (1935). *Analyse des Willens* [The analysis of willing]. Berlin: Urban & Schwarzenberg.

Alloy, L. B., & Abramson, L. Y. (1979). Judgment of contingency in depressed and nondepressed students: Sadder but wiser? *Journal of Experimental Psychology: General, 108,* 441-485.

Alloy, L. B., & Abramson, L. Y. (1982). Learned helplessness, depression and the illusion of control. *Journal of Personality and Social Psychology, 42,* 1114-1126.

Alloy, L. B., & Abramson, L. Y. (1988). Depressive realism: Four theoretical perspectives. In L. B. Alloy (Ed.), *Cognitive processes in depression* (pp. 223-265). New York: Guilford Press.

Anderson, J. R. (1982). Acquisition of cognitive skill. *Psychological Review, 89,* 369-406.

Anderson, J. R. (1987). Skill acquisition: Compilation of weak-minded problem solutions. *Psychological Review, 94,* 192-210.

Atkinson, J. W. (1957). Motivational determinants of risk-taking behavior. *Psychological Review, 64,* 359-372.

Atkinson, J. W. (1964). *An introduction to motivation.* Princeton, NJ: Van Nostrand.

Atkinson, J. W. (1974). Strength of motivation and efficiency of performance. In J. W. Atkinson and J. O. Raynor (Eds.), *Motivation and achievement* (pp. 193-218). Washington, DC: V. H. Winston.

Atkinson, J. W., & Birch, D. (1970). *The dynamics of action.* New York: Wiley.

Atkinson, J. W., & Reitman, W. R. (1956). Performance as a function of motive strength and expectancy of goal attainment. *Journal of Abnormal and Social Psychology, 53,* 361-366.

Bargh, J. A. (1989). Conditional automaticity: Varieties of automatic influence in social perception and cognition. In J. S. Uleman & J. A. Bargh (Eds.), *Unintended thought* (pp. 3-51). New York: Guilford Press.

Bargh, J. A., & Thein, R. D. (1985). Individual construct accessibility, person memory, and the recall-judgment link: The case of information overload. *Journal of Personality and Social Psychology, 49,* 1129-1146.

Baron, J. (1988). *Thinking and deciding.* New York: Cambridge University Press.

Beck, A. T. (1967). *Depression: Clinical, experimental, and theoretical aspects.* New York: Hoeber.

Beck, A. T. (1976). *Cognitive therapy and the emotional disorders.* New York: International Universities Press.

Beckmann, J., & Gollwitzer, P. M. (1987). Deliberative versus implemental states of mind: The issue of impartiality in pre- and postdecisional information processing. *Social Cognition, 5,* 259-279.

Birnbaum, M. H., & Mellers, B. A. (1983). Bayesian inference: Combining base rates with opinions of sources who vary in credibility. *Journal of Personality and Social Psychology, 45,* 792-804.

Bobrow, D. G., & Norman, D. A. (1975). Some principles of memory schemata. In D. G. Bobrow & A. Collins (Eds.), *Representation and understanding* (pp. 131-149). New York: Academic Press.

Bobrow, D. G., & Winograd, T. (1977). An overview of KRL, a knowledge representation language. *Cognitive Science, 1,* 3-46.

Boring, E. G. (1950). *A history of experimental psychology.* New York: Appleton-Century-Crofts.

Brehm, J. W. (1956). Postdecision changes in the desirability of alternatives. *Journal of Abnormal and Social Psychology, 52,* 384-389.

Brehm, J. W., & Cohen, A. R. (1962). *Explorations in cognitive dissonance.* New York: Wiley.

Brehm, J. W., Wright, R. A., Solomon, S., Silka, L., & Greenberg, J. (1983). Perceived difficulty, energization, and the magnitude of goal valence. *Journal of Experimental Social Psychology, 19,* 21-48.

Brickman, P. (1987). *Commitment, conflict, and caring.* Englewood Cliffs, NJ: Prentice-Hall.

Brock, T. C., & Balloun, J. L. (1967). Behavioral receptivity to dissonant information. *Journal of Abnormal and Social Psychology, 6,* 413-428.

Brock, T. C., & Fromkin, H. L. (1968). Cognitive tuning set and behavioral receptivity to discrepant information. *Journal of Personality, 36,* 108-125.

Brockner, J., & Rubin, J. Z. (1985). *Entrapment in escalating conflicts: A social psychological analysis.* New York: Springer.

Bruner, J. S. (1957). On perceptual readiness. *Psychological Review, 64,* 123-152.

Bruner, J. S., & Goodman, C. C. (1947). Value and need as organizing factors in perception. *Journal of Abnormal and Social Psychology, 42,* 33-44.

Buchanan, B. (1974). Building organizational commitment: The socialization of managers in work organizations. *Administrative Science Quarterly, 19,* 533-546.

Carver, C. S., & Scheier, M. F. (1981). *Attention and self-regulation: A control-theory approach to human behavior.* New York: Springer.

Case, R., Kurland, D. M., & Goldberg, J. (1982). Operational efficiency and the growth of short-term memory span. *Journal of Experimental Child Psychology, 33,* 386-404.

Chapman, D. W. (1932). Relative effects of determinate and indeterminate *Aufgaben. American Journal of Psychology, 44,* 163-174.

Chi, M. T. H. (1976). Short-term memory limitations in children: Capacity or processing deficits? *Memory and Cognition, 4,* 559-572.

Cohen, A. R. (1961). Cognitive tuning as a factor affecting impression formation. *Journal of Personality, 29,* 235-245.

Csikszentmihalyi, M. (1975). *Beyond boredom and anxiety.* San Francisco: Jossey-Bass.

Davidson, J. R., & Kiesler, S. B. (1964). Cognitive behavior before and after decisions. In L. A. Festinger (Ed.), *Conflict, decision, and dissonance* (pp. 45-61). Stanford, CA: Stanford University Press.

Dellarosa, D., & Bourne, L. E. (1984). Decision and memory: Differential retrievability of consistent and contradictory evidence. *Journal of Verbal Learning and Verbal Behavior, 23,* 669-682.

Dempster, F. N. (1985). Short-term memory development in childhood and adolescence. In C. J. Brainerd (Ed.), *Basic processes in memory development* (pp. 209-248). New York: Springer.

Emmons, R. A. (1989). The personal striving approach to personality. In L. A. Pervin (Ed.), *Goal concepts in personality and social psychology* (pp. 87-126). Hillsdale, NJ: Erlbaum.

Ericsson, K. A., & Simon, H. A. (1980). Verbal reports as data. *Psychological Review, 87,* 215-251.

Farrell, D., & Rusbult, C. E. (1981). Exchange variables as predictors of job satisfaction, job commitment, and turnover: The impact of rewards, costs, alternatives, and investments. *Organizational Behavior and Human Performance, 28,* 78-95.

Feather, N. T. (1967). Valence of outcome and expectation of success in relation to task difficulty and perceived locus of control. *Journal of Personality and Social Psychology, 7,* 372-386.

Festinger, L. A. (1942). A theoretical interpretation of shifts in level of aspiration. *Psychological Review, 49,* 235-250.

Festinger, L. A. (Ed.). (1964). *Conflict, decision, and dissonance.* Stanford, CA: Stanford University Press.

Fischhoff, B., Slovic, P., & Lichtenstein, S. (1977). Knowing with certainty: The appropriateness of extreme confidence. *Journal of Experimental Psychology: Human Perception and Performance, 3,* 552-564.

Frey, D. (1986). Recent research on selective exposure to information. In L. Berkowitz (Ed.), *Advances in experimental social psychology* (Vol. 19, pp. 41-80). Orlando: Academic Press.

Gallistel, C. R. (1980). *The organization of action: A new synthesis.* Hillsdale, NJ: Erlbaum.

Gallistel, C. R. (1985). Motivation, intention and emotion: Goal-directed behavior from a cognitive-neuro-ethological perspective. In M. Frese & J. Sabini (Eds.), *Goal-directed behavior: The concept of action in psychology* (pp. 48-65). Hillsdale, NJ: Erlbaum.

Gerard, H. B. (1967). Choice difficulty, dissonance, and the decision sequence. *Journal of Personality, 35,* 91-108.

Gibson, J. J. (1941). A critical review of the concept of set in contemporary experimental social psychology. *Psychological Bulletin, 38,* 781-817.

Gollwitzer, P. M. (1987). The implementation of identity intentions: A motivational-volitional perspective on symbolic self-completion. In F. Halisch & J. Kuhl (Eds.), *Motivation, intention and volition* (pp. 349-369). Heidelberg: Springer-Verlag.

Gollwitzer, P. M. (1990). *Abwägen und Planen als Bewußtseinslagen* [Deliberating and planning as mind-sets]. Göttingen: Hogrefe.

Gollwitzer, P. M., & Heckhausen, H. (1987). *Breadth of attention and the counterplea heuristic: Further evidence on the motivational and volitional mind-set distinction.* Unpublished manuscript, Max-Planck-Institut für psychologische Forschung, Munich.

Gollwitzer, P. M., & Heckhausen, H., & Ratajczak, H. (1990). From weighing to willing: Approaching a change decision through pre- or postdecisional mentation. *Organizational Behavior and Human Decision Processes, 45,* 41-65.

Gollwitzer, P. M., & Heckhausen, H., & Steller, B. (1989). *Deliberative and implemental mind-sets: Cognitive tuning toward congruous thoughts and information.* Unpublished manuscript, Max-Planck-Institut für psychologische Forschung, Munich.

Gollwitzer, P. M., & Kinney, R. F. (1989). Effects of deliberative and implemental mind-sets on illusion of control. *Journal of Personality and Social Psychology, 56,* 531-542.

Gollwitzer, P. M., & Wicklund, R. A. (1985). The pursuit of self-defining goals. In J. Kuhl & J. Beckmann (Eds.), *Action control: From cognition to behavior* (pp. 61-85). Heidelberg: Springer-Verlag.

Hacker, W. (1985). Activity: A fruitful concept in industrial psychology. In M. Frese & J. Sabini (Eds.), *Goal-directed behavior: The concept of action in psychology* (pp. 262-283). Hillsdale, NJ: Erlbaum.

Hagen, J. W., & Hale, G. A. (1973). The development of attention in children. In A. D. Pick (Ed.), *Minnesota Symposium on Child Psychology* (Vol. 7, pp. 117-140). Minneapolis: University of Minnesota Press.

Heckhausen, H. (1977). Achievement motivation and its constructs: A cognitive model. *Motivation and Emotion, 1,* 283-329.

Heckhausen, H. (1987a). Intentionsgeleitetes Handeln und seine Fehler [Action slips]. In H. Heckhausen, P. M. Gollwitzer, & F. E. Weinert (Eds.), *Jenseits des Rubikon: Der Wille in den Humanwissenschaften* (pp. 143-175). Heidelberg: Springer-Verlag.

Heckhausen, H. (1987b). Wünschen-Wählen-Wollen [Wishing-weighing-willing]. In H. Heckhausen, P. M. Gollwitzer, & F. E. Weinert (Eds.), *Jenseits des Rubikon: Der Wille in den Humanwissenschaften* (pp. 3-9). Heidelberg: Springer-Verlag.

Heckhausen, H., & Gollwitzer, P. M. (1986). Information processing before and after the formation of an intent. In F. Klix & H. Hagendorf (Eds.), *In memoriam Hermann Ebbinghaus: Symposium on the structure and function of human memory* (pp. 1071-1082). Amsterdam: Elsevier/North-Holland.

Heckhausen, H., & Gollwitzer, P. M. (1987). Thought contents and cognitive functioning in motivational versus volitional states of mind. *Motivation and Emotion, 11*, 101-120.

Heckhausen, H., & Kuhl, J. (1985). From wishes to action: The dead ends and short-cuts on the long way to action. In M. Frese & J. Sabini (Eds.), *Goal-directed behavior: The concept of action in psychology* (pp. 134-159). Hillsdale, NJ: Erlbaum.

Higgins, E. T., & Bargh, J. A. (1987). Social cognition and social perception. *Annual Review of Psychology, 38*, 369-425.

Higgins, E. T., & King, G. (1981). Accessibility of social constructs: Information-processing consequences of individual and contextual variability. In N. Cantor & J. F. Kihlstrom (Eds.), *Personality, cognition, and social interaction* (pp. 69-121). Hillsdale, NJ: Erlbaum.

Higgins, E. T., McCann, C. D., & Fondacaro, R. (1982). The communication game: Goal-directed encoding and cognitive consequences. *Social Cognition, 1*, 21-37.

Higgins, E. T., Rholes, W. S., & Jones, C. R. (1977). Category accessibility and impression formation. *Journal of Experimental Social Psychology, 13*, 141-154.

Hillgruber, A. (1912). Fortlaufende Arbeit und Willensbetätigung [Continuous work and willing]. *Untersuchungen zur Psychologie und Philosophie, 1*(6).

Hoch, S. J. (1985). Counterfactual reasoning and accuracy in predicting personal events. *Journal of Experimental Psychology: Learning, Memory, and Cognition, 11*, 719-731.

Humphrey, G. (1951). *Thinking*. London: Methuen.

Insko, C. A., Worchel, S., Folger, R., & Kutkus, A. (1975). A balance theory interpretation of dissonance. *Psychological Review, 82*, 169-183.

Janis, I. L., & Mann, L. (1968). A conflict theory approach to attitude change and decision making. In A. Greenwald, T. Brock, & T. Ostrom (Eds.), *Psychological foundations of attitudes* (pp. 327-360). New York: Academic Press.

Jecker, J. D. (1964). The cognitive effects of conflict and dissonance. In L. A. Festinger (Ed.), *Conflict, decision, and dissonance* (pp. 21-30). Stanford, CA: Stanford University Press.

Jones, E. E., & Gerard, H. B. (1967). *Foundations of social psychology*. New York: Wiley.

Kanter, R. M. (1972). *Commitment and community: Communes and utopias in sociological perspective*. Cambridge, MA: Harvard University Press.

Kelley, H. H. (1983). Love and commitment. In H. H. Kelley, E. Berscheid, A. Christensen, J. H. Harvey, T. L. Huston, G. Levinger, E. McClintock, L. A. Peplau, & D. R. Peterson (Eds.), *Close relationships* (pp. 265-314). San Francisco: W. H. Freeman.

Kiesler, L. A. (1971). *The psychology of commitment*. New York: Academic Press.

Klinger, E. (1977). *Meaning and void: Inner experience and the incentives in people's lives*. Minneapolis: University of Minnesota Press.

Kornadt, H. J. (1988). Motivation und Volition: Anmerkungen und Fragen zur wiederbelebten Willenspsychologie [Motivation and volition: Comments on the revived psychology of willing]. *Archiv für Psychologie, 140*, 209-222.

Kuhl, J. (1983). *Motivation, Konflikt und Handlungskontrolle*. [Motivation, conflict, and action control]. Heidelberg: Springer-Verlag.

Kuhl, J. (1984). Volitional aspects of achievement motivation and learned helplessness: Toward a comprehensive theory of action control. In B. A. Maher (Ed.), *Progress in experimental personality research* (Vol. 13, pp. 99-171). New York: Academic Press.

Kukla, A. (1972). Foundations of an attributional theory of performance. *Psychological Review, 79*, 454-470.

Langer, E. J. (1975). The illusion of control. *Journal of Personality and Social Psychology, 32*, 311-328.

Leventhal, H. (1962). The effects of set and discrepancy on impression change. *Journal of Personality, 30*, 1-15.

Lewin, K. (1926). Vorsatz, Wille und Bedürfnis [Intention, will, and need]. *Psychologische Forschung, 7*, 330-385.

Lewin, K. (1936). *Principles of topological psychology.* New York: McGraw-Hill.

Lewin, K., Dembo, T., Festinger, L. A., & Sears, P. S. (1944). Level of aspiration. In J. M. Hunt (Ed.), *Personality and the behavior disorders* (pp. 333-378). New York: Ronald Press.

Luchins, A. S. (1942). Mechanization in problem solving. *Psychological Monographs, 54,* 1-95.

Lund, M. (1985). The development of investment and commitment scales for predicting continuity of personal relationships. *Journal of Social and Personal Relationships, 2,* 3-23.

Mann, L., Janis, I. L., & Chaplin, R. (1969). Effects of anticipation of forthcoming information on predecisional processes. *Journal of Personality and Social Psychology, 11,* 10-16.

Martin, D. J., Abramson, L. Y., & Alloy, L. B. (1984). Illusion of control for self and others in depressed and nondepressed college students. *Journal of Personality and Social Psychology, 46,* 125-136.

McClelland, D. C. (1980). Motive dispositions. In L. Wheeler (Ed.), *Review of personality and social psychology* (Vol. 1, pp. 10-41). Beverly Hills, CA: Sage.

Meyer, W. U. (1973). *Leistungsmotiv und Ursachenerklärung von Erfolg and Mißerfolg* [Achievement motive and attributions for success and failure]. Stuttgart: E. Klett.

Michotte, A. E., & Prüm, E. (1910). Étude expérimentale sur le choix volontaire et ses antécédents immédiats. [The immediate antecedents of the act of choice]. *Archives de Psychologie, 10,* 119-299.

Miller, P. H., & Weiss, M. G. (1981). Children's attention allocation, understanding of attention, and perförmance on the central incidental learning task. *Child Development, 52,* 1183-1190.

Mischel, W. (1983). Delay of gratification as process and as person variable in development. In D. Magnusson & V. P. Allen (Eds.), *Human development: An interactional perspective* (pp. 149-165). New York: Academic Press.

Mowday, R. T., Porter, L. W., & Steers, R. M. (1982). *Employee-organization linkages: The psychology of commitment, absenteeism, and turnover.* New York: Academic Press.

Nisbett, R. E., Fong, G. T., Lehman, D. R., & Cheng, P. W. (1987). Teaching reasoning. *Science, 238,* 625-631.

Nisbett, R., & Ross, L. (1980). *Human inference: Strategies and shortcomings of social judgment.* Englewood Cliffs, NJ: Prentice-Hall.

Norman, D. A., & Bobrow, D. G. (1976). On the role of active memory processes in perception and cognition. In C. N. Cofer (Ed.), *The structure of human memory* (pp. 114-132). San Francisco, W. H. Freeman.

Norman, D. A., & Bobrow, D. G. (1979). Descriptions: An intermediate stage in memory retrieval. *Cognitive Psychology, 11,* 107-123.

Olson, J. M., & Zanna, M. P. (1979). A new look at selective exposure. *Journal of Experimental Social Psychology, 15,* 1-15.

O'Reilly, C. O., III, & Chatman, J. (1986). Organizational commitment and psychological attachment: The effects of compliance, identification, and internalization on prosocial behavior. *Journal of Applied Psychology, 71,* 492-499.

Pervin, L. A. (Ed.). (1989). *Goal concepts in personality and social psychology.* Hillsdale, NJ: Erlbaum.

Pietromonaco, P., & Rook, K. (1987). Decision style in depression: The contribution of perceived risks vs. benefits. *Journal of Personality and Social Psychology, 52,* 399-408.

Posner, M. I., & Warren, R. E. (1972). Traces, concepts and conscious constructions. In A. W. Melton & E. Martin (Eds.), *Coding processes in human memory* (pp. 25-44). Washington, DC: V. H. Winston.

Rabkin, E. S. (1979). *Fantastic worlds: Myths, tales and stories.* Oxford: Oxford University Press.

Raynor, J. O. (1969). Future orientation and motivation of immediate activity: An elaboration of the theory of achievement motivation. *Psychological Review, 76,* 606-610.

Rosenblatt, P. C. (1977). Needed research on commitment in marriage. In G. Levinger & H. L. Rausch (Eds.), *Close relationships: Perspectives on the meaning of intimacy* (pp. 73-86). Amherst: University of Massachusetts Press.

Ruble, D. N., & Stangor, C. (1986). Stalking the elusive schema: Insights from developmental and social psychological analyses of gender schemas. *Social Cognition, 4,* 227-261.

Rumelhart, D. E. (1975). Notes on a schema for stories. In D. G. Bobrow & A. M. Collins (Eds.), *Representation and understanding* (pp. 211-236). New York: Academic Press.

Rumelhart, D. E. (1977). Understanding and summarizing brief stories. In D. LaBerge & J. Samuels (Eds.), *Basic processes in reading and comprehension* (pp. 265-303). Hillsdale, NJ: Erlbaum.

Salancik, G. R. (1977). Commitment and the control of organizational behavior and belief. In B. M. Staw & G. R. Salancik (Eds.), *New directions in organizational behavior* (pp. 1-54). Chicago: St. Clair Press.

Schwartz, B. (1988). The experimental synthesis of behavior: Reinforcement, behavioral stereotypy, and problem solving. In G. H. Bower (Ed.), *The psychology of learning and motivation: Advances in research and theory* (Vol. 22, pp. 93-135). New York: Academic Press.

Selz, O. (1910). Die experimentelle Untersuchung des Willensaktes. *Zeitschrift für Psychologie, 37*, 241-270.

Semmer, N., & Frese, M. (1985). Action theory in clinical psychology. In M. Frese & J. Sabini (Eds.), *Goal-directed behavior: The concept of action in psychology* (pp. 296-310). Hillsdale, NJ: Erlbaum.

Sigwart, C. (1889). *Der Begriff des Wollens und sein Verhältnis zum Begriff der Ursache* [The concept of willing vs. the concept of motive]. Freiburg: J. C. B. Mohr.

Slovic, P., Lichtenstein, S., & Fischhoff, B. (1988). Decision making. In R. C. Atkinson, R. J. Hernstein, G. Lindzey, & R. D. Luce (Eds.), *Stevens' handbook of experimental psychology: Learning and cognition* (Vol. 2, pp. 673-738). New York: Wiley.

Smith, E. R., Branscombe, N. R., & Borman, C. (1988). Generality of the effects of practice on social judgment tasks. *Journal of Personality and Social Psychology, 54*, 385-395.

Smith, E. R., & Lerner, M. (1986). Development of automatism of social judgments. *Journal of Personality and Social Psychology, 50*, 246-259.

Sorrentino, R. M., & Short, J. (1986). Uncertainty orientation, motivation, and cognition. In R. M. Sorrentino & E. T. Higgins (Eds.), *Handbook of motivation and cognition: Foundations of social behavior* (Vol. 1, pp. 379-403). New York: Guilford Press.

Srull, T. K. (1981). Person memory: Some tests of associative storage and retrieval models. *Journal of Experimental Psychology: Human Learning and Memory, 7*, 440-463.

Srull, T. K. (1984). Methodological techniques for the study of person memory and social cognition. In R. S. Wyer & T. K. Srull (Eds.), *Handbook of social cognition* (Vol. 2, pp. 1-72). Hillsdale, NJ: Erlbaum.

Srull, T. K., & Wyer, R. S. (1979). The role of category accessibility in the interpretation of information about persons: Some determinants and implications. *Journal of Personality and Social Psychology, 37*, 1660-1672.

Srull, T. K., & Wyer, R. S. (1986). The role of chronic and temporary goals in social information processing. In R. M. Sorrentino & E. T. Higgins (Eds.), *Handbook of motivation and cognition: Foundations of social behavior* (Vol. 1, pp. 503-549). New York: Guilford Press.

Toda, M. (1976). The decision process. A perspective. *International Journal of General Systems, 3*, 79-88.

Tversky, A., & Kahnemann, D. (1973). Availability: A heuristic for judging frequency and probability. *Cognitive Psychology, 5*, 207-232.

Tversky, A., & Kahnemann, D. (1974). Judgment under uncertainty: Heuristics and biases. *Science, 185*, 1124-1131.

Vallacher, R. R., & Wegner, D. M. (1987). What do people think they're doing? *Psychological Review, 94*, 3-15.

Vazquez, C. V. (1987). Judgments of contingency: Cognitive biases in depressed and nondepressed subjects. *Journal of Personality and Social Psychology, 52*, 419-431.

von Cranach, M. (1982). The psychological study of goal-directed action: Basic issues. In M. von Cranach & R. Harré (Eds.), *The analysis of action* (pp. 35-73). Cambridge, England: Cambridge University Press.

Walster, E., & Festinger, L. (1964). Decisions among imperfect alternatives. In L. A. Festinger (Ed.), *Conflict, decision, and dissonance* (pp. 131-145). Stanford, CA: Stanford University Press.

Watt, H. J. (1905). Experimentelle Beiträge zu einer Theorie des Denkens [Experiments on a theory of thinking]. *Archiv für die gesamte Psychologie, 4,* 289–436.

Weiner, B. (1974). *Achievement motivation and attribution theory.* Morristown, NJ: General Learning Press.

Wicklund, R. A. (1986). Orientation to the environment versus preoccupation with human potential. In R. M. Sorrentino & E. T. Higgins (Eds.), *Handbook of motivation and cognition: Foundations of social behavior* (Vol. 1, pp. 64–95). New York: Guilford Press.

Wicklund, R. A., & Brehm, J. W. (1976). *Perspectives on cognitive dissonance.* Hillsdale, NJ: Erlbaum.

Wicklund, R. A., & Frey, D. (1981). Cognitive consistency: Motivational versus non-motivational perspectives. In J. P. Forgas (Ed.), *Social cognition: Perspectives on everyday understanding* (pp. 141–163). London: Academic Press.

Wicklund, R. A., & Gollwitzer, P. M. (1982). *Symbolic self-completion.* Hillsdale, NJ: Erlbaum.

Wicklund, R. A., & Ickes, W. J. (1972). The effect of objective self-awareness on predecisional exposure to information. *Journal of Experimental Social Psychology, 8,* 378–387.

Woodworth, R. S., & Schlosberg, H. (1954). *Experimental psychology.* New York: Holt, Rinehart & Winston.

Yerkes, R. M., & Dodson, J. D. (1908). The relation of strength of stimulus to rapidity of habit formation. *Journal of Comparative Neurology and Psychology, 18,* 459–482.

Zajonc, R. B. (1960). The process of cognitive tuning in communication. *Journal of Abnormal and Social Psychology, 61,* 159–167.

Zukier, H. (1986). The paradigmatic and narrative modes in goal-guided inference. In R. M. Sorrentino & E. T. Higgins (Eds.), *Handbook of motivation and cognition: Foundations of social behavior* (Vol. 1, pp. 465–502). New York: Guilford Press.

CHAPTER 3

Auto-Motives

Preconscious Determinants of Social Interaction

JOHN A. BARGH
New York University

Habit covers a very large part of life, and one engaged in studying the objective manifestations of mind is bound at the very outset to define clearly just what its limits are.—*James (1890, p. 104)*

I can control something that is self-controlled—if I can control the states of the world that cause it, in controlling itself, to act.—*Dennett (1984, p. 56)*

THE QUESTION OF CONTROL OVER SOCIAL THOUGHT AND BEHAVIOR

How much control does one exercise over one's own thought and behavior in social situations? This important and intriguing question has guided a considerable amount of research since it was posed by Langer (1978; see Uleman & Bargh, 1989). To ask whether we as individuals control our own thought and behavior supposes that other agents of control are possible. Thus, one approach to the question is to consider what other agents of control may exist, and the extent of their influence.

One possibility is that to some extent social behavior and cognition are under the direct control of the environment (Bargh, 1984). That is, information present in the social environment may activate internal memory representations that then influence the interpretation of that information, or perhaps even act upon it, such as to make and store judgments or impressions, or make and carry out behavioral decisions. Because these operations on the environmental input occur without active, intentional conscious involvement, or awareness of the extensive processing taking place, they are called "preconscious" processes (see Bargh, 1989, for a review).

Automatic Influences in Social Perception and Judgment

How long is the reach of these environmentally driven influences? Are they limited to social perception, or can they guide actual social behavior? Stimulated by Langer's (1978) position that one's behavior in complex social interactions is often under the control of environmental cues, such that behavioral responses do not require active conscious involvement, my colleagues and I embarked on research testing the existence and then the limits of the social environment's direct control over thought and behavior. This research has shown that social information activates internal memory representations without the person's awareness of the presence of the information in the environment (Bargh, 1982), and that these activated representations subsequently influence the interpretation of behavioral information and the outcome of social judgment processes (Bargh, Bond, Lombardi, & Tota, 1986; Bargh & Pietromonaco, 1982). Moreover, these preconscious activation effects occur even under conditions of information overload (Bargh & Thein, 1985; Bargh & Tota, 1988), and when the subject is actively attempting to prevent them from occurring (Bargh & Pratto, 1986).

Other lines of research have documented the unintentional, preconscious activation of social stereotypes by salient, differentiating environmental features such as age, race, and gender (e.g., Brewer, 1988; Devine, 1989; McArthur & Friedman, 1980; Mills & Tyrrell, 1983; Pratto & Bargh, in press). There is also a growing body of evidence that social stimuli are evaluated preconsciously; that is, they are classified as "good" or "bad," and this evaluation then remains active in memory to influence responses to the stimulus (Bargh, Chaiken, Govender, & Pratto, 1990; Bargh, Litt, Pratto, & Spielman, 1989; Fazio, Sanbonmatsu, Powell, & Kardes, 1986). Still other studies have shown that social behaviors are preconsciously classified in terms of the traits they exemplify (e.g., Winter & Uleman, 1984), and that these activated trait-related representations are likely then to be used in a default manner in ascribing causality for the behavior (i.e., in making dispositional attributions when attentional resources are not sufficient to accomplish the more effortful task of making a situational attribution; see Gilbert, 1989; Gilbert, Pelham, & Krull, 1988).

Responses to the Environment Require an Intention

But there are indications that there is a limit to the extent of preconscious determination of social cognition and behavior, and that this is at the stage of *responding* to the environment, be it in the form of judgments or decisions, or in terms of behavior (verbal and nonverbal) itself. That is, preconscious processing of environmental information appears to be bounded, the restriction being that although responses may be strongly or even exclusively influenced by preconscious analyses, the making of the response itself requires an intervening intention (see Bargh, 1989). For instance, it has been argued that social judgments and causal attributions (Smith, 1984, p. 403; Smith & Miller, 1983; Winter, Uleman, & Cunniff, 1985) and behavior (Langer, 1978) are produced directly by environmental stimuli without the need of an intervening conscious intent, and the evidence is that these effects do not occur without an intention that they do (see Bargh, 1984, 1989; Higgins & Bargh, 1987, pp. 376–378). Also, although subjects who were chronically sensitive to certain dimensions on social behavior were more likely to notice them and use them in judgments (Bargh et al., 1986; Bargh & Thein, 1985; Higgins, King, & Mavin, 1982), and those subjects whose attitude toward an activity had been made more accessible were more or less likely (depending on the valence of their attitude) to engage in that activity (Fazio, Powell, & Herr, 1983), those judgments and behavior were always *intended* by the subjects in those studies.

There are several lines of evidence supporting the existence of the apparent asymptote for preconscious control at the point of responding to the environment. First, the forms of preconscious social information processing documented thus far—stereotype and trait construct activation, for example—can be *prevented* from influencing responses, given sufficient motivation and effort (Bargh, 1989; Devine, 1989; Fiske, 1989). It has been well documented that current conscious purposes are capable of overriding automatically suggested responses if the two are in conflict (Bargh, 1984; Logan, 1980; Neely, 1977; Posner & Snyder, 1975). For example, in the Bargh (1982) dichotic listening study, the presence in the unattended channel of stimuli relevant to a subject's self-concept did activate the corresponding mental constructs (as indicated by measures of spare processing capacity), demonstrating preconscious, unintended activation of the self-concept by relevant information in the environment. However, this activation did *not* interfere with the subject's conscious and intended task of shadowing the attended channel.

Moreover, the tendency to spontaneously encode verbally presented behaviors in terms of trait concepts (e.g., Winter & Uleman, 1984) disappears when the subject's processing goal does not require comprehension of the meaning of the behavior (Moskowitz & Uleman, 1987; Uleman, 1987). Thus, when pursuing a goal for which spontaneous trait influences are not useful (as they are useful in comprehending a behavior), subjects do not make them. In addition, although there is converging evidence as to the ability of one's chronically accessible, frequently applied social trait constructs to become activated automatically in the mere presence of relevant information, in all studies showing an influence of these automatically activated structures on actual *responses* (judgments, attention allocation, memory; Bargh et al., 1986; Bargh & Thein, 1985; Higgins et al., 1982), subjects had the intentional goal of forming an impression of the target person.

Studies utilizing the Stroop paradigm (e.g., Bargh & Pratto, 1986; Pratto & John, 1989) also demonstrate uncontrollable activation effects by obtaining longer color-naming latencies for stimuli predicted to automatically attract processing resources, such as those corresponding to negative personality traits or to the subjects' chronically accessible social constructs. Yet at the same time, subjects rarely make mistakes in their intended task of correctly naming the colors of the stimulus words. Such studies show that even preconscious processes that do strongly suggest a behavioral response appropriate for the current task (e.g., the word "GREEN" in blue ink in the Stroop task) can be and are typically inhibited from determining the response if they conflict with the response called for by a subject's current goal. This holds true even when the automatic response is the usual and habitual one for that situation and the goal response is novel (Logan & Zbrodoff, 1979; Neely, 1977; on the general point that automatic processes can be overridden by acts of control, see Logan, 1989; Posner & Snyder, 1975; Uleman, 1989).

Finally, many social-cognitive processes that have been claimed to occur automatically have been shown instead to require the existence of a specific intention or goal state. We (Bargh & Tota, 1988) found, in fact, that even in the case of the initial automatic activation of chronic constructs, different constructs may become active for depressed individuals, depending on whether the subject is actively thinking about the self or about the average other person. Similarly, Paulhus and Levitt (1987) showed that the trait concepts subjects endorsed as self-descriptive became increasingly positive as attentional load was increased; thus, when the ability to engage in deliberate, strategic responding was precluded, the default set of constructs automatically ready under the goal of self-presentation were considerably more positive (see also Paulhus, Graf, & Van Selst, 1989). Such findings of *goal-dependent* automaticity (Bargh, 1989), especially in the case of responses (as opposed to measures of cognitive activity alone), underscore the importance of the current processing goal in the making of responses to the environment.

Social Cognition and Interaction Are Goal-Directed

As to whether the social environment directly controls behavior, there exists no evidence in favor of—but compelling logical arguments against—the notion that social-interactive behavior can occur without an interposed intent or goal that it occur (see Bargh, 1989; Fiske, 1989). Behavioral responses in routine social interactions are highly dependent on consciously made choices and decisions during the course of the interaction (Abelson, 1980; Fiske, 1989; Gollwitzer, Chapter 2, this volume; Miller, Galanter, & Pribram, 1960; Norman & Shallice, 1986; Shallice, 1972). Automatic, preconscious influences on behavioral decisions certainly exist, and because of their implicit nature great confidence and weight may be placed on them (Bargh, 1989; Jacoby & Kelley, 1987), but the decisions themselves are made intentionally and in the service of the current goal.

Ever since the work of Kulpe, Ach, and Watt of the Würzburg school at the turn of the century, it has been known that the goal in place makes a tremendous difference in determining what information is attended to, how it is interpreted, and how it is acted upon. The Würzburg researchers observed that the subject's task goal, or *Aufgabe*, created a "determining tendency" that then automatically resulted in the desired response with no intervening conscious intent necessary (see Boring, 1950, pp. 402–406; see also Gollwitzer, Chapter 2, this volume; Zajonc, 1960). Neisser (1967) concluded that the current intent or goal was a primary determinant of cognition and behavior:

> In accounting for the course of thought and action, there has been repeated reference to the subject's motives and expectations. . . . To know what the subject

will think of next [requires] a detailed understanding of what he is trying to do, and why. (pp. 304-305)

Social psychologists have long recognized the power of the current goal state to determine what situational stimuli will be attended and what meaning they will have for the individual. Lewin (1935) argued that "a strongly accented goal so transforms the situation that practically all objects acquire a reference to this goal" (p. 102). The influence of goals and motives on perception was, of course, a major theme of the New Look research (see reviews by Allport, 1955; Bruner, 1957). The perceiver's current goals and physiological needs were considered a primary determinant of the accessibility of perceptual categories, and hence of perceptual selectivity and categorization of inputs. Jones and Thibaut (1958), in their pioneering paper on the consequences of interaction goals for social perception, put the point most directly:

> If we can successfully identify the goals for which an actor is striving in the interaction situation, we can begin to say something about the cues to which he will attend, and the meaning he is most likely to assign them. (p. 152)

The last decade has seen a resurgence of research on the influences of information-processing goals (see Srull & Wyer, 1986, for a review). Briefly, these studies have shown that what is attended to among the different behaviors of a target person, the organization of that information in memory, and the amount of that information accessible to recall are all quite different for subjects trying to form an impression of the target than for those trying to remember the information for a subsequent memory test (Cohen & Ebbesen, 1979; Hamilton, Katz, & Leirer, 1980; Srull & Brand, 1983; Wyer & Gordon, 1982). Subjects encountering information (e.g., about a house) with different purposes (e.g., mentally assuming the role of a burglar vs. a home buyer) notice and remember different features (Anderson & Pichert, 1978; Wyer, Srull, Gordon, & Hartwick, 1982). One's mental organization of person information is altered by the nature of the audience to which one communicates that information—namely, whether one believes the audience's opinion of the target to be favorable or unfavorable (Higgins & McCann, 1984; Higgins & Rholes, 1978).

Motivational influences have received increased research attention as well. Persuasion researchers have documented that the particular features of a persuasive appeal that are attended to and have an influence on attitude change vary as a function of the processing strategy adopted by the subject, which in turn is a function of the personal importance of the message topic (Chaiken, 1980; Petty, Cacioppo, & Goldman, 1981; see review by Chaiken, Liberman, & Eagly, 1989). Moreover, the self-concept itself appears to be malleable in the face of motivational influences such as self-presentation (Jones, Rhodewalt, Berglas, & Skelton, 1981; Kunda & Sanitoso, 1989; Rhodewalt & Agustsdottir, 1986).

Motivation to be accurate in perceiving other people has been found to overcome some very strong automatic tendencies, such as stereotyping, the fundamental attribution error, and the influence of prior expectancies. Impression formation processes are different, depending on whether one's own important outcomes depend on the other person; such outcome dependency has been shown to lead to increased effort expended in the judgmental process and to greater accuracy as well (e.g., Erber & Fiske, 1984; Neuberg & Fiske, 1987). If a subject anticipates interacting with the target person he or she is judging, more information about the person is stored in memory, and it is also better organized (Devine, Sedikides, & Fuhrman, 1989); the motivating effect of anticipated interaction is quite pronounced in younger children, resulting in a considerable increase in their use of psychological concepts in thinking about other children (Feldman & Ruble, 1988). The powerful and difficult-to-overcome influence of salient information on social judgments (such as when a target person's features differ from those of the majority of the group being perceived; see Taylor & Fiske, 1978) can be overcome to an extent if it matters to the self-interest of the subject (Borgida & Howard-Pitney, 1983). Knowing that one is *accountable* for one's judgment about the attitudes and beliefs of another person has been found to overcome the "fundamental" attribution error of not taking situational constraints into account (Tetlock, 1985), and encouragement to form accurate impressions overcomes the influence of negative initial expectancies in impression formation (Neuberg, 1989). Finally, racial and other stereotypes can be overruled in the judgment process if the subject's values motivate him or her to counteract the stereotypic influence (Devine, 1989; Fiske, 1989).

Where Do Goals Come From?

Recently, detailed models of social cognition and personality have been developed that recognize this accumulation of evidence by including the current processing goal as a major determining factor of the course of thought and judgment (e.g., Cantor & Kihlstrom, 1987; Smith, 1984; Wyer & Srull, 1986). However, in recognizing the influence of goals, these models leave open the question of where the goal itself comes from on a moment-to-moment basis. A similar difficulty exists with previous cognitive models, as well as with most current artificial intelligence models that include a goal state as a determining factor (e.g., Miller et al., 1960; Newell & Simon, 1972; see critical review by Wilensky, 1983). The goal in these models is a given entity, a starting point for the model, which takes things from there. (The treatments of plans and goals by Miller et al., 1960, and by Schank & Abelson, 1977, do contain considerable attention to the matter of the original source of goals for the individual—in values, roles, and aspirations—but no specification of what determines which particular goal will be in place at any particular point in time.) This is not to suggest that these models are compromised by this lack of specification—only that their predictive ability, as Neisser (1967, p. 305) anticipated, is limited, as is the extent to which they capture the essence of naturalistic social cognition. As Wilensky (1982) put it,

> Conventional [artificial intelligence] models by and large do not deal with this issue of where goals come from. . . . In the real world, at least as much work is involved in determining what one wants to do as in determining how to do it. (p. 13)

By including the "goal box" or "executive process" only as an exogenous variable in models of cognition and action, and by leaving the question open as to where the goals themselves come from, one quickly runs into the classical "problem of volition" (see historical review by Kimble & Perlmuter, 1970), or what Neisser (1967, p. 292) called the "problem of the executive." That is, by not specifying why and when we have the goals we do, explanatory appeals must be made to nonobservable concepts, such as "consciousness," the "will," of "intention." Typically, the "executive process" selects the current goal and chooses among available alternative actions. But who *is* this executive making the choices and selecting the goals? "Is there a little man in the head, a *homunculus?* . . . Such explanations seem to lead only to an infinite regress" (Neisser, 1967, p. 295).

The "soul" or "homunculus" problem in accounting for voluntary, intended thought and behavior has, of course, been around for a long time; Sechenov (1935), James (1890), and Miller et al. (1960), among others, have wrestled with it. In their review, Kimble and Perlmuter (1970) point out that "the central problem in accounting for voluntary behavior is finding a cause for it" (p. 364).

The Incredible Shrinking Little Person in the Head

Needless to say, the reader will not find a solution to this age-old problem in this chapter. But he or she will find a proposal for one way to reduce the contents of the "black box" that currently contains the executive processes supplying individuals with processing goals and action plans—a proposal codified from many related but partial previous proposals. The general strategy is to shrink the domain of the unknown in the "black box" and bring ever more of its workings out into the specified open (see the cogent and entertaining discussions of this solution to the homunculus problem by Dennett, 1978, and Uleman, 1989).

At the opening of the 1957 science fiction film *The Incredible Shrinking Man*, the protagonist finds himself trapped in a radioactive mist. This, of course, results in a syndrome previously unheard of in the annals of medicine or science: Our hero gradually but inexorably shrinks until he eventually disappears and becomes one with the universe. Just such a fate is to be desired for the homunculus or "little person in the head" who, in the guise of "executive" or "control" processes, directs the rest of a model that *is* specified (see Dennett, 1978; Kimble & Perlmuter, 1970; Neisser, 1967). I argue here for one approach to shrinking the domain of the homunculus: To wit, much goal-setting activity may not be under "executive" control after all, but instead may be initiated by patterns of environmental features.

AUTOMATIC ACTIVATION OF MOTIVES AND GOALS

The evidence reviewed earlier indicated that responses to the environment—be they behaviors, decisions, or judgments—are goal-directed. Thus, if there does exist any control of responses by the social environment, it follows that it must be via an automatic pathway through the particular goal or intention representation that will produce that behavior. In other words, if one grants that responses to the environment require an intervening goal and intent, the only way it is possible for direct environmental control over responses to occur is for the environment itself to activate that goal or intent. This formulation supposes that goals and intents are represented in the mind in the same fashion as are social constructs, stereotypes, and schemas. The probability that such social representations become activated directly by environmental information is a joint function of their applicability to the information and their accessibility in memory (Higgins, 1989; Higgins & Bargh, 1987). Just as other chronically accessible social representations do, then, chronic goals and intents, and the procedures (Smith, 1984) and plans (Miller et al., 1960; Wilensky, 1983) associated with them, may become directly and automatically linked in memory with representations of environmental features to which they are frequently and consistently associated (see Bargh, 1984; Posner, 1978). As a consequence, these chronic goals and intents may become active automatically upon the activation of the relevant feature representations.

Therefore, the mechanism proposed here by which the social environment may control judgments, decisions, and behavior is the formation of direct and automatic mental links between representations of motives and goals in memory (and consequently the goals and plans associated with them) and the representations of the social situations in which those motives have been frequently pursued in the past. The result of this automatic associative link is that the motive–goal–plan structure becomes activated whenever the relevant triggering situational features are present in the environment. The activated goals and plans then presumably guide the social cognition and interaction of the individual, without the person's intention or awareness of the motive's guiding role.[1]

There are two fundamental components to the proposed process. First, there is an automatic, preconscious activation of situational motives and goals by the patterns of environmental stimuli to which they have become associated. Second, these activated goal structures guide social perception, judgment, and behavior in response to subsequent features of the situation, without the person knowing of this influence. In the next section, I marshal support for the existence and operation of these two component processes. Following that is a discussion of how this "auto-motive" model may account for observed phenomena in social perception and interaction.

Situations Directly Activate Intentions

There are three basic routes by which situational features may automatically activate motives and goals (see Figure 3.1). First, a motive or goal frequently and

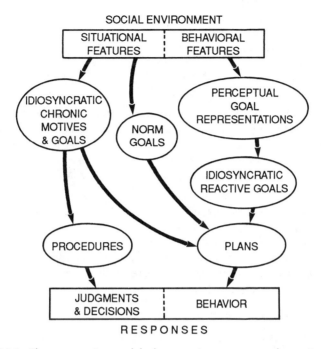

SOCIAL ENVIRONMENT

FIGURE 3.1 The auto-motive model of automatic responses to the environment.

consistently activated in that general type of situation (e.g., a self-presentational goal at a party) may be activated by the generic features of that situation (see Schank & Abelson, 1977). Second, the societal or cultural norms for appropriate behavior in that type of situation may be directly activated by situational features, and these norms in turn may directly activate intentions and goals to behave in normative ways. Finally, the third possible route to behavioral intention representations is not triggered by global features of the situational setting, but by the perceived goals and intents of the people one is interacting with within the situation. These *reactive* goals are thus linked with the goal representation relevant for the other's behavior, and not to the representation of the situation (i.e., a pan-situational automatic route to interaction goal setting).

The strength or diagnosticity of the environmental information needed to automatically activate a goal representation is likely to differ among the three routes shown in Figure 3.1. It is assumed that features associated with frequently encountered situations (e.g., work settings, dates, home, shopping) will most usually be unambiguous and clearly relevant to a single situational representation, so that the accessibility of the situational representation will not play much of a role in whether the features will activate the representation directly. There also should be minimal individual differences in whether the situational representation will be activated directly by the features of the setting, as the representations of such frequently encountered situations should be highly chronically accessible for most people. Because the pathway from the environmental features to the situational representation (for common situations) is assumed to be automatic for most people, the situational representation is not included as a variable in the diagram of Figure 3.1.

The interplay of applicability and accessibility is much more critical for the remaining pathway to automatic goal activation, that from behavioral features through perceptual goal categories to one's own response goals (see Figure 3.1). Behavioral information is likely to be potentially relevant to several different underlying goals for the actor, and so what one perceives the goal of the actor to be will be highly dependent on the relative accessibilities of the various goal representations applicable to the behavioral features. Once the behavior of the actor is categorized in terms of a goal, the activation of the "reactive goal" is assumed to follow directly and immediately. Thus, the goal that the perceiver adopts automatically in response to the perceived goal of the target will largely be a function of the relative accessibility of the various perceptual goal representations applicable to the behavior. Considerable individual differences in the accessibility of perceptual goal constructs are expected, as have been obtained in the case of trait construct accessibility (Higgins et al., 1982).

Automatic Activation of Situation-Specific Motives and Goals

Several theories of intentional behavior have, in fact, posited an automatization of behavior through the development of an automatic associative link between situational features and behavioral intentions. Lewin's (e.g., 1935) field theory considered behavior to be "steered' by the valences, or learned functional possibilities, of the objects in the environment by activating behavioral goals associated with them (pp. 49–50). Valences of environmental objects were described as deriving "from the fact that the object is a means to the satisfaction of a need" (p. 78). Thus environmental features had their effect as "field forces" on an individual's behavior in Lewin's theory by their continual activation of goal and need representations. Ach (1935; see also Heckhausen & Beckmann, 1990) referred to a process of *volutionale Objektion* by which intentions repeatedly carried out in a given situation come to be activated upon the mere perception of the situational features. It can be said that the early German will psychology embraced the principle of the close connection between the perception of an environmental object and the activation of motives and goals previously associated with it (see also Gollwitzer, Chapter 2, this volume).

Later treatments of intentional behavior in the information-processing tradition have been quite explicit in postulating a direct link between environmental features and behavioral goals. Miller et al. (1960), in proposing their cybernetic "test–operate–test–exit" (TOTE) model of plan-driven behavior, drew a parallel between innate animal instincts and habitual, overlearned plans:

> Ethologists have much to say about the stimulus control of behavior, about the recognition by the animal of the conditions appropriate for executing a Plan.

> Habits and skills [in humans] are Plans that were originally voluntary but that
> have become relatively inflexible, involuntary, automatic. . . . The description of
> the conditions under which various skilled components will be triggered, or
> released, is much the same in both cases. (pp. 75, 82)

Norman and Shallice (1986; see also Shallice, 1972) have developed a detailed model of the interplay between goal or action schemas, and the environmental conditions to which they respond. Their model provides an account of
how well-learned action sequences—for example, those involved in driving a
car—can be accomplished without the need for much attentional or intentional
involvement, once the initial "source" goal (e.g., to drive home from work) has
been set. Component "subschemas" of the larger action structure (e.g., those
involved in turning, stopping, and steering) operate autonomously in response to
relevant environmental input. Neisser (1967, p. 92) and Kahneman (1973, p. 70)
have also argued that well-learned actions can be controlled directly by preconscious mechanisms.

Hence, in Norman and Shallice's (1986) model, environmental stimuli can
control behavior, but only given that the overarching source goal has been
activated (e.g., the intention to drive home). The activation for the source goal
itself is said to come either from a "supervisory attentional system" (SAS;
Norman & Shallice, 1986, p. 6), clearly the source of intentional and conscious
control, or from "motivational factors" (p. 7) that are said to bias the SAS
"toward the long-term goals of the organism by activating source schemas" (p. 7).

Although there is no explicit link between environmental stimuli and the
activation of a source goal schema in their model, Norman and Shallice (1986)
claim that it accounts for a certain type of "action slip" or unintended behavior
called a "capture error" (Norman, 1981). Such unintended acts occur when the
environmental cues relevant for a habitual action "capture" an individual's behavior, even though his or her intention is currently otherwise this particular time
(e.g., when a bus driver pulls over at a bus stop while driving the family car).
These capture errors occur only when insufficient attention is being paid to the
intended action, allowing the behavioral goal to be usurped by a highly accessible,
automatically suggested behavioral response associated with those environmental
conditions. The fact that greater concentration on the unintended act would
prevent these usurpations is consistent with the evidence cited earlier that consciously held goals are able to override and inhibit automatically suggested, even
habitual, responses.

An important difference between these positions and the present argument
is that all of them are concerned with the production of specific actions without
the need for attentional monitoring. In contrast, I am suggesting that the higher-
order goals and motives themselves can be activated automatically and then guide
behavior. This is accomplished through the same mechanism advocated by Miller
et al. (1960) and Norman and Shallice (1986)—the automatic activation of a goal
intention—but I am arguing that higher-order, more abstract goals and plans

than those discussed by Miller et al. and Norman and Shallice (i.e., those involved in social interactions) can become automatically activated as well.

Wilensky (1983), in his information-processing approach to planning, has provided a detailed model of how the environment directly sets goals within the individual. In his model, the "planner's" control structure contains a "goal detector" that is sensitive to the presence of information relevant to a stored goal. This information may concern an internal state, such as hunger or fatigue, or an external state that is relevant to a strongly held value or a currently operating goal or plan. The component of the goal detector specifically in charge of monitoring the environment, termed the "noticer," contains descriptions of situations relevant to goals in its knowledge base. It is continually vigilant for the occurrence of these situations, and reports them as they occur to the goal detector. Wilensky (1983) explicitly calls for direct links between environmental features and the behavioral plans associated with them:

> If a standard plan is associated with a goal that occurs in a particular situation, it would be more efficient to associate this plan directly with that situation and select the plan at the same time the goal is detected. This would permit the planner to "short-circuit" part of the planning algorithm and suggest a plan immediately upon noticing a significant situation. (pp. 24-25)

In other words, the situational features will activate the goal; the person will "notice" this significant situation and be aware of the goal to be attained; and a plan will be automatically (given the activation of the goal) ready for use.

Reactive Goals

There is a second possible route from the social environment to goals, and that is as a consequence of the direct activation of goals in the course of understanding the behavior of others in the situation. There may be motives and goals automatically set in motion by the perceived goals of another, in reaction to the other's intentions and the potential consequences of those for oneself. Simon (1967) recognized the need for quick goal setting in response to others' behavior in social interactions:

> The most active part of the environment of man, and the part most consequential to him, consists of living organisms, particularly other men. Hence, a large part of the complexity of goals arises from the need, while accomplishing tasks, to attend to the responses of other human beings and to do this in real time. (p. 37)

There are two steps to the process proposed here by which such reactive goals are set: (1) the activation of the goal representation relevant to the other's behavior in the course of understanding it, and (2) the consequent automatic activation of one's own goal in reaction to the perceived intent of other.

Schank and Abelson (1977) developed a model of the comprehension and understanding of stories in terms of the scripts, plans, and goals of the actor. Thus, people were said to understand others' and their own behavior in terms of what usually occurs within given situations, and the intentions and goals for which the behavior is enacted.

Brewer and his colleagues (Brewer & Dupree, 1983; Lichtenstein & Brewer, 1980) have obtained evidence suggesting that people naturally understand social behavior in terms of the intentions and goals of the actor. When action descriptions were presented to subjects in an "in-order-to" relation to each other, they were recalled much better than the same actions not organized explicitly in terms of plans. Moreover, over time those actions not important to the overall plan were more likely to be forgotten, and what subjects retained best in memory was abstract information about the target person's overall intentions.

Trzebinski (e.g., 1989) has also stressed the importance of "action-oriented" representations in one's understanding of the social environment. In fact, he argues that "categories of actors, their goals, and conditions and means for the goal realizations" (p. 364) are the chief principles by which one's social knowledge is organized. Similarly, Read and Miller (1989) contend that "our knowledge of goals and the plans needed to achieve them is used both to plan our behavior and to understand and explain other's behavior" (p. 436). Like Schank and Abelson (1977) and Wilensky (1983), Trzebinski and Read and Miller consider goal and intention concepts to be the usual means by which an individual categorizes his or her social reality.

Thus, there seems to be general agreement that familiar situational features automatically activate representations of behavioral goals, plans, and intentions that have been repeatedly active within those situations, in the service of comprehending the situation and of suggesting behavioral responses to it. Of course, that goal and motive structures are used in understanding the behavior of others has been recognized by achievement motivation researchers for some time, as shown by their use of projective techniques in which the subject's stories about the motives of others in an ambiguous scenario are assumed to reflect the subject's own chronic motives (McClelland, Atkinson, Clark, & Lowell, 1953; Sorrentino & Higgins, 1986).

Once activated, the perceived goal of the other may then activate a reactive goal of one's own that has been frequently and consistently operative in response to such goals. For example, the perception that one is being ignored by another person in a small group may trigger a reactive goal of publicly ignoring that person in return (a "tit-for-tat" reactive goal). Importantly, this type of automatic goal activation cuts across situations, as it is linked to behavior patterns (perceived goals) of others that may occur in many different situations. Research by Buss, Gomes, Higgins, and Lauterbach (1987) has documented such reactive goals in response to the manipulative behavior of a relationship partner. Couples tended to respond in consistent ways to each other's manipulative tactics (e.g., charm, or the dreaded "silent treatment"); for example, the use of a given tactic tended to produce the same tactic in response, and nonreciprocal response tendencies (e.g., reacting to coercion with whining or a similar "regression" tactic) were also found. Importantly, stable individual differences in preferred tactics in responding to perceived manipulativeness were found to be associated with personality traits such as arrogance and agreeability. I return in a later section to the types of reactive goals that are likely candidates to be automatically activated by social-behavioral information.

Situational Norms ("Settings")

Situational features may also automatically activate behavioral goals that correspond to the appropriate or normative behaviors within the situation. The natural course of comprehending a situation involves the activation of a representation of the situation stored in memory, and this representation includes the normative features of that situation (see Cantor, Mischel, & Schwartz, 1982; Fiske & Taylor, 1984; Higgins & Bargh, 1987). Situational features activate situational frames (Goffman, 1974; Minsky, 1975) that provide the implicit knowledge necessary for guiding one's own situationally appropriate behavior.

The chronic, implicit application of situational knowledge is demonstrated by the greater attention immediately allocated to a feature or event that is inconsistent with that knowledge, whether it be a tricycle in the kitchen sink (Friedman, 1979), counternormative social behavior (Fiske, 1980), or unusual physical appearance (McArthur, 1981); it is also demonstrated by the different causal reasoning processes triggered as a function of the perceived normality of the conditions that produced the event (Hilton & Slugoski, 1986). That situational norms are well-learned behavioral guides that we apply effortlessly and automatically, both in understanding and in producing behavior, is noncontroversial (see Barker & Wright, 1955; Schank & Abelson, 1977).

Goals May Operate Outside of Awareness

A goal can play an essential role in the psychological situation
without being clearly present in consciousness.—*Lewin* (*1936, p. 19*)

The next part of the present argument is that motives and goals activated automatically by situational features will then operate outside of awareness to guide behavior. Consequently, although the person is certainly aware of his or her behavior and the specific plan of which it is a part (as well as other aspects of the situation), he or she is not aware of the guiding motive, so that control over the influence of the environment over behavior via the motive or goal is not possible (see Bargh, 1989, especially pp. 39–40; Dennett, 1984; Uleman, 1989). This postulate is consistent with recent research utilizing Lewin's concept of the psychological situation (Higgins, Bond, Klein, & Strauman, 1986; Strauman & Higgins, 1987); this research has demonstrated motivational and emotional consequences of the current situational context, the influence of which the person is unaware.

The auto-motive model hypothesizes that chronically accessible goals and motives become active automatically upon the mere presence of relevant environmental information, in the same fashion as chronically accessible social constructs have been found to become automatically activated (see Bargh, 1984; 1989; Higgins, 1989). Furthermore, just as a person is not aware of the influence of his or her accessible social constructs on the interpretation of relevant information input

(Bargh, 1984; Higgins & King, 1981), so too the person may not be aware of the subsequent influence of the activated goal on perception, judgment, and behavior.

One's lack of awareness of the influence of the activated goal or motive that causes the activation of the specific plan or action schema guiding the behavior or judgment process is analogous to a situation in which a light reflects off many surfaces prior to the one at which a person looks. The person is phenomenally aware of the light "coming from" that final surface, but not at all of the actual origin and course of that light source. The full moon is also an apparent origin of light, because the sun (the actual origin) is not observable in the sky. To put it another way, an individual is often aware of only the endpoint of a causal chain, not of all the necessary steps along the chain (see, e.g., James, 1890, pp. 116–117). Similarly, people appear to be unaware of the sources of their arousal or excitation levels (Zillman, 1978) or knowledge accessibility levels (Higgins, 1990), and phenomenally experience only the final outcome level.

In a related line of research, Marcel (1983) has argued that one is first conscious of a stimulus in terms of the most abstract representation automatically activated in perceiving it. For example, one is immediately aware of one's father *as* father; only then can strategic processing consider him in terms of other representations (male, about 60, Republican, chess player, etc.). The auto-motive model varies slightly from Marcel's (1983) position: Here an individual is said to be aware of the final representation activated in the automatic pathway from pattern detectors to action systems, which are not necessarily the most abstract representation relevant to the stimulus, as called for in Marcel's theory. The lack of awareness postulated here of the processing influence of an automatically activated goal or motive can also be considered as another instance of one's more general lack of awareness of the operation of a cognitive process, and general awareness of the output of those processes (see Ericsson & Simon, 1984; Nisbett & Wilson, 1977).

This state of awareness of action but not of the motivational basis for it is also consistent with the Norman and Shallice (1986) model, which is concerned principally with the roles of awareness and attention in the control of action. In that model, a person is aware of the overarching motive or intent behind a behavior plan if conscious control processes (i.e., those comprising the SAS) themselves activate the source schema for the goal-directed behavior. If the SAS is not the cause of the activation of the source schema, but instead the cause is the triggering environmental feature, then one "does experience the response as proceeding with 'an awareness of determination', even if it is not immediately preceded by any experience of intention to act" (p. 2).

Automatically Activated Goals and Plans

Miller et al. (1960, p. 82) likened habitual, automatically triggered plans to the instincts of lower animals, but instincts that "man wires in deliberately to serve his own purposes" (p. 89). They were referring to the development of complex, desired skills (see also Newell & Rosenbloom, 1981) that, at a higher level of inclusion, are nonetheless under intentional control. The automatically activated goals and motives proposed here are similar to Miller et al.'s (1960) "acquired instincts," except that they are hypothesized to be wired in *un*intentionally by the person.

From the case of well-learned, complex skills, such as the hackneyed example of driving a car (or the equally valid but more interesting case of *selling* one; Simon, 1976), it is clear that goal-directed behavior sequences can operate autonomously and without the need for conscious involvement (Norman & Shallice, 1986): Until one learns to drive (or sell) cars well, the separate component operations all require conscious control individually. This function of frequent experience to eventually reduce the attentional demands of a given process to (near) zero has long been known as the "law of habit" (e.g., Boring, 1950, p. 310; James, 1890, pp. 104–127). A complex behavioral sequence formerly thought of by the individual as a combination of several different actions becomes, with sufficient experience, subjectively experienced as a whole—and no longer as an activity itself (e.g., driving the car), but in terms of the intent or purpose involved (e.g., going to work; Wegner & Vallacher, 1986). So it is certainly the case that a frequently enacted behavioral plan becomes capable of operating autonomously and outside of awareness (Miller et al., 1960).

Can Goals and Intentions Operate Outside of Awareness?

These examples of behavior without conscious guidance nonetheless require an overarching intention or goal that the behavior be produced. In the case of the automatized subgoals involved in driving, their operation in controlling perceptual–motor activity requires the conscious higher-order intent of "going to work" or "visiting Aunt Martha." Once that intentional goal has been set and committed to (see Gollwitzer, Chapter 2, this volume), the process can run off automatically (i.e., intended goal-dependent automaticity; Bargh, 1989). But is there any evidence suggesting that the instigating intentions or goals *themselves* may operate outside of awareness?

Libet (1985) has argued provocatively from electroencephalographic (EEG) evidence that the readiness potential associated with a spontaneous, voluntary motor movement *precedes* the conscious awareness of the intention to move. His data were consistent in showing that the readiness potential shifted about a half-second *before* the subject's initial awareness of wanting to move. Libet (1985) concluded that the "cerebral initiation of a spontaneous voluntary act begins unconsciously" (p. 529). This conclusion echoes William James's (1890, p. 109) analysis of the origin of voluntary acts: that the *first* occurrence of each and every action must be impulsive or reflexive, and only after it has occurred for the first time for the individual can it then be brought under voluntary control. Interestingly, Libet (1985) also obtained evidence that the ultimate decision to act could be (consciously) controlled prior to the actual movement (see also Logan & Cowan, 1984), so that, in summary, "the role of conscious will would be not to initiate a specific voluntary act but rather to select and control volitional outcome" (Libet, 1985, p. 529).

A second (and less controversial) line of support involves the well-known "tip-of-the-tongue" phenomenon (Brown & McNeill, 1986; Norman & Bobrow, 1976; Yaniv & Meyer, 1987). One tries hard to remember something, feels as though the information is there somewhere in memory, and eventually gives up and moves on to other purposes. Later, in the middle of an unrelated activity, the sought-for information "pops" into awareness. The unfulfilled goal has continued to operate outside of awareness.

This tendency of unsatisfied goals to continue operating in the quest for their desired end state, even when the goal is no longer the current conscious purpose, has been noted by many theorists and incorporated into their models (see Anderson, 1983, p. 156; Klinger, 1975; Lewin, 1928; Mandler, 1975; Martin & Tesser, 1989; Norman & Shallice, 1986; Shallice, 1972). Just as with the development of skill and habit, what appears to be necessary for the "postconscious" operation of a goal (see Bargh, 1989) is extended frequent or recent residence in consciousness, both of which work to increase the goal's state of activation to a level sufficient for operation without attentional support (Higgins, 1989; Higgins, Bargh, & Lombardi, 1985). Examples of the frequency factor are a mother's sensitivity to the sounds of her infant in another room (Klinger, 1975) and the appearance of solutions to difficult problems in dreams and at moments when one is not thinking about the problem (see Ghiselin, 1952, for many anecdotes from the memoirs of famous creative figures in history). The tip-of-the-tongue phenomenon is an example of the recency factor, as is the reappearance in awareness of the original thread of a conversation after an interesting digression. Moreover, thoughts related to unresolved difficulties (e.g., Martin & Tesser, 1989; Tait & Silver, 1989) or "current concerns" (Klinger, 1975) tend to appear in consciousness unbidden, in the same way as does stored knowledge that was on the tip of one's tongue.

In this tendency to remain active for long periods of time outside of awareness, motive and goal representations appear to be fundamentally different from other memory nodes and cognitive structures, which rapidly decay once activated (Anderson, 1983; Kuhl, 1986). In Anderson's (1983, pp. 156–170) ACT* associative network model of memory, for example, goal nodes are considered to be constant and strong sources of spreading activation while active, and not to stop being sources until deliberately changed. Kuhl (1986) has argued cogently that this difference in persistence has consequences for other basic operational differences between cognitive and motivational mental processes—for example, in the buildup of a cumulative, increasingly strong motivational tendency across situations in which the goal or motive has not been expressed (Kuhl & Blankenship, 1979). The point to be stressed here is that there is ample support from motivational as well as cognitive theory and research for the proposition that motives and goals are capable of operating outside of awareness. The dynamic properties (persistence, cumulation) just described are also relevant for the question of where goals come from when *not* triggered by environmental stimuli; this question is discussed later.

Automatically Activated Goals Guide Thought and Behavior

Lewin (1935) opposed purely associative, stimulus–response approaches to behavior on the grounds that associative connections between the representation of the stimulus and the effector units controlling behavior were not sufficient to generate behavior:

> The experimental investigation of habits (association) has shown that the couplings created by habit are never, as such, the motor of a psychical event.. . . Rather, in order that the bound or coupled complex move . . . energy capable of doing work must be set free. (pp. 44–45)

Thus, what was needed over and above associative connections was the *energy* to drive the action system. In the auto-motive model, the motive or intention is hypothesized to correspond to a memory representation that is a persistent and strong *source* of activation (as in Anderson's [1983] ACT* model), resulting in perseveration effects and activation durations longer than those for nongoal memory nodes (see also Kuhl, 1986).

Motives and intentions have associated with them stored plans and response production systems that guide and produce actual judgment and behavior (Miller et al., 1960; Norman & Shallice, 1986; Schank & Abelson, 1977; Wilensky, 1983). For frequently used behavioral plans, these action systems become compiled or proceduralized (see Smith, 1984), such that once the overarching goal or implemental intention representation is activated, the thought process or behavioral response is produced. Buss et al. (1987), for example, have found specific manipulation tactics to be used consistently with specific interaction goals; when a subject's goal was to get the relationship partner to do something, the charm tactic was employed, and when the goal was to get the partner to *stop* doing something, coercion or the silent treatment was more frequently used.

Gollwitzer (Chapter 2, this volume; see also Heckhausen, 1987) presents a detailed model of the steps involved from having the goal of achieving a certain outcome, to producing a specific behavior in the service of that goal. His work has shown that manipulations designed to induce subjects to form a specific behavioral ("implemental") intention resulted in considerably higher rates of subsequently engaging in that behavior, even if the subjects had no previous wish or need to perform that behavior.

Goals and Plans Operate on Current Environmental Input

A final point is that once the compiled plan is set into motion by the activated motive–intention representation, it operates interactively with the environment (Norman & Shallice, 1986; Schank & Abelson, 1977). That is, once set in motion, judgment processes or interactive behaviors are not conducted without any regard to feedback or cues from the environment. Rather, the plan is conceptualized as a cybernetic system that sensitizes the individual to expected occurrences in the environment (e.g., likely reaction to his or her own behavior), preconsciously interprets the meaning of those environmental events, and readies appropriate responses so long as the feedback fits the goal–plan structure for that situation. Such feedback systems have long been a staple of proposed planning and action system mechanisms (Carver & Scheier, 1981; Miller et al., 1960; Norman & Shallice, 1986; Schank & Abelson, 1977; Wilensky, 1983).

Thus far, I have proposed four steps involved in the preconscious activation of motives and intents by situational features: (1) that patterns of environmental features automatically activate mental representations of those motives and goals chronically associated with them; (2) that these motives and goals are not available to awareness, even though active (just as preconsciously activated chronically accessible constructs are not available to awareness); (3) that the activation of these motives and goals activates in turn their corresponding specific behavioral plans and implemental intentions; (4) and that these plans and intentions then interact with environmental information to be expressed in behavior, given the appropriate opportunity (i.e., relevant environmental information; Gollwitzer, Chapter 2, this volume; Norman & Shallice, 1986). These postulates have previously been proposed singly and in slightly different versions in many motivational and cognitive models, and are supported by a considerable array of evidence.

CHRONICALLY ACCESSIBLE MOTIVES AND SOCIAL INTERACTION GOALS

Not all goals and motives a person may have are capable of direct environmental activation. In the same way that a person's chronically accessible trait constructs are preconsciously activated by relevant environmental input, whereas his or her inaccessible constructs are not (Bargh & Pratto, 1986; Bargh & Thein, 1985), so too only an individual's chronically accessible goals and motives should be capable of being preconsciously activated.

The notion that individuals possess chronic goals that they pursue in social interactions is not new, and recently these chronic goals have been proposed to be a major source of personality differences (e.g., Cantor & Kihlstrom, 1987; Emmons, 1989; Higgins, 1990; Miller & Read, 1987). What the auto-motive concept adds to this idea is that these chronic goals behave like any other chronic social concept and become directly activated by the environment (Bargh, 1984), through the activation of the environmental representations to which they are linked.

This proposal also has implications for how chronic motivations may *develop*. As a consequence of the motive's or goal's being paired repeatedly with certain social situations, the representation of that situation and that of the motive or goal become ever more strongly linked in memory (see Bargh, 1984; Fazio, 1986; Higgins, 1987). The increasing accessibility, or ease of activation, that results from the frequent associative pairing (Higgins & King, 1981) should make that particular goal increasingly likely to become activated relative to other potentially relevant goals for that situation, just as an accessible category is more likely to capture information relevant to several categories (Bruner, 1957). Just as accessible attitudes have been argued to be more likely to influence behavior than less accessible attitudes (Fazio, 1986), so too accessible motives and goals should be more likely to influence behavior. In this cyclic, snowballing manner, accessible motives may become even more accessible (given continued exposure to the relevant environmental features), until the link between them and the situational features is automated (Bargh, 1984).

Chronic Motivations

What kinds of social motives would be likely to become automated in this way? The first likely candidates are, of course, the chronic motivations and orientations postulated to drive cognition and behavior across a variety of situations, such as need for achievement (Atkinson & Feather, 1966), authoritarianism (Adorno, Frenkel-Brunswik, Levinson, & Sanford, 1950), chronic self-consciousness (Fenigstein, Scheier, & Buss, 1975), need for structure and fear of invalidity (Kruglanski & Freund, 1983), need for cognition (Cacioppo & Petty, 1982), and control motivation (Pittman & D'Agostino, 1985). In addition, Cantor and Langston (1989, p. 132) have suggested that some strategies (not all of them adaptive) that individuals chronically employ in accomplishing important "life tasks" are conducted without awareness or intention (e.g., self-handicapping, defensive pessimism). Emmons (1989) has proposed that people continually strive toward three basic needs—safety and control, social belongingness, and self-esteem and competence—and that an individual possesses implicit, preconsciously activated beliefs about how to satisfy these needs (e.g., "To be competent, I must become independent from my parents").

Chronic Goals

There has been surprisingly little research to date on the role of chronically accessible or situationally activated social goals in perception and behavior (Pervin, 1989; for an exception involving both chronic and situational goals, see Higgins & McCann, 1984). Srull and Wyer (1986), in their review of research into the roles of both chronic and temporary goals in social information processing, devoted the vast majority of the review to the influence of temporary goals. The only direct support presented for the hypothesis that chronically held goals are preconsciously activated (as opposed to studies demonstrating preconscious processing of emotional material; see Kuhl, 1986, on the distinction) came from the classic studies by Bruner (1951) and Postman, Bruner, and McGinnies (1948). Both studies showed powerful effects of the subject's predetermined value orientations on perception; the Postman et al. (1948) study demonstrated greater sensitivity by subjects to stimuli congruent with their important values, in much the same way that one is more sensitive to the presence of stimuli relevant to one's chronically accessible social constructs (Bargh & Pratto, 1986).

It would seem to be a highly promising bridge between motivation and cognition to develop the notion of chronically accessible social interaction goals more completely. Although temporary goal states have received by far the most research attention to date, it is important for the study of personality in particular to focus on stable, enduring determinants of behavior (Emmons, 1989). Similarly, the well-documented importance of temporary processing goals on the outcome of social memory and judgment (Srull & Wyer, 1986) underscores the importance of studying chronic links between situations and those processing goals. Differences in the accessibilities of different goals should result in differences in the likelihood of their activation and application in relevant situations, and so one obvious avenue of research would be to extend the study of chronically accessible social trait constructs (see Bargh, 1989, and Higgins, 1989, for reviews) to the case of cognitive and behavioral goals. Paradigms utilized in that research could be applied to study what goals and motives are chronically accessible to an individual with specific social situations (e.g., Bargh & Pratto, 1986; Higgins et al., 1982; Sorrentino & Higgins, 1986).

A fruitful starting point for this research would be the existing literature on social interaction goals (see review by McCann & Higgins, 1988). There is certainly no shortage of ideas concerning the variety of goals one can have in a social situation. As Schank and Abelson (1977) noted, many goal taxonomies have been proposed in the past (e.g., Allport, Vernon, & Lindzey, 1951; Murray, 1938; for more contemporary proposals see Emmons, 1989; Read & Miller, 1989), and "if one were to set out to list all the different kinds of things that could be desired, there would be no end to it" (Schank & Abelson, 1977, p. 112). Still, as the question of automatic social goal activation is an empirical one, consideration of the types of goals and motives hypothesized to exist in these models and theories is a useful beginning.

Jones and Thibaut (1958) listed many kinds of possible interaction goals and described how they would result in attention to and use of different informational features within that situation. Entirely different "inferential sets" were hypothesized to become activated by these different interaction goals. For example, a goal of "determining what the other person [is] like" should focus the perceiver on the target's personality as well as attributional processing of the causes behind the target's behavior; a goal of applying social control should lead to a "situation-matching" set in which situational norms are the important processing and evaluation structures (p.177). The type of goals that guide "most of our interactions, and the social inference activities deriving from them" (p. 164) were said to be "value-expressive" sets, in which the actor attempts to gratify a personal need. Four main types of value-expressive goals were hypothesized; these are presented in Table 3.1.

Jones and Thibaut (1958) then carried their analysis a step further, and speculated on the aspects of the other's personality to which the goal-driven actor would be the most sensitive. These are given alongside the four value-expressive goal types in Table 3.1. What is important about the Jones and Thibaut analysis for present purposes is the conceptual linkage of subsystems of social trait constructs as activated by various interaction goals—the notion that one's set of accessible trait constructs can be a function of one's goal within the interaction;

TABLE 3.1   Jones and Thibaut's (1958) Linkages between Value-Expressive Social Interaction Goals and Perceptual Trait Construct Sensitivities

Goal	Traits
I. Gaining information about the shared environment	Reliability, candor, objectivity, expertise
II. Gaining support and validation for one's own beliefs and attitudes from the other	Attitude positions on relevant, important issues
III. Gaining social approval from the other	Friendliness, acceptance, tolerance, supportiveness
IV. Accomplishing some external goal through the interaction	Cooperativeness, dependability, hard work

different sets for different goals, leading potentially to quite different evaluations of the target (e.g., the case of an unfriendly expert; see also Carlston, 1980).[2] In positing goal specificity in construct accessibility, Jones and Thibaut (1958) anticipated the concept of goal-dependent automaticity (Bargh, 1989; Bargh & Tota, 1988): Depending on the individual's processing goal, different sets of social constructs become automatically activated.

Predicting Goals from Situational Features

Recent work has described a great variety of information-processing and social-interactive goals and motives (e.g., Cantor & Kihlstrom, 1987; Emmons, 1989; Read & Miller, 1989; Srull & Wyer, 1986): information acquisition, impression formation, self-presentation and impression management, ingratiation, entertainment, comprehension, pleasing others, competing, gaining power. The goals so identified vary in their level of abstraction–concreteness (Emmons, 1989; Gollwitzer, Chapter 2, this volume; Martin & Tesser, 1989; Miller et al., 1960; Schank & Abelson, 1977; Wilensky, 1983), with some goals highly situation-specific (e.g., "having to be right" in an argument or a friendly discussion, despite the cost to other relationship goals) and others related to deeply held values more likely to operate across situations (e.g., a concern with equity of treatment in any social exchange situation; see Tyler, 1987).

Thus, an individual's chronically accessible goals may be dependent for their covert activation and operation on environmental features specific to a particular social situation or on features characteristic of a variety of social situations. The influence on behavior will be more pervasive and cross-situational if that goal develops an automatic link to the (perceived) repeatedly recurring features.

It should be possible to test for links between specific social situations and specific motives and goals by first conceptualizing both the situation and the goal in terms of the same underlying variables of feature representations, social constructs, and their relative accessibilities in memory (Bargh, Lombardi, &

Higgins, 1988; Higgins, 1990). Next, the nature of the subject's situational representations should be assessed (e.g., Cantor, 1982; Cantor et al., 1982). Finally, the relation of these situational features to identifiable chronic motivational states and possible situational goals should be examined—for example, by using the questionnaire method of Buss et al. (1987) to inquire into the interactional patterns and individual characteristics of partners in established work, social, or intimate relationships. The automaticity of the associations between situational features and goals could then be assessed with any of the variety of standard methods for assessing associative links in memory and their strength and automaticity (e.g., priming, memory load, speeded response; see Bargh, 1988, 1989). For example, after a subject's chronic goal within a situation has been identified, it might be possible to activate that goal by presenting the triggering features outside of the subject's awareness (Bargh & Pietromonaco, 1982; Neuberg, 1988), or when the subject's attentional capacity is fully loaded (Bargh & Thein, 1985), and then to test for goal-related behavior in a goal-relevant setting.

Reactive Goals in Social Interaction

To pursue this logic a bit further, one might ask *which* features will be the most likely to recur repeatedly across many different situations. Of course, in a shared culture, there are norms of behavior that may apply in most social settings; as already discussed, these normative guidelines will serve both as implicit expectancies for others' behavior and as scripts for one's own (Higgins, 1990; Schank & Abelson, 1977; Wilensky, 1983). Moreover, a person's role and status in a situation induce both constraints on his or her behavior and also appropriate goals to pursue within the situation (e.g., subordinates should be deferential to their superordinates; see Schank & Abelson, 1977, pp. 132-138). But what about individual variability around these cultural and sociostructural main effects?

One's set of chronically accessible social constructs is presumed to reflect regularities in features of social behavior that one idiosyncratically encounters across situations (Bargh, 1984; Higgins & King, 1981). That is, chronic constructs develop to represent those patterns of behavior one has frequently and consistently perceived in one's environment. Such constructs have been found to become automatically activated in the presence of relevant stimuli even when attention is in short supply or focused elsewhere (Bargh & Pietromonaco, 1982; Bargh & Thein, 1985), and their activation is uncontrollable, even when it conflicts with the current processing goal (Bargh & Pratto, 1986). Thus the activation of chronically accessible constructs is entirely preconscious and not dependent on the particular processing goal in place.

In other words, the types of social behavior one perceives across many different social situations are likely to be those corresponding to one's chronic constructs; this information is perceived automatically, no matter what. And because an individual acts on a perceived and not an objective world (e.g., Kelly, 1955; Lewin, 1935), the individual will be *reacting* to these particular types of behavior frequently and across situations. Consistent with this reasoning, Fiske,

Neuberg, Beattie, and Milberg (1987) showed that social perceivers' evaluations and impressions of a target person were dependent on the fit between the target's characteristics and the content of the perceivers' social categories (e.g., for occupations): When the feature–category fit was good (as compared to when it was not), subjects' evaluations and impressions were more of a function of the category features and less of the target's individuating attributes. That is, subjects' reactions to the target person were triggered in the high-fit case by the target's category-relevant features, and not by other relevant information.

Given the frequency with which an individual is presumed to perceive these types of social behavior, it would make functional sense for him or her to possess plans for responding to them. It would be inefficient and antagonistic to the usual need for quick action (Rothbart, 1981) to have to come up repeatedly with a behavioral plan in response to recurring features of the environment. These reactive plans are especially needed and therefore likely to exist in connection with negatively evaluated forms of behavior—for example, when the other's behavior threatens a valued state, possession, or goal of one's own. "Reactance" behavior (Brehm, 1966) can be seen as an example of this; the individual quickly reacts against a perceived loss of freedom. The notion of the "control motive," as developed by Pittman and his colleagues (e.g., Pittman & D'Agostino, 1985; Pittman & Pittman, 1980), is another good example: Unexpected events within situations are hypothesized to trigger a motive to regain (predictive) control through increased cognitive analysis of the situation. One may also have reactive goals triggered by perceived manipulativeness on the part of another, in response to nontrivial favors (Langer, Blank, & Chanowitz, 1978), perceived competitiveness or hostility, and so on. All of these goals would fall under Schank and Abelson's (1977) heading of "preservation goals," designed to protect valued aspects of the status quo; to the extent that reactive goals seek specifically to thwart the goals of the other person, they constitute what Schank and Abelson (1977) referred to as "anti-plans" (pp. 115–116).

Not all reactive goals are anti-plans, just as not all chronically accessible constructs are negatively valenced (see norms in Higgins et al., 1982). One may be chronically sensitive to kindness or honesty, and react (for example) with a stored goal and plan of attempting to establish a friendship—or, perhaps less ambitiously, to have a pleasant social encounter. (Our figmentary "one" need not always be such a saint, however; one may instead react to another's kindness or cooperation with a selfish, greedy, or competitive "taking advantage" plan.)

An empirical illustration of possibly automated reactive goals is provided in a study by Neuberg (1988). In the experimental situation, subjects were subliminally primed with competition-related or neutral words, and then played a Prisoner's Dilemma game on a computer with a (fictitious) partner. Subjects were classified as to whether they had competitive or cooperative behavioral predispositions, based on their initial move in the game, which was made prior to their partner's. The effect of priming on subjects' behavior in the Prisoner's Dilemma game (in which one can respond to one's partner's first move in either a competitive or a cooperative manner) depended on their behavioral predisposition: For the dispositionally competitive but not the dispositionally cooperative subjects, the competitive primes increased the incidence of competitive behavior in reaction to the partner's first move; moreover, competitive subjects primed with competition-related stimuli behaved more competitively than did the competition-primed cooperative subjects. To put these results in terms of the present discussion, the environmental information (competition primes) activated reactive interactional goals (to behave competitively) only for subjects who chronically had such goals (the dispositionally competitive subjects).

Neuberg's (1988) findings illustrate how accessible social constructs may be activated outside of awareness by relevant environmental information and a reactive goal set in place by this automatically made interpretation. Reactive goals tied to an individual's chronically accessible constructs would appear to be a promising avenue in the search for those individual differences in goals and resultant behavior that are stable and consistent across situations.

Automatic versus Conscious Sources of Situational Goals

Which Motives and Goals Will Become Automated?

The varieties of social interaction goals and motives postulated by Jones and Thibaut (1958), Read and Miller (1989), and others can be sorted as to which of two possible ways they are likely to become activated to direct decisions and behavior: either automatically by the presence of relevant environmental features, or deliberately and consciously in the course of a controlled planning process. In general, from the work already reviewed here, it would seem that the more abstract and less concrete the goal—that is, the broader the array of behaviors that will satisfy it—the less likely it will be for that goal to become capable of direct activation by the environment. This is because the "longer" a cognitive pathway is (i.e., the more links it contains), the less likely it is to become automated; the more abstract a representation, the greater the number of analytic steps both between it and the relevant environmental feature detectors on the one hand, and the action effector units on the other (see Bargh, 1984).

A second and related point is that the broader the range of situations relevant to a motive or goal, the more likely it will be that other goals and motives will be active instead in those situations at other times. Because the development of automatic pathways requires a high degree of consistency of pathway activation between the two representations in question, as well as sufficient frequency of activation (Posner, 1978; Schneider & Fisk, 1982; Schneider & Shiffrin, 1977), there is a greater likelihood of inconsistency or unreliability in the association between any one of those situations and that particular motive or goal. For example, it may be that Jack always has an impression management goal (e.g., Schlenker, 1980) operative when being introduced to someone for the first time. Thus we would expect that an automatic pathway would develop between the particular features of social introduction situations and the goal of impression management, and perhaps also to particular action plans within that goal (e.g., to make witty remarks). It is also likely that Jack has the goal of impression management within many other social situations, such as when interacting with colleagues at work or being at home with his family, but that other goals can also exist within those situations (e.g., getting the job done at work, exerting some-times unpopular authority over his children). So it is unlikely (and it makes no functional sense) for the impression management goal to be *automatically* acti-vated in response to situational features unless those features have reliably resulted in that goal—and no other goal—in the past. In Jack's case, it may be that impression management is cued by two reliable features of situations: the pres-ence of others with whom he is not yet acquainted, and the presence of others who are of higher status than himself. For Jill, on the other hand, it may be that the only reliable feature cue is the presence of others whom she respects.

In the case of chronic motivations, however, such as need for achievement (Atkinson & Feather, 1966), or chronic values, such as truth (Allport et al., 1951) or justice (Tyler, 1987), it may be that automatic connections exist because such a wide variety of situations can directly activate the motive or goal. My point here is simply that for any given individual, there will be a greater number of automatic pathways between environmental features and specific, behavioral goals than between environmental features and abstract motives and values; at the same time, however, such direct links certainly may exist at all levels of abstraction.

Proactive ("Conscious") Goals

Our little person in the head, while perhaps somewhat diminished if the present analysis is valid, is hardly in danger of extinction just yet. Relatively novel situations abound in which some flexible and quick thinking and planning are needed (Schank & Abelson, 1977, p. 97). Moreover, people's goals are not always reactive to the situation, but may instead be *proactive* attempts to achieve a desired outcome. We can seek out and enter situations in the service of these proactive goals (Miller et al., 1960, p. 90). Goals and plans are very frequently deliberate, conscious constructions for the purpose of satisfying a consciously known value or need; these "value-expressive" goals were argued by Jones and Thibaut (1958) to be the most frequent type a person has in social interactions (see also Emmons, 1989, p. 119; Weiner, 1986). Other sources of deliberate goal setting are those required for the pursuit of "life tasks" (Cantor & Kihlstrom, 1987) and for coping with an unresolved problem (e.g., Martin & Tesser, 1989).

But we *can* shrink the little person even further than the auto-motive concept accomplishes by itself. Motives and goals that have been persistently pursued, but not satisfied, tend to persevere as tendencies outside of awareness (e.g., Kuhl, 1986; Lewin, 1935, p. 60; Shallice, 1972; Wilensky, 1983); they enter into consciousness when there is no current focal goal, or there is one but not that much effort is being expended on it (Atkinson & Birch, 1970; Martin & Tesser, 1989; Norman & Shallice, 1986). That is, these motives and goals capture awareness and the current goal state, depending on their strength and the strength of the current goal. Strengths of goals are functions both of the amount of tendency that has accumulated over time (Atkinson & Birch, 1970; Kuhl, 1986) and of the priority or precedence relations among the goals (Schank & Abelson,

1977; Wilensky, 1983). For example, biological needs generally take precedence over achievement-related goals, which in turn dominate entertainment goals, but the satisfaction of a given goal reduces its strength so that lower-priority goals may take command (see the lucid discussion of major goal types and their precedence relations in Schank & Abelson, 1977, pp. 111-119). Martin and Tesser (1989) hypothesize that this tendency of unsatisfied goal states to capture the stream of consciousness at relatively unguarded moments is the cause of uncontrollable ruminations about negative life events (see also Klinger, 1975; Tait & Silver, 1989).

Therefore, direct control over the setting of the current goal, with all of its ramifications for behavior and the outcome of cognitive processing, can be due either to frequently appearing situational features, or to predictable qualities of goal strengths and their interactions (see Atkinson & Birch, 1970; Kuhl & Atkinson, 1984; Schank & Abelson, 1977; Wilensky, 1983).

CONCLUSIONS: "BUT IS IT *INTENTIONAL*?"

The question of the degree of control one has over one's thought and behavior in social interactions has been stimulating research for the past decade. Direct environmental control (i.e., preconscious effects) has been demonstrated to occur principally for social perception, and in two main forms: interpretation/categorization of social information (including stereotype activation) and evaluation of it (see Bargh, 1989, pp. 11-14, for a review). There is a firm basis for the conclusion that social judgment and behavior can be influenced by these automatic perceptual processes; however, other evidence suggests that ultimate control over judgment and behavior is invested in the current intention and goal (see Fiske, 1989; Logan & Cowan, 1984). Preconscious influences over social perception have been likened to the "power behind the throne" of intentionally made decisions; automatically made interpretations and evaluations may heavily influence the decision, but the throne of intent has the ultimate say (Bargh, 1989, pp. 38-40).

But there is an implicit assumption behind this contrast between preconscious and automatic processes on the one hand, and goal-directed processes on the other; this is that goals are always placed there by deliberate and controlled means. However, why cannot the goal *itself* be preconsciously and directly activated by environmental features? Motives, goals, and plans are all mental representations; there is no theoretical reason why the mechanisms of automatic pathway development (Newell & Rosenbloom, 1981; Posner, 1978) should not apply to them as well as to any other representation. It has been the purpose of this chapter to marshal the evidential as well as the theoretical support for the hypothesis that features of the social environment may automatically activate those goal representations frequently and consistently paired with them, and that these goals may then operate without the individual's awareness of their operation.

The question of the extent to which a person is in control in social interactions is one for which an actuarial answer, in terms of the proportion of social interactions or of the number of waking hours during which the person is actively and consciously guiding thought and behavior, may or may not be possible (Bargh, 1984; Fiske, 1989). The present approach—to hypothesize automatic pathways linking representations of the environment to motive and goal representations— takes a different tack. This hypothesis is certainly testable, and it transforms the issues of whether the activation of influential goals is under a person's direct and deliberate control or is under the direct control of the environment, and how typical these two sources of goal activation are in social interaction settings, into empirical ones. If there turns out to be no support for direct environmental activation, this would suggest that goals are largely generated internally in the service of higher-order needs, motives, and values. Either way, research on the possible existence of such "auto-motives" would bear directly on the important question that has opened this chapter.

Automaticity and Free Will

As I write, it is the 200th anniversary of the storming of the Bastille and the start of the French Revolution. Naturally, what come to mind (other than cake) are the concepts of freedom and liberty, and in the present context the concept of free will. If a goal is activated unintentionally and then guides behavior, is the resultant behavior intentional or unintentional? Speaking of cake, can we have our automaticity and our free will too?

The behavior that occurs as a consequence of an automatically activated goal is certainly *purposive* as it is directed toward a goal, though the goal itself is in this case not accessible to the individual. Libet (1985) has argued that to be goal-directed and to be intentional are two different things. Pervin (1989, p. 476) has pointed out that Piaget (1952) had earlier made a similar distinction. Children were said to be capable of goal-directed behavior in response to the immediate environment before they develop the capacity for intentional behavior, which involves the creation of goals in the absence of goal-relevant external events. This distinction fits the present arguments quite well; the label of "intentional" should be reserved for the case in which the guiding goal itself is intentionally activated (see also Norman & Shallice, 1986; Uleman, 1989).

Control as Achieving Desired Change

To argue that automatic goal activation results in unintended thought and behavior may raise in many readers' minds the specter of determinism—of human beings as ant-like automata controlled by the environment. As Dennett (1984) shows, the problem we have with the concept of determinism is largely due to a confusion of control with causation. "Control" typically refers to the ability of agent A to drive agent B into a state that A *wants* B to be in (Dennett, 1984, p. 52). Similarly, Uleman (1989) argues that the concept of control "requires a standard or goal in terms of which something is regulated or guided . . . and a controlling process operates to reduce the discrepancy" (p. 430), meaning that the controlling agent is pursuing a goal of its own. To say that the environment does the controlling is therefore disturbing to us because "it hints subliminally at the dark idea that the environment *wants* us to do this and that, and acting on the desire, *makes* us do what it wants" (Dennett, 1984, p. 57; emphasis in original). Dennett (1984, p. 59; emphasis in original) concludes that the environment does not "control" us because "the environment is not designed to *tell* us what to do; we are designed to *figure out* from the indifferent environment what to do."

But is the *social* environment "indifferent" to what we do? The idea of the environment's having "desires" and "wishes" for our behavior does not sound as silly when we are discussing a social environment filled with people and institutions that *do* have desires and wants, that *are* constantly attempting to get us to behave in ways advantageous to them (and maybe or maybe not advantageous to us as well).

Yet, for direct environmental control over one's decisions and behavior to occur, the environmental agent (e.g., a person, an advertisement) must intend to activate one's chronically accessible motives and goals; this means that the agent *must know what those are.* Knowledge is power, and "foreknowledge is what permits control" (Dennett, 1984, p. 54). And in some cases perhaps this foreknowledge does exist—most likely in intimate (or parent–child) relationships, when, for example, one partner knows that making the other feel guilty results in the desired behavior (e.g., acquiescence). Cases in which the environmental agent does not know the individual's chronic goals but makes a good guess based on general cultural tendencies include U.S. state lottery advertisements that appeal directly to greed as a motivation that will override any rational estimation of probable return on the bet amount, and the actions of skilled salespeople who know well the motivating effect on public behavioral commitment, such as in the "foot-in-the-door" technique (Freedman & Fraser, 1966). And as Dennett (1984) has argued in one of the quotes opening this chapter, one can control someone else if one can control the causes of the other's behavior.

For the most part, however, we are aware in such situations that an attempt to manipulate or persuade us is being or probably will be made; we can be on our guard when in the automobile showroom and skeptical when encountering ads. It is only when we are unaware of the activation of a motive or goal that we cannot counter its influence (Bargh, 1989); in obvious persuasion situations, we may not *know* that certain of our motives have been activated, but we can assume they have been and can take this into account when making decisions. Dennett (1984) notes that attempts by others to control us

> are precisely the sort of activities we human beings dislike, resent, and seek to avoid. We don't like being controlled by others in this sort of way, so apparently we do feel that we are controlled (to some extent) by such activities. (p. 57)

In other words, people know they can be controlled without being aware of how; this is known as "being manipulated."

It is the cases such as intimate relationships in which direct control by the environment is likeliest, because here the agent *has* the particular knowledge (from experience) of the chronic motivations of the partner, and also the power of the activated motive (e.g., to avoid guilt feelings) or goal (e.g., to stay in the relationship—a power device more likely to be employed by men against women than vice versa; see Hatfield, Traupmann, Sprecher, Utne, & Hay, 1984). These cases of intended activation of one's chronic motivations and goals by an environmental agent, with foreknowledge of what those chronic goals are, are probably limited to the case of intimate relationships, and as such would constitute an important feature distinguishing intimate from other social-interactive behavior (see, e.g., Derlega, 1984; Kelley et al., 1983).

Aside from these cases of extensive foreknowledge, however, the social environment does not know what one's chronic goals are, and so does not "wish" to activate them. Hence, although the environmental features may *cause* the goal-directed behavior, they do not generally *control* it in the sense of intended, desired causation. And if the frightening part of the concept of environmental control over one's behavior lies in the implication that one's behavior conforms to the desires of an agent other than oneself, then seeing the environment as generally an indifferent cause in cases of automatic motive activation defuses the issue. For if the desire for the automated behavior to occur is not outside the person, it is surely *within*—for there is no other player left on the field. Who else put that goal or motive in place in that situation so frequently and intentionally in the past, so that it eventually became automated?

Therefore, automatic goal structures are not operating to satisfy the desires of the social environment, but are active *in the service of the individual.* Ultimate "control" in the sense of desired causation is back in the hands of the person whose motives they are; they are not anyone else's. Even though chronically accessible goals and motives result in unintentional (albeit goal-directed) decisions and behavior, in the final analysis they are acting in the individual's own interest and values. This would be demonstrated by the very fact of the automation itself: The motive or goal would have had to be frequently and consistently *chosen* by the individual in response to that situation in the past, to the point where the choice was so regular and reliable that there was no longer any need to make it through an act of will.

Acknowledgments

This chapter was written while I was a Research Fellow of the Alexander von Humboldt Foundation at the Universität Mannheim, West Germany. Preparation of the chapter also was supported in part by National Institute of Mental Health Grant No. MH-43265. My thanks to Tory Higgins, Peter Gollwitzer, and Steve Neuberg for their insightful and extensive comments on an earlier version.

Notes

1. Although there are superficial similarities between this proposal and the concepts of "mindlessness" and of "ecological perception" or "direct perception," there are fundamental differences as

well. "Mindless" social-interactive behavior is hypothesized to be driven by situational cues with minimal conscious involvement (e.g., Langer, 1978; Langer, Blank, & Chanowitz, 1978). The "automotive" model presented here proposes that motives and goals are preconsciously activated and then guide behavior. The social-interactive behavior that results is thus very much goal-directed and purposive, whereas "mindlessness" refers to a mental state of low effort, low involvement, and disengagement from the present environment (Langer, 1978). Actually, the automatically motivated behavior described here fits better with the opposite concept of "mindfulness," because whereas one is not aware of the guiding intent or goal, one's behavior is goal-directed and responsive to the contingencies of the environment.

The ecological perception view (e.g., McArthur & Baron, 1983) argues that social stimuli directly suggest behavioral responses to the perceiver. However, it also contends that these behavioral possibilities are intrinsic to the stimuli themselves, following Gibson's (e.g., 1966) notion of "affordances." The present position, on the other hand, is closer to Lewin's (e.g., 1936) conception of the determining influence of the entire *field* of situational and personal influences over goal setting and behavior. Another clear difference is that the ecological approach to social perception and behavior asserts that social judgments and causal attributions are made directly upon perception of a behavioral event, whereas the present view is that these cognitive activities are entirely goal-dependent and are not driven solely by the stimulus, outside of its situational context.

2. It should be noted that no claim is being made here as to the validity of Jones and Thibaut's (1958) analysis of the particular trait dimensions associated with the particular goals they describe; the point being made here is that the authors associated different sets of perceptual constructs with different interaction goals. Also, it should be noted that Jones and Thibaut (1958) did not explicitly take a stand as to whether these sets of constructs are reflexively or automatically activated as a direct consequence of the interaction goal, but the tenor of their discussion is that the use of the goal-associated constructs is reflexive, given the goal.

References

Abelson, R. P. (1980). Psychological status of the script concept. *American Psychologist, 36*, 715–729.

Ach, N. (1935). Analyse des Willens. In E. Abderhalden (Ed.), *Handbuch der biologishen Arbeitsmethoden* (Vol. 6, Part E). Berlin: Urban & Schwarzenberg.

Adorno, T. W., Frenkel-Brunswik, E., Levinson, D. J., & Sanford, R. N. (1950). *The authoritarian personality*. New York: Harper & Row.

Allport, F. H. (1955). *Theories of perception and the concept of structure*. New York: Wiley.

Allport, G. W., Vernon, P., & Lindzey, G. (1951). *A study of values*. Boston: Houghton Mifflin.

Anderson, J. R. (1983). *The architecture of cognition*. Cambridge, MA: Harvard University Press.

Anderson, R. C., & Pichert, J. W. (1978). Recall of previously unrecallable information following a shift in perspective. *Journal of Verbal Learning and Verbal Behavior, 17*, 1–12.

Atkinson, J. W., & Birch, D. (1970). *The dynamics of action*. New York: Wiley.

Atkinson, J. W., & Feather, N. T. (1966). *A theory of achievement motivation*. New York: Wiley.

Bargh, J. A. (1982). Attention and automaticity in the processing of self-relevant information. *Journal of Personality and Social Psychology, 43*, 425–436.

Bargh, J. A. (1984). Automatic and conscious processing of social information. In R. S. Wyer, Jr., & T. K. Srull (Eds.), *Handbook of social cognition* (Vol. 3, pp. 1–43). Hillsdale, NJ: Erlbaum.

Bargh, J. A. (1988). Automatic information processing: Implications for communication and affect. In L. Donohew, H. E. Sypher, & E. T. Higgins (Eds.), *Communication, social cognition, and affect* (pp. 9–37). Hillsdale, NJ: Erlbaum.

Bargh, J. A. (1989). Conditional automaticity: Varieties of automatic influence in social perception and cognition. In J. S. Uleman & J. A. Bargh (Eds.), *Unintended thought* (pp. 3–51). New York: Guilford Press.

Bargh, J. A., Bond, R. N., Lombardi, W. J., & Tota, M. E. (1986). The additive nature of chronic and temporary sources of construct accessibility. *Journal of Personality and Social Psychology, 50*, 869–878.

Bargh, J. A., Chaiken, S., Govender, R., & Pratto, F. (1990). *The generality of the automatic attitude activation effect*. Unpublished manuscript, New York University.

Bargh, J. A., Litt, J., Pratto, F., & Spielman, L. A. (1989). On the preconscious evaluation of social stimuli. In A. F. Bennett & K. M. McConkey (Eds.), *Cognition in individual and social contexts: Proceedings of the XXIV International Congress of Psychology* (Vol. 3, pp. 357-370). Amsterdam: Elsevier.

Bargh, J. A., Lombardi, W. J., & Higgins, E. T. (1988). Automaticity of chronically accessible constructs in person × situation effects on person perception: It's just a matter of time. *Journal of Personality and Social Psychology, 55*, 599-605.

Bargh, J. A., & Pietromonaco, P. (1982). Automatic information processing and social perception: The influence of trait information presented outside of conscious awareness on impression formation. *Journal of Personality and Social Psychology, 43*, 437-449.

Bargh, J. A., & Pratto, F. (1986). Individual construct accessibility and perceptual selection. *Journal of Experimental Social Psychology, 22*, 293-311.

Bargh, J. A., & Thein, R. D. (1985). Individual construct accessibility, person memory, and the recall-judgment link: The case of information overload. *Journal of Personality and Social Psychology, 49*, 1129-1146.

Bargh, J. A., & Tota, M. E. (1988). Context-dependent automatic processing in depression: Accessibility of negative constructs with regard to self but not others. *Journal of Personality and Social Psychology, 54*, 925-939.

Barker, R. G., & Wright, H. F. (1955). *Midwest and its children: The psychological ecology of an American town*. New York: Row, Peterson.

Borgida, E., & Howard-Pitney, B. (1983). Personal involvement and the robustness of perceptual salience effects. *Journal of Personality and Social Psychology, 45*, 560-570.

Boring, E. G. (1950). *A history of experimental psychology* (2nd ed.). New York: Appleton-Century-Crofts.

Brehm, J. W. (1966). *A theory of psychological reactance*. New York: Academic Press.

Brewer, M. B. (1988). A dual process model of impression formation. In T. K. Srull & R. S. Wyer, Jr. (Eds.), *Advances in social cognition* (Vol. 1, pp. 1-36). Hillsdale, NJ: Erlbaum.

Brewer, W. F., & Dupree, D. A. (1983). Use of plan schemata in the recall and recognition of goal-directed actions. *Journal of Experimental Psychology: Learning, Memory, and Cognition, 9*, 117-129.

Brown, R., & McNeill, D. (1966). The "tip of the tongue" phenomenon. *Journal of Verbal Learning and Verbal Behavior, 5*, 325-337.

Bruner, J. S. (1951). Personality dynamics and the process of perceiving. In R. R. Blake & G. V. Ramsey (Eds.), *Perception: An approach to personality* (pp. 121-147). New York: Ronald Press.

Bruner, J. S. (1957). On perceptual readiness. *Psychological Review, 64*, 123-152.

Buss, D. M., Gomes, M., Higgins, D. S., & Lauterbach, K. (1987). Tactics of manipulation. *Journal of Personality and Social Psychology, 52*, 1219-1229.

Cacioppo, J. T., & Petty, R. E. (1982). The need for cognition. *Journal of Personality and Social Psychology, 42*, 116-131.

Cantor, N. (1982). Perceptions of situations: Situation prototypes and person-situation prototypes. In D. Magnusson (Ed.), *The situation: An interactional perspective* (pp. 229-244). Hillsdale, NJ: Erlbaum.

Cantor, N., & Kihlstrom, J. F. (1987). *Personality and social intelligence*. Englewood Cliffs, NJ: Prentice-Hall.

Cantor, N., & Langston, C. A. (1989). Ups and downs of life tasks in a life transition. In L. A. Pervin (Ed.), *Goal concepts in personality and social psychology* (pp. 127-168). Hillsdale, NJ: Erlbaum.

Cantor, N., Mischel, W., & Schwartz, J. (1982). A prototype analysis of psychological situations. *Cognitive Psychology, 14*, 45-77.

Carlston, D. E. (1980). The recall and use of traits and events in social inference processes. *Journal of Experimental Social Psychology, 16*, 303-329.

Carver, C. S., & Scheier, M. F. (1981). *Attention and self-regulation: A control theory approach to human behavior.* New York: Springer.

Chaiken, S. (1980). Heuristic versus systematic information processing and the use of source versus message cues in persuasion. *Journal of Personality and Social Psychology, 39,* 752-766.

Chaiken, S., Liberman, A., & Eagly, A. (1989). Heuristic and systematic information processing within and beyond the persuasion context. In J. S. Uleman & J. A. Bargh (Eds.), *Unintended thought* (pp. 212-252). New York: Guilford Press.

Cohen, C. E., & Ebbesen, E. B. (1979). Observational goals and schema activation: A theoretical framework for behavior perception. *Journal of Experimental Social Psychology, 15,* 305-329.

Dennett, D. C. (1978). *Brainstorms: Philosophical essays on mind and psychology.* Cambridge, MA: MIT Press.

Dennett, D. C. (1984). *Elbow room: The varieties of free will worth wanting.* Cambridge, MA: MIT Press.

Derlega, V. (Ed.). (1984). *Communication, intimacy, and close relationships.* New York: Academic Press.

Devine, P. G. (1989). Stereotypes and prejudice: Their automatic and controlled components. *Journal of Personality and Social Psychology, 56,* 5-18.

Devine, P. G., Sedikides, C., & Fuhrman, R. W. (1989). Goals in social information processing: The case of anticipated interaction. *Journal of Personality and Social Psychology, 56,* 680-690.

Emmons, R. A. (1989). The personal striving approach to personality. L. A. Pervin (Ed.), *Goal concepts in personality and social psychology* (pp. 87-126). Hillsdale, NJ: Erlbaum.

Erber, R., & Fiske, S. T. (1984). Outcome dependency and attention to inconsistent information. *Journal of Personality and Social Psychology, 47,* 709-726.

Ericsson, K., & Simon, H. A. (1984). *Protocol analysis.* New York: Cambridge University Press.

Fazio, R. H. (1986). How do attitudes guide behavior? In R. M. Sorrentino & E. T. Higgins (Eds.), *Handbook of motivation and cognition: Foundations of social behavior* (Vol. 1, pp. 204-243). New York: Guilford Press.

Fazio, R. H., Powell, M. C., & Herr, P. M. (1983). Toward a process model of the attitude-behavior relation: Accessing one's attitudes upon mere observation of the attitude object. *Journal of Personality and Social Psychology, 44,* 723-735.

Fazio, R. H., Sanbonmatsu, D. M., Powell, M. C., & Kardes, F. R. (1986). On the automatic activation of attitudes. *Journal of Personality and Social Psychology, 50,* 229-238.

Feldman, N. S., & Ruble, D. N. (1988). The effect of personal relevance on psychological inference: A developmental analysis. *Child Development, 59,* 1339-1352.

Fenigstein, A., Scheier, M. F., & Buss, A. H. (1975). Public and private self-consciousness: Assessment and theory. *Journal of Consulting and Clinical Psychology, 43,* 522-527.

Fiske, S. T. (1980). Attention and weight in person perception: The impact of negative and extreme behavior. *Journal of Personality and Social Psychology, 38,* 889-906.

Fiske, S. T. (1989). Examining the role of intent: Toward understanding its role in stereotyping and prejudice. In J. S. Uleman & J. A. Bargh (Eds.), *Unintended thought* (pp. 253-283). New York: Guilford Press.

Fiske, S. T., Neuberg, S. L., Beattie, A. E., & Milberg, S. J. (1987). Category-based and attribute-based reactions to others: Some informational conditions of stereotyping and individuating processes. *Journal of Experimental Social Psychology, 23,* 399-427.

Fiske, S. T., & Taylor, S. E. (1984). *Social cognition.* Reading, MA: Addison-Wesley.

Freedman, J. L., & Fraser, S. C. (1966). Compliance without pressure: The foot-in-the-door technique. *Journal of Personality and Social Psychology, 4,* 195-202.

Friedman, A. (1979). Framing pictures: The role of knowledge in automatized encoding and memory for gist. *Journal of Experimental Social Psychology, 38,* 889-906.

Ghiselin, B. (Ed.). (1952). *The creative process.* New York: New American Library.

Gibson, J. J. (1966). *The senses considered as perceptual systems.* Boston: Houghton Mifflin.

Gilbert, D. T. (1989). Thinking lightly about others: Automatic components of the social inference process. In J. S. Uleman & J. A. Bargh (Eds.), *Unintended thought* (pp. 189-211). New York: Guilford Press.

Gilbert, D. T., Pelham, B. W., & Krull, D. S. (1988). On cognitive busyness: When person perceivers meet persons perceived. *Journal of Personality and Social Psychology, 54,* 733-740.

Goffman, E. (1974). *Frame analysis.* New York: Harper & Row.

Hamilton, D. L., Katz, L. B., & Leirer, V. O. (1980). Cognitive representation of personality impressions: Organizational processes in first impression formation. *Journal of Personality and Social Psychology, 39,* 1050-1063.

Hatfield, E., Traupman, J., Sprecher, S., Utne, M., & Hay, J. (1984). Equity and intimate relations: Recent research. In W. Ickes (Ed.), *Compatible and incompatible relationships* (pp. 1-27). New York: Springer.

Heckhausen, H. (1987). Wunschen-Wahlen-Wollen. In Heckhausen, H., P. M. Gollwitzer, & F. E. Weinert (Eds.), *Jenseits des Rubicon: Der Wille in den Humanwissenschaften.* Heidelberg: Springer-Verlag.

Heckhausen, H. & Beckmann, J. (1990). Intentional action and action slips. *Psychological Review, 97,* 36-48.

Higgins, E. T. (1987). Self-discrepancy: A theory relating self and affect. *Psychological Review, 94,* 319-340.

Higgins, E. T. (1989). Knowledge accessibility and activation: Subjectivity and suffering from unconscious sources. In J. S. Uleman & J. A. Bargh (Eds.), *Unintended thought* (pp. 75-123). New York: Guilford Press.

Higgins, E. T. (1990). Personality, social psychology, and person–situation relations: Standards and knowledge activation as a common language. In L. A. Pervin (Ed.), *Handbook of personality: Theory and research* (pp. 301-338). New York: Guilford Press.

Higgins, E. T., & Bargh, J. A. (1987). Social perception and social cognition. *Annual Review of Psychology, 38,* 369-425.

Higgins, E. T., Bargh, J. A., & Lombardi, W. (1985). The nature of priming effects on categorization. *Journal of Experimental Psychology: Learning, Memory, and Cognition, 11,* 59-69.

Higgins, E. T., Bond, R. N., Klein, R., & Strauman, T. (1986). Self-discrepancies and emotional vulnerability: How magnitude, accessibility, and type of discrepancy influence affect. *Journal of Personality and Social Psychology, 51,* 5-15.

Higgins, E. T., & King, G. (1981). Accessibility of social constructs: Information processing consequences of individual and contextual variability. In N. Cantor & J. F. Kihlstrom (Eds.), *Personality, cognition, and social interaction* (pp. 69-121). Hillsdale, NJ: Erlbaum.

Higgins, E. T., King, G. A., & Mavin, G. H. (1982). Individual construct accessibility and subjective impressions and recall. *Journal of Personality and Social Psychology, 43,* 35-47.

Higgins, E. T., & McCann, C. D. (1984). Social encoding and subsequent attitudes, impressions, and memory: "Context-driven" and motivational aspects of processing. *Journal of Personality and Social Psychology, 47,* 26-39.

Higgins, E. T., & Rholes, W. S. (1978). "Saying is believing": Effects of message modification on memory and liking for the person described. *Journal of Experimental Social Psychology, 14,* 363-378.

Hilton, D. J., & Slugoski, B. R. (1986). Knowledge-based causal attribution: The abnormal conditions focus model. *Psychological Review, 93,* 75-88.

Jacoby, L. L., & Kelley, C. M. (1987). Unconscious influences of memory for a prior event. *Personality and Social Psychology Bulletin, 13,* 314-336.

James, W. (1890). *The principles of psychology* (Vol. 1). New York: Holt.

Jones, E. E., Rhodewalt, F., Berglas, S., & Skelton, J. A. (1981). Effects of strategic self-presentation on subsequent self-esteem. *Journal of Personality and Social Psychology, 41,* 407-421.

Jones, E. E., & Thibaut, J. W. (1958). Interaction goals as bases of inference in interpersonal perception. In R. Taguiri & L. Petrullo (Eds.), *Person perception and interpersonal behavior* (pp. 151-178). Stanford, CA: Stanford University Press.

Kahneman, D. (1973). *Attention and effort.* Englewood Cliffs, NJ: Prentice-Hall.

Kelley, H. H., Berscheid, E., Christensen, A., Harvey, J. H., Huston, T. L., Levinger, G., McClintoch, E., Peplau, L. A., & Peterson D. (Eds.). (1983). *Close relationships.* San Francisco: W. H. Freeman.

Kelly, G. A. (1955). *The psychology of personal constructs*. New York: Norton.

Kimble, G. A., & Perlmuter, L. C. (1970). The problem of volition. *Psychological Review*, 77, 361-384.

Klinger, E. (1975). Consequences of commitment to and disengagement from incentives. *Psychological Review*, 82, 1-25.

Kruglanski, A. W., & Freund, T. (1983). The freezing and unfreezing of lay-inferences: Effects on impressional primacy, ethnic stereotyping, and numerical anchoring. *Journal of Experimental Social Psychology*, 19, 448-468.

Kuhl, J. (1986). Motivation and information processing: A new look at decision making, dynamic change, and action control. In R. M. Sorrentino & E. T. Higgins (Eds.), *Handbook of motivation and cognition: Foundations of social behavior* (Vol. 1, pp. 404-434). New York: Guilford Press.

Kuhl, J., & Atkinson, J. W. (1984). Perspectives in human motivational psychology: A new experimental paradigm. In V. Sarris & A. Parducci (Eds.),,, *Perspectives in psychological experimentation*. Hillsdale, NJ: Erlbaum.

Kuhl, J., & Blankenship, V. (1979). The dynamic theory of achievement motivation: From episodic to dynamic thinking. *Psychological Review*, 86, 141-151.

Kunda, Z., & Sanitoso, R. (1989). Motivated changes in the self-concept. *Journal of Experimental Social Psychology*, 25, 272-285.

Langer, E. J. (1978). Rethinking the role of thought in social interaction. In J. H. Harvey, W. J. Ickes, & R. F. Kidd (Eds.), *New directions in attribution research* (Vol. 2, pp. 36-58). Hillsdale, NJ: Erlbaum.

Langer, E. J., Blank, A., & Chanowitz, B. (1978). The mindlessness of ostensibly thoughtful action: The role of "placebic" information in interpersonal interaction. *Journal of Personality and Social Psychology*, 36, 635-642.

Lewin, K. (1928). Wille, Volsatz, und Bedurfnis. *Psychologische Forschung*, 7, 330-385.

Lewin, K. (1935). *A dynamic theory of personality: Selected papers*. New York: McGraw-Hill.

Lewin, K. (1936). *Principles of topological psychology*. New York: McGraw-Hill.

Libet, B. (1985). Unconscious cerebral initiative and the role of conscious will in voluntary action. *Behavioral and Brain Sciences*, 8, 529-566.

Lichtenstein, E. H., & Brewer, W. F. (1980). Memory for goal-directed events. *Cognitive Psychology*, 12, 412-445.

Logan, G. D. (1980). Attention and automaticity in Stroop and priming tasks: Theory and data. *Cognitive Psychology*, 12, 523-553.

Logan, G. D. (1989). Automaticity and cognitive control. In J. S. Uleman & J. A. Bargh (Eds.), *Unintended thought* (pp. 52-74). New York: Guilford Press.

Logan, G. D., & Cowan, W. B. (1984). On the ability to inhibit thought and action: A theory of an act of control. *Psychological Review*, 91, 295-327.

Logan, G. D., & Zbrodoff, N. J. (1979). When it helps to be misled: Facilitative effects of increasing the frequency of conflicting stimuli in a Stroop-like task. *Memory and Cognition*, 7, 166-174.

Marcel, A. J. (1983). Conscious and unconscious perception: An approach to the relations between phenomenal experience and perceptual processes. *Cognitive Psychology*, 15, 238-300.

Mandler, G. (1975). *Mind and emotion*. New York: Wiley.

Martin, L. L., & Tesser, A. (1989). Toward a motivational and structural theory of ruminative thought. In J. S. Uleman & J. A. Bargh (Eds.), *Unintended thought* (pp. 306-326). New York: Guilford Press.

McArthur, L. Z. (1981). What grabs you? The role of attention in impression formation and causal attribution. In E. T. Higgins, C. P. Herman, & M. P. Zanna (Eds.), *Social cognition: The Ontario Symposium* (Vol. 1, pp. 201-246). Hillsdale, NJ: Erlbaum.

McArthur, L. Z., & Baron, R. (1983). Toward an ecological theory of social perception. *Psychological Review*, 90, 215-238.

McArthur, L. Z., & Friedman, S. (1980). Illusory correlation in impression formation: Variations in the shared distinctiveness effect as a function of the distinctive person's age, race, and sex. *Journal of Personality and Social Psychology*, 39, 615-624.

McCann, C. D., & Higgins, E. T. (1988). Motivation and affect in interpersonal relations: The role of personal orientations and discrepancies. In L. Donohew, H. E. Sypher, & E. T. Higgins (Eds.), *Communication, social cognition, and affect* (pp. 53–79). Hillsdale, NJ: Erlbaum.

McClelland, D., Atkinson, J. W., Clark, R. A., & Lowell, E. L. (1953). *The achievement motive.* New York: Appleton-Century-Crofts.

Miller, G. A., Galanter, E., & Pribram, K. (1960). *Plans and the structure of behavior.* New York: Holt.

Miller, L. C., & Read, S. J. (1987). Why am I telling you this? Self-disclosure in a goal-based model of personality. In V. J. Derlega & J. Berg (Eds.), *Self-disclosure: Theory, research, and therapy.* New York: Plenum.

Mills, C. J., & Tyrrell, D. J. (1983). Sex-stereotypic encoding and release from proactive interference. *Journal of Personality and Social Psychology, 45,* 772–781.

Minsky, M. (1975). A framework for representing knowledge. In P. Winston (Ed.), *The psychology of computer vision* (pp. 211–277). New York: McGraw-Hill.

Moskowitz, G. B., & Uleman, J. S. (1987, August). *The facilitation and inhibition of spontaneous trait inferences.* Paper presented at the 95th annual convention of the American Psychological Association, New York.

Murray, H. (1938). *Explorations in personality.* New York: Oxford University Press.

Neely, J. H. (1977). Semantic priming and retrieval from lexical memory: Roles of inhibitionless spreading activation and limited-capacity attention. *Journal of Experimental Psychology: General, 106,* 225–254.

Neisser, U. (1967). *Cognitive psychology.* New York: Appleton-Century-Crofts.

Neuberg, S. L. (1988). Behavioral implications of information presented outside of conscious awareness: The effect of subliminal presentation of trait information on behavior in the Prisoner's Dilemma game. *Social Cognition, 6,* 207–230.

Neuberg, S. L. (1989). The goal of forming accurate impressions during social interactions: Attenuating the impact of negative expectancies. *Journal of Personality and Social Psychology, 56,* 374–386.

Neuberg, S. L., & Fiske, S. T. (1987). Motivational influences on impression formation: Outcome dependency, accuracy-driven attention, and individuating processes. *Journal of Personality and Social Psychology, 53,* 431–444.

Newell, A., & Rosenbloom, P. S. (1981). Mechanisms of skill acquisition and the law of practice. In J. R. Anderson (Ed.), *Cognitive skills and their acquisition* (pp. 1–55). Hillsdale, NJ: Erlbaum.

Newell, A., & Simon, H. A. (1972). *Human problem solving.* Englewood Cliffs, NJ: Prentice-Hall.

Nisbett, R. E., & Wilson, T. D. (1977). Telling more than we can know: Verbal reports on mental processes. *Psychological Review, 84,* 231–259.

Norman, D. A. (1981). Categorization of action slips. *Psychological Review, 88,* 1–15.

Norman, D., A., & Bobrow, D. G. (1976). On the role of active memory processes in perception and cognition. In C. N. Cofer (Ed.), *The structure of human memory* (pp. 114–132). San Francisco: W. H. Freeman.

Norman, D. A., & Shallice, T. (1986). Attention to action: Willed and automatic control of behavior. In R. J. Davidson, G. E. Schwartz, & D. Shapiro (Eds.), *Consciousness and self-regulation: Advances in research and theory* (Vol. 4, pp. 1–18). New York: Plenum.

Paulhus, D. L., Graf, P., & Van Selst, M. (1989). Attentional load increases the positivity of self-presentation. *Social Cognition, 7,* 389–400.

Paulhus, D. L., & Levitt, K. (1987). Desirable responding triggered by affect. *Journal of Personality and Social Psychology, 52,* 245–259.

Pervin, L. A. (1989). Goal concepts: Themes, issues, and questions. In L. A. Pervin (Ed.), *Goal concepts in personality and social psychology* (pp. 473–479). Hillsdale, NJ: Erlbaum.

Petty, R. E., Cacioppo, J. T., & Goldman, R. (1981). Personal involvement as a determinant of argument-based persuasion. *Journal of Personality and Social Psychology, 41,* 847–855.

Piaget, J. (1952). *The origins of intelligence in children.* New York: International Universities Press.

Pittman, T. S., & D'Agostino, P. R. (1985). Motivation and attribution: The effects of control deprivation on subsequent information processing. In J. Harvey & G. Weary (Eds.), *Attribution: Basic issues and applications* (pp. 117–141). New York: Academic Press.

Pittman, T. S., & Pittman, N. L. (1980). Deprivation of control and the attribution process. *Journal of Personality and Social Psychology, 39,* 377-389.

Posner, M. I. (1978). *Chronometric explorations of mind.* Hillsdale, NJ: Erlbaum.

Posner, M. I., & Snyder, C. R. R. (1975). Attention and cognitive control. In R. L. Solso (Ed.), *Information processing and cognition: The Loyola Symposium* (pp. 55-85). Hillsdale, NJ: Erlbaum.

Postman, L., Bruner, J. S., & McGinnies, E. (1948). Personal values as selective factors in perception. *Journal of Abnormal and Social Psychology, 43,* 142-154.

Pratto, F., & Bargh, J. A. (in press). Stereotyping based on apparently individuating information: Trait and global components of sex stereotypes under attention overload. *Journal of Experimental Social Psychology.*

Pratto, F., & John, O. P. (1989). *The attention-grabbing power of negative information about people.* Unpublished manuscript, University of California-Berkeley.

Read, S. J., & Miller, L. C. (1989). Inter-personalism: Toward a goal-based theory of persons in relationships. In L. A. Pervin (Ed.), *Goal concepts in personality and social psychology* (pp. 413-472). Hillsdale, NJ: Erlbaum.

Rhodewalt, F., & Agustsdottir, S. (1986). Effects of self-presentation on the phenomenal self. *Journal of Personality and Social Psychology, 50,* 47-55.

Rothbart, M. (1981). Memory processes and social beliefs. In D. L. Hamilton (Ed.), *Cognitive processes in stereotyping and intergroup behavior* (pp. 145-181). Hillsdale, NJ: Erlbaum.

Schank, R. C., & Abelson, R. P. (1977). *Scripts, plans, goals, and understanding.* Hillsdale, NJ: Erlbaum.

Schlenker, B. R. (1980). *Impression management: The self concept, social identity, and interpersonal relations.* Monterey, CA: Brooks/Cole.

Schneider, W., & Fisk, A. D. (1982). Degree of consistent training: Improvements in search performance and automatic process development. *Perception and Psychophysics, 31,* 160-168.

Schneider, W., & Shiffrin, R. M. (1977). Controlled and automatic human information processing: I. Detection, search, and attention. *Psychological Review, 84,* 1-66.

Sechenov, I. M. (1935). *Collected works.* Moscow: State Publishing House.

Shallice, T. (1972). Dual functions of consciousness. *Psychological Review, 79,* 383-393.

Simon, H. A. (1967). Motivational and emotional controls of cognition. *Psychological Review, 74,* 29-39.

Smith, E. R. (1984). Model of social inference processes. *Psychological Review, 91,* 392-413.

Smith, E. R., & Miller, F. D. (1983). Mediation among attributional inferences and comprehension processes: Initial findings and a general method. *Journal of Personality and Social Psychology, 44,* 492-505.

Sorrentino, R. M., & Higgins, E. T. (1986). Motivation and cognition: Warming up to synergism. In R. M. Sorrentino & E. T. Higgins (Eds.), *Handbook of motivation and cognition: Foundations of social behavior* (Vol. 1, pp. 3-19). New York: Guilford Press.

Srull, T. K., & Brand, J. F. (1983). Memory for information about persons: The effect of encoding operations on subsequent retrieval. *Journal of Verbal Learning and Verbal Behavior, 22,* 219-230.

Srull, T. K., & Wyer, R. S., Jr. (1986). The role of chronic and temporary goals in social information processing. In R. M. Sorrentino & E. T. Higgins (Eds.), *Handbook of motivation and cognition: Foundations of social behavior* (Vol. 1, pp. 503-549). New York: Guilford Press.

Strauman, T. J., & Higgins, E. T. (1987). Automatic activation of self-discrepancies and emotional syndromes: When cognitive structures influence affect. *Journal of Personality and Social Psychology, 53,* 1004-1014.

Tait, R., & Silver, R. C. (1989). Coming to terms with major negative life events. In J. S. Uleman & J. A. Bargh (Eds.), *Unintended thought* (pp. 351-382). New York: Guilford Press.

Taylor, S. E., & Fiske, S. T. (1978). Salience, attention, and attribution: Top of the head phenomena. In L. Berkowitz (Ed.), *Advances in experimental social psychology* (Vol 11, pp. 249-288). New York: Academic Press.

Tetlock, P. E. (1985). Accountability: A social check on the fundamental attribution error. *Social Psychology Quarterly, 48,* 227-236.

Trzebinski, J. (1989). The role of goal categories in the representation of social knowledge. In L. A. Pervin (Ed.), *Goal concepts in personality and social psychology* (pp. 363-412). Hillsdale, NJ: Erlbaum.

Tyler, T. R. (1987). Conditions leading to value-expressive effects in judgments of procedural justice: A test of four models. *Journal of Personality and Social Psychology, 52,* 333-344.

Uleman, J. S. (1987). Consciousness and control: The case of spontaneous trait inferences. *Personality and Social Psychology Bulletin, 13,* 337-354.

Uleman, J. S. (1989). A framework for thinking intentionally about unintended thoughts. In J. S. Uleman & J. A. Bargh (Eds.), *Unintended thought* (pp. 425-449). New York: Guilford Press.

Uleman, J. S., & Bargh, J. A. (Eds.). (1989). *Unintended thought.* New York: Guilford Press.

Wegner, D. M., & Vallacher, R. R. (1986). Action identification. In R. M. Sorrentino & E. T. Higgins (Eds.), *Handbook of motivation and cognition: Foundations of social behavior* (Vol. 1, pp. 550-582). New York: Guilford Press.

Weiner, B. (1986). Attribution, emotion, and action. In R. M. Sorrentino & E. T. Higgins (Eds.), *Handbook of motivation and cognition: Foundations of social behavior* (Vol. 1, pp. 281-312). New York: Guilford Press.

Wilensky, R. (1983). *Planning and understanding.* Reading, MA: Addison-Wesley.

Winter, L., & Uleman, J. S. (1984). When are social judgments made? Evidence for the spontaneousness of trait inferences. *Journal of Personality and Social Psychology, 47,* 237-252.

Winter, L., Uleman, J. S., & Cunniff, C. (1985). How automatic are social judgments? *Journal of Personality and Social Psychology, 49,* 904-917.

Wyer, R. S., Jr., & Gordon, S. E. (1982). The recall of information about persons and groups. *Journal of Experimental Social Psychology, 18,* 128-164.

Wyer, R. S., Jr., & Srull, T. K. (1986). Human cognition in its social context. *Psychological Review, 93,* 322-359.

Wyer, R. S., Jr., Srull, T. K., Gordon, S. E., & Hartwick, J. (1982). Effects of processing objectives on the recall of prose material. *Journal of Personality and Social Psychology, 43,* 674-688.

Yaniv, I., & Meyer, D. E. (1987). Activation and metacognition of inaccessible stored information: Potential bases for incubation effects in problem solving. *Journal of Experimental Social Psychology: Learning, Memory, and Cognition, 13,* 187-205.

Zajonc, R. B. (1960). The process of cognitive tuning in communication. *Journal of Abnormal and Social Psychology, 61,* 159-167.

Zillman, D. (1978). Attribution and misattribution of excitatory reactions. In J. H. Harvey, W. J. Ickes, & R. F. Kidd (Eds.), *New directions in attribution research* (Vol. 2, pp. 335-368). Hillsdale, NJ: Erlbaum.

CHAPTER 4

Inhibition of Internally Cued Behavior

JANET POLIVY

University of Toronto

This chapter is a preliminary attempt to outline a model that integrates feelings arising from or accompanied by sensations inside the body with cognitions and behaviors. These feelings include emotions as well as other internal sensations (hunger, thirst, sleepiness, need to urinate or defecate, sexual arousal, cravings for drugs, etc.). Specifically, I argue that such internal sensations are cues for behavior; they may be interpreted cognitively and then acted on either appropriately (in accordance with the internal feeling) or inappropriately (by inhibiting the appropriate behavior, or attempting to substitute an alternative behavior). The appropriateness of the overt response will produce correspondingly positive or negative effects on the individual's comfort and well-being. This is obviously not an innovation in psychological theorizing. Schachter and Singer (1962), Freud (1930/1989), and McDougall (1908), among others, have all proposed similar models. However, the connection between internal sensations and behavior has been somewhat neglected recently; in particular, the effects of ignoring or inhibiting behavioral responses to such cues have not been delineated. The focus of this chapter is thus on the effects of suppressing internally cued behavior, in an attempt to determine whether the effects are general across behaviors and cues, or specific to particular types of activities or sensations.

The notion that inhibiting internally cued behavior is likely to cause problems (negative effects) for the individual can be traced back to Freud's (1930/1989) discussion of id urges, as well as Breuer and Freud's (1893–1895/1955) classic theory of hysteria and catharsis. Freud also pointed out the potential negative societal consequences of indiscriminate gratification of internal urges: A world in which we all gratified each id urge would be chaotic and dangerous (much like visiting New York City!). More recently, psychologists have described negative consequences of inhibiting cognitive and behavioral responses to emotionally traumatic events (Pennebaker, 1985) and of restraining emotional actions, leading to incomplete emotional experiences (Nichols & Efran, 1985). Moreover, inhibiting thoughts (Wegner, Schneider, Carter, & White, 1987) or behaviors (Pennebaker, 1985) in general may be difficult and costly for the individual.

MOTIVATIONAL UNDERPINNINGS: INSTINCT AND DRIVE

A basic proposition of this model is that ignoring internal signals for behavior or inhibiting the "appropriate" behavioral response produces discomfor and/or distress, cognitive disruption, and (in at least some cases) maladaptive behavior or behavioral excess. Moreover, this is the case for almost any internal drive, activation, or "feeling." This does not necessarily imply that the organism seeks a homeostatic, tensionless state, nor is it an argument for pure hedonism. As Weiner (1989) has pointed out, neither of these motivational goals is sufficient to explain the majority of human behavior.

Responding "appropriately" or in accordance with emotional or other internal cues for behavior is likely to be more comfortable in most situations than attempting to behave in a way other than that signaled by our bodies. In other words, inhibiting the "natural" or "appropriate" response to an internal signal for behavior is likely to lead to discomfort, since the activation signaled by the "feeling" has not been expressed or relieved. This may not, however, be either the most comfortable or hedonistic response the person could make, or the most tension-reducing. For example, there may be external pressures to behave in a different fashion that must be resisted, as when a male in our society feels sad and cries. Although crying is the behavior cued by the feeling of sadness, social sanctions against the expression of emotion, particularly crying, by males discourage such behavior. Most males in our society would thus attempt to inhibit their tears rather than face the embarassment of crying in public.

This model accords with the Freudian notion of id energy and its need for discharge, and with other early instinct theories of motivation and behavior (e.g., McDougall, 1908) as well. According to McDougall, when an instinct is provoked by the environment, the organism is impelled to act by the emotional state aroused by the instinct. McDougall believed, however, that learning can modify the behavioral response to an instinct-aroused emotion, and that the individual exerts free will in deciding whether or not to behave in response to the emotion. In either theory, instincts act to guide behavior to satisfy bodily needs and maintain the individual in a purposive fashion.

Drives replaced instincts in psychological theorizing after the 1920s and 1930s, at which time drives were defined as intense internal forces that motivate behavior. As Klein (1982) points out, the concept of drive was similar to that of instincts in its impulsive or urge-like aspect, but removed the idea of purposiveness. Hull (1943) maintained that an organism becomes more active when it is in a state of biological need, and that this higher level of activity increases the likelihood of the animal's performing a behavior that will eliminate the need. Through such reductions of need, which are reinforcing and increase the strength of the connection between the stimuli present at the time and the response that results in the reduction in need, the organism learns to behave in different ways in response to different environmental cues. Drive itself was held to be nonspecific, acting only to energize habitual behaviors. The environmental stimuli present presumably determine which habit (or behavior) is elicited when the drive motivates the organism to act.

Finally, drives can be acquired and are not necessarily based solely upon biological needs. Theorists such as Lewin began as early as the 1930s to focus discussions of motivation on psychological needs and their associated "tensions." For example, one of Lewin's students demonstrated that interrupted activities are remembered better than are completed ones, presumably because the tension generated by beginning the task is not fully discharged until the task is completed. (This is, of course, the Ziegarnik effect, named after the student who first demonstrated it.) According to Lewin, the residual tension associated with the incomplete task is what causes it to be remembered. Indeed, subsequent experiments demonstrated that subjects chose to do the interrupted tasks when free to do whatever they liked; substitute tasks could prevent this if they were similar to the original task, and repeated performance of the task removed its attraction for the subjects (Cofer, 1972). Stopping or inhibiting performance thus does seem to generate some sort of tension or urge to achieve completion.

The present theory is thus in many ways a combination of classical instinct and drive theories. The individual is motivated to act or behave by internal cues, which may be instinctual, psychological, or learned (as in drive theory), and which signal the organism to behave in a particular manner (more as in instinct theory, though learning may certainly play a role in determining the "appropriate" response to a given cue). The internal cues have elements of both a purposive, functionalistic specificity (e.g., the cue for eating is different in many ways from that for smoking a cigarette, for having sex, etc.) and a nonspecific, general, energizing quality (e.g., the consequences of not behaving in accordance with a cue are to a large extent similar, regardless of what the particular cue was). Interrupting or inhibiting a motivated behavior has consequences for the individual. Finally, the ultimate goal of the organism is reasonably hedonistic, in that it is to behave in such a way as to optimize one's experiential state, although this does not seem to mean responding to the most salient external rewards and punishments or seeking a tension-free homeostasis, as was previously postulated.

THE COSTS OF INHIBITING BEHAVIORS

Pennebaker (1985) reviews compelling evidence that inhibiting behavior is arousing, stressful, and related to ill health. He demonstrates that inhibiting emotional behavior, either through (individual differences in) lack of facial expressiveness or through intentional efforts to deceive, results in heightened physiological activation as measured by heart rate, skin conductance, respiration rate, and similar measures. Specifically, Gray (1975) showed in animals that inhibitory processes activated different brain regions than did excitatory ones. Fowles (1980) took this further and suggested that inhibition and excitation result in different kinds of autonomic activity. Pennebaker (1985) interprets these publications as indicating a physiological mechanism for the effects of inhibition of behaivor. Accordingly, he did a study showing that lying (inhibiting a truthful response) is associated with elevated skin conductance (Pennebaker & Chew, 1985).

In a similar vein, a body of emotion research indicates a negative correlation between facial expressiveness and indices of physiological arousal: Inhibitors (who are less expressive) have more autonomic arousal (Adelmann & Zajonc, 1989). For example, Lanzetta and Kleck (1970) videotaped subjects who were receiving electric shocks, and had judges view the tapes and attempt to discriminate shock from nonshock trials on the basis of subjects' facial expressiveness. In addition, subjects' galvanic skin responses (GSRs) were measured. The least facially responsive subjects had the greatest GSRs. Similarly, Buck (1977) investigated preschoolers' responses to slides and found higher skin conductance associated with lower expressiveness.

Taking this even further, Pennebaker (1985) cites research showing that individuals with a repressive coping style or personality (i.e., repressors, as opposed to sensitizers) demonstrate elevated cancer rates, high blood pressure, and general physical disorders. For example, a study of women diagnosed with breast cancer indicated that the more overtly hostile and emotional patients had a better prognosis than did repressors (Derogatis, Abeloff, & Melisaratos, 1979). Similarly, traumas that are less likely to be discussed with others (e.g., rape) have been shown to be associated with more health problems following the trauma than are socially acceptable and discussable traumas (e.g., the death of a loved one). Conversely, talking about a trauma (thus expressing the emotion connected to it to at least some degree) seems to be associated with less subsequent distress and disease (Pennebaker & O'Heeron, 1984).

Correspondingly, "expressed emotion" (i.e., chronic levels of hostile and/or intrusive emotional provocation from close family members) has been shown to correlate positively with schizophrenic relapse rate, poor diabetic control, obesity, and neurotic depression (Koenigsberg & Handley, 1986). Presumably, the victims of this chronic "expressed emotion" are unable to express (sufficiently?) their own emotional responses, and instead relapse into illness. For example, Hooley (1986) rated spouses of depressed patients for expressed emotion and then observed each patient and spouse interacting as they discussed a low-conflict issue. Spouses higher in expressed emotion were more negative toward their depressed partners on both verbal and nonverbal measures. The patients, however, were not more negative than those interacting with spouses low in expressed emotion, but rather behaved in a more neutral, less self-disclosing manner. The high expressed emotion of the spouses was thus associated with less expressive behavior from the depressed patients.

There has also been a history of clinical research and theorizing about the negative effect on affective experience of inhibiting behaviors inconsistent with one's self-concept (e.g., Rogers, 1961). Individuals who deny experiences, ignore their natural impulses (or organismic valuing process), and inhibit appropriate behavioral responses develop conditions of worth that constrict behavior still further. The ultimate results of such denial and inhibition are anxiety and neurosis (Rogers, 1961).

Hunger provides a general illustration of the model being proposed. The internal signals of gastric contractions and conditioned hormonal secretions are felt and interpreted (cognitively) by the individual as hunger. The appropriate behavioral response (simply put) is to eat, which is what most people do when they are hungry. When this is done, the arousal or drive engendered by the internal sensations of hunger is relieved, and the individual feels "satisfied" and, presumably, comfortable. However, having made a cognitive decision to lose weight, some individuals try to ignore hunger signals and inhibit their eating behavior. Such individuals are what we call "restrained eaters" (e.g., Herman & Polivy, 1988).

Our research on such restrained eaters (or dieters) shows that chronic restrained eating seems to produce increased emotionality and distractibility (Herman & Polivy, 1988; Polivy & Herman, 1987). Dieters get more upset than do nondieters when confronted with an emotional provocation (e.g., Polivy, Herman, & Warsh, 1978), and their performance on cognitive tasks (such as proofreading) deteriorates rapidly and drastically under conditions of distraction (e.g., Herman, Polivy, Pliner, Munic, & Threlkeld, 1978). Restrained eaters also spend more time thinking about food and eating and pay more attention to information connected to food and weight than to other information (King, Polivy, & Herman, in press), selectively retaining in memory the former over the latter. It is also interesting that anecdotal and other descriptions of dieters tend to mention their preoccupation with both their diets and food in general (e.g., recipes), to the exclusion of potentially more important concerns (e.g., Polivy & Herman, 1987). Furthermore, the most extreme dieters, anorexia nervosa and bulimia nervosa patients, show many of these same characteristics—often in exaggerated degrees, such as the often-mentioned preoccupation or obsession with food said to characterize these patients (e.g., Garfinkel & Garner, 1982; Polivy & Herman, 1987).

There is also evidence that restrained eating is physiologically stressful or arousing (e.g., elevated free fatty acid levels in the bloodstream; Hibscher & Herman, 1977). Although overweight is often cited as a health risk, arguments have been made that dieting is really responsible for some of the disorders seemingly caused by overweight. Dieting itself has been held responsible for such physical problems as postural hypotension, gall bladder disease, coronary problems, weakness, fatigue, and sometimes death (see Polivy & Herman, 1983, 1985b, and Wooley & Wooley, 1984, for full discussions). Finally, restrained eaters are also susceptible to bouts of excessive or even binge eating, particularly of proscribed, "fattening" foods (Polivy & Herman, 1985b, 1987). Thus, inhibiting the appropriate response to hunger (eating) actually leads to excessive eating, as well as to emotional and cognitive disruption.

More generally, there is evidence that inhibiting any behavior that is internally cued or desirable may frequently result in the opposite of the intended suppression, actually promoting behavioral excess. This is true for other behaviors in addition to inhibited eating. Marlatt's research on the "abstinence violation effect" (e.g., Marlatt & Gordon, 1985) indicates that such behavioral excess or bingeing often follows suppression of alcohol drinking or cigarette smoking. Once inhibited individuals violate their prohibition by having one alcoholic drink or cigarette, or one piece of fattening food, their behavior seems to rebound against the suppression, resulting in an overexpression of the forbidden act. Inhibiting appetitive behaviors thus seems to cause behavioral hyperreactivity. The end result of attempted suppression is often both discomfort and overindulgence in the proscribed behavior

After prolonged use of drugs such as alcohol or nicotine, many individuals develop a physiological need for or dependence upon the drug (e.g., Herman & Kozlowski, 1979; Jaffe & Jarvik, 1978; Marlatt, 1985). When they abstain from the drug in question long enough that their blood levels decline below a critical threshold (withdrawal), they develop a desire or craving for the drug (like hunger for food). If they react "appropriately" to this internal signal and ingest a suitable amount of the drug, the distress of withdrawal is alleviated, and they feel comfortable again. If, however, the addict tries to inhibit drug ingestion (i.e., to stop drinking or smoking), withdrawal continues and its symptoms increase. This discomfort may last hours, days, or months as the user's body readjusts physiologically to the absence of the drug. There have been suggestions that in some individuals the body never returns completely to its pre-drug-use state, and the rapid return to previous levels of usage after a relapsed quitting episode attests to this (e.g., Herman & Kozlowski, 1979). The discomfort of drug withdrawal often seems to involve symptoms similar to the side effects of dieting: Abstinent smokers and alcoholics report heightened emotionality (particularly irritability, nervousness, and depression), obsessive thoughts about cigarettes or alcohol, and general distractibility and inability to concentrate (see, e.g, Ludwig & Stark, 1974; Shiffman, 1979). Moreover, the most frequently cited triggers for smoking relapse (or a smoking binge) are negative affect or stress, and the example of others—two common triggers for overeating in dieters (Shiffman, Read, Maltese, Rapkin & Jarvik, 1985). Similarly, for drinking binges, negative affect, stress, failure, and having already begun drinking (i.e., consuming a preload) are among the most frequent precipitators (Ludwig & Stark, 1974). The costs of inhibiting appetitive behaviors such as eating, alcohol drinking, and cigarette smoking are thus similar, and the behavioral excess characterizing the failure of suppression has similar triggers.

Solomon and Corbit's (1974) "opponent process theory" offers a general mechanism and explanation for such opposite behaviors. The theory is based on the assumption that any intense affective state produces an oppositely valenced emotion as well, which may be accompanied by corresponding physiological changes (Solomon, 1980). For example, Solomon (1980) describes the reaction of a baby given a nipple providing a sweet liquid. The baby will suck happily. If the nipple is withdrawn after a minute, the baby will cry for several minutes. The distress is presumably indicative of a negative state produced by the previous induction of a positive state; if there had been no nipple presented in the first place, the baby would not be crying at this time. In a similar manner, parachute jumpers who feel nervous before a jump report feeling elated after the jump, presumably as a result of the contrast between their initial fear and current relief. Thus, a motivated activity presumably provokes a positive affective response, whereas abstaining from the activity produces a negative one. Engaging in the behavior again alleviates the negative response, provoking an even stronger positive reinforcement and an opposing stronger negative response to "withdrawal." In fact, this is how Solomon (1980) explains opiate addiction, and it clearly applies well to other behaviors.

Pennebaker (1985) argues in a similar fashion about a different class of behaviors—namely, expressive behaviors. He maintains that traumatic events involving the inhibition of behavior are likely to be the objects of ruminative obsession for as much as years afterward. In addition to such cognitive preoccupation, these events seem to be related to the development of a variety of major and minor diseases, as discussed above. Pennebaker proposes that the inhibition of an ongoing behavior, as well as the obsessive thoughts about it afterward, produces physiological activation that may result in stress-related diseases over the long term. Pennebaker concludes that confiding in or telling someone about the inhibition or traumatic event allows it to be cognitively reorganized so that it can be integrated by the individual. I would argue, however, that the benefits of such confiding, like catharsis, accrue from the active behavioral expression of the inhibited emotions, rather than from a cognitive reorganization of them. This implies that mere nonemotional recounting of the trauma is not sufficient to alleviate the "distress," and that some sort of expressing of the affect involved may be necessary. This is obviously an empirical question that future research may resolve.

THE DIFFICULTY OF INHIBITING STIMULATED BEHAVIORS

The inhibition of any behavior or even a thought requires effort. This effect is illustrated by the joke George Burns is purported to have played on his friend Jack Benny (R. M. Sorrentino, personal communication, 1989). Benny was having a party and had arranged for Jeanette MacDonald to sing at the party. The day before the party, Burns called Benny and told him that whatever he did, he must not laugh when Jeanette sang. Burns called Benny two more times before the party and repeated his injunction not to laugh during the singing. Finally, Jeanette began to sing, and Benny broke into a fit of laughter and fell to the floor. Wegner et al. (1987) demonstrated this more scientifically in the laboratory. Subjects asked to suppress a thought ("Do not think about a white bear") wound up thinking about it almost half as often as subjects explicitly instructed to think about it as much as possible. Moreover, in a within-subjects design, suppression of a thought was followed by an increased level of that thought in a sort of cognitive rebound. The authors concluded that attempted thought suppression has the paradoxical effect of producing a preoccupation with the inhibited thought, which is expressed both immediately by intrusions of the forbidden thought and in a delayed manner by an increase in the thought when the prohibition is lifted.

Telling subjects to think of a particular distractor when the prohibited thought intrudes ("Think about a red Volkswagen instead") did not reduce the number of intrusions, but did eliminate the rebound effect when expression was allowed. (The distractor might have been more effective if it had not been made contingent upon the occurrence of the prohibited thought.) Even with a strategy to help them, subjects were unable to suppress a simple thought (Wegner et al., 1987).

Similarly, as mentioned above, restrained eaters or dieters seem to have difficulty suppressing their eating in many situations. In our laboratory, my colleagues and I have demonstrated that dieters who eat a high-calorie "preload" such as a large milkshake or a big piece of cake are likely to eat excessively in subsequent "taste-rating" tasks, though they eat sparingly when not preloaded (see Herman & Polivy, 1988, for a review). It appears to be enough that dieters perceive the preload as high-calorie or "fattening," regardless of its actual caloric level, for dieting to be abandoned and overeating to occur (e.g., Knight & Boland, 1989; Polivy, 1976; Spencer & Fremouw, 1979). Similarly, restrained eaters who knowingly drink alcohol (Polivy & Herman, 1976) or are upset emotionally, particularly by an ego threat of some sort (Herman, Heatherton & Polivy, 1989; Herman, Polivy, Lank, & Heatherton, 1987), overeat (relative to nondieters or calm, sober dieters). This tendency toward rebound or excessive eating, and inability to maintain suppressed eating levels, compounds the negative sequelae of chronic restrained eating discussed in the preceding section.

Before these characteristics were associated with restrained eaters, many of these qualities (emotionality, distractibility, improper regulation of food intake) were shown to characterize a group of subjects who were described as externally bound and insensitive to their internal states. Schachter's work on obese subjects focused on these aspects of what was called the "externality" of the obese (Schachter, 1971; Schachter & Rodin, 1974). In other words, obese subjects failed to act in accordance with their internal states, and were also found to be hyper-emotional and distractible. Since a prominent internal state for most people is hunger, since obese people have an obvious motive for trying to suppress their hunger (given our society's derogation of overweight and preference for thinness), and since in fact most overweight people are restrained eaters (Herman & Polivy, 1980), this may well be another instance of the difficulty and side effects of inhibiting internally motivated behavior.

In fact, dieting in the obese population is a notoriously ineffective activity. This is demonstrated not only by the constant presence of diet books on best-seller lists and by the multibillion-dollar diet industry, but by statistics on weight loss programs for overweight patients (when statistics are made available at all). Not only is the dropout rate high for most treatments, but as Stunkard (1975) has so often been quoted as saying, of the obese who enter treatment, "most will not lose much weight and of those who do lose weight, most will regain it." Current reviews of the literature on weight loss in overweight individuals reach similar conclusions: Losing weight and maintaining the loss seem to be virtually impossible for most of the overweight population (e.g., Wadden & Stunkard, 1987). Despite intense societal pressures to be thin and sanctions against fatness (e.g., Polivy, Garner, & Garfinkel, 1986), and their own desperate desire to lose weight, obese people are notoriously poor at restraining their eating sufficiently to enable them to normalize their weight. Average weight has actually increased between 1960 and 1980, despite the tremendous increase in dieting (Foreyt, 1987). Apparently it is difficult to inhibit eating behavior.

Taking this one step further, Rothenberg (1986) points out that desire for or attempts at control of various aspects of one's feelings or behavior constitute a central facet of obsessive–compulsive psychiatric illness, and he argues that the eating disorders of anorexia nervosa and bulimia nervosa are actually variants of obsessive–compulsive disorder. He further argues that the hysterical or conversion disorders so common in Freud's time and so rare today were products of their social milieu (wherein the societal emphasis was on inhibition of sexual thoughts and behaviors), whereas eating disorders reflect current society's "focus on food, dieting and body shape" (p. 45). Thus, the attempts of Victorian men and women (especially women) to ignore or suppress their sexual feelings instead of expressing them can be seen as having provoked the widespread incidence of hysterical and conversion disorders discussed and analyzed by Freud (and generally characterized by emotional distress and obsessive thoughts about sex), whereas the current cultural pursuit of thinness and consequent suppression of eating have provoked the widespread incidence of eating disorders (generally characterized by emotional distress and obsessive thoughts about food).

The response of individuals to long-term use of (and addiction to) drugs such as alcohol and nicotine (in cigarettes) also fits within this framework. In addition to the development of dependence and withdrawal as discussed earlier, failed attempts to stop drug use are often followed by short-term binges or episodes of excessive usage (Bensley, Kuna, & Steele, 1988; Marlatt & Gordon, 1985). As indicated above, the period of active inhibition is characterized by discomfort, emotionality (specifically irritability, in most cases), and cravings for the drug, which often give rise to preoccupations with the drug and its use. In other words, trying to inhibit one's dependence on alcohol or nicotine results in side effects similar to those of inhibiting other (non-drug-related but internally instigated) behaviors. Probably because of this, inhibiting one's use of such substances is also notoriously difficult to achieve (e.g., Hunt & Matarazzo, 1973; Marlatt & Gordon, 1985; Shiffman et al., 1985). As with obesity and weight loss, most people who quit smoking eventually relapse (75-80% in the first 6 months; Hunt & Matarazzo, 1973), and 50-60% of abstinent alcoholics relapse within the first 3 months (Hunt, Barnett, & Branch, 1971). Inhibiting physiologically based behavior thus seems to be extremely difficult.

EMOTION AS A BEHAVIORAL CUE

In the present conceptual framework, emotions may be seen as internally cued motivators. It has long been argued that emotions serve a communicative function, informing others of an individual's state of mind or reaction to the current situation (e.g., Andrew, 1965; Darwin, 1872/1965; Ekman, Friesen, & Ellsworth, 1972). The ability of individuals in various cultures to encode and decode affective responses has been well studied and repeatedly demonstrated (see, e.g., Ekman & Oster, 1979, for a review). The function of emotion for the individual emoter has been less well investigated, though. This is somewhat surprising, given the insistence of investigators such as Tomkins (e.g., 1978), who has maintained for many years that the communicative function of emotion is secondary to its motivating purpose for the individual. The model presented here also suggests that the function of emotion for the individual is as a motivator to behave in a manner that will be most comfortable and adaptive for the person.

Recently, Oatley and Johnson-Laird (1987) have proposed a cognitive theory of the emotions. They state that emotions act as an internal communicator that changes the relative priority of goals, as well as an external communicator for adjusting social relations. Thus, when plans are being achieved successfully, the emotion elicited is happiness, and the effect on the individual is to continue current activity patterns, modifying behavior only as it becomes necessary. A failure of an important plan or loss of a goal leads to sadness, which results in the individual's ceasing activity or searching for a new plan or focus. Oatley and Johnson-Laird propose that there are five basic emotions—happiness, sadness, fear/anxiety, anger, and disgust—which operate cognitively in this fashion.

Similarly, Nichols and Efran (1985) describe emotions as responses to goal-directed actions that are somehow incomplete or unfinished. They maintain that emotions represent "blocked actions" (p. 55). It is not possible to experience emotion intensely in the midst of important activity; the emotion occurs either in anticipation of or following the event. They illustrate this by pointing out that fear tends to occur in dangerous situations only after there is no possibility of productive action.

This concept is also similar to Tomkins's (1978) discussion of "backed-up affect." Tomkins suggests that most societies "suppress the free vocalization of affect" (p. 208) through systematic suppression (holding one's breath, among other things) and transformation, creating stress or backed-up affect, which may contribute to psychosomatic disease. As examples, he cites an elevation in blood pressure caused by unexpressed rage, and evidence found for suppressed distress in psychosomatic asthma patients.

The model presented herein posits a behavioral theory of both emotion and general motivation along the lines of such a goal-related theory. In such a behavioral model, emotions may be seen as a guide to behavior or action for the individual, as well as a means of communicating appropriate reactions to observers. If an individual ignores his or her emotions, there will be negative consequences. The affect the person feels may thus give feedback about salient aspects of the situation that need attention, and also cue the individual about how to respond behaviorally. Thus, to illustrate, someone who feels happy should continue to behave as he or she has been doing, so as to maintain the positive aspects of the situation; someone who feels sad should withdraw or seek comfort; someone who feels fearful or anxious should attempt to reduce the threat or escape the fear-inducing situation; someone who feels anger should strike out or fight back at the offending stimulus; and someone who feels disgusted should reject or push away the stimulus (and so on throughout the emotional lexicon). Performing the behaviors indicated by the affect should presumably relieve the discomfort of negative emotional arousal and maintain pleasurable affect. The goal in this model, then, is to respond in the manner indicated by the particular emotion, so as to maximize comfort and minimize distress. The specific emotion serves as a guide indicating which behavior will most efficiently provide this outcome at the present time (although for negative emotions such as anger, societal complications often make it difficult to see exactly what behavior will both express the affect and promote comfort). Affect is thus a guide, but not an explicit blueprint: Anger can be expressed by a firm statement that one is displeased and will not tolerate the situation as it stands, or by yelling and throwing things. How the affect is expressed is determined by the individual and the situation.

To use a more concrete example, an individual who has been criticized may feel the emotion of sadness, in which case he or she would look for comfort or withdraw from the criticizer (and this may or may not involve displaying or expressing sadness by crying). If the individual is successful at expressing sadness and withdraws or receives comfort, presumably the sad feeling will be alleviated and comfort will be achieved. On the other hand, someone who reacts emotionally to criticism by feeling angry would defend himself or herself and perhaps try to stop the criticizer (and again, this may or may not involve yelling or some other open manifestation of anger). Again, to the extent that the individual is successful at expressing the anger, the criticizer should cease criticizing, allowing the individual's anger to be replaced by a more positive feeling (of vindication, relief, or whatever, as long as the conflict is resolved, not escalating). This model thus builds on Tomkins's and on Oatley and Johnson-Laird's theorizing, suggesting that emotions are meant to guide behavior.

If, indeed, emotions are meant to guide our behavior, then inhibiting them should have both behavioral and perhaps further affective consequences. The extensive literature on catharsis of emotions indicates that it is indeed beneficial for individuals to express their emotions (e.g., Nichols, 1974; Nichols & Zax, 1977; Quanty, 1976; Scheff, 1979), and possibly harmful (e.g., see Pennebaker, 1985, for a review) to suppress them. Although controversy has raged since the times of Plato and Aristotle over whether catharsis purges people's passions or provokes them (Nichols & Efran, 1985), it seems that if the emotion is expressed behaviorally, one's level of emotional arousal is reduced (e.g., Baron, 1977). The benefits of catharsis, then, may stem not merely from the reliving or experiencing of strong emotions, but from an accompanying appropriate behavioral expression of such feelings. In fact, Nichols and Efran (1985) argue that catharsis actually is the *completion* of a previously interrupted (or restrained) emotional experience, and is the "expression" of a feeling rather than its "expulsion." They thus come close to the present thesis, but although they regard the experience of emotion as having two components (one of which is acting or doing), they stop short of describing the affective response as being primarily meant to elicit appropriate behaviors (as, for instance, Tomkins asserts), with negative consequences for the individual when these are not performed.

In general, then, one might expect that individuals who suppress their emotional responses and inhibit emotionally appropriate behaviors will feel worse than those who behave in accordance with their feelings. For example, if it is deemed inappropriate or "unmanly" to feel sad, some males may try to inhibit their sad affect, with the result that they do not behave "sadly" in a sad situation. Assuming that behaving sadly is the necessary or appropriate response in some psychophysiological sense, males should experience more discomfort in sad situations to the extent that they inhibit their sadness behaviorally (and perhaps cognitively, by, e.g., refusing to recognize their affect as sadness).

Preliminary data from our own laboratory support this notion, though in a somewhat indirect manner. When describing how they would respond to male and female faces portraying emotions, subjects were less likely to interpret the sad male's expression as sadness than the sad female's, and they were more likely to see the male's sadness as a desire for solitude (Polivy, Krames, & Bycio, 1988). Further testing is needed to confirm that this is a general response not limited to the particular subjects and stimuli in this initial study. If confirmed, however, this would suggest that others do not recognize sadness in males, supporting the social sanction against sadness in males. Of course, this is still a step away from a demonstration that males inhibit or do not recognize sadness in themselves.

THE ROLE OF COGNITION

Cognition has a variety of potential roles in such a model. The emotional response may be simultaneous with cognitions, in that one may feel angry simultaneously with perceiving that one is being criticized in a hostile manner or "attacked." The emotional response may precede cognitions, such that one feels sad immediately without knowing precisely why. Or the emotional response may follow and depend upon the cognitions, such that one feels angry only upon realizing that one is not wrong. However, cognitions may actually alter the initial emotional response, and thus determine the ultimate affective (and behavioral) responses (as when one talks oneself into feeling angry when one's initial response was really anxiety, and then one behaves angrily and fights back). Cognitions may thus mediate between a situation and the emotional and behavioral responses to that stimulus (see, e.g., Hoffman, 1986, for a thorough review of the relation between affect and cognition, as well as a discussion of how cognition may influence affect and vice versa).

This raises some questions about the effect of cognitively altering the affective response, and hence the behavioral response, on the ultimate outcome for the individual's state of mind. Does direct expression of the appropriate emotion provide the best "outcome" for the individual? A recent study on emotion and psychotherapy may offer some relevant data addressing this issue (Polivy, Howard, Marziali, & Yoken, 1988). Patients entering brief (12-session) outpatient psychotherapeutic treatment for nonpsychotic disorders were assessed at the beginning, middle, and end of therapy with a questionnaire measuring their self-predictions of complex emotional responses to a variety of emotion-inducing events. The patients' responses at each time were compared to the responses of a normal control group. It was found that although the patients' response patterns differed from the normal group's at the beginning of therapy, by the end of treatment they no longer differed from those of the normal group; in addition, the patients' final patterns were significantly different from their initial pretreatment responses. Initially, patients reported more emotion overall, with only happiness being reported to the same extent as normals reported it, though only anger, fear, and loneliness showed statistically significant differences. Over the course of therapy, patients' overall responses became identical to normals', with anger and anxiety changing significantly over time, and a marginal change in overall emotional intensity. Thus, in the course of psychotherapy, patients changed with respect to how they expected to respond to emotional events: They became more "normal" in their response patterns, particularly with respect to negative emotions. One might interpret this to mean that psychological distress (before therapy) was associated with inappropriate emotional responding, particularly more negative emotionality. Over the course of therapy, as patients worked through the sources of their distress, they may have learned more appropriate emotional responding; alternatively, they may no longer have "needed" to respond inappropriately.

Another possibility is suggested by Higgins's work on self-evaluation and self-discrepancies (e.g., Higgins, Strauman, & Klein, 1986). For example, if patients prior to therapy were using unrealistically high standards to evaluate themselves and their performance in various situations, they would be more likely to experience negative affect and to experience it more intensely in more situations, as was the case with the patient group in this study. Therapy may have helped patients develop more realistic guides for self-evaluation, with the result that their self-images improved, leading to more positive attributions for their behaviors and more positive affects associated with various situations.

Whatever the process, psychological distress was associated with inappropriate emotional response patterns at the beginning of the study, and improved psychological functioning at the end of therapy (as confirmed by several measures at termination) was associated with more normal emotional responding. This implies that responding inappropriately (or in a manner different from what is "normal") to emotions may lead or contribute to distress. Appropriate expression of emotions, on the other hand, seems to be connected to an improved psychological state.

Pilot data from a short-term study also support this view (Polivy, 1988). Subjects made to feel angry but forced to behave in a quiet, constrained manner (e.g., threading needles, gently tossing bean bags so as not to tip precariously perched bowls) reported feeling worse (more depressed) than angry subjects made to perform more violent tasks (hammering nails, throwing bean bags at plastic bowling pins to knock them over). Follow-up work will attempt to assess both emotional discomfort when affect cannot be expressed "appropriately," and the sort of cognitive disruption characteristic of the inhibition of other behaviors (e.g., obsessive thoughts about the inhibited behavior, distractibility).

CONCLUSIONS ABOUT THE INHIBITION OF BEHAVIOR

The attempt to inhibit internally cued or motivated behaviors seems to have predictable costs for the individual—heightened emotionality and distress, cognitive disruption, behavioral excess once the prohibition is temporarily lifted, and possible illness or disease in the long term. Whether the behavior involves an expressive motive (such as expression of emotion) or an appetitive motive (either acquired, such as smoking cigarettes or drinking alcohol, or innate, such as hunger), its suppression seems to have similar outcomes. The widely recognized difficulty of inhibiting most internally cued behavior may reflect these common unpleasant sequelae of attempted restraint. Certainly individuals who forgo such suppression of their "feelings" are more comfortable, at least in the short term. When the behavior in question is socially or medically unacceptable, the individual is faced with a dilemma: to express the behavior and feel comfortable but guilty, or to strive for acceptability and experience the negative effects of inhibition. When the behavior is known to have deleterious long-term effects, as in the case of smoking cigarettes or abusing alcohol, there may be sufficient motivation for the individual to accept the penalties of "withdrawal" and hope to achieve abstinence or behavioral control despite the odds. In cases where the long-term danger is less obviously present (if at all), such as expressing emotions or restraining eating in order to lose weight (which may not do anything to protect one against the supposed health risks of obesity), the costs of behavioral inhibition may be simply excessive.

This preliminary analysis has raised the possibility that a wide range of internally motivated behaviors may serve the common purpose of maintaining the individual at some optimal level of physical and psychological comfort, and that attempting to suppress any of these behaviors may have common consequences for the individual. This thesis clearly needs further examination. If it continues to hold up, however, it has implications for both the study of normal behavior and the treatment of psychological distress. Researchers studying the inhibition of a particular behavior should recognize the more general phenomena attendant upon suppressing any internally cued action. Therapists may find it useful to help patients to identify their feelings more accurately and act to express them appropriately. In general, the optimal response seems to be to "trust your feelings."

References

Adelmann, P. K., & Zajonc, R. B. (1989). Facial efference and the experience of emotion. *Annual Review of Psychology, 40,* 249-280.

Andrew, R. J. (1965). The origin of facial expressions. *Scientific American, 213,* 88-94.

Baron, R. A. (1977). *Human aggression.* New York: Plenum.

Bensley, L. S., Kuna, P. H., & Steele, C. M. (1988). The role of external responsiveness in drinking restraint. *Cognitive Therapy and Research, 12,* 261-278.

Breuer, J., & Freud, S. (1955). Studies on hysteria. In J. Strachey (Ed. and Trans.), *The standard edition of the complete psychological works of Sigmund Freud* (Vol. 2, pp. 1-305). London: Hogarth Press. (Original work published 1893-1895)

Buck, R. (1977). Nonverbal communication of affect in preschool children: Relationships with personality and skin conductance. *Journal of Personality and Social Psychology, 35,* 225-236.

Cofer, C. N. (1972). *Motivation and emotion.* Glenview, IL: Scott, Foresman.

Darwin, C. (1965). *The expression of the emotions in man and animals.* Chicago: University of Chicago Press. (Original work published 1872)

Derogatis, L. R., Abeloff, M. D., & Melisaratos, N. (1979). Psychological coping mechanisms and survival time in metastatic breast cancer. *Journal of the American Medical Association, 242,* 1504-1508.

Ekman, P., Friesen, W. V., & Ellsworth, P. (1972). *Emotion in the human face.* New York: Pergamon Press.

Ekman, P., & Oster, H. (1979). Facial expressions of emotion. *Annual Review of Psychology, 30,* 527-554.

Foreyt, J. P. (1987). Issues in the assessment and treatment of obesity. *Journal of Consulting and Clinical Psychology, 55,* 677-684.

Fowles, D. C. (1980). The three arousal model: Implications of Gray's two-factor theory for heart rate, electrodermal activity, and psychopathy. *Psychophysiology, 17,* 87-104.

Freud, S. (1989). Civilization and its discontents. In P. Gay (Ed.), *The Freud reader* (pp. 722-771). New York: W. W. Norton. (Original work published 1930)

Garfinkel, P. E., & Garner, D. M. (1982). *Anorexia nervosa: A multidimensional perspective.* New York: Brunner/Mazel.

Gray, J. (1975). *Elements of a two-process theory of learning.* New York: Academic Press.

Herman, C. P., Heatherton, T. F., & Polivy, J. (1989). *Distress and eating in restrained and unrestrained eaters.* Manuscript submitted for publication.

Herman, C. P., & Kozlowski, L. T. (1979). Indulgence, excess, and restraint: Perspectives on consummatory behavior in everyday life. *Journal of Drug Issues, 2,* 185-196.

Herman, C. P., & Polivy, J. (1980). Restrained eating. In A. Stunkard (Ed.), *Obesity* (pp. 208-225). Philadelphia: W. B. Saunders.

Herman, C. P., & Polivy, J. (1988). Studies of eating in normal dieters. In B. T. Walsh (Ed.), *Eating behavior in eating disorders* (pp. 95-112). Washington, DC: American Psychiatric Press.

Herman, C. P., Polivy, J., Lank, C., & Heatherton, T. F. (1987). Anxiety, hunger and eating. *Journal of Abnormal Psychology, 96,* 264-269.

Herman, C. P., Polivy, J., Pliner, P., Munic, D., & Threlkeld, J. (1978). Distractibility in dieters and nondieters: An alternative view of "externality." *Journal of Personality and Social Psychology, 36,* 536-548.

Hibscher, J., & Herman, C. P. (1977). Obesity, dieting, and the expression of "obese" characteristics. *Journal of Comparative and Physiological Psychology, 91,* 374-380.

Higgins, E. T., Strauman, T., & Klein, R. (1986). Standards and the process of self-evaluation: Multiple affects from multiple stages. In R. M. Sorrentino & E. T. Higgins (Eds.), *Handbook of motivation and cognition: Foundations of social behavior* (Vol. 1, pp. 23-63). New York: Guilford Press.

Hoffman, M. L. (1986). Affect, cognition, and motivation. In R. M. Sorrentino & E. T. Higgins (Eds.), *Handbook of motivation and cognition: Foundations of social behavior* (Vol. 1, pp. 244-280). New York: Guilford Press.

Hooley, J. M. (1986). Expressed emotion and depression: Interactions between patients and high- versus low-expressed-emotion spouses. *Journal of Abnormal Psychology, 95,* 237-246.

Hull, C. L. (1943). *Principles of behavior.* New York: Appleton.

Hunt, W. A., Barnett, L. W., & Branch, L. G. (1971). Relapse rates in addiction programs. *Journal of Clinical Psychology, 27,* 455-456.

Hunt, W. A., & Matarazzo, J. D. (1973). Three years later: Recent developments in the experimental modification of smoking behavior. *Journal of Abnormal Psychology, 81,* 107-114.

Jaffe, J. H., & Jarvik, M. E. (1978). Tobacco use and tobacco use disorder. In M. A. Lipton, A. DiMascio, & K. F. Killam (Eds.), *Psychopharmacology: A generation of progress.* New York: Raven Press.

King, G., Polivy, J., & Herman, C. P. (in press). Dietary restraint, weight and distortions in person memory. *International Journal of Eating Disorders.*

Klein, S. B. (1982). *Motivation: Biosocial approaches.* Toronto: McGraw-Hill.

Knight, L., & Boland, F. (1989). Restrained eaters: What are they trying to avoid? *Journal of Abnormal Psychology, 98,* 412-420.

Koenigsberg, H. W., & Handley, R. (1986). Expressed emotion: From predictive index to clinical construct. *American Journal of Psychiatry, 143,* 1361-1373.

Lanzetta, J. T., & Kleck, R. E. (1970). Encoding and decoding of nonverbal affect in humans. *Journal of Personality and Social Psychology, 16,* 12-19.

Ludwig, A. M., & Stark, L. H. (1974). Alcohol craving: Subjective and situational aspects. *Quarterly Journal of Studies on Alcohol, 35,* 370-373.

Marlatt, G. A. (1985). Relapse prevention: Theoretical rationale and overview of the model. In G. A. Marlatt & J. R. Gordon (Eds.), *Relapse prevention* (pp. 3-70). New York: Guilford Press.

Marlatt, G. A., & Gordon, J. R. (Eds.). (1985). *Relapse prevention.* New York: Guilford Press.

McDougall, W. (1908). *An introduction to social psychology.* London: Methuen.

Nichols, M. P. (1974). Outcome of brief cathartic psychotherapy. *Journal of Consulting and Clinical Psychology, 42,* 403-410.

Nichols, M. P., & Efran, J. S. (1985). Catharsis in psychotherapy: A new perspective. *Psychotherapy, 22*(Spring), 46-58.

Nichols, M. P., & Zax, M. (1977). *Catharsis in psychotherapy.* New York: Gardner Press.

Oatley, K., & Johnson-Laird, P. N. (1987). Towards a cognitive theory of the emotions. *Cognition and Emotion, 1,* 29-50.

Pennebaker, J. W. (1985). Traumatic experience and psychosomatic disease: Exploring the roles of behavioural inhibition, obsession, and confiding. *Canadian Psychology, 26,* 82-95.

Pennebaker, J. W., & Chew, C. H. (1985). Behavioral inhibition and electrodermal activity during deception. *Journal of Personality and Social Psychology, 49,* 1427-1433.

Pennebaker, J. W., & O'Heeron, R. C. (1984). Confiding in others and illness rates among spouses of suicide and accidental death. *Journal of Abnormal Psychology, 93,* 473-476.

Polivy, J. (1976). Perception of calories and regulation of intake in restrained and unrestrained subjects. *Addictive Behaviors, 1,* 237-244.

Polivy, J. (1988). [Initial emotion, behavioral suppression of expression, and facial affect.] Unpublished data.

Polivy, J., Garner, D. M., & Garfinkel, P. E. (1986). Thinness and social behavior. In C. P. Herman, M. P. Zanna, & E. T. Higgins (Eds.), *Physical appearance, stigma, and social behavior: The Ontario Symposium* (Vol. 3, pp. 89-112). Hillsdale, NJ: Erlbaum.

Polivy, J., & Herman, C. P. (1976). Effects of alcohol on eating behavior: Influences of mood and perceived intoxication. *Journal of Abnormal Psychology, 85,* 601-606.

Polivy, J., & Herman, C. P. (1983). *Breaking the diet habit: The natural weight alternative.* New York: Basic Books.

Polivy, J., & Herman, C. P. (1985a). Dieting and binging: A causal analysis. *American Psychologist, 40,* 193-201.

Polivy, J., & Herman, C. P. (1985b). Dieting as a problem in behavioral medicine. In E. S. Katkin & S. B. Manuck (Eds.), *Advances in behavioral medicine* (pp. 1-38). New York: SAI.

Polivy, J., & Herman, C. P. (1987). The diagnosis and treatment of normal eating. *Journal of Consulting and Clinical Psychology, 55*, 635-644.

Polivy, J., Herman, C. P., & Warsh, S. (1978). Internal and external components of emotionality in restrained and unrestrained eaters. *Journal of Abnormal Psychology, 87*, 497-504.

Polivy, J., Howard, K. I., Marziali, E., & Yoken, C. (1988). *Learning what to feel: Effects of psychotherapy on patients' self-reports of emotional responses.* Manuscript in preparation.

Polivy, J., Krames, L., & Bycio, P. (1988). *The communicative value of facial expressions of emotion.* Manuscript in preparation.

Quanty, M. B. (1976). Aggression catharsis: Experimental investigations and implications. In R. G. Geen & E. C. O'Neal (Eds.), *Perspectives on aggression* (pp. 99-132). New York: Academic Press.

Rogers, C. R. (1961). *On becoming a person.* Boston: Houghton Mifflin.

Rothenberg, A. (1986). Eating disorder as a modern obsessive–compulsive syndrome. *Psychiatry, 49*, 45-53.

Schachter, S. (1971). Some extraordinary facts about obese humans and rats. *American Psychologist, 26*, 129-144.

Schachter, S., & Rodin, J. (1974). *Obese humans and rats.* Potomac, MD: Erlbaum.

Schachter, S., & Singer, J. E. (1962). Cognitive, social, and physiological determinants of emotional state. *Psychological Review, 69*, 379-399.

Scheff, T. J. (1979). *Catharsis in healing, ritual, and drama.* Berkeley: University of California Press.

Shiffman, S. (1979). The tobacco withdrawal syndrome. In N. M. Krasnegor (Ed.), *Cigarette smoking as a dependence process.* Washington, DC: U.S. Government Printing Office.

Shiffman, S., Read, L., Maltese, J., Rapkin, D., & Jarvik, M. E. (1985). Preventing relapse in ex-smokers: A self-management approach. In G. A. Marlatt & J. R. Gordon (Eds.), *Relapse prevention* (pp. 472-520). New York: Guilford Press.

Solomon, R. L. (1980). The opponent-process theory of acquired motivation: The costs of pleasure and the benefits of pain. *American Psychologist, 35*, 691-712.

Solomon, R. L., & Corbit, J. D. (1974). An opponent-process theory of motivation: I. Temporal dynamics of affect. *Psychological Review, 81*, 119-145.

Spencer, J. A., & Fremouw, W. J. (1979). Binge eating as a function of restraint and weight classification. *Journal of Abnormal Psychology, 88*, 262-267.

Stunkard, A. J. (1975). From explanation to action in psychosomatic medicine: The case of obesity. *Psychosomatic Medicine, 37*, 195-236.

Tomkins, S. S. (1978). Script theory: Differential magnification of affects. In R. A. Dienstbier (Ed.), *Nebraska Symposium on Motivation* (Vol. 26, pp. 201-236). Lincoln: University of Nebraska Press.

Wadden, T. A., & Stunkard, A. J. (1987). Psychopathology and obesity. In R. J. Wurtman & J. J. Wurtman (Eds.), *Human obesity* (pp. 55-65). New York: New York Academy of Sciences.

Wegner, D. M., Schneider, D. J., Carter, S. R., III, & White, T. L. (1987). Paradoxical effects of thought suppression. *Journal of Personality and Social Psychology, 53*, 5-13.

Weiner, B. (1986). Attribution, emotion, and action. In R. M. Sorrentino & E. T. Higgins (Eds.), *Handbook of motivation and cognition: Foundations of social behavior* (Vol. 1, pp. 281-312). New York: Guilford Press.

Wooley, S. C., & Wooley, O. W. (1984). Should obesity be treated at all? *Research Publications of the Association of Research into Nervous and Mental Disease, 62*, 185-192.

PART II

Affect, Value, and Inference as Sources of Action

CHAPTER 5

Bridging the Gap between Values and Actions

Recent Applications of the Expectancy-Value Model

NORMAN T. FEATHER

The Flinders University of South Australia

In this chapter, I describe three recent studies in which the relations between the values that people hold and their actions in defined situations were investigated within the framework of "expectancy-value theory." This general approach to the analysis of behavior attempts to relate a person's actions to the perceived attractiveness or aversiveness of expected outcomes (Feather, 1982c). What a person does in a situation is assumed to relate to the expectations that the person holds and to the subjective value of the outcomes that may occur following the action. The expectations encompass beliefs about whether a particular action can be performed to some required standard that defines a successful outcome, and beliefs about the various positive and negative consequences that may follow the outcome. These two kinds of expectations can be distinguished at a conceptual level (Bandura, 1986a), but there continues to be debate about whether they are completely independent or interrelated (e.g., Bandura, 1986b; Eastman & Marzillier, 1984; Feather, 1986c).[1]

The expectancy-value approach provides a means of bridging the gap between knowing and doing. It has had wide application in psychology. Many years ago, I noted that the analysis of behavior in terms of expected outcomes and consequences had been applied to areas as diverse as level of aspiration behavior, social learning and clinical psychology, achievement motivation, SEU (subjectively expected utility) decision theory, the principles of performance, and the study of object preference (Feather, 1959). Over the intervening years this conceptual approach has been refined in various ways and continues to have wide application, with extensions and liberalization of the approach being most evident in recent work in human motivation and the dynamics of action (Brown & Veroff, 1986; Feather, 1982c; Kuhl, 1985).

Applications of the approach that relate to motivational psychology typically allow for the influence of relatively stable personality dispositions or motives in the models that are presented. The initial theory of achievement motivation

(Atkinson & Feather, 1966) included motives to achieve success and to avoid failure in the equations that were used to define approach and avoidance tendencies, and more recent theoretical statements continue to allow for individual differences in the strength of needs and motives (e.g., Brown & Veroff, 1986; Kuhl & Atkinson, 1986).

In my recent research, I have assumed that the class of motives includes values as well as needs, and that an important function of both needs and values is to induce "valences" (or subjective values) on events and objects within the psychological environment—so that, for example, food becomes more attractive for a hungry person, and social arrangements that foster equality between the sexes become more attractive for individuals who assign higher importance to equality within their value systems. These assumptions enable one to develop new ways of analyzing the relations between values and actions, using the basic ideas of expectancy–value theory. Before I turn to this analysis, however, it will be useful to consider some recent discussions both from cognitive-developmental theory and from social learning theory concerning relations between moral reasoning and behavior. Both approaches raise issues that are relevant to the analysis to be presented subsequently.

MORAL REASONING AND BEHAVIOR

In recent discussions, both Kohlberg and Candee (1984) and Rest (1979, 1983) have attempted to draw out the processes that link moral behavior to moral reasoning. The concept of morality that is involved in these discussions is one that relates to an ethic of rights, concerned with justice and fairness. Rest (1979) notes a number of reasons why people may not practice what they preach, and these are elaborated in a subsequent analysis of four major components of morality. These components involve (1) interpreting the situation in terms of how people's welfare might be affected by one's possible actions; (2) determining what the ideal moral course of action would be; (3) deciding which course of action to take, having weighed the possible outcomes of different courses of action; and (4) executing and implementing what one intends to do.

Rest's (1983) discussion of each of these components raises some useful points. Of particular interest is his acknowledgment that the final action taken may involve an interplay of many kinds of values, moral values being only one kind, and his further observation that implementing an intention involves the operation of ego strength and self-regulation. These ideas are compatible with recent theoretical analyses relating to motivation and volition (e.g., Heckhausen, 1986b; Kuhl, 1985, 1986, 1987). They set the investigation of moral reasoning and moral behavior in a much wider context. They also imply that a failure to behave morally can result from a deficiency in any one or more of the four components. For example, a person may misinterpret a situation where moral action is needed, may be inadequate in moral reasoning, may be influenced by other values in deciding what to do, or may lack the will to act upon the decision that has been taken.

Kohlberg and Candee (1984) refer to Brown and Herrnstein's (1975) discussion of observed discrepancies between verbally expressed moral values and actual behavior, or what Brown and Herrnstein term "talking on the high road and acting on the low road" (p. 289). Brown and Herrnstein (1975) resolve this paradox by assuming that whereas moral judgment may develop according to principles of cognitive conflict and movement through stages, moral behavior may be governed more by principles of social learning and reinforcement. Kohlberg and Candee (1984) disagree with this analysis and prefer to see moral development as a single-track process, both causing moral action and arising out of moral action itself. Thus, "there is a unitary developmental process involved in the development of both judgment and action" (p. 506). One has to discover how individuals define their own moral judgments and principles, and to consider the form taken by a person's moral reasoning as distinct from its content. These comments are not surprising, given Kohlberg's firm adherence over the years to a cognitive-developmental approach involving a concern with the structure of moral judgment and the successive transformations that occur in the way moral reasoning is organized in the course of development.

What is new is the presentation of a model of moral judgment and moral action in which Kohlberg and Candee (1984) identify four major steps: (1) interpretation of the situation, in which one's moral stage and social perspective taking have important roles; (2) decision making, in which a moral choice concerning what is fair and right is made; (3) a further judgment concerning one's responsibility and obligation to take moral action; and (4) ego controls that enable follow-through to the execution and implementation of the moral action. Kohlberg and Candee indicate that the interrelated set of events is similar to the four-component model presented by Rest (1983), but somewhat more specific in its focus. Kohlberg and Candee use the model to develop theoretical propositions that are then examined in relation to the available literature on moral reasoning and moral action. One implication of the Kohlberg and Candee analysis is that there should be more consistency between moral reasoning and moral action at higher moral stages. There is insufficient space here to describe the full development of these ideas, but it should be evident that they represent an extension of previous theoretical statements. Kohlberg and Candee also note that the model they present is compatible with other models presented by Blasi (1980) and by Locke (1983).

Note that the cognitive-developmental approach is only one perspective on the relation between moral thought and moral action. It has been subject to detailed criticism, especially by theorists who emphasize the molding effects on behavior of social learning and reinforcement (e.g., Bandura, 1986a; Mischel & Mischel, 1976). These critics point to countless examples from history where atrocities were justified by invoking high moral principles such as universal right, equality, freedom, and social equity. Indeed, Mischel and Mischel (1976) quote

Pascal's comment that "Evil is never done so thoroughly or so well as when it is done with a good conscience" (p. 107). The social learning approaches emphasize such factors as past learning in social contexts; the effects of role models; the individual's ability to self-regulate and monitor behavior in relation to internal standards and social influences; the capacity for individuals to discriminate between situations and to generalize past learning; the effects of cognitive expectancies in the initiation and maintenance of action sequences; and the role of self-generated affective consequences.

These various factors are discussed in considerable detail in Bandura's (1986a) latest work from a social-cognitive viewpoint. Bandura (1986a) accepts that developmental trends exist in moral reasoning and judgment, as they do in everything else, but comments that "the conditions of social learning are much too varied to produce uniform moral types" (p. 493). He goes on to argue that in social-cognitive theory,

> how moral thought affects conduct is not entirely an intrapsychic affair . . . it involves a reciprocality of influence between thought, conduct, and social factors. . . . The process of self-regulation, which involves moral standards, judgments, and self-regulated affective consequences, operates interactively within a network of social influences. (p. 497)

Bandura (1986a) emphasizes the role of value preferences and evaluative standards as internal sources of guidance that enable people to "give direction to their lives and to derive satisfactions from what they do" (p. 323). He indicates that learning from others is a central basis for developing and modifying values and standards. On this basis, one would expect some value preferences and evaluative standards to be idiosyncratic (based upon learning experiences specific to the individual), some to be shared within a group or culture (based upon common learning experiences at the group or cultural level), and some to be universal (based upon learning experiences that all individuals share). Both Kohlberg (1969) and Rokeach (1973) take a universalistic stance in discussions of their respective approaches, Kohlberg arguing for a set of universal stages and Rokeach for a set of universal values. I have assumed in my own theorizing that there exist universal values with a common core of meaning, but that values also have more specific connotations, depending upon individual, group, and cultural experiences (Feather, 1986a, 1988c).

Mischel and Mischel (1976) also present a wide-ranging discussion of their cognitive–social learning approach to morality and self-regulation. They distinguish between moral competence and moral conduct, and argue that "a comprehensive psychological approach to morality needs to include the individual's conceptions of what he 'should' do (his moral judgments, good–bad evaluations) as well as the moral conduct and self-regulatory behaviors required to achieve moral ideals" (p. 85). Their discussion of moral conduct and self-regulation emphasizes expected response consequences (an individual's specific expectancies about the consequences of different behavioral possibilities within a situation) and subjective values relating to possible outcomes. These subjective values can be positive or negative; they refer to stimuli that "have acquired the power to induce positive or negative emotional states in the person and to function as incentives or reinforcers for his behavior" (p. 91). The affective value (or valence) of a stimulus is assumed to depend on the exact conditions under which the stimulus occurs, and is influenced by both person and situation variables. Behavioral choices are then assumed to be guided by the subject's own behavior–outcome expectancies and by the subjective (perceived) value of potential outcomes. In addition, Mischel and Mischel (1976) discuss variables concerned with self-regulation that enable an individual to carry moral conduct through to its final goal (e.g., by relating progress to self-imposed standards and self-produced consequences).

The Mischel and Mischel (1976) analysis is similar to my own theoretical position, because it combines social learning concepts with cognitive variables that emphasize expectancies and subjective values. Before I present my approach, however, I consider one outcome of moral development that appears to be generally accepted, regardless of whether the theoretical emphasis is on cognitive development or social learning—namely, that developmental trends exist in the emergence of value priorities. My discussion of this point focuses on the likelihood that the so-called moral stages described by Kohlberg (1969, 1976) and Rest (1979, 1983) are associated with different value preferences.

MORAL STAGES AND VALUE PREFERENCES

Discussions of moral reasoning in the Kohlberg tradition are primarily concerned with the form and structure of thought rather than with its content. The major interest is in how people justify decisions about justice and fairness in relation to levels of moral maturity, and the fine-grained analysis of value content is of less concern (Feather, 1988b). The assumption by Kohlberg (1969, 1976) that stages of moral reasoning fit together in a fixed developmental sequence has been the subject of much criticism (e.g., Locke, 1979), as has the male-centered bias within the theory that appears in its focus on an ethic of rights rather than an ethic of responsibility and concern for others (Gilligan, 1982), despite evidence of gender differences in values (Feather, 1987).

There have also been attempts to link different stages of moral judgment with different value preferences. There are at least two reasons for expecting links between values and stages of moral judgment. First, stage theories of moral development assert that there is a shift to different value criteria as individuals move through successive stages toward more universal and principled modes of moral reasoning. Kohlberg's (1969, 1976) influential theory describes six moral stages that involve different criteria for moral judgment. Stages 1 and 2 are defined as preconventional and are concerned with avoiding punishment and physical damage; with obedience for its own sake; and with self-interest, instrumental purpose, and exchange. Stages 3 and 4 are concerned with conventional moral reasoning, in which one tries to live up to others' expectations, fulfills one's duties, and upholds the law. Stages 5 and 6 are concerned with principled moral reasoning, in which there is recognition of the need for a wider social contract, the equality of human rights, and respect for the dignity of individuals.

There is a second reason for expecting relations between moral judgments and particular values. It can be argued that moral judgments and value preferences both depend upon a person's socialization experiences. The values that people develop and the way in which they go about resolving moral conflicts can both be seen as partly determined by what they have learned in the past, especially in social situations (e.g., Bandura, 1986a; Mischel & Mischel, 1976). The form of socialization will vary according to a range of factors, including a person's culture, location in the social structure, membership and reference groups, gender, work environment, and mass media exposure—all of which are factors that help to shape one's personal and social identity. As an example, it has been argued that moral judgments and political attitudes may represent partially overlapping domains, both presumably relating to socialization experiences. Thus, Emler, Renwick, and Malone (1983) have asserted that individual differences in moral reasoning among adults can be interpreted as "variations on a dimension of politico-moral ideology and not as variations on a cognitive-developmental dimension" (p. 1075).

In a recent study (Feather, 1988b), I related stages of moral judgment as defined by the Defining Issues Test (DIT; Rest, 1979, 1983) to value priorities as assessed by the Rokeach Value Survey (RVS; Rokeach, 1973) and to general conservatism as assessed by the Conservatism Scale (Wilson, 1973; Wilson & Patterson, 1968). The stages identified by the DIT are very similar to those presented by Kohlberg. One can obtain a measure of the relative importance that a subject gives to Stage 5 and Stage 6 items from the DIT (i.e., the two principled stages). This measure, called the P index, indicates the degree to which a subject's moral judgments involve more abstract principles of procedural justice, rationality, and impartiality, as compared with judgments that reflect earlier stages of moral development. The scoring procedure for the DIT also allows one to obtain separate scores for stages that are below the stages of principled moral judgment. I obtained a score for each subject that related to Stage 4 moral judgment, the morality of law and duty to the social order.

I found statistically significant positive correlations between the P index and the relative importance assigned by subjects to the following values from the RVS: inner harmony and being broad-minded and logical. Negative correlations were obtained between the P index and the relative importance assigned to being clean and obedient. There were statistically significant positive correlations between Stage 4 moral judgment and the relative importance assigned to salvation and obedience, and negative correlations between Stage 4 moral judgment and the relative importance assigned to excitement, love, pleasure, open-mindedness, and imagination. Stage 4 scores and Conservatism Scale scores were positively correlated ($r = .27$, $p < .01$).

Thus, principled moral judgment was positively associated with terminal and instrumental values from the RVS that concerned harmony, logic, and open-minded inquiry, and negatively associated with values that concerned cleanliness and obedience. Principled moral thinking as exemplified by DIT responses to the moral dilemmas therefore involved a greater commitment to values concerned with the virtues of harmony, reason, and tolerance, and a downgrading of values concerned with deference to conventional authority and rules of conduct. In contrast, Stage 4 moral judgment was linked to conservative values, with a higher regard for obedience and respect for authority and less emphasis on a life of pleasure and excitement, on love and intimacy, and on imaginative and open-minded ways of thinking.

These differences can be restated by using Schwartz and Bilsky's (1987, in press) classification of motivational domains, which are assumed to encompass the universal types of motivational concerns that values express. In terms of this classification, the results suggest that principled moral thinkers can be seen as placing more emphasis on values falling within motivational domains concerned with maturity and self-direction, and less emphasis on values within the domain of restrictive conformity. Stage 4 moral thinkers can be seen as placing more emphasis on values falling within the domains of security and restrictive conformity, and less emphasis on values that fall within the domains of self-direction, maturity, and enjoyment.

I find it more plausible to assume that these different value preferences influence the nature of thinking and the direction that thought takes, rather than that the form of thought somehow determines the content of values. Both the emergence of values and higher levels of cognitive development would be influenced by socialization processes and by particular learning experiences. They would also be constrained by biological givens and by maturational processes. But there is plenty of evidence to show that values play a key role in the choices that individuals make, in the plans that guide their behavior, in the way they justify their decisions, and in the way they structure their beliefs and attitudes (Feather, 1975, 1979, 1984, 1987; Rokeach, 1973, 1979). I refer to some of this evidence later in this chapter, especially in relation to behavior. Values also change in relative importance as individuals move through the life cycle and take on new roles and responsibilities as they grow older (Feather, 1975, 1980; Rokeach, 1973). Thus, I prefer to see values as variables that help to shape or structure thought across the life span, rather than as variables that follow transformations in the formal structure of thought.

In a functional sense, values may be seen to express both motivational concerns and societal demands. This view is central to Rokeach's theoretical analysis of values; it is also prominent in my own work (Feather, 1975, 1986c, 1987) and in the Schwartz and Bilsky (1987, in press) analysis of the universal content and structure of values. One implication of the results that I have just presented is that different levels of moral reasoning may be linked not only to different value preferences, but also to different kinds of motivation.

In the present volume (Chapter 6), Sorrentino, Raynor, Zubek, and Short reinterpret cognitive-developmental theories in terms of an analysis of a theory of personality functioning and change that involves the concepts of information value, affective value, the psychological career, and stages of striving. Their theory reflects an elaboration of the expectancy–value approach to the analysis of action (Feather, 1982c) and takes account of individual differences in resultant information and affective value. Sorrentino et al. give particular emphsis in their chapter to individual differences in resultant information value, which they investigate in terms of differences in uncertainty orientation (see also Sorrentino & Short, 1986). Uncertainty-oriented individuals are assumed to be primarily motivated by a need to seek clarity through the mastery of uncertainty. In contrast, certainty-oriented individuals are assumed to be motivated by a need to maintain clarity by adhering to what is already known. Thus, uncertainty-oriented individuals tend to be open-minded and curious about new and possibly inconsistent information. Certainty-oriented individuals tend to prefer the familiar and predictable, to have an authoritarian and dogmatic way of knowing, and to have a low tolerance of ambiguity.

These individual-difference variables remind me of variables that I introduced in an earlier analysis of information-seeking behavior, where I assumed that seeking information can be related to motives to achieve consistency and to avoid inconsistency; expectations about the likelihood of achieving consistency and avoiding inconsistency; and the positive and negative incentive values of consistency and inconsistency. These variables were assumed to combine to determine action tendencies to seek information that leads to consistency and to avoid information that leads to inconsistency. Seeking out consistent or inconsistent information was assumed to reflect the effects of these two tendencies as well as other extrinsic tendencies (see Feather, 1967a, 1969, for a fuller discussion).

The Sorrentino et al. discussion (Chapter 6) is relevant because they propose that uncertainty-oriented individuals prefer principled moral thinking, whereas certainty-oriented individuals prefer conventional moral solutions. It is reasonable to assume that the values that I found to be associated with principled moral thinkers and with Stage 4 moral thinkers in the study previously described (Feather, 1988b) would also discriminate between uncertainty-oriented and certainty-oriented individuals, especially given the fact that uncertainty orientation is assessed via a projective measure of n Uncertainty linked with low scores on an authoritarianism scale. Thus, I would expect uncertainty-oriented individuals to assign less importance to values concerned with restrictive conformity and security and to show other value differences when compared with certainty-oriented individuals, who are likely to be more conservative and authoritarian in their attitudes and less tolerant of ambiguity. I have previously described value differences relating to differences in conservatism, intolerance of ambiguity, and Protestant ethic values that are also consistent with the prediction just made (Feather, 1971b, 1979, 1984).

In summary, I would see the so-called stages of moral reasoning described by Kohlberg (1969, 1976) and Rest (1979, 1983) as associated with different value preferences that are complexly determined by a variety of factors. The values themselves express basic motivational concerns as well as societal demands, and they influence the ways of thinking about problems that individuals adopt. My concern in the remainder of this chapter, however, is less with the nature of thought and more with the analysis of behavior. The bridge that I construct to link values and actions involves an elaboration of expectancy–value theory, to which I now turn.

VALUES, VALENCES, AND EXPECTATIONS

My interest in conceptualizing relations between values and actions extends beyond moral values (however they may be defined) to the wider domain of human values. Rokeach (1973, 1979) provides illuminating discussions of the concept of "value" and the ways in which a person's value systems might be assessed. Rokeach (1979) conceives of values as

> cognitive representations of human needs on the one hand and of societal demands on the other. They take the psychological form of prescriptive or prospective beliefs about the desirable means and ends of action. They are organized hierarchically to serve as standards or criteria . . . that the socialized self—a self born with biological needs continuously shaped by societal demands—employs to judge the efficacy of itself not only as a competent self . . . but also as a moral self. (p. 295)

My treatment of values owes much to Rokeach, but has unique aspects as well (Feather, 1975, 1986c). This is apparent in the following statement (Feather, 1982d), where values are conceived of as

> organized summaries of experience that capture the focal, abstracted qualities of past encounters, that have a normative or oughtness quality about them, and that function as criteria or frameworks against which present experience can be tested. . . . But they are not affectively neutral abstract structures. They are tied to our feelings and can function as general motives. (p. 275)

Values can be conceptualized as part of the class of general motives, just as needs also fall within this class. In this regard I differ from McClelland (1985), who argues that it is important to separate motives and values (see also Veroff, 1986). McClelland believes that motives are best measured by coding motivational concerns in associative thought or fantasy; they are not necessarily conscious, and so may not be identified by persons as part of their self-image. Values, on the other hand, are conscious and are intimately tied to a person's view of self. Projective measures of motives, such as *n* Achievement and *n* Power, are essentially uncorrelated with questionnaire measures of values. Moreover, motives are assumed to play a greater role in operant behaviors, whereas values are better predictors of cognitive choices. Thus, "motives are more important for predicting what a person will spontaneously do, whereas values are more important for determining what [the person] will cognitively decide should be done" (McClelland, 1985, p. 536).

My own preference is to consider needs and values as having some distinctive characteristics, but as also having a degree of functional and conceptual overlap (Feather, 1986c). The differences relate to the fact that values are tied to a normative base involving a dimension of goodness–badness. No necessary connection seems to exist, however, between needs and normative evaluations of goodness and badness. It is clear that "The desired is not always the desirable; goodness and badness are not identical to pleasure and pain; sometimes 'want' and 'ought' coincide, but by no means always; and action often takes place in the absence of conscious evaluation" (Feather, 1975, p. 300). Values are more verbalizable and closer to conscious levels of awareness than many underlying needs, and they are also an integral part of the self-concept (McClelland, 1985; Rokeach, 1973).

Despite these differences between values and needs, I believe that it is useful to consider them both as instances of the general class of motives. As motives, both needs and values can be assumed to influence a person's subjective definition of a situation, so that objects, activities, and states of affairs within the immediate situation are seen as having positive valence (they become attractive) or negative valence (they become aversive), to use Lewin's (1936) terminology.

Needs and values therefore function to induce valences. They influence a person's cognitive–affective appraisal of a situation in relation to both means and ends. The possible actions that can be performed, and the outcomes and consequences that can follow from these actions, become linked to the affective system. Some become invested with positive or negative affect, and some remain neutral. A hungry person sees food as attractive; a fearful person constructs a world fraught with danger. A person for whom equality is an important value sees social arrangements that are aimed at reducing inequalities as attractive; a student who values being logical perceives academic courses that call for expressive and divergent modes of thought as undesirable and to be avoided. In each of these cases, actions and possible outcomes become invested with positive or negative affect within the constructed map of a person's anticipations, depending upon the dominant needs and values.

The precise way in which this process occurs awaits more detailed analysis, but recent contributions from cognitive psychology that emphasize links between affect and cognition may provide some answers (Feather, 1986b). I refer to some of these contributions later in this chapter. One can assume that specific features of a situation key into a person's motive and value structures, and that once the connection is made, "the affective system is recruited in such a way as to provide an added dimension to cognitive appraisal, one that involves anticipations of positive and negative affect associated with the different actions and outcomes that are available within the defined situation" (Feather, 1986c, p. 154).

The assumption that values can induce valences that are coordinated to experienced and anticipated positive and negative affect associated with actions and outcomes provides only part of the theoretical network necessary for predicting relations between values and actions. A basic tenet of the expectancy–value approach to the psychology of motivation is that the prediction of action must take expectations or subjective probabilities into account as well as valences. I assume that these expectations encompass both efficacy expectations and expectations that concern outcome-related consequences.

One can elaborate the concept of expectation even further, as Heckhausen (1977, 1986a) has done in relating expectations to a four-stage sequence of events: the initial situation as perceived, the person's own action, the outcome of the action or situation, and the consequences of the outcome. In Heckhausen's view, the anticipated outcome is the pivotal point in the building of expectancies. For Heckhausen (1986a), an "outcome" is any "motive-relevant alteration of the initial situation that remains at least temporarily . . . having no incentive value in itself" (p. 447). It is assumed to acquire incentive value as a result of its potential consequences. The same outcome may give rise to several kinds of consequences and to different consequences for different individuals. Heckhausen (1986a) points out that individuals can influence outcomes (e.g., by ability or effort), but many consequences of outcomes cannot be influenced directly by the actor because they depend upon the responsiveness of the environment. Moreover, the distinction between outcome and consequences enables one to determine the degree to which actions are intrinsically or extrinsically motivated, depending on the extent to which the consequence is endogenous to the action or exogenous to the action and its outcome (e.g., Kruglanski, 1975).

Heckhausen defines four different kinds of expectancies in terms of how the outcome relates to the other three stages in the sequence. These four kinds of expectancies are "situation–outcome expectancies," "action–outcome expectancies," "action × situation–outcome expectancies," and "outcome–consequence expectancies." Heckhausen believes that the first two types of expectancies have typically been confounded in motivational theory (e.g., by Tolman), and that the fourth type was neglected until it became an important focus of instrumentality theories dealing with job satisfaction and work motivation (e.g., Mitchell, 1982; Vroom, 1964).

Most expectancy–value models have focused upon action–outcome expectancies, to use Heckhausen's (1977) term. These are defined in the single case by a person's subjective estimate of the likelihood that a given action will lead to a specified outcome within the immediate situation that provides the context for action. "Efficacy expectancies" refer to the "conviction that one can successfully execute the behavior required to produce the outcomes" (Bandura, 1977, p. 193). An efficacy expectation can be seen as belonging to the same family of concepts that include perceived competence, person as "origin," perceived control, mastery, the concept of "can," and self-concept of ability. Heckhausen (1986a) equates self-efficacy with what he calls an action–outcome expectancy and distinguishes it from an outcome–consequence expectancy. This latter expectancy is seen by Heckhausen as equivalent to what Bandura (1977) terms an "outcome expectancy," defined as "a person's estimate that a given behavior will lead to certain outcomes" (p. 193). Heckhausen notes that Bandura does not distinguish between an action outcome and its consequences, but uses the term "outcome" in the sense of a consequence of an action outcome (e.g., the social reactions, personal benefits, and self-satisfactions that might follow from achieving a high level of performance in a competition). However, Bandura (1986b) does assert the necessity of distinguishing between the specifying criteria of a performance level and the consequences of achieving that performance level.[2]

Applications of expectancy–value models usually assume that subjects are able to execute the response that is required, and they focus upon the implication relations that are involved in action–outcome expectancies (i.e., on the perceived likelihood that actions will lead to outcomes). Bandura (1977) is correct, however, in drawing attention to the importance of perceived self-efficacy as an important aspect of expectations, even though in a recent statement (Bandura, 1986b) he asserts:

> Because self-percepts of efficacy are formed through acts of self-appraisal based on multidimensional information, perceived self-efficacy is more closely allied to the field of human judgment than to the subject of expectancy, which refers to an anticipation that something is likely to happen. (p. 362)

Expectations about what leads to what in a defined situation, however, also involve judgments about likelihood, and they are also based upon multiple sources of information (Feather, 1982a, 1986c; Weiner, 1980, 1986a).

I accept, however, that one can distinguish conceptually between efficacy beliefs that are linked to the self-system and beliefs that concern the consequences of expected performances or outcomes, even though these two types of beliefs may often be intertwined and are not always easy to disentangle at an empirical level (Eastman & Marzillier, 1984; Bandura, 1986a, 1986b, 1988; Feather, 1986c; Heckhausen, 1986a). As Bandura (1988) states, "People act on their beliefs about what they can do, as well as their beliefs about the likely effects of various actions. The effects of outcome expectancies on performance motivation are partly governed by self-beliefs of capabilities" (p. 39).

Clearly, there have been important developments in the conceptual analysis of expectations in recent years. We need further exploration of the implications of distinctions that have been made between different types of expectation in regard to human behavior (choice, performance, and persistence). We also require more analysis of other questions, including the determinants of expectations; the implications of specifying expectations along dimensions such as strength, magnitude, and generality; the interrelationships between different types of expectations; the degree to which expectations are connected to the self-system; the process by which expectations become chained together and refined; their relationship to other concepts in the literature, such as schemas, scripts, and plans; the extent to which expectations involve conscious experience and cognitive content; and the ways in which expectations might be measured (Feather, 1982a, 1982b, 1986c).

Within expectancy-value theory, valences and expectations in combination are assumed to guide actions. Thus, whether a person has a tendency to act in a particular direction will depend on that person's expectation about whether he or she can perform the action to the required standard, on a further set of expectations about the potential consequences of the action, and on the valences (or subjective values) associated with the activity and with the anticipated action outcome. Those actions will be preferred that can be coordinated to the dominant motivational or action tendencies that relate to a combination of these expectations and valences. Usually, the combination is assumed to be a multiplicative one.

The preceding analysis presents in skeletal form the theoretical framework that I have used to model relations between values and actions. I now turn to three recent studies in which this form of analysis was applied.

THREE STUDIES

Participating in Social Movements

James Newton and I investigated differences between individuals in regard to their willingness to join a social movement organization (Feather & Newton, 1982). We presented subjects enrolled in a first-year course in introductory psychology at Flinders University with detailed descriptions of two social movement organizations. The first organization was called the "Movement to Promote Community Standards," and the second was called the "Campaign to Safeguard Individual Rights." These two organizations were contrasted in the values they were said to promote. The Movement was described as a more traditional, conservative organization, and the Campaign was presented as being much more liberal in its stance toward individual rights and social issues. The description of each organization was presented in the form of a pamphlet, which subjects read before giving their responses; these descriptions occurred in counterbalanced order in the questionnaires that contained them.

After reading each description, subjects were asked to check specific actions that they would be willing to volunteer to undertake in support of each organization (they were asked to assume that they had 10 hours of free time each week). The list included such actions as signing a petition to be sent to the proper authorities, handing out pamphlets on street corners, and participating in peaceful rallies and marches. The number of actions that they checked was the first measure of willingness to assist the organization. A second measure used was the number of hours subjects said that they would be prepared to contribute to the organization (again, under the assumption that they had 10 hours of uncommitted time available).

Our subjects also completed Form D of the RVS (Rokeach, 1973), ranking the 18 terminal values and the 18 instrumental values in order of importance for themselves in accordance with the usual instructions. Rokeach's list of terminal values contains such values as equality, freedom, family security, and social recognition; the instrumental list contains such values as being ambitious, courageous, loving, and self-controlled. The terminal values are assumed to represent general goals; the instrumental values are thought to represent ways of behaving or modes of conduct.

We also obtained a measure of attitude toward each organization ("To what extent do you personally agree or disagree with the views expressed in the pamphlet published by this organization?"), and a measure of expectancy of success ("How helpful do you think your own personal efforts will be as a contribution to the organization's success?").

It was assumed that aspects of the description of the social movement organization would have positive or negative valence, depending upon the value priorities held by each person. For example, subjects who assigned a great deal of importance to being ambitious and obedient and to salvation would be expected to see statements that described the organization as supporting "hard work and investment," "respect for legitimate authority," and "decent standards of morality" as attractive (or as having positive valence). Other aspects of the pamphlet that criticized "progressive intellectuals" and deplored a "misguided obsession with civil liberties" would be expected to have negative valence for people who ranked such values as freedom and being broad-minded and intellectual high in relative importance within their own value priorities.

Newton and I did not measure the actual pattern of valences elicited by each pamphlet. Clearly, this should be done in future research. Instead, we assumed that each subject's attitude toward the organization would reflect a cognitive integration of the positive and negative valences relating to the descriptive statement for that organization. Thus, the resultant affective reaction that defined a person's overall attitude was conceived of as an integration of valences, or experienced and anticipated positive and negative affective charges, that referred to specific features of the organization; these valences, in turn, were thought of as being determined by underlying general value priorities, according to a sequence that moved from values to induced valences to the overall attitude.

Some support for this sequence came from the fact that the values from Rokeach's lists related to the attitude measures in the direction that one would predict. For example, those subjects who expressed more agreement with the views in the pamphlet that concerned the conservative "Movement to Promote Community Standards" tended to rank salvation, family security, and being obedient, polite, and self-controlled as more important values, and mature love, equality, a world of beauty, freedom, and being broad-minded, imaginative, and intellectual as less important values, when compared with those subjects whose attitude toward the Movement was less favorable. Previous studies of conservatism have found similar relations between value priorities and conservative attitudes (Feather, 1979).

The results of the study showed that there were statistically significant positive correlations between both action measures and the measures of attitude and expectancy. Thus, favorable attitudes and positive expectancies predicted action when taken independently of each other (see Table 5.1). A hierarchical

TABLE 5.1 Correlations Relating Action Measures to Attitude, Expectancy, and Their Multiplicative Combinations

	Action measures				
	Number of volunteer actions for Movement or Campaign			Number of volunteer hours for Movement or Campaign	
Independent variables	n	r	r^2	r	r^2
Movement					
Attitude	134	.616	.380	.495	.245
Expectancy	127	.341	.116	.309	.095
Attitude × expectancy	127	.673	.452	.579	.335
Campaign					
Attitude	134	.466	.217	.369	.136
Expectancy	133	.340	.115	.302	.091
Attitude × expectancy	133	.487	.237	.411	.169

Note. Expectancy and attitude toward the Movement were not significantly correlated ($r = .123$), but expectancy and attitude toward the Campaign were significantly correlated in the positive direction ($r = .246$, $df = 131$, $p < .01$). All correlations in this table are statistically significant, most of them at a high level ($p < .001$). From "Values, Expectations, and the Prediction of Social Action: An Expectancy-Valence Analysis" by N. T. Feather and J. W. Newton, 1982, *Motivation and Emotion*, 6, 217–244. Copyright 1982 by Plenum Publishing Corp. Reprinted by permission.

multiple-regression analysis showed that adding expectancy to attitude led to statistically significant increases in the amount of variance in the action measures that could be accounted for (see Table 5.2). Thus, an additive combination of attitude and expectancy led to a better prediction of each behavioral variable than did either attitude or expectancy considered alone. The further addition of the attitude × expectancy product led to statistically significant increments in the variance for the Movement measures but not for the Campaign measures. This product term was included because in expectancy-value models, behavioral measures are typically related to the product of expectations and subjective values (valences) rather than to their sum.

We also conducted a follow-up study in which the degree of commitment to action was increased by presenting a pamphlet under more realistic conditions (Feather & Newton, 1982). Subjects were led to believe that they were volunteering for action with a genuine organization that would contact them personally. Thus, the questions concerned actual commitments rather than hypothetical commitments. The results lent further support to our analysis of the conditions under which values relate to overt action.

Note that the theoretical approach that has been described is similar in some ways to that used by Fishbein and Ajzen (1975) in their analysis of attitude-behavior relations, but with some distinctive differences (Feather & Newton, 1982, pp. 240–241). One major difference is that we did not include a normative component in the conceptual analysis, believing that it should be possible to model compliance with social norms by using the expectancy–value framework rather than by adding a separate term to the equation. For example, one might assume that needs for social approval and affiliation induce valences on selected outcomes (e.g., having the approval of significant others). One could then derive action tendencies that relate to these valences, weighted by the relevant expectations. The final resultant action tendency would then represent a sum of a number of component tendencies, each modeled in expectancy–value terms (i.e., the same form of theoretical analysis would be used throughout). The question of how theories of motivated action can take account of normative and group pressures is an important one that requires further attention. Certainly these kinds of pressures have to be considered. In many cases, they override the individual preferences that would be expressed if these pressures were absent.

Looking for Employment

Findings from a major longitudinal study of young people leaving school in metropolitan Adelaide provide further information that is relevant to the expectancy–value formulation. This study was conducted in collaboration with another colleague, Gordon O'Brien. Students in the final three grades of high school were first tested in 1980 while they were still at school, and then followed up in 1981

TABLE 5.2   Multiple Correlations (*R*'s) and Proportions of Variance Explained (*R²*'s) from Hierarchical Multiple-Regression Analyses Predicting Action Measures from Attitude and Expectancy

	Action measures					
	Number of volunteer actions for Movement or Campaign			Number of volunteer hours for Movement or Campaign		
Independent variables	*R*	*R²*	*R² change*	*R*	*R²*	*R² change*
Movement						
Step 1. Attitude	.616	.380	.380***	.495	.245	.245***
Step 2. Expectancy	.672	.451	.071***	.554	.307	.062***
Step 3. Attitude × expectancy	.689	.474	.023*	.583	.340	.032*
Campaign						
Step 1. Attitude	.466	.217	.217***	.369	.136	.136***
Step 2. Expectancy	.521	.271	.054**	.429	.184	.048**
Step 3. Attitude × expectancy	.525	.275	.004	.432	.186	.003

Note. From "Values, Expectations, and the Prediction of Social Action: An Expectancy-Valence Analysis" by N. T. Feather and J. W. Newton, 1982, *Motivation and Emotion*, 6, 217-244. Copyright 1982 by Plenum Publishing Corp. Reprinted by permission.
    *$p < .05$; **$p < .01$; ***$p < .001$.

and 1982 when they were either students, employed, or unemployed. Control groups were included in the investigation to permit us to check the effects of both repeated testing and general social change. The main variables included in the questionnaires were measures of self-concept, values, external control, job need, affect and psychological well-being, job confidence, attributions for unemployment, and the attribution dimensions of internality, stability, globality, personal uncontrollability, and external uncontrollability (Feather & O'Brien, 1986a, 1986b).

Most relevant are the results from two groups of unemployed subjects (Feather & O'Brien, 1987). One group was unemployed in 1981; the other was unemployed in 1982. The results of a factor analysis involving the 1982 sample revealed a set of interpretable factors, including two that were used to define expectancy and valence. The first of these factors was called Control–Optimism, because it linked confidence about finding a job with feelings of control and self-efficacy. Five variables were used to define this factor. These variables were feeling that one has some control over being unemployed, feeling confident about finding the job one really wants in the near future, feeling confident about finding any kind of job in the near future, believing that the cause of one's present unemployment may not be present in the future, and believing that one can change the cause of one's present unemployment. This factor was taken to reflect subjects' expectations of finding employment, fusing confidence about finding a job with beliefs that one is not helpless but can exert control and change the underlying causes that influence outcomes. The second factor was called Job Valence, and it was defined by three variables. These variables involved a measure of how much one needs a job and two measures of how depressed or disappointed one feels about being unemployed. This factor, therefore, was seen as fusing need for a job with depressed feelings. The two factors that were obtained were similar to the Helpless–Pessimism and Employment Importance factors obtained in an independent factor-analytic study with schoolchildren (Feather, 1986b). Thus, conceptually and empirically, we were on firm ground in proceeding to the next step of the investigation, in which job-seeking behavior was related to the expectation and valence measures.

Job-seeking behavior was measured by an item that has been used in a previous study of unemployment (Feather, 1982e). Subjects were asked how frequently they looked for a job. They could check one of six responses: "Not looking for a job," "When I feel like it," "Monthly," "Weekly," "Every couple of days," and "Daily." The questionnaire also contained a number of measures of work values. I report results here for only one of these, the Mirels and Garrett (1971) Protestant Ethic Scale, which was modeled on Weber's (1905/1976) classic analysis of the work ethic. Items on this scale emphasize the virtues of industriousness, asceticism, and individualism (Feather, 1984).

Finally, the questionnaire also included items concerned with the social class of the family (income and education of parents), degree of social support received from parents, job history (number of jobs applied for since becoming unemployed, duration of unemployment measured in weeks), teachers' ratings of academic potential, and the usual background and demographic items.

TABLE 5.3 Correlations between Variables for 1981 and 1982 Unemployed Respondents

Variable	Control-Optimism	Job Valence	Support	Duration unemployed	Job applications	Sex of respondent	Work ethic	Job seeking
Control-Optimism	—	-.26***	.12*	-.26***	-.20***	-.04	.06	-.07
Job Valence	-.04	—	.07	.11*	.16**	-.00	.19***	.40***
Support	.14	.20*	—	-.08	-.01	.16**	.12*	.04
Duration unemployed	-.19*	.14	-.09	—	.45***	.01	.03	.15**
Job applications	-.13	.08	-.13	.28**	—	.06	-.06	.28***
Sex of respondent	-.01	.23**	.21*	.10	.08	—	-.05	-.02
Work ethic	.27**	.31***	.17	-.13	-.10	.12	—	.11*
Job seeking	-.17	.30***	-.11	.18*	.26**	.04	-.06	—

Note. Tests of significance are two-tailed. Sex of respondent was coded as follows: 1 = male, 2 = female. Correlations for the 1982 sample are above the diagonal; correlations for the 1981 sample are below the diagonal. From "Looking for Employment: An Expectancy-Valence Analysis of Job-Seeking Behaviour among Young People" by N. T. Feather and G. E. O'Brien, 1987, *British Journal of Psychology*, 78, 251–272. Copyright 1987 by the British Psychological Society. Reprinted by permission.

*p < .05; **p < .01; ***p < .001.

The complete findings from this study are reported elsewhere (Feather & O'Brien, 1987). Table 5.3 presents the intercorrelations between the major variables for the 1981 and 1982 samples separately. Note that we found statistically significant positive correlations for both samples between Job Valence and job-seeking behavior, but Control–Optimism and job-seeking behavior were unrelated. Job Valence and work ethic were positively correlated in both samples, and these correlations were also statistically significant.

Figure 5.1 presents the results of a path analysis for the 1982 sample. Table 5.4 reports the results of a hierarchical multiple-regression analysis for both samples, in which an even wider range of variables was considered in relation to job-seeking behavior. Neither set of findings altered the conclusions derived from the simple correlations—namely, that job-seeking behavior was positively related to Job Valence but unrelated to Control–Optimism, and that values linked to the work ethic predicted Job Valence. Figure 5.1 also shows that frequency of current job-seeking behavior was predicted by the number of job applications respondents reported making since they became unemployed; that there was a negative relation between Control–Optimism and length of unem-

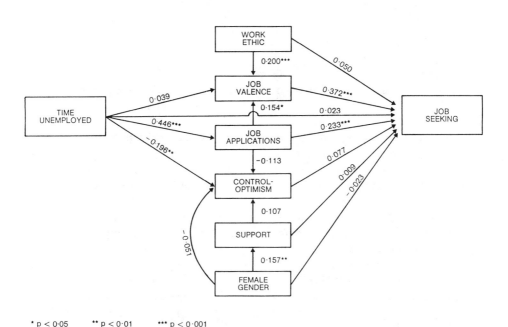

* p < 0·05   ** p < 0·01   *** p < 0·001

FIGURE 5.1 Path diagram linking job-seeking behavior to time unemployed, work ethic, Job Valence, job applications, Control–Optimism, support, and female gender. The numbers on the lines are standardized beta coefficients. From "Looking for Employment: An Expectancy–Valence Analysis of Job-Seeking Behaviour among Young People" by N. T. Feather and G. E. O'Brien, 1987, *British Journal of Psychology, 78,* 251–272. Copyright 1987, by the British Psychological Society. Reprinted by permission.

TABLE 5.4   Multiple Correlations (*R*'s) and Proportions of Variance Explained (*R²*'s) from Hierarchical Multiple-Regression Analyses Predicting Job Seeking

		1982 sample: Job seeking			1981 sample: Job seeking		
Step	*Independent variable*	*R*	*R²*	*R² change*	*R*	*R²*	*R² change*
1.	Social class + academic potential + age + sex	.089	.008	.008	.085	.007	.007
2.	Support	.101	.010	.002	.136	.019	.011
3.	Work ethic	.143	.020	.010	.143	.020	.002
4.	Length unemployed + job applications	.330	.109	.088***	.292	.086	.065*
5.	Control-Optimism	.330	.109	.000	.315	.099	.014
6.	Job Valence	.471	.222	.113***	.440	.194	.094**
7.	Control-Optimism × Job Valence	.477	.228	.006	.445	.198	.004

Note. From "Looking for Employment: An Expectancy-Valence Analysis of Job-Seeking Behaviour among Young People" by N. T. Feather and G. E. O'Brien, 1987, *British Journal of Psychology, 78,* 251-272. Copyright 1987 by the British Psychological Society. Reprinted by permission.
*p < .05; **p < .01; ***p < .001.

ployment (more weeks out of a job being associated with lower Control-Optimism); and that female respondents reported more parental support than male respondents. These results are discussed in more detail in the original report (Feather & O'Brien, 1987).

Note that in this study of job-seeking behavior, the assumption that values influence valences was tested directly and was confirmed. But the results were only partially consistent with the expectancy–value analysis: Although the measure of valence predicted job-seeking behavior, the measure of expectation did not. This negative result for the expectation variable is surprising; possible reasons for it are given in the original published report (Feather & O'Brien, 1987) and in my recent book concerned with the psychological impact of unemployment (Feather, 1989). The negative finding may reflect problems of measurement or complexities that are introduced when ongoing behavior involves real-life events (see also Mineka & Hendersen, 1985). Once one moves outside the laboratory to investigate the stream of behavior as it occurs in everyday life, variables such as our Control-Optimism factor may be involved in complex ways with changes in other variables, such as coping styles, cognitive–affective appraisals, motivational forces, and the self-concept. Theoretical models and research procedures that deal with changing processes, with the dynamics of action, with patterns of self-beliefs, and with action control may then become more appropriate as aids to understanding the behavior that is being considered (e.g., Atkinson & Birch, 1970; Heckhausen, Schmalt, & Schneider, 1985; Higgins, Tykocinski, & Vookles, in press; Kuhl, 1986; Weiner, 1986a, 1986b). For example, recent theoretical analyses of relations among the self-concept, affect, and motivation (Higgins et al., in press) and of the role of causal attributions in relation to motivation and emotion (Weiner, 1986a, 1986b) may help to explain a turning away from job seeking on the part of some unemployed individuals. Following Higgins et al. (in press), it could be argued that dejection-related emotions following from chronic unfulfilled hopes or from a chronic failure to realize positive potential may be associated with low motivation to look for a job. Weiner's (1986a, 1986b) analysis implies that negative emotions associated with causal attributions to internal and stable causes (such as lack of ability), combined with low expectancies, may lead to reduced motivation to seek employment. I have discussed these two approaches, along with other theoretical ideas that are relevant to understanding the psychological effects of unemployment, in my recent book (Feather, 1989).

Some variables that account for individual differences in responses in constrained laboratory settings may become much less important sources of variance in real-life contexts, where there is a wider set of influences and where actions occur in relation to the realities of situational constraints, social norms, task requirements, and other imposed conditions. For example, various external pressures (e.g., from parents) may push young people to look for employment even when they have very low expectations of success. Any tendency in young unemployed people to scale down job-seeking behavior because of low expectations may then be counteracted by their compliance with normative pressures to look for a job.

The failure to find the predicted positive relation between the Control-Optimism factor and job-seeking behavior could also be interpreted as due to an application of the expectancy-value analysis that was too general as far as coordinating definitions were concerned. It could be argued that we would be more likely to find relations involving the expectation variable if the expectations were related to specific behaviors linked to particular outcomes instead of to a person's general Control-Optimism about finding a job. Most laboratory studies that employ expectancy-value theory specify the alternative behaviors and potential outcomes in detail, as when a study of choice, performance, or persistence is conducted under controlled conditions. We were limited in how much information we were able to ask for about our variables, because we had to keep our questionnaire to a reasonable length. A more molecular investigation of expectations and valences might have provided better support for the theoretical ideas that we were testing. Despite these limitations, however, some of our predictions were confirmed.

Enrolling in University Courses

The final study to be described here was concerned with enrollment decisions made by university students at Flinders University (Feather, 1988d). I was interested in linking students' enrollment in humanities, social science, and science courses to measures of the perceived attractiveness-aversiveness of mathematics and English (valence measures) and to measures of self-concepts of ability for mathematics and English (expectancy measures). I expected that students who placed higher value on mathematics and who had higher self-concepts of ability for mathematics would be more likely to enroll in science versus social science versus humanities courses, in that order, and that students who placed higher value on English and who had higher self-concepts of ability for English would be more likely to enroll in humanities versus social sciences versus science courses, in that order. In each case, a person's decision to enroll in a course would be related to the subjective value or valence assigned to a key requirement of success (mathematics or English) and to the person's expectation that he or she could work at mathematics or English successfully.

In line with previous investigations (e.g., Eccles, Adler, & Meece, 1984), I also expected to find evidence of gender differences in the subjective value assigned to mathematics and English, with male students placing more value on mathematics when compared with female students, and female students placing more value on English.

Finally, I expected to find that the subjective value or valence of mathematics and English would be related to the personal values held by the students. It was hypothesized that the extent to which a student valued mathematics would be related to personal values linked with convergent and controlled modes of thought that emphasize logic and the following of rules, and that higher subjective value placed on English would relate to personal values linked with expressive and prosocial concerns. Again, therefore, I was interested in investigating the relation between general values and more specific valences.

These hypotheses were tested by using data obtained from students beginning a first-year course in introductory psychology at Flinders University. The students completed a questionnaire administered to them prior to commencement of their course. They indicated which school of the university they had enrolled in; on this basis, they were classified as humanities, social sciences, or science students. Measures of self-concepts of ability were obtained by combining information about perceived past grades in either mathematics or English with students' own ratings of their ability to do well at mathematics or English. These self-concept-of-ability measures involved beliefs about what each person was capable of doing, rather than beliefs about the possible consequences of success or failure. Hence, they tapped efficacy expectations rather than outcome–consequence expectations (Bandura, 1986a).

The measures of valence were based on a conceptual analysis of subjective task value by Eccles et al. (1983), in which task value was conceptualized in terms of four major components: attainment value, intrinsic value or interest, utility value, and cost. The value that a person places on enrolling in mathematics, for example, would depend upon how important it is for the person to do well in mathematics; how much enjoyment he or she gets out of engaging in the activity; the extent to which working at mathematics is instrumental to reaching a range of long- and short-term goals; and the cost of engaging in the activity in relation to what is lost, given up, or suffered. Three items for mathematics and three items for English when designed to cover the first three of these four components, and responses to each respective set of items were combined to provide measures of mathematics valence and English valence.

General values were assessed by asking students to rate the importance of each of the 18 instrumental values from Form D of the RVS (Rokeach, 1973). A factor analysis of the intercorrelations between ratings across subjects for the 18 values showed that there were three readily interpretable factors, and these were employed to provide three derived scales. The first derived scale was called Restrictive Control, and it involved five values (clean, obedient, polite, responsible, and self-controlled). The second derived scale, called Prosocial Concern, involved three values (forgiving, helpful, and loving). The third derived scale, titled Intellectual Orientation, involved two values (intellectual and logical). These three value composites were used in testing the predictions that related the subjective value or valence of mathematics and English to personal values.

The correlations obtained between the major variables supported the main predictions (Feather, 1988d). These correlations are reported in Table 5.5. Table 5.6 and Figure 5.2 present the results of more detailed analyses (hierarchical multiple regression, path analysis) involving a wider range of variables. It can be seen in Figure 5.2 that mathematics ability and mathematics valence predicted course enrollment; that Restrictive Control predicted mathematics valence; that Prosocial Concern predicted English valence; that female gender predicted both mathematics valence and English valence (in opposite directions); that female gender predicted Prosocial Concern; and that ability and valence measures were positively associated. English valence predicted course enrollment, but English ability and course enrollment were not linked together in these wider analyses. The regression analyses showed that a multiplicative combination of mathematics ability and mathematics valence made a statistically significant contribution to the variance in course enrollment when added to the regression equation (Table 5.6).

These findings, along with others, are reported and discussed in more detail in the original report (Feather, 1988d). The results involving mathematics ability and mathematics valence provided stronger support for the expectancy–value analysis than those relating to English, after other variables were taken into account in the path analysis and in the hierarchical multiple-regression analysis. Like the results of the unemployment study, results from this investigation again provided direct evidence to support the assumption that general values influence specific valences. Finally, the findings indicated gender differences that were generally in line with results obtained previously (e.g., Eccles et al., 1984; Feather, 1987).

WIDER IMPLICATIONS

What are the wider implications of these studies? It should be clear that the hypotheses that were tested represent a significant advance on simple ideas that values will directly determine action. Instead, these hypotheses were developed

TABLE 5.5 Correlations between Variables

Variable	Correlations							
	EA	MV	EV	RC	IO	PC	Sex	Course enrollment
Mathematics ability (MA)	.03	.40***	-.13**	-.01	.07	.00	.01	.29***
English ability (EA)		-.20***	.45***	-.08	.04	.06	.08	-.19***
Mathematics valence (MV)			-.05	.21***	.11*	.05	-.10*	.22***
English valence (EV)				.07	.03	.23***	.17***	-.40***
Restrictive Control (RC)					.32***	.41***	-.02	.02
Intellectual Orientation (IO)						.19***	-.01	.06
Prosocial Concern (PC)							.13**	-.04
Sex of subject								-.10*

Note. Correlations are based on pairwise deletion of missing cases. The *n*'s for the correlations ranged from 434 to 443. Tests of significance are two-tailed. Sex of subject was coded as follows: 1 = male, 2 = female. Course enrollment was coded as follows: 1 = humanities, 2 = social sciences, 3 = sciences. From "Values, Valences, and Course Enrollment: Testing the Role of Personal Values within an Expectancy-Value Framework" by N. T. Feather, 1988, *Journal of Educational Psychology, 80,* 381–391. Copyright 1988 by the American Psychological Association. Reprinted by permission.
*p < .05; **p < .01; ***p < .001.

TABLE 5.6   Multiple Correlations (R's) and Proportions of Variance Explained (R²'s) from Hierarchical Multiple-Regression Analyses Predicting Course Enrollment

		Course enrollment		
Step	*Independent variables*	R	R^2	R^2 change
1.	Social class + age + sex	.227	.052	.052***
2	Restrictive Control + Intellectual Orientation + Prosocial Concern	.245	.060	.009
3.	Mathematics valence	.319	.102	.042***
4.	Mathematics ability	.368	.135	.033***
5.	Mathematics ability × mathematics valence	.394	.155	.020**
1.	Social class + age + sex	.277	.052	.052***
2	Restrictive Control + Intellectual Orientation + Prosocial Concern	.245	.060	.009
3.	English valence	.439	.193	.132***
4.	English ability	.439	.193	.000
5.	English ability × mathematics valence	.448	.201	.008
1.	Social class + age + sex	.227	.052	.052***
2	Restrictive Control + Intellectual Orientation + Prosocial Concern	.245	.060	.009
3.	Mathematics valence + English valence	.478	.229	.168***
4.	Mathematics ability + English ability	.501	.252	.023**
5.	Mathematics ability × mathematics valence + English ability × English valence	.521	.271	.020**

Note. From "Values, Valences, and Course Enrollment: Testing the Role of Personal Values within an Expectancy-Value Framework" by N. T. Feather, 1988, *Journal of Educational Psychology*, *80*, 381-391. Copyright 1988 by the American Psychological Association. Reprinted by permission. *$p < .05$; **$p < .01$; ***$p < .001$.

within the framework of a long-established motivational approach, expectancy-value theory, with the added assumption that a person's general values can induce valences both on alternative ways of behaving and on expected outcomes. Taken as a whole, the results of the three studies provide encouraging support for this approach, and they do so in three quite different contexts: assisting a social movement organization, seeking employment, and choosing an academic course. Each study raises particular issues that are relative to that investigation; these have been discussed more fully in the individual reports (Feather, 1988d; Feather & Newton, 1982; Feather & O'Brien, 1987). The conceptual leverage provided by the expectancy-value approach provides a new agenda for the analysis of relations

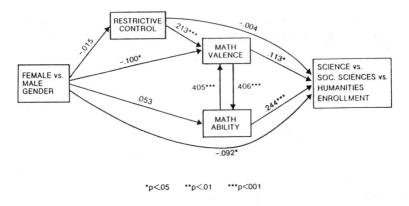

*p<.05   **p<.01   ***p<001

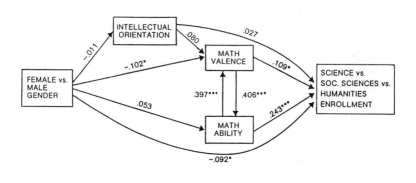

*p<.05   **p<.01   ***p<001

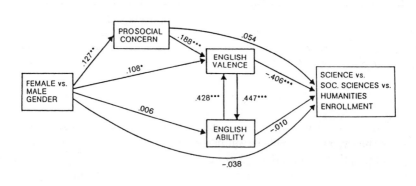

*p<.05   **p<.01   ***p<001

FIGURE 5.2 Path diagram linking course enrollment to valence, ability, values, and sex of student. The numbers on the lines are standardized beta coefficients. From "Values, Valences, and Course Enrollment: Testing the Role of Personal Values within an Expectancy-Value Framework" by N. T. Feather, 1988, *Journal of Educational Psychology, 80,* 381–391. Copyright 1988 by the American Psychological Association. Reprinted by permission.

between values and actions—one that links this analysis with theoretical developments from the psychology of motivation.

How do the present ideas relate to the moral reasoning and social learning forms of analysis described at the beginning of this chapter? The theoretical basis for the three studies clearly differs from the general approach adopted by Kohlberg and Candee (1984) and Rest (1983) in their discussions of moral judgment and moral action. The analysis is concerned with motivational rather than developmental issues. It takes account of individual differences in specific values, whereas central to moral judgment theory is the form of reasoning that individuals employ when they respond to moral dilemmas. Nevertheless, a conceptual analysis in terms of expectations and valences does not neglect the effects of the past in shaping a person's abilities, motives, and beliefs. Indeed, there is a long research tradition associated with Atkinson, McClelland, and their colleagues that is concerned with how motives such as the needs for achievement, affiliation, and power develop (e.g., Atkinson & Birch, 1978; McClelland, 1985; Veroff, 1986); there is a similar interest in the development of expectations (e.g., Feather, 1982a, 1982b; Weiner, 1980). In addition, recent extensions to the analysis of cumulative achievement explicitly deal with relations between past events and present conditions (Atkinson, 1974; Revelle, 1986). Despite this, the major emphasis in a motivational analysis is on how present behavior can be accounted for in terms of immediate conditions that involve the person and the situation. The analysis of developmental outcomes has somewhat secondary status when the focus is on what Lewin (1936) would call the present field.

The theoretical formulation that I have presented shares some common ground with Bandura's social-cognitive theory. Bandura's wide-ranging theory is more than a theory of motivation, because it addresses issues concerned with learning and cognition and the complex interactions among thought, affect, action, and environmental influences. However, Bandura's (1986a, 1988) emphasis on the motivational impact of goal structures and the role of self-evaluation, perceived self-efficacy, and self-set standards is compatible with the expectancy–value approach and with other analyses of goal-directed behavior (e.g., Locke, Motowildo, & Bobko, 1986). Thus, expectancies are central concepts both in expectancy–value theory and in Bandura's (1986a) social-cognitive theory; moreover, both forms of analysis recognize the ongoing nature of behavioral events and the modifications that occur in the light of experience. This latter emphasis becomes most apparent in expectancy–value theory when the theory is coordinated with recent developments that are concerned with the dynamics of action and the processes underlying change in activity (e.g., Kuhl & Atkinson, 1986).

Bandura (1986a), however, gives less attention to the valence concept, preferring to emphasize the importance of feelings of self-dissatisfaction as a motivator of enhanced effort when standards are not met in the course of task performance (e.g., Bandura & Cervone, 1983). Thus, people are represented as acting to reduce negative states that are the products of comparisons in which self-standards are central and the subjective reality falls short of those standards. As I have noted in a previous discussion (Feather, 1986c), this way of thinking seems to ignore the positive side of human action—the fact that much of a person's behavior "can be seen as directed toward immediate and long-term goals that arouse anticipations of positive affect" (p. 149). It may well be the case that social-cognitive theory can meet this point by a more detailed conceptual analysis of the status of incentive motivators. Note that other investigators have recently proposed outcome value or outcome importance as an additional component of a self-efficacy model (Maddux, Norton, & Stoltenberg, 1986; Manning & Wright, 1983; Teasdale, 1978). A formal integration of the valence variable into self-efficacy theory would create even more common ground between Bandura's (1986a) social-cognitive approach and expectancy–value theory, though some important differences would still remain.

One apparent difference is the lack of interest in relatively stable personality variables shown by social-cognitive theory. There may be several reasons for this lack of interest. It may reflect a belief that specific situational variables and individual learning experiences have a much more important status in the prediction of behavior than variables that define relatively stable differences in personality; it may reflect a skepticism that these personality differences can be identified and measured reliably; it may reflect a belief that it is a better strategy to look for general principles than to incorporate personality variables into theoretical models from the very start (e.g., Weiner, 1980, 1986b). The present approach explicitly allows for the incorporation of needs and values into the theoretical analysis, mainly as variables that influence the valences of events and outcomes.

FUTURE DEVELOPMENTS

How might the value–action model that I have presented be further developed? A number of general points are suggested by the three studies I have described. They relate to the conceptual analysis of expectations and valences, to the interrelations between expectations and valences, to the activation of values, and the role of volition.

Conceptual Analysis of Expectations and Valences

As noted previously, there is a need to distinguish between different types of expectation (e.g., efficacy and outcome-consequence expectations), both conceptually and at the level of measurement; it must be recognized, however, that disentangling expectations and their dimensions may not be an easy task in some contexts. In measuring expectations, one probably needs to give more attention to the particular behavior that has to be performed and to the specific outcomes and consequences that might occur (e.g., to how an unemployed person handles an interview for a specified job) than to less defined actions and outcomes (e.g., to finding employment in general).

More theoretical attention should also be paid to the nature and determinants of valences. I have conceptualized the valences of possible activities and outcomes in terms of anticipated positive and negative affects, but we need more conceptual analysis of how links with the affective system are made, whether on the basis of past learning or built-in mechanisms. The wider analysis of valences is a neglected area in psychology, crying out for attention (Feather, 1986c). Expectancy–value theory has provided conceptual analyses of valences (e.g., Feather, 1986c; Heckhausen, 1977; Mitchell, 1982; Rotter, 1954, 1982; Vroom, 1964), and there have been contributions from other theoretical frameworks as well (e.g., Wright, Contrada, & Patane, 1986). I have assumed that the valences of events and outcomes are influenced by general personality dispositions (needs and values), but they are not the only influences (Feather, 1982a, 1982b). Other variables also have effects (e.g., the objective characteristics of possible outcomes, the difficulty of a task, the expected consequences that follow a particular outcome, the amount of personal control that one can exert, moods and other states of the person). We can list various factors that influence the subjective attractiveness and aversiveness of objects and events, but we are still a long way from having a comprehensive theory about the processes that determine valences or demand characteristics in particular situations.

Recent contributions at the interface of cognition and affect should add to our knowledge. For example, Hoffman (1986) has discussed various modes of information processing that generate affective responses to an event:

> (1) direct affective response to the physical or sensory aspects of a stimulus (sight, sound, smell, feel); (2) affective responses to the match between the physical or sensory aspects of a stimulus and an internal representation or schema; and (3) affective responses to the meaning of a stimulus beyond its physical and sensory aspects (its causes, consequences, implications for the self. (p. 245)

The second and third modes appear to be most relevant in the present context. For example, information that is consistent with an underlying value schema would be expected to generate positive affect; events that are categorized as exemplars of a particular value should evoke more positive affect than those that are not categorized as exemplars. Hoffman (1986) also considers preparatory transformations of a stimulus that lead to the generation of affect, and discusses the ways in which affect elicited through any of the models influences subsequent information processing.

Fiske and Pavelchak (1986) have also discussed the generation of affective responses in terms of information-processing models, distinguishing between category-based and piecemeal-based responses. Their analysis draws on the concepts of category and schema and on the effects of successful versus unsuccessful categorization. They relate their analysis to research in person perception and social cognition.

Weiner's (1986a) theoretical analysis of attribution, emotion, and motivation also gives affect a central place in relation to outcomes and causal attributions. His approach implies that the anticipated affect associated with an outcome relates to how a person might construe the causes of the outcome. Potential success at a task might generate more anticipated positive affect, for example, if the individual were to construe success at the task as indicating a high level of skill rather than as due to the fact that the task is easy.

The recent development by Higgins (1987) of self-discrepancy theory also has implications for the analysis of affect. Discrepancies that involve relations among the "actual" self, the "ought" self, and the "ideal" self, and that take account of the person's own perspective and the perspective of significant others, are assumed to be related to different kinds of affect. For example, a discrepancy between the actual/own self-concept and the ideal/own self-guide (a particular kind of self-directive standard) is predicted to make the person more vulnerable to dejection-related emotions such as disappointment and dissatisfaction. A discrepancy between the actual/own self-concept and the ought/own self-guide (another kind of self-directive standard) is predicted to make the person more vulnerable to agitation-related emotions, especially guilt, self-contempt, and uneasiness. Recent extensions of the theory have incorporated the "can" self and the "future" self, and the relations between different configurations of actual self, ideal self, can self, and future self have been elaborated (Higgins et al., in press).

These various approaches demonstrate a lively interest in the analysis of cognition and affect; they have obvious relevance for the analysis of the concept of valence, given that the positive and negative valences of objects and events are assumed to be linked to the cognitive, affective, and motivational systems.

Interrelations between Expectations and Valences

We need more analysis of the interrelations between expectations and valences. When are these variables independent, and when are they related either positively or negatively? I discussed this issue many years ago in relation to the range of expectancy–value models that was available at that time (Feather, 1959). In a more recent review of expectancy–value models (Feather, 1982a), I concluded that

> there was agreement that valences and expectations would not be independent in situations where success and failure could be evaluated against standards of excellence and where outcomes were relevant to a person's self-concept insofar as perceptions of ability, skill, and effort were concerned. (p. 57)

In these situations, success would be seen as more attractive (or more positively valent) for more difficult levels of a task where expectations of success would be lower, and failure would be seen as more aversive (or more negatively valent) for easier levels of a task where expectations of success would be higher. This kind of assumption was made by Atkinson (1958) in his theory of achievement motivation, and earlier by Lewin, Dembo, Festinger, and Sears (1944) in their analysis of level of aspiration behavior (see other discussions by Feather, 1982b; Heckhausen et al., 1985; Kuhl, 1982).

Note, however, that the results of the study of choice of academic courses (Feather, 1988d) showed that the valence of mathematics or English was positively related to a student's self-concept of ability in mathematics or English (see Figure 5.2). Thus, those who assigned higher value to mathematics or English also tended to have higher self-concepts of ability at mathematics or English, respectively. These results could be taken to indicate that those who like working at a task tend to do better at it, or that those who perform well as a task come to value it more. In regard to achievement motivation theory, however, these results could also be taken to imply a positive relation between expectations and valences: Higher expectations of success at a task might be associated with higher subjective task value.

Do these results contradict the assumptions made in achievement motivation theory that expectations and valences are negatively related—that the positive valence of success and the negative valence of failure are inverse functions of the corresponding subjective probabilities of success and failure (Atkinson & Feather, 1966; Feather, 1982a)? I do not believe so. One needs to understand the intervening processes that link expectations and valences. The way in which an individual explains success or failure would seem to be especially important (Weiner, 1986a, 1986b). For example, negative relations between expectations and valences in achievement-related situations may reflect the fact that success at a task is more attractive when it can be attributed to high ability (as would be the case if it were known that most others fail at the task) and failure at a task is more aversive when it signals low ability (as would be the case if it were known that most others succeed at the task). These negative relations would then be genotypically similar to the positive relations between ability and valence found in the study of academic choice (Feather, 1988d). Both types of relation can be seen as evidence for the proposition that actions and outcomes that reflect ability and skill are positively valued, and, more generally, for the proposition that the valence of activities and outcomes depends in part upon the extent to which these activities are seen to involve valued attributes of the self. This interpretation is clearly consistent with the line of argument that I have presented in this chapter.

Valences can also have an effect on expectations; that is, the influence can work in the opposite direction. For example, a person may be more unduly optimistic about his or her chances of success when a large reward is at stake than when the reward is small. These effects of valence on subjective probability are more likely to occur when cues about subjective probabilities are conflicting, ambiguous, or ill defined, and when a person's expectations are not solidly grounded in relation to a consistent past record of success and failure. That is, motivational factors have more impact when expectations are not or cannot be firmly based (Feather, 1967b).

We also need to investigate the conditions that affect the relative weights assigned to expectations and valences in determining motivational or action tendencies. The usual assumption is that these variables combine multiplicatively to determine action tendencies, but it is possible that expectations and valences have different weights, depending upon individuals and situations. Kuhl (1982,

1986), in discussing applications of a method called "logical statement analysis," has observed that subjects' behavior does not always seem to be a function of the conjunction of expectancy and valence (the logical analogue of a multiplicative relationship). Kuhl (1986) states:

> Some subjects seem to base their decisions entirely on value-related information, ignoring the subjective chances of success, at least in some situations. Others focus on expectancy-related information. . . . Some subjects even combine expectancy- and value-related information disjunctively. (p. 410)

Kuhl (1986) notes that similar individual differences regarding the type of information that affects motivation have been found in achievement-related contexts (see Raynor & McFarlin, 1986; Sorrentino & Short, 1986). Whether one is influenced mainly by expectations or by valences may also depend upon the nature of the situation. For example, where situations are structured at a wishful level, individuals may attend more to the subjective values or valences of possible events and discount the subjective probabilities. Realistic expectations may become more important in situations where the stakes are high and where mistakes could be very costly (Feather, 1959, 1982a).

Activation of Values

We need more theoretical analysis of how needs and values are engaged in a situation. For example, what makes some values rather than others salient at a particular time? As noted elsewhere (Feather, 1986c), cognitive models that deal with information processing, affective networks, and attitude accessibility may provide theoretical leads for a detailed answer to this question.

Fazio (1986) has described a process model that is applied to the question of how attitudes guide behavior. He argues that a person's social behavior largely depends upon his or her perceptions in the immediate situation in which the attitude object is encountered. These perceptions involve perceptions of both the attitude object and the context or situation (see also Rokeach, 1972). These two components make up a person's definition of an event, and this definition is assumed to be crucial in the attitude–behavior link. Fazio (1986) assumes that an individual's attitudes will influence this definition—an assumption that has a long history in attitude theory (Allport, 1935; Katz, 1960; Smith, Bruner, & White, 1956). Fazio (1986) notes, however, that the way a person defines an event is also influenced by his or her knowledge of what behaviors are or are not normatively appropriate. Subjective norms may influence a person's definition of the situation and subsequent behavior in such a way as to override immediate perceptions of attitude-linked objects. One may disapprove of the manner in which a waiter delivers service in a restaurant, but may still provide a tip because social norms dictate this form of behavior.

Attitudes can only play a role in influencing a person's definition of an event if these attitudes are activated from memory. As Fazio (1986) points out, "Unless the attitude is accessed from memory, it cannot produce selective perception of the object in the immediate situation. The individual may never consider the attitude object in evaluative terms" (p. 212). Fazio (1986) discusses variables that influence whether individuals will access their attitudes upon encountering an attitude object. This activation may occur because of the presence of some situational cue that is relevant to the attitude. It may also depend upon the strength of the attitude, where strength is defined in terms of the strength of the association between the attitude object and an affectively based evaluation (positive or negative). Fazio (1986) observes:

> Even without prompting from situational cues . . . the attitudes of people for whom the object–evaluation association is strong may be activated when they encounter the attitude object and may affect their perceptions of and behavior toward the object. A relatively weak association, on the other hand, may mean that the attitude is never activated in the encounter with the object; hence, behavior occurs without any guidance from the attitude. (p. 214)

Fazio (1986) describes experiments from his own program of research that generally support the process approach. These studies have examined the effects on attitude accessibility of direct or indirect experience with the attitude object; the use of a "priming" paradigm for investigating attitude activation; parallels between response latency to an attitudinal inquiry and the likelihood of spontaneous activation; the role of selective attention in the attitude-to-behavior process; and other topics. Fazio (1986) also relates his approach to other attempts to model attitude–behavior relations that involve more controlled forms of information processing (e.g., the theory of reasoned action developed by Ajzen & Fishbein, 1980), in contrast to his own emphasis on more automatic forms of processing. He concludes that a more comprehensive model would integrate his approach with approaches that assume more controlled processes. Thus, he suggests the following (Fazio, 1986):

> An integrative model might involve the possibility of the present automatic process if the attitude is activated from memory upon mere observation of the attitude object. If the attitude is not activated automatically, then a more controlled process . . . may still produce attitude–behavior consistency, provided that some situational variable (such as highly consequential decision settings) motivates the individual to retrieve from memory and carefully consider his or her attitudes. If the object–evaluation association is too weak for automatic activation to occur, and if the situation does not motivate a controlled analysis, then attitudes cannot be expected to motivate behavior. (p. 238)

I have given some attention to Fazio's analysis of attitude-to-behavior relations, because in some ways it resembles my own approach to bridging the gap between values and actions. I could also have drawn parallels with self-discrepancy theory (Higgins, 1987, 1989), because the self-guides that form part of that theory are valued end states that function as standards for the actual self to meet. Higgins assumes that as cognitive structures they function according to the same accessibility and activation factors that characterize any other knowledge structure. He also considers self-guides to be motivational variables, in the sense that wholistic patterns between the self-concept and self-guides have affective and motivational significance. In my analysis, however, I am much more concerned with the content and structure of values, with positive affect as well as negative affect, and with integrating values into the expectancy–value framework than I am with the effects of self-discrepancies.

As noted previously, I assume that the values that people hold are tied to an affective base. Indeed, I have related values to my earlier analysis of abstract structures (Feather, 1971a), conceived as underlying schemas against which incoming information can be tested. Abstract structures are residues or summaries of past experience that provide continuity and meaning under changing environmental circumstances. They are organized cognitive structures, and they are relatively stable. But they are also susceptible to change as the person encounters new and discrepant information that cannot readily be interpreted in terms of existing abstract structures.

In the earlier article (Feather, 1971a), I considered the question of how individuals resolve discrepancies between abstract structures and the perceived information that comes from the immediate situation in relation to theoretical analyses of communication effects, causal attributions, and attitude-related recall. Later I discussed the concepts of values and value systems as examples of abstract structures that are tied to an affective base (Feather, 1975). Values, for example, have a number of defining characteristics that distinguish them from other concepts such as needs and attitudes (Feather, 1975; Rokeach, 1973). As a general belief about what is or is not desirable, however, a value can also be conceptualized as an abstract structure or concept involving an associative network that is tied to our feelings. Each of us, for example, has a concept of what freedom means and how desirable freedom is. This concept derives its meaning from the network of associations in which it is embedded—a network that involves not only relatively neutral cognitive associations, but affective associations as well. We can feel emotional about freedom, approve of those who support freedom, and disapprove of those who oppose freedom.

I would argue that values are more readily activated in a situation if they are strongly held values and if there are cues in the situation that trigger them off. For example, when equality is a very important value within a person's value system, it may be activated with relative ease, and the person may become sensitive to many different forms of equalities and inequalities within situations. The value is readily activated because it is strong; once activated, it has widespread effects on how the person defines situations. As a further example, freedom as a value will be more readily elicited in situations where there are threats to freedom than in situations where such threats do not exist. In this case, relevant cues in the situation are an important basis for the activation of the value, and the value may be elicited even though it may be less important than other values that remain latent. This type of analysis has obvious similarities to Fazio's (1986) discussion of the activation of attitudes.

My approach, however, goes back a further step, because I see values as more general concepts than attitudes. Unlike attitudes, they are not tied to specific objects, but they transcend objects and situations. They are fewer in number than a person's attitudes; moreover, in contrast to attitudes, they function as standards or criteria. Values also occupy a more central position in relation to self-conceptions than attitudes do. These and other differences have been discussed in the value literature (Feather, 1975; Rokeach, 1973). They imply a form of hierarchical organization with values at a deeper and more abstract level than attitudes (see also Homer & Kahle, 1988). As I have indicated earlier in this chapter, I assume that values function like motives to induce valences on objects and events; hence, they are central to how a person defines situations in terms of cognitive–affective appraisals. The valences or affective evaluations that are attached to different objects and events within the immediate situation define the more specific attitudes that people hold toward these objects and events (Feather & Newton, 1982). As noted previously, these valences are influenced by a number of variables, not only by a person's needs and values. Finally, the valences and expectations in combination are assumed to influence the particular actions that are taken within defined situations.

It will be evident that my approach overlaps with Fazio's (1986) process model but has its own distinctive features. I have attempted to incorporate ideas both from cognitive theory and from value–attitude theory into the framework of expectancy-value theory, a basic approach to the analysis of motivated behavior. My approach links with cognitive theory in that values are conceived as abstract structures and are tied to a motivation–affective base with all that this entails. It converges with attitude theory in the sense that valences can be conceptualized as attitudes toward objects and events that involve positive or negative evaluations. To say that an object, event, or activity is attractive or aversive is to say that one has an affectively charged positive or negative attitude toward it. The attitudes that I deal with in the present analysis, however, are keyed to the momentary situation, and they are not necessarily stable (although they can be so). They may change from situation to situation and from time to time as they are influenced by the variables that determine positive and negative valences at any given moment. Because of this, it is useful to maintain the distinction between attitudes and valences in the language that we employ, with "attitudes" referring to the more stable orientations and "valences" to the attractive and aversive features of the momentary situation. The determinants of valences extend beyond a person's needs and values to encompass other variables as well, some of which I have mentioned in the earlier discussion (e.g., the perceived consequences of outcomes, the causal attributions that a person makes, the objective characteristics of objects and events).

In a general sense, however, it can be said that the present analysis links induced attitudes to personally held general values and that these positive and negative attitudes toward objects and events, together with cognitive beliefs or expectancies, are assumed to influence the action that is taken.

The Role of Volition

A final comment is suggested by the emphasis given by both Kohlberg and Candee (1984) and Rest (1983) to self-regulation in their analyses of links between moral judgment and moral action. This emphasis is compatible with new developments in the psychology of motivation that stress the role of volition. For example, Kuhl (1985, 1987) argues that action tendencies wax and wane in the dynamic flow of behavior, even when the expectancies and valences associated with them remain constant (see also Kuhl & Atkinson, 1986; Kuhl & Blankenship, 1979). Kuhl distinguishes between an intention and a motivational tendency. An intention is defined as "an activated plan to which an actor has committed herself or himself" (Kuhl, 1987, p. 282). Converting a motivational tendency to an intention thus requires an act of will and the linking of the action tendency to a plan that can be accessed from memory. Once activated, an intention is maintained and protected according to processes of action control. Thus, according to Kuhl (1987),

> People do not always act according to their current hierarchy of motivational tendencies. Somebody who has just decided to stop smoking might still feel a stronger urge to smoke than to chew gum, but he or she may end up enacting the initially weaker motivational tendency (i.e., chewing gum) as a result of a superordinate control process which gradually changes the relative strengths of the two competing action tendencies in favor of the intentional commitment. (p. 281)

Kuhl (1987) presents a model of action control that involves a motivation system and three memory systems (action memory, semantic memory, emotional memory). He also describes a dimension of action orientation versus state orientation along which individuals may vary: Action-oriented people are more likely to focus on a fully developed and realistic action plan, and state-oriented people are more likely to focus on past, present, or future states (especially unrealistic goals). These orientations are assumed to define the flexibility or rigidity of the motivational maintenance system that is involved in action control.

These ideas and other related discussions (e.g., Heckhausen, 1986b; Heckhausen & Gollwitzer, 1987) mark a renewed interest in the psychology of volition, and they suggest that volition should be distinguished from motivation. If one accepts this distinction, then some new directions emerge in the conceptual analysis of relations between values and actions. Most important, perhaps, is the need to analyze a person's degree of commitment to a planned course of action and the ways in which a course of action is protected and maintained once initiated. Such analyses should provide deeper understanding of the conditions under which dominant motivational tendencies linked to values are in fact acted upon.

CONCLUSION

It is evident that there is plenty of scope for further development of the motivational approach that I have outlined in the present chapter. But the results of the three studies that I have discussed show that it is a feasible approach for analyzing relations between values and actions. Applications of this approach that go beyond the laboratory should recognize the wider set of conditions that apply in real-life contexts, where actions occur in relation to the realities of situational constraints, social norms, group pressures, task requirements, and other imposed conditions. It is also important to recognize that a great deal of behavior occurs without much thought about expected consequences. Research on judgment conducted in recent years indicates that the routine use of convenient heuristics may circumvent more rational forms of judgment based upon conscious reflection (e.g., Kahneman, Slovic, & Tversky, 1982; Nisbett & Ross, 1980).

I return, however, to my conviction that much of human behavior can be seen in relation to means-end structures that involve beliefs about the implications of events—beliefs extending beyond present actions to the potential outcomes of these actions and to the possible future consequences of the outcomes. Thus, I assume that people possess cognitive structures that concern the implications of their actions, both now and in the future. These implication structures may not always be well defined; they may be in error; and one would expect them to vary in detail from person to person. But they are assumed to exist and, along with subjective values, valences, or utilities, to be important determinants of goal-directed behavior.

Notes

1. This chapter is an expanded and revised version of an earlier article (Feather, 1988a). The "value" aspect of the expectancy-value approach refers to incentive values and not to the values that people hold. Indeed, a major focus of this chapter is to discuss relations between human values and subjectively perceived incentive values. In order to avoid confusion, I refer in some of my recent publications to the "expectancy-valence model," where the term "valence" refers to the perceived attractiveness (positive valence) or aversiveness (negative valence) of actions or outcomes. Because the term "expectancy-value" has wider currency, I use it in the present chapter, but it has the same meaning as "expectancy-valence."

2. The term "outcome expectancy" has been used in two different ways, and it is important to note these differences. In the expectancy-value approach, an outcome expectation relates to response-outcome contingencies within a defined situation. These expectancies are action-outcome expectancies, to use Heckhausen's (1977, 1986a) term. The history of this concept has been discussed by Atkinson (1982). Action-outcome expectancies have received a great deal of attention in the literature over many years. They are a major focus of my book on expectations and actions (Feather, 1982c). As used by Bandura (1977, 1986a), however, the term "outcome expectancy" refers to an outcome-consequence expectancy, again to use Heckhausen's (1977, 1986a) term. The focus is on what the outcome leads to, rather than on what the action leads to. To avoid confusion in the future, investigators should refrain from using the term "outcome expectancy" and instead should distinguish clearly between action-outcome expectancies and outcome-consequence expectancies.

References

Ajzen, I., & Fishbein, M. (1980). *Understanding attitudes and predicting social behavior.* Englewood Cliffs, NJ: Prentice-Hall.

Allport, G. W. (1935). Attitudes. In C. Murchison (Ed.), *Handbook of social psychology* (pp. 798–844). Worcester, MA: Clark University Press.

Atkinson, J. W. (1958). *Motives in fantasy, action, and society.* Princeton, NJ: Van Nostrand.

Atkinson, J. W. (1974). Motivational determinants of intellective performance and cumulative achievement. In J. W. Atkinson & J. O. Raynor (Eds.), *Motivation and achievement* (pp. 389–410). New York: Wiley.

Atkinson, J. W. (1982). Old and new conceptions of how expected consequences influence actions. In N. T. Feather (Ed.), *Expectations and actions: Expectancy-value models in psychology* (pp. 17–52). Hillsdale, NJ: Erlbaum.

Atkinson, J. W., & Birch, D. (1970). *The dynamics of action.* New York: Wiley.

Atkinson, J. W., & Birch, D. (1978). *An introduction to motivation.* New York: Van Nostrand.

Atkinson, J. W., & Feather, N. T. (1966). *A theory of achievement motivation.* New York: Wiley.

Bandura, A. (1977). Self-efficacy: Toward a unifying theory of behavioral change. *Psychological Review, 84,* 191–215.

Bandura, A. (1986a). *Social foundations of thought and action.* Englewood Cliffs, NJ: Prentice-Hall.

Bandura, A. (1986b). The explanatory and predictive scope of self-efficacy theory. *Journal of Social and Clinical Psychology, 4,* 359–373.

Bandura, A. (1988). Self-regulation of motivation and action through goal systems. In V. Hamilton, G. H. Bower, & N. H. Frijda (Eds.), *Cognitive perspectives on emotion and motivation* (pp. 37–61). Dordrecht, The Netherlands: Martinus Nijhoff.

Bandura, A., & Cervone, D. (1983). Self-evaluative and self-efficacy mechanisms governing the motivational effects of goal systems. *Journal of Personality and Social Psychology, 45,* 1017–1028.

Blasi, A. (1980). Bridging moral cognition and moral action: A critical review of the literature. *Psychological Bulletin, 88,* 1–45.

Brown, D. R., & Veroff, J. (Eds.). (1986). *Frontiers of motivational psychology: Essays in honor of John W. Atkinson.* New York: Springer-Verlag.

Brown, R., & Herrnstein, R. J. (1975). *Psychology.* London: Methuen.

Eastman, C., & Marzillier, J. S. (1984). Theoretical and methodological difficulties in Bandura's self-efficacy theory. *Cognitive Therapy and Research, 8,* 213–229.

Eccles, J., Adler, T. E., Futterman, R., Goff, S. B., Kaczala, C. M., Meece, J. L., & Midgley, C. (1983). Expectancies, values, and academic behaviors. In J. Spence (Ed.), *Achievement and achievement motivation* (pp. 75–146). San Francisco: W. H. Freeman.

Eccles, J., Adler, T., & Meece, J. L. (1984). Sex differences in achievement: A test of alternate theories. *Journal of Personality and Social Psychology, 46,* 26–43.

Emler, N., Renwick, S., & Malone, B. (1983). The relationship between moral reasoning and political orientation. *Journal of Personality and Social Psychology, 45,* 1073–1080.

Fazio, R. H. (1986). How do attitudes guide behavior? In R. M. Sorrentino & E. T. Higgins (Eds.), *Handbook of motivation and cognition: Foundations of social behavior* (Vol. 1, pp. 204–243). New York: Guilford Press.

Feather, N. T. (1959). Subjective probability and decision under uncertainty. *Psychological Review, 66,* 150–164.

Feather, N. T. (1967a). An expectancy–value model of information-seeking behavior. *Psychological Review, 74,* 342–360.

Feather, N. T. (1967b). Level of aspiration and performance variability. *Journal of Personality and Social Psychology, 6,* 37–46.

Feather, N. T. (1969). Preference for information in relation to consistency, novelty, intolerance of ambiguity, and dogmatism. *Australian Journal of Psychology, 21,* 235–249.

Feather, N. T. (1971a). Organization and discrepancy in cognitive structures. *Psychological Review, 78,* 355–379.

Feather, N. T. (1971b). Value differences in relation to ethnocentrism, intolerance of ambiguity, and dogmatism. *Personality: An International Journal, 2*, 349-366.

Feather, N. T. (1975). *Values in education and society.* New York: Free Press.

Feather, N. T. (1979). Value correlates of conservatism. *Journal of Personality and Social Psychology, 37*, 1617-1630.

Feather, N. T. (1980). Values in adolescence. In J. Adelson (Ed.), *Handbook of adolescent psychology* (pp. 247-294). New York: Wiley.

Feather, N. T. (1982a). Actions in relation to expected consequences: An overview of a research program. In N. T. Feather (Ed.), *Expectations and actions: Expectancy-value models in psychology* (pp. 53-95). Hillsdale, NJ: Erlbaum.

Feather, N. T. (1982b). Expectancy-value approaches: Present status and future directions. In N. T. Feather (Ed.), *Expectations and actions: Expectancy-value models in psychology* (pp. 395-420). Hillsdale, NJ: Erlbaum.

Feather, N. T. (Ed.). (1982c). *Expectations and actions: Expectancy-value models in psychology.* Hillsdale, NJ: Erlbaum.

Feather, N. T. (1982d). Human values and the prediction of action: An expectancy-valence analysis. In N. T. Feather (Ed.), *Expectations and actions: Expectancy-value models in psychology* (pp. 263-289). Hillsdale, NJ: Erlbaum.

Feather, N. T. (1982e). Unemployment and its psychological correlates: A study of depressive symptoms, self-esteem, protestant ethic values, attributional style, and apathy. *Australian Journal of Psychology, 34*, 309-323.

Feather, N. T. (1984). Protestant ethic, conservatism, and values. *Journal of Personality and Social Psychology, 46*, 1132-1141.

Feather, N. T. (1986a). Cross-cultural studies with the Rokeach Value Survey: The Flinders program of research on values. *Australian Journal of Psychology, 38*, 269-283.

Feather, N. T. (1986b). Employment importance and helplessness about potential unemployment among students in secondary schools. *Australian Journal of Psychology, 38*, 33-44.

Feather, N. T. (1986c). Human values, valences, expectations and affect: Theoretical issues emerging from recent applications of the expectancy-value model. In D. R. Brown & J. Veroff (Eds.), *Frontiers of motivational psychology: Essays in honor of John W. Atkinson* (pp. 146-172). New York: Springer-Verlag.

Feather, N. T. (1987). Gender differences in values: Implications of the expectancy-value model. In F. Halisch & J. Kuhl (Eds.), *Motivation, intention, and volition* (pp. 31-45). New York: Springer-Verlag.

Feather, N. T. (1988a). From values to actions: Recent applications of the expectancy-value model. *Australian Journal of Psychology, 40*, 105-124.

Feather, N. T. (1988b). Moral judgment and human values. *British Journal of Social Psychology, 27*, 239-246.

Feather, N. T. (1988c). The meaning and importance of values: Research with the Rokeach Value Survey. *Australian Journal of Psychology, 40*, 377-390.

Feather, N. T. (1988d). Values, valences, and course enrollment: Testing the role of personal values within an expectancy-value framework. *Journal of Educational Psychology, 80*, 381-391.

Feather, N. T. (1989). *The psychological impact of unemployment.* New York: Springer-Verlag.

Feather, N. T., & Newton, J. W. (1982). Values, expectations, and the prediction of social action: An expectancy-valence analysis. *Motivation and Emotion, 6*, 217-244.

Feather, N. T., & O'Brien, G. E. (1986a). A longitudinal analysis of the effects of different patterns of employment and unemployment on school-leavers. *British Journal of Psychology, 77*, 459-479.

Feather, N. T., & O'Brien, G. E. (1986b). A longitudinal study of the effects of employment and unemployment on school-leavers. *Journal of Occupational Psychology, 59*, 121-144.

Feather, N. T., & O'Brien, G. E. (1987). Looking for employment: An expectancy-valence analysis of job-seeking behaviour among young people. *British Journal of Psychology, 78*, 251-272.

Fishbein, M., & Ajzen, I. (1975). *Belief, attitude, intention, and behavior: An introduction to theory and research.* Reading, MA: Addison-Wesley.

Fiske, S. T., & Pavelchak, M. A. (1986). Category-based versus piecemeal-based affective responses: Developments in schema-triggered affect. In R. M. Sorrentino & E. T. Higgins (Ed.), *Handbook of motivation and cognition: Foundations of social behavior* (Vol. 1, pp. 167-203). New York: Guilford Press.

Gilligan, C. (1982). *In a different voice: Psychological theory and women's development.* Cambridge, MA: Harvard University Press.

Heckhausen, H. (1977). Achievement motivation and its constructs: A cognitive model. *Motivation and Emotion,* 1, 283-329.

Heckhausen, H. (1986a). Achievement and motivation through the life span. In A. B. Sörenson, F. E. Weinert, & L. R. Sherrod (Eds.), *Human development and the life course: Multidisciplinary perspectives* (pp. 445-466). Hillsdale, NJ: Erlbaum.

Heckhausen, H. (1986b). Why some time out might benefit achievement motivation research. In J. H. L. van den Bercken, T. C. M. Bergen, & E. E. J. De Bruyn (Eds.), *Achievement and task motivation* (pp. 7-39). Lisse, The Netherlands: Swets & Zeitlinger.

Heckhausen, H., & Gollwitzer, I. (1987). Thought contents and cognitive functioning in motivational vs. volitional states of mind. *Motivation and Emotion,* 11, 101-120.

Heckhausen, H., Schmalt, H. D., & Schneider, K. (1985). *Achievement motivation in perspective.* New York: Academic Press.

Higgins, E. T. (1987). Self-discrepancy: A theory relating self and affect. *Psychological Review,* 94, 319-340.

Higgins, E. T. (1989). Knowledge accessibility and activation: Subjectivity and suffering from unconscious sources. In J. S. Uleman & J. A. Bargh (Eds.), *Unintended thought* (pp. 75-123). New York: Guilford Press.

Higgins, E. T., Tykocinski, O., & Vookles, J. (in press). Patterns of self-beliefs: The psychological significance of relations among the actual, ideal, ought, can, and future selves. In J. M. Olson & M. P. Zanna (Eds.), *Self-inference processes: The Ontario Symposium* (Vol. 6). Hillsdale, NJ: Erlbaum.

Hoffman, M. L. (1986). Affect, cognition, and motivation. In R. M. Sorrentino & E. T. Higgins (Eds.), *Handbook of motivation and cognition: Foundations of social behavior* (Vol. 1, pp. 244-280). New York: Guilford Press.

Homer, P. M., & Kahle, L. R. (1988). A structural equation test of the value–attitude–behavior hierarchy. *Journal of Personality and Social Psychology,* 54, 638-646.

Kahneman, E., Slovic, P., & Tversky, A. (Eds.). (1982). *Judgment under uncertainty: Heuristics and biases.* New York: Cambridge University Press.

Katz, D. (1960). The functional approach to the study of attitudes. *Public Opinion Quarterly,* 24, 163-204.

Kohlberg, L. (1969). Stage and sequence: The cognitive-developmental approach to socialization. In D. A. Goslin (Ed.), *Handbook of socialization theory and research* (pp. 347-380). Chicago: Rand McNally.

Kohlberg, L. (1976). Moral stages and moralization: The cognitive-developmental approach. In T. Lickona (Ed.), *Moral development and behavior: Theory, research, and social issues* (pp. 31-53). New York: Holt, Rinehart & Winston.

Kohlberg, L., & Candee, D. (1984). The relationship of moral judgment to moral action. In L. Kohlberg (Ed.), *The psychology of moral development: The nature and validity of moral stages* (pp. 498-581). New York: Harper & Row.

Kruglanski, A. W. (1975). The endogenous-exogenous partition in attribution theory. *Psychological Review,* 82, 387-406.

Kuhl, J. (1982). The expectancy–value approach within the theory of social motivation: Elaborations, extensions, critique. In N. T. Feather (Ed.), *Expectations and actions: Expectancy–value models in psychology* (pp. 125-160). Hillsdale, NJ: Erlbaum.

Kuhl, J. (1985). Volitional mediators of cognition-behavior consistency: Self-regulatory processes and action versus state orientation. In J. Kuhl & J. Beckmann (Eds.), *Action control: From cognition to behavior* (pp. 101-128). New York: Springer-Verlag.

Kuhl, J. (1986). Motivation and information processing: A new look at decision making, dynamic change, and action control. In R. M. Sorrentino & E. T. Higgins (Eds.), *Handbook of motivation and cognition: Foundations of social behavior* (Vol. 1, pp. 404-434). New York: Guilford Press.

Kuhl, J. (1987). Action control: The maintenance of motivational states. In F. Halisch & J. Kuhl (Eds.), *Motivation, intention, and volition* (pp. 279-291). New York: Springer-Verlag.

Kuhl, J., & Atkinson, J. W. (1986). *Motivation, thought, and action.* New York: Praeger.

Kuhl, J., & Blankenship, V. (1979). The dynamic theory of achievement motivation: From episodic to dynamic thinking. *Psychological Review, 86,* 141-151.

Lewin, K. (1936). *Principles of topological psychology.* New York: McGraw-Hill.

Lewin, K., Dembo, T., Festinger, L., & Sears, P. S. (1944). Level of aspiration. In J. McV. Hunt (Ed.), *Personality and the behavior disorders,* (Vol. 1, pp. 333-378). New York: Ronald Press.

Locke, D. (1979). Cognitive states or developmental phases: Critique of Kohlberg stage-structural theory of moral reasoning. *Journal of Moral Education, 8,* 168-181.

Locke, D. (1983). Doing what comes morally. *Human Development, 26,* 11-25.

Locke, E. A., Motowildo, S. J., & Bobko, P. (1986). Using self-efficacy theory to resolve the conflict between goal-setting theory and expectancy theory in organizational behavior and industrial/organizational psychology. *Journal of Social and Clinical Psychology, 4,* 328-338.

Maddux, J. E., Norton, L. W., & Stoltenberg, C. D. (1986). Self-efficacy expectancy, outcome expectancy, and outcome value: Relative effects on behavioral intentions. *Journal of Personality and Social Psychology, 51,* 783-789.

Manning, M. M., & Wright, T. L. (1983). Self-efficacy expectancies, outcome expectancies, and the persistence of pain control in childbirth. *Journal of Personality and Social Psychology, 45,* 421-431.

McClelland, D. C. (1985). *Human motivation.* Glenview, IL: Scott, Foresman.

Mineka, S., & Hendersen, R. W. (1985). Controllability and predictability in acquired motivation. *Annual Review of Psychology, 36,* 495-529.

Mirels, H. L., & Garrett, J. B. (1971). The Protestant ethic as a personality variable. *Journal of Consulting and Clinical Psychology, 36,* 40-44.

Mischel, W., & Mischel, H. N. (1976). A cognitive social-learning approach to morality and self-regulation. In T. Lickona (Ed.), *Moral development and behavior: Theory, research, and social issues* (pp. 84-107). New York: Holt, Rinehart & Winston.

Mitchell, T. R. (1982). Expectancy–value models in organizational psychology. In N. T. Feather (Ed.), *Expectations and actions: Expectancy–value models in psychology* (pp. 293-312). Hillsdale, NJ: Erlbaum.

Nisbett, R., & Ross, L. (1980). *Human inference: Strategies and shortcomings of social judgment.* Englewood Cliffs, NJ: Prentice-Hall.

Raynor, J. O., & McFarlin, D. B. (1986). Motivation and the self-system. In R. Sorrentino & E. T. Higgins (Ed.), *Handbook of motivation and cognition: Foundations of social behavior* (Vol. 1, pp. 315-349). New York: Guilford Press.

Rest, J. R. (1979). Development in judging moral issues. Minneapolis: University of Minnesota Press.

Rest, J. R. (1983). Morality. In J. H. Flavell & E. M. Markman (Vol. Eds.), *Handbook of child psychology* (4th ed.): *Vol. 3. Cognitive development* (pp. 556-627). New York: Wiley.

Revelle, W. (1986). Motivation and efficiency of cognitive performance. In D. R. Brown & J. Veroff (Eds.), *Frontiers of motivational psychology: Essays in honor of John W. Atkinson* (pp. 107-131). New York: Springer-Verlag.

Rokeach, M. (1972). *Beliefs, attitudes, and values.* San Francisco: Jossey-Bass.

Rokeach, M. (1973). *The nature of human values.* New York: Free Press.

Rokeach, M. (1979). Some unresolved issues in theories of beliefs, attitudes, and values. In M. M. Page (Ed.), *Nebraska Symposium on Motivation* (Vol. 27, pp. 261-304). Lincoln: University of Nebraska Press.

Rotter, J. B. (1954). *Social learning and clinical psychology.* Englewood Cliffs, NJ: Prentice-Hall.

Rotter, J. B. (1982). Social learning theory. In N. T. Feather (Ed.), *Expectations and actions: Expectancy–value models in psychology* (pp. 241-260). Hillsdale, NJ: Erlbaum.

Schwartz, S. H., & Bilsky, W. (1987). Toward a psychological structure of human values. *Journal of Personality and Social Psychology, 53,* 550-562.

Schwartz, S. H., & Bilsky, W. (in press). Toward a theory of the universal content and structure of values: Extensions and cross-cultural replications. *Journal of Personality and Social Psychology.*

Smith, M. B., Bruner, J. S., & White, R. W. (1956). *Opinions and personality.* New York: Wiley.

Sorrentino, R., & Short, J. (1986). Uncertainty orientation, motivation, and cognition. In R. Sorrentino & E. T. Higgins (Eds.), *Handbook of motivation and cognition: Foundations of social behavior* (Vol. 1, pp. 379-403). New York: Guilford Press.

Teasdale, J. D. (1978). Self-efficacy: Toward a unifying theory of behavioural change? In S. Rachman (Ed.), *Advances in behaviour research and therapy* (Vol. 1, pp. 211-215). Oxford: Pergamon Press.

Veroff, J. (1986). Contextualism and human motives. In D. R. Brown & J. Veroff (Eds.), *Frontiers of motivational psychology: Essays in honor of John W. Atkinson* (pp. 132-143). New York: Springer-Verlag.

Vroom, V. H. (1964). *Work and motivation.* New York: Wiley.

Weber, M. (1976). *The Protestant ethic and the spirit of capitalism* (T. Parsons, Trans.). London: George Allen & Unwin. (Original work published 1904-1905)

Weiner, B. (1980). *Human motivation.* New York: Holt, Rinehart & Winston.

Weiner, B. (1986a). *An attributional theory of motivation and emotion.* New York: Springer-Verlag.

Weiner, B. (1986b). Attribution, emotion, and action, In R. M. Sorrentino & E. T. Higgins (Eds.), *Handbook of motivation and cognition: Foundations of social behavior* (Vol. 1, pp. 281-312). New York: Guilford Press.

Wilson, G. D. (Ed.). (1973). *The psychology of conservatism.* New York: Academic Press.

Wilson, G. D., & Patterson, J. R. (1968). A new measure of conservatism. *British Journal of Social and Clinical Psychology, 7,* 264-269.

Wright, R. A., Contrada, R. J., & Patane, M. J. (1986). Task difficulty, cardiovascular response, and the magnitude of goal valence. *Journal of Personality and Social Psychology, 51,* 837-843.

CHAPTER 6

Personality Functioning and Change
Informational and Affective Influences on Cognitive, Moral, and Social Development

RICHARD M. SORRENTINO
University of Western Ontario
JOEL O. RAYNOR
JO MARIE ZUBEK
State University of New York at Buffalo
JUDITH-ANN C. SHORT
Victoria Hospital

Since the emergence of Piaget's theory of cognitive development, developmental psychology has been roughly divided into two camps, the organismic-structural tradition and the mechanistic-functional tradition. According to Fischer and Silvern (1985),

> Scholars working in the organismic-structural tradition find that development occurs in universal stages, which reflect the structure of thought that lies behind the diversity of manifest behavior. Scholars working in the mechanistic-functional tradition find development (or more commonly, learning) in manifest behavior, which varies widely across diverse environments and functions. Observations made by the methods of the one approach are easily discounted as irrelevent by proponents of the other (p. 618)

Following their review of the literature, Fischer and Silvern (1985) conclude that evidence exists to support both approaches. They argue that what is needed is research showing an integration of these two approaches. It is our belief that the theory of personality functioning and change (Raynor, 1982; Raynor & McFarlin, 1986), coupled with developments regarding research on uncertainty orientation (see Sorrentino & Roney, 1989a; Sorrentino & Short, 1986), can provide the basis for such an integration. Our viewpoint is consistent with contemporary approaches to cognitive development, which attempt to reconcile organismic-structural approaches with mechanistic-functional approaches (e.g., Fischer & Silvern, 1985). It is also consistent with the recent literature arguing for an interaction between emotional and cognitive development (e.g., Case, Hayward, Lewis, &

Hurst, 1988) and for the importance of social life phases in determining age-related changes in social cognition (Higgins & Eccles-Parsons, 1983).

What distinguishes our approach from previous ones is that we believe we have found a fundamental organismic variable (i.e., uncertainty orientation) that governs cognitive, moral, and ego-identity development. Furthermore, we can specify more precisely under what conditions motivational and environmental forces will enhance or inhibit development of various stages or levels in each of these areas.

In this chapter, our focus is on preadolescence through adulthood rather than on early childhood. Emphasis is placed on understanding changes at later stages of these developmental sequences; from concrete to formal operational thought, from conventional to postconventional moral reasoning, and from ego diffusion to ego identity.[1]

We propose that as a consequence of past experience, people emerge from childhood with markedly different expectations about themselves and the world around them. These expectations systematically affect their movement or lack of movement into later stages of development. People move toward or away from these stages, depending upon the informational value and affective value they perceive in situations related to these stages. Before presenting these implications, we briefly describe the theory and update research on uncertainty orientation relevant to the issues at hand.

A THEORY OF PERSONALITY FUNCTIONING AND CHANGE

Our theory of personality functioning and change (Raynor, 1982; Raynor & McFarlin, 1986) postulates that the concept of "value" is of functional significance. It assumes that people are motivated to maximize positive value and to minimize negative value. The maximization of positive value and minimization of negative value are the basic functions of personality. Adaptive behavior is the result of a person's constant striving in accordance with these two principles.

There are two primary kinds of value, "information value" and "affective value." Information value refers to the cognitive functioning of personality—knowing or being confused. Affective value refers to the emotional functioning of personality—feeling good or feeling bad. Thus, people are assumed to be motivated to find out or maintain clarity about themselves or the environment, and to feel good. They are also motivated to avoid confusion and feeling bad.

The theory of personality functioning and change distinguishes between the behavioral system and the self-system. Value in the behavioral system refers to the attractiveness or repulsiveness of informational and affective consequences of actions. Outcomes of action are sources of value in the behavioral system. Maximizing positive value and minimizing negative value in this system are functions of personality that do not require phenomenal awareness. However, as the value of outcomes becomes greater, phenomenal awareness increases.

Value in the self-system refers to the degree of clarity or confusion about perceived self-images, attributes, and abilities (information value) and self-esteem or esteem income derived from self-perceptions (affective value). Self-images, attributes, and abilities are sources of value in the self-system. Functioning in the self-system is dependent upon emergence of the capacity to answer the question "Who am I?" When a particular self-image becomes a source of value, that self-image comes to serve as a basis for perceived self-identity and leads to phenomenal self-awareness. When a self-image loses its value, it no longer serves as a basis for perceived self-identity. Some people derive little value from the self-system, and therefore questions about "Who am I?" have little psychological importance. For them, the self-system is irrelevant, and value in the behavioral system determines thought and action.

The Psychological Career

Value in a Psychological Career

Value in a psychological career refers to self-system value determined by the outcomes of action. The "psychological career" is the integrative concept invoked when a person derives value simultaneously from the behavioral system and the self-system. For example, a factory worker (though this is certainly not true of all factory workers) might perceive his or her occupation only in terms of the behavioral system. An academic (though, again, this is certainly not true of all academics) might perceive his or her occupation as critical to self-definition. Only the latter case would be considered a psychological career.

The psychological career, then, represents a link between action and perceived self-definition. It is a behavioral opportunity for perceived self-identity. It is pursued when outcomes of action become valuable (important) for self-identity (information value) and self-enhancement (affective value). The person is motivated to find out "who I am" and to "feel good about me." When action outcomes no longer provide sufficient value, they no longer define self-image, and functioning occurs only in the behavioral system. Many of us have colleagues who seem no longer to care about their careers and have taken up goat farming, pottery, or banjo picking as their primary preoccupation.

Stages of Striving in a Psychological Career

Early-stage striving is termed "becoming," since the predominant sources and amounts of value are in the anticipated future. The person is primarily motivated to attain a future self-image defined by the final outcome along a path. Late-stage striving is termed "having been," since the person is primarily motivated to reattain a past self-image defined by previous outcomes along that path. Evaluation of immediate outcomes and personal attributes can occur at any stage of striving. The person is motivated to assess perceived self-images, attributes, and abilities, in order to be clear and not confused, and to feel good and not feel bad.

Value as a Determinant of Action

Our theory reflects an elaboration of expectancy–value theory of action (Feather, 1982; Raynor & Entin, 1982) to deal with personality functioning and change. Positive value instigates thought or action to attain an anticipated outcome, reattain a recalled outcome, or maintain an outcome presently being experienced. Negative value inhibits thought or action concerning an anticipated or retrospected outcome, or instigates thought or action to remove an outcome presently being experienced. The amount of value and its expectancy or subjective probability of being experienced or removed combine multiplicatively to determine aroused motivation.

Resultant tendency to think or act is a function of the difference between motivation to think or act and motivation to resist thought or action. Resultant tendency to maintain or remove a source of value being experienced is a function of the difference between motivation to maintain and motivation to remove it.

The difference between total positive and total negative value determines resultant value, which determines thought or action if expectancy is held constant. Resultant value can involve positive and negative affective and information value in any combination. Positive and negative value can operate independently. A source of value may be entirely positive, entirely negative, or both positive and negative. It may be entirely affective, entirely informational, or both affective and informational. A person may think or act to maximize positive value, minimize negative value, or simultaneously maximize positive and minimize negative value (see Raynor & McFarlin, 1986, for a more extended treatment of these assumptions).

A good example of this is achievement behavior. It can be a source of positive or negative affective value (feeling good about success, feeling bad about failure). It can be a source of positive or negative information value (maintaining or attaining clarity about one's ability, introducing ambiguity or confusion about one's ability). Fear of failure and desire to succeed can operate independently, as can attaining clarity or avoiding confusion. Whether one is motivated to approach or avoid, or think or act, in an achievement-oriented situation will be some resultant combination of these forces.

Individual Differences in Resultant Value

People for whom affective value is strong and information value is weak are dominated by affective value. Feeling good is the primary goal, and feeling bad is the primary threat. Those for whom information value is strong and affective value is weak are dominated by information value. Attaining or maintaining clarity (or knowing) is the primary goal, and being confused is the primary threat.

Resultant Affective Value

Individual differences in resultant affective value as they relate to achievement have been systematically investigated in research on achievement motivation (Atkinson & Feather, 1966; Atkinson & Raynor, 1974; Raynor & Entin,

1982). Attempts to interpret the achievement motive in terms of self-assessment (information value) instead of affective value (Trope, 1975; Weiner, 1972) have been discounted in our research (Sorrentino & Hewitt, 1984; Sorrentino & Roney, 1986; Sorrentino, Short, & Raynor, 1984). Success-oriented individuals (i.e., persons who score relatively high on the projective measure of *n* Achievement and low in test anxiety) have a motivation to achieve that is stronger than their motivation to avoid failure. Their resultant affective value is assumed to be positive for outcomes in the achievement domain involving standards of good performance. Failure-threatened individuals (i.e., persons who score relatively low on *n* Achievement and high in test anxiety) have stronger motivation to avoid failure than motivation to achieve. Their resultant affective value is assumed to be negative. Since the motive to succeed and the motive to avoid failure are independent, people can have equal strengths of both motives. Their resultant affective value is near zero.

Resultant Information Value

Individual differences in resultant information value have recently been investigated in terms of differences in "uncertainty orientation" (see Sorrentino & Short, 1986). Uncertainty orientation reflects the degree to which situations of uncertainty or certainty arouse resultant information value that is positive, negative, or near zero.

Uncertainty-oriented individuals (i.e., persons who score relatively high on our projective measure of *n* Uncertainty [Sorrentino, Hanna, & Roney, in press] and low in authoritarianism [Byrne & Lamberth, 1971]) are assumed to be primarily motivated to seek clarity through mastery of uncertainty, whereas certainty-oriented individuals (i.e., persons who score relatively low in *n* Uncertainty and high in authoritarianism) are motivated to maintain clarity by adhering to what is already known (Raynor & McFarlin, 1986; Sorrentino & Short, 1986).[2] The uncertainty-oriented are curious about the unknown, are open to new and possibly inconsistent information, and have a high tolerance for ambiguity. They experience positive information value from the process of thinking, discovering, and finding out. They derive little cognitive satisfaction from knowing without working through the challenge of uncertainty. This cognitive functioning is consistent with the notion of "human the scientist" and hypothetical–deductive reasoning (see Roney & Sorrentino, 1989a, described below).

The certainty-oriented are assumed to be dominated by a need to ignore changes to existing cognitions, and by a need to maintain clarity. They are attracted to the familiar and predictable, have an authoritarian and dogmatic way of knowing, and have a low tolerance for ambiguity. They experience positive information value from the product of thinking—knowledge—but are threatened by the process of thought in any situation where there is confusion about the self or the environment. Their cognitive functioning features adherence to a particular viewpoint and resistance to alternatives or change. Uncertainty is to be avoided. It provides negative information value. The certainty-oriented are motivated to remove uncertainty when it is experienced. The characteristics of uncertainty-oriented and certainty-oriented persons resemble those of open-minded and closed-minded individuals, respectively (Rokeach, 1960).

Uncertainty orientation is assumed to be time-linked. The uncertainty-oriented seek out new ideas and explore previously unknown possibilities. They are presumed to be future-oriented. The certainty-oriented cling to previously established ideas and are threatened by the uncertainty of the unknown. They are presumed to be past-oriented.

Current Research

Recent findings support much of the above-described viewpoint. In two recent studies (Roney & Sorrentino, 1989a), for example, theoretical and scientific reasoning was among the highest values for uncertainty-oriented persons, but among the lowest for certainty-oriented persons. This research also verified our assumption that uncertainty-oriented persons will be more likely than certainty-oriented persons to compare themselves with others, regardless of the relative importance of the value. Both of these studies were derived from the Sorrentino and Hewitt (1984) study, which showed that certainty-oriented persons would not engage in activity that would resolve uncertainty about an important ability. This was true even where the information was potentially positive (of course, these persons also would not look at potentially negative information). They simply did not want to engage in uncertain situations even if their action could resolve the uncertainty. Apparently, finding out something new about the self may lead to greater uncertainty in the future; a person may be forced to re-evaluate his or her circumstances. He or she may ask, "Given that I have this new and important ability, what do I do now?" or "How does this affect my career, my social relations, and so on?" Uncertainty-oriented persons will engage in activity that will provide either type of information.

We have also questioned whether self-discrepancy theory (Higgins, Strauman, & Klein, 1986) applies only to uncertainty-oriented individuals, as they should be more tied up in the self than certainty-oriented persons. So far, we have found that uncertainty-oriented persons do have larger self-discrepancies of all types (i.e., ideal–own, ideal–other, ought–own, ought–other), and that they experience more negative affect (possibly because of these discrepancies), than certainty-oriented persons (Roney & Sorrentino, 1989b). We have also found that Higgins et al. (1986) were correct in their prediction that experiencing ideal–own discrepancies should lead to increases in performance and experiencing ought–other discrepancies should lead to decreases in performance. However, this again only applies to uncertainty-oriented persons (Sorrentino & Roney, 1989b). Certainty-oriented persons probably "tune out" from these discrepancies rather than face the uncertainty involved in reducing them (see below for further discussion).

Individual Differences in Affective and Information Value

Although one might expect information value and affective value to combine additively, this does not appear to be the case, at least with regard to achievement-oriented situations. In six different studies reported in three sources (Roney & Sorrentino, 1989b; Sorrentino & Roney, 1986; Sorrentino et al., 1984), we have found that information value appears to influence affective value. That is, differences in expected performance due to achievement-related motives (i.e., better performance by success-oriented persons that by failure-threatened persons) are greatest in situations relevant to the individuals' mode of uncertainty orientation. Thus, for uncertainty-oriented persons, expected differences due to achievement-related motives are greatest where the persons have an opportunity to find out about the self or the behavioral system. For certainty-oriented persons, these differences are greatest in situations where the persons can maintain clarity about the self or the behavioral system. In situations not relevant to uncertainty orientation (i.e., where there is little opportunity to find out for the uncertainty-oriented persons, or there is the possibility of confusion for the certainty-oriented persons), either there is no difference in behavior as a function of achievement-related motives, or, as is often the case, the failure-threatened persons outperform the success-oriented persons.[3]

We believe that our theory of personality functioning and change can help us understand this phenomenon. Recall that if a situation offers high information value, a person is motivated to think or act. If, however, it has little positive information value or negative information value, there is resistance to thought or action. In the former case, a success-oriented person is positively motivated and a failure-threatened person is negatively motivated, because information value is high. In the latter case, positive motivation is diminished, but so is fear of failure. Not thinking about the situation will simultaneously diminish achievement motivation and reduce anxiety. As Atkinson and Birch (1978) have demonstrated with their theory of the dynamics of action, it then becomes theoretically possible for failure-threatened persons to outperform success-oriented persons.[4]

We have dwelled on this issue for an important reason. We believe that the theory helps us reconcile the discrepancy between the apparent avoidance behavior of certainty-oriented persons in some situations (e.g., Sorrentino & Hewitt, 1984) and their apparent lack of negative affect in others (e.g., Sorrentino et al., 1984). Briefly, when given the opportunity to avoid confusion (such as not to engage in activity that will tell them something about the self or the environment), certainty-oriented persons will do so. However, when they are placed in an activity they cannot avoid, there is resistance to thought. Thus the success-oriented persons no longer have pride of accomplishment in mind, and the failure-threatened persons are no longer concerned with shame over failure. The latter can have the paradoxical effect of improving performance if the persons normally suffer from anxiety or fear of failure. However, it does diminish the performance of success-oriented persons.

Although discussion of this research is beyond the bounds of the present chapter, it appears that a situation is first assessed for information value. If it has positive information value (providing clarity for an uncertainty-oriented person, maintaining clarity for a certainty-oriented person), then affectve arousal (approach and avoidance behavior) due to achievement-related motives occurs. However, affective value (feeling good or feeling bad) is diminished in situations that do not have positive information value. Regardless of the theoretical underpinnings of this phenomenon, it is important for the reader to note that people will approach or avoid a situation depending upon the information value it provides for them. If forced to undertake activity with little or negative information value, they may resist thought or action.

This interactive view of information value and affective value continues to receive support from current research. Both a field study and a laboratory experiment (Roney & Sorrentino, (1989b) found that expected differences in performance due to achievement-related motives were greatest in situations relevant to subjects' uncertainty orientation. Hence, on a complex arithmetic ability task (Study 1) and on final examination grades in an introductory psychology course (Study 2), uncertainty-oriented persons showed expected performance differences due to their achievement-related motives only where there was a self-discrepancy (cf. Higgins et al., 1986), and certainty-oriented persons showed these differences where there was no self-discrepancy.

Finally, this notion that motivation will be greatest in situations relevant to one's uncertainty orientation has carried over into the field of attitude change and persuasion. In two studies (Sorrentino, Bobocel, Gitta, Olson, & Hewitt, 1988), it was found, as we have argued, that uncertainty-oriented persons systematically processed information more and relied on heuristics less as personal relevance increased. Certainty-oriented persons, however, actually decreased their use of systematic processing and increased their usage of heuristic devices as personal relevance increased. Personal relevance should have high positive information value for uncertainty-oriented persons (finding out more about the self), and they should process systematically. For certainty-oriented persons, however, personal relevance should contain high negative information value (revealing new information about the self), and they should revert to more automatic forms of processing information. Additional evidence from thought-listing data suggested that both uncertainty-oriented and certainty-oriented persons resisted or ignored systematic processing of information in situations that did not have positive information value (see Sorrentino et al., 1988).

Summary

We are accruing a strong body of evidence indicating that finding out new things about the self or the environment has high positive information value for uncertainty-oriented persons and high negative information value for certainty-oriented persons. Conversely, maintaining clarity or avoiding confusion has high positive information value for certainty-oriented persons, but little positive value for uncertainty-oriented persons. In addition, when one actually engages in achievement behavior, affective value will systematically interact with information value. Here, arousal or resistance to achievement-oriented activity will depend on that activity's relevance to information value. This would seem to have important implications for current theories of developmental psychology, to which we now turn.

A REINTERPRETATION OF STAGE THEORIES OF DEVELOPMENT

Our motivational perspective has provided the basis for rethinking the traditional distinction between developmental and motivational approaches to the study of the same phenomena. Motivational psychology provides the principle of the contemporaneous determinants of action to view a person's behavior at a given point in time (e.g., Atkinson & Birch, 1978). Developmental psychology provides a means of conceptualizing change over time (e.g., Erikson, 1968; Kohlberg, 1973; Piaget, 1972), as can be seen in Table 6.1. Our position integrates these two viewpoints from the motivational perspective.

Stability and Change from the Motivational and Stage Theory Perspectives

A stage theory view of adult development considers individual differences in cognitive, moral, and ego functioning in terms of movement through an invariant sequence that is equivalent for all persons. People at later stages are assumed to possess modes of thinking and patterns of responding that differ qualitatively from those at earlier stages. The stage perspective assumes that change is necessary and inevitable.

The motivational perspective derives rather than assumes stability or change in thought or action. The occurrence or experience of common stages may depend upon the nature and direction of motivational arousal. The factors that influence action at a particular time, and change or stability in these over time, are the variables that determine stability or change in overt or covert behavior. From the motivational perspective, adulthood should not be viewed in terms of invariant stages or progression. Individual differences in personal characteristics, life circumstances that determine perceived path characteristics, and the outcomes of actions are assumed to determine different patterns of motivation over time.

Our approach, then, is similar to the collaborative approach advocated by Fischer and Silvern (1985). These authors point out that competence-performance approaches do try to reconcile organismic-structural frameworks with mechanistic-functional frameworks. However, they do so by giving each one responsibility for a different aspect of behavior; hence, they isolate rather than take advantage of the information from each other. Fischer and Silvern advocate, instead, that an approach is needed that conjoins organism and environment in its central methods and explanatory constructs: "Our favorite metaphors for that conjoining are transaction and collaboration. People transact with their environment or collaborate with it; they work with and affect it, and it works with and affects them" (1985, p. 643).

TABLE 6.1 Stage Theories of Cognitive Development, Moral Development, and Ego Identity

Age	Piaget	Kohlberg	Erikson
0–1	Sensorimotor stage		Trust vs. mistrust
1–2			
2–3			Autonomy vs. shame or doubt
3–4		Level 1. Preconventional morality	Initiative vs. guilt
4–5	Preoperational stage	Stage 1. Punishment-obedience	
5–6		Stage 2. Naive hedonism or instrumental orientation	
6–7			
7–8			
8–9	Concrete operational stage	Level 2. Conventional morality[a]	Competence vs. authority
9–10		Stage 3. "Good boy" or "good girl" orientation	
10–11		Stage 4. Authority- and social-order-maintaining morality	
11–12			
12–13			
13–14	Formal operational stage	Level 3. Postconventional morality[b]	Identity vs. role confusion
		Stage 5. Morality of contract, social rights, and democratically accepted law	Stages of adulthood
		Stage 6. Morality of individual principles of conscience	

[a] Ages when Stage 3 and Stage 4 begin to exceed Level 1.
[b] Ages when Stage 5 and Stage 6 begin to exceed (Stage 5) or approach (Stage 6) Level 1.

We are also in line with the "how" as opposed to the "can" distinction advocated by Higgins and Wells (1986): "The 'how' approach emphasizes the structures and processes that actually underlie people's social judgments, rather than people's capacity to fulfil prescribed processing requirements" (p. 203). We do not doubt that certainty-oriented persons have the capacity to achieve higher levels of development. However, their methods of processing information, combined with motivational and situational determinants, may delay their progress toward that goal. They may even prevent the persons from ever experiencing higher levels.

Figure 6.1 illustrates the three stage theories described in Table 6.1 from our motivational perspective. Note that the figure depicts people moving upward *or* downward through the various stages of development. It also depicts our hypothesis that only uncertainty-oriented persons reach the final stages hypothesized by stage theorists. Certainty-oriented persons take longer to achieve lower levels, and they may never achieve higher levels. Figure 6.1 does not depict upward and downward movement that should also occur as a function of important motivational determinants (e.g., achievement-related motives, affiliation-related motives) that interact with specific situational components.

Cognitive Development

Piaget's theory proposes a progression of four stages of cognitive development (Piaget, 1972; Piaget with Inhelder, 1969). Sensorimotor intelligence is characterized by gradual movement, starting at birth, from reflexive to intentional re-

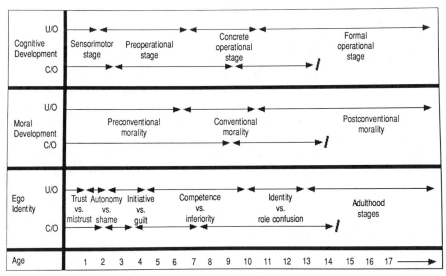

FIGURE 6.1 Uncertainty-oriented (U/O) and certainty-oriented (C/O) persons according to a cognitive–motivational theory of development.

sponses. Preoperational thought is characterized by intuitive reasoning. Concrete operational thought involves the capacity to reason inductively in terms of the real and the experienced. Ideally, cognitive development progresses to the stage of formal operations, characterized by hypothetical thinking and deductive logic. We focus here on the transition from concrete to formal operations, since its occurrence is posited from late childhood onward.

Concrete versus Formal Thought

Those who reach the stage of formal operations are described as being in "intellectual high gear" (Houston, Bee, Hatfield, & Rimm, 1979); their thinking extends beyond reasoning about the actual to reasoning about the possible. They devise hypotheses, deduce their logical consequences, and search for logical consistencies and inconsistencies. They use a methodical approach to problem solving by isolating variables and systematically testing all possible solutions. For them, dealing with the unexperienced is an enjoyable process (Kagan & Havemann, 1976). The relationship of formal thought to the ideals of scientific inquiry is apparent.

People who are at the stage of concrete operations apply rules and concepts to that which is real or has been experienced. They lack the capacity to organize systematically the imagined or the unexperienced into a logical system (Bee, 1981) and do not consider possibilities on a theoretical plane (Houston et al., 1979). They do have the capacity to transfer old knowledge and methods to similar situations, and to reason inductively from the specific to the general. They do not, however, have the capacity to reason in the abstract.

Uncertainty Orientation and Cognitive Level

In our view, uncertainty-oriented persons should use formal thinking. They anticipate positive information value from the process of knowing and find cognitive satisfaction in the process of discovery (e.g., Roney & Sorrentino, 1989b). They are attracted to hypothetical–deductive thinking, which provides them with an opportunity to maximize positive information value. The certainty-oriented should use concrete thought and should not engage in formal thinking. Searching for consistencies and inconsistencies and dealing with the abstract involve experiencing ambiguity, confusion, and uncertainty. The certainty-oriented obtain greater positive information value from knowing than from finding out, and prefer that which is familiar and predictable to that which is unknown and uncertain.[5] They are attracted to thinking that deals with the real and the experienced—that is, concrete operational thought—rather than with the hypothetical.

The certainty-oriented and closed-minded are conceptually similar. Closed-mindedness is negatively correlated with tolerance for ambiguity (Chabassol & Thomas, 1975; Shaffer & Hendrick, 1974). The closed-minded have difficulty synthesizing new beliefs into a belief system (Rokeach, 1960). The concrete thinker has similar difficulty organizing what is imagined or possible into a system (Bee, 1981).

The Emergence of Formal Thought

Formal operations emerge "as the individual is faced with excessive complexity and is forced to consider hypothetical attributes before finding new types of solutions" (Clayton & Overton, 1976, p. 238). Piaget (1972) suggests that all normal people reach formal thought if social environment and experiences are nourishing and stimulating, and if the opportunity is available for spontaneous activity. In our view, an enriched environment can only be appreciated by uncertainty-oriented persons as it provides the opportunity to find out new things about the self or environment. Certainty-oriented persons, however, will not engage in this opportunity. An enriched environment, therefore, should simultaneously cultivate formal thinking and further uncertainty orientation for the incipient uncertainty-oriented; it would do little, however, to cultivate either for the certainty-oriented.

If the development of uncertainty orientation precedes the development of formal thought, then the certainty-oriented may fail to acquire formal operations, regardless of increased environmental stimulation. Alternatively, the development of uncertainty orientation may require formal thinking. The two variables should be positively correlated. The direction of developmental influence between formal thinking and uncertainty orientation is not clear now. There is, however, some evidence consistent with the notion that uncertainty orientation is related to both the desire or capacity to appreciate new environments, and the opportunity to experience new environments. This comes from a study by Kelman and Barclay (1963). These investigators classified subjects according to whether they had high or low psychological capacity (intolerance of ambiguity) and high or low opportunity (e.g., socioeconomic status, rural vs. urban background, education level). They found, as they predicted, that subjects with a high psychological capacity and high opportunity to experience enriched environments had the lowest authoritarianism scores; subjects low on both dimensions had the highest. Thus, there does appear to be a relation between the opportunity and the capacity to appreciate new environments on one of our component measures of uncertainty orientation (i.e., authoritarianism).

EXPERIMENTAL ATTEMPTS TO STIMULATE FORMAL THOUGHT   Tomlinson-Keasey (1972) tried to increase cognitive level by individually tailored training in thinking. Significant increases occurred, but did not generalize to new tasks. In our view, although both uncertainty- and certainty-oriented persons would be able to learn a specific method of thinking, only uncertainty-oriented persons would generalize such a method to new tasks requiring formal thought. The certainty-oriented, in adhering to what is already known, would only replicate the training procedure, thus failing to show generalization required by formal logical thought. The uncertainty-oriented would show generalization. However, data analysis, without taking into account differences in uncertainty orientation, could reduce or eliminate overall generalization. This would depend upon the proportions of uncertainty- and certainty-oriented subjects in the sample.

This generalization interpretation is consistent with the apparent "black-and-white" thinking found on the part of certainty-oriented persons (Roney &

Sorrentino, 1987). In this study, subjects were asked to describe traits characteristic of persons in different occupations. Certainty-oriented persons were less likely than uncertainty-oriented persons to generalize personality traits of people in one occupation (e.g., secretary) to people in another (e.g., doctor). Although one might argue that this indicates more complex reasoning in the Piagetian sense by certainty-oriented persons (Higgins, personal communication, 1989), we believe that it is more likely to indicate such persons' inability to employ accommodative strategies in going from one abstract category to another. Thus, for the certainty-oriented person, secretaries are stereotypical in one way and doctors are stereotypical in another.[6] Indeed, we have argued that this inability may be one of the underlying causes of prejudice in certainty-oriented or authoritarian persons (Roney & Sorrentino, 1987).

ASSESSMENT AND FUNCTIONING OF FORMAL OPERATIONAL THOUGHT

Formal thought is most commonly assessed by physical and logical–mathematical tasks. However, these tasks may fail to provide an adequate assessment of logical functioning in adults. The problem is that uncertainty-oriented persons probably have a higher capacity for formal thought than certainty-oriented persons. Such tasks are also what may be called "achievement-oriented"; that is, the person knows that he or she is being evaluated on a skilled task, and feels responsible for the outcome (see Atkinson & Raynor, 1974; McClelland, 1961). Recall that information value appears to determine affective arousal as a result of achievement-related motives. If the situation is relevant to a person's uncertainty orientation, then the person will either be positively motivated to succeed or negatively motivated to avoid failure. If situations requiring formal thought are relevant for the uncertainty-oriented person, then that person will perform better only if he or she is also success-oriented. If failure-threatened, he or she will perform worse in that situation. Hence, although the latter person may have the ability to perform well, he or she will be inhibited in such situations. By looking only at information value, Piagetians may misclassify many people who have actually reached the level of formal operations, but are incapacitated by the achievement tasks administered to them.

Piaget (1972) acknowledges that physical and logical–mathematical tasks may apply to schoolchildren but may not generalize beyond this age group. People may reason hypothetically in particular areas of specialization. However, when faced with experimental situations, "their lack of knowledge or the fact that they have forgotten certain ideas . . . [may] give the appearance of being at the concrete level" (Piaget, 1972, p. 10). Piaget (1972) also suggests that formal thinking may be manifested in different areas for different people; for example, they may reach formal operations in areas particular to their interests or careers. However, he provides no systematic principles to account for such selectivity. We are saying much the same thing, except that we can provide systematic principles to account for such selectivity.

In our view, motivational variables may determine the pursuit of psychological careers in different substantive areas. These areas in turn may provide varying knowledge of and ability to perform logical thought, making comparison of these people's formal scores misleading. This may also explain the apparent selective use of formal thinking. The uncertainty-oriented, success-oriented person should seek clarity through mastering uncertainty in occupational activity by using propositional thought. As an example, consider a psychological career in basic science, where persons see themselves as rational thinkers, handling new and unknown phenomena by systematic principles of logic. Conversely, the certainty-oriented, success-oriented person should attempt to maintain clarity and avoid confusion in occupational activity by using concrete thought—doing to new things what has been done to old things (Houston et al., 1979). Consider an occupational career in applied technology, where persons see themselves as problem solvers, using previously acquired knowledge to yield a required product.

So far, we have only talked about uncertainty orientation in terms of the person who is also success-oriented. Failure-threatened, uncertainty-oriented persons will probably choose occupational careers that are not achievement-oriented (e.g., unskilled labor, politics).[7] Thus, they may not develop formal thought in achievement domains, but may do so in other areas (e.g., social relationships, influence situations).

People may use a form of logic in real life that differs from Piagetian logic (Berzonsky, Weiner, & Raphael, 1975). Alternatively, formal thought may be available to some, but as adults they may tend toward concrete thinking as a means of either attaining clarity or avoiding negative affect. This interpretation is consistent with the Berzonsky et al. (1975) view that formal thinking may be a potential competency, but that its use, once acquired, depends on other variables. An important and perhaps necessary variable for the use of formal thinking may be our informational variable, uncertainty orientation. This must, of course, be considered in conjunction with important affective variables, such as achievement, affiliation, and power motivation.

Cognitive Functioning in Middle and Late Adulthood

People who are uncertainty-oriented but lack opportunities to master uncertainty may fail to use formal thought in early adulthood, but may do so later if such opportunities become available. In late-stage striving, uncertainty orientation and hence formal thought may (1) decline because future opportunities to engage in uncertain situations are lacking or the uncertain situations become affectively aversive (e.g., constant failure); or (2) remain high because affective value is sustained or because a search for valued future goals turns certain paths into uncertain ones.

Clayton and Overton (1976) found no difference in the use of formal thought between institutionalized and noninstitutionalized elderly persons. This finding is consistent with the second suggestion above. It implies that uncertainty orientation is relatively stable throughout life, and that the uncertainty-oriented remain future-oriented, regardless of type of setting. We expect little change in cognitive functioning of the certainty-oriented at different stages of striving. They should continually try to maintain or reattain clarity obtained by adherence to the concrete, known, and previously experienced.

Moral Development

Kohlberg (1969, 1973) proposes six stages of moral development, which represent three distinct levels of reasoning (see Table 6.1). Moral development represents structural transformation or a change in the form of thinking rather than in its content. It results from disequilibrium experienced when the existing mode of thought proves inadequate for dealing with ethical conflict. The stages are universal and occur in an invariant sequence in which each higher stage reintegrates the thinking of the previous stage. Movement in the sequence is always progressive, never regressive, except for conditions of extreme trauma (Kohlberg & Hersh, 1977). People employ the highest level of moral thought available to them (Kohlberg, 1973; Kohlberg & Hersh, 1977).

At the preconventional level, morality is externally determined by the avoidance of punishment and deference to those with superior power (Stage 1), and by hedonistic emphasis on personal gain (Stage 2). The conventional level stresses conformity and loyalty to the family and the priority of interpersonal relationships (Stage 3). It also stresses conformity and loyalty to the larger society, the fulfillment of duties, and unquestioning obedience to the law (Stage 4). In the transition from conventional to principled thought (Stage 4½), the person is characterized by egoism and skepticism. He or she questions the validity of earlier moral reasoning (e.g., obedience to the law). The postconventional or principled level involves an emphasis on basic nonrelative values. These include liberty, the belief that laws are a service to society and subject to change (Stage 5), the pre-eminence of self-chosen ethical principles, and the domination of conscience in making moral decisions (Stage 6).[8] The principled moral level is considered to be a "more sophisticated and mature" moral orientation. This is because it "allows for the resolution of the conflicts and inconsistencies present in earlier stages" (Gutkin & Suls, 1979, p. 435).

It is assumed that moral development is related to cognitive stage development. Both logical and moral thought are "schemata which develop a set of general structural characteristics representing successive forms of psychological equilibrium" (Kohlberg & Gilligan, 1971, p. 1069). Formal operational thought is necessary but not sufficient for higher moral reasoning.

Assessment of Moral Level and Cultural Value

Moral level is generally assessed by classifying a subject's responses to hypothetical moral dilemmas on the basis of reasoning used to arrive at solutions rather than on that of content. In our view, this assessment may be confounded by a person's beliefs that a type of reasoning is "good" or "bad"—that is, by individual cultural value. If establishing one's own convictions and following the dictates of conscience are seen as "good" (positive cultural value), and unquestioning obedience to authority and the law are seen as "bad" (negative cultural value), we predict that the choice of moral solutions will be consistent with these cultural values. Gutkin and Suls (1979) found that subjects who valued an "ethics of personal conscience" (which emphasizes personal notions of morality; Hogan, 1970) obtained high scores on a measure of principled morality. Those who valued an "ethics of social responsibility" were rated as conventional moral reasoners. This type of ethics emphasizes the legal system and the general welfare; it often involves a distrust of personal notions of morality (Hogan, 1970). These findings are consistent with our view that people's cultural values concerning the type of moral reasoning may affect and confound their scores on a measure of moral level. Similar arguments have been made by Edwards (1981), Miller (1984), and Rogoff and Morelli (1989).

Moral Reasoning and Personality Functioning

Kohlberg (1973; see also Kohlberg & Hersh, 1977) has proposed that people prefer a solution at the "highest" available level of moral thought. In our view, people use a type of moral thinking whose outcomes maximize positive and minimize negative value. The uncertainty-oriented should prefer principled moral thinking. Its process of acquisition provides positive information value by forcing recognition of the relativism of beliefs, the mutability of the law, and the pre-eminence of abstract principles rather than concrete rules.

The certainty-oriented should prefer conventional moral solutions. They should resist principled thinking because the process of acquisition provides negative information value. Thus, although principled moral reasoning could lead to resolution of the conflicts and inconsistencies present in earlier stages (Gutkin & Suls, 1979), certainty-oriented persons, ironically, never achieve this level. Instead, they avoid confusion in the moral realm by stressing duty as defined by authority, family, or the law (conventional reasoning). They may also avoid confusion by a reliance on the certainty of reward or punishment (preconventional reasoning). If the certainty of reward or punishment is greater than that provided by conventional views, the certainty-oriented should use preconventional reasoning, even though the next "higher" level is available. Since the expectancy of gaining clarity is usually higher when morality is based on adherence to parents, authorities, or the law, we generally expect a positive correlation between certainty orientation and conventional moral reasoning. The certainty-oriented should prefer the conventional level rather than the "higher" principled level, in order to maintain clarity and avoid the confusion of postconventional relativism.[9]

Changes in Level of Moral Reasoning

Reversals in the stage of moral reasoning have been found (Arbuthnot, 1975; Holstein, 1976; Kramer, 1986; Turiel, 1966). Arbuthnot (1975) used role play and discussion to investigate progression through moral stages and found that Stage 4 subjects showed substantial movement in *both* directions. We suggest that the Stage 4 subjects who moved "forward" were the uncertainty-oriented, attracted to mastering uncertainty offered by postconventional reasoning. It is less clear why subjects moved backward unless they were actually at Stage 4½, which involves challenging unquestioned obedience to the law. We would expect that exposure to such uncertainty would move the certainty-oriented "back" toward conventional reasoning, in order to remove the confusion posed by the moral dilemma.

Rate of Progression in Moral Reasoning

A consistent finding in moral progression research is that there is a "ceiling effect," with more upward movement among lower- than among higher-stage subjects (Arbuthnot, 1975; Blatt, 1970; Holstein, 1976; Keasey, 1973; Tracy & Cross, 1973; Turiel, 1965). Tracy and Cross (1973), for example, stimulated moral progression through a role-playing exercise. They found that Level 1 (preconventional) subjects increased substantially in moral reasoning, but that Level 2 (conventional) subjects did not. We suggest that more upward movement occurred from the lower level because most people will move from Level 1 to Level 2. However, only uncertainty-oriented persons will move to Level 3. For certainty-oriented persons, conventional adherence to authority (Level 2) usually provides greater subjective probability to clarity over the more uncertain rewards and punishments involved in preconventional moral reasoning (Level 1). However, progression from Level 2 (conventional) to Level 3 (principled) should occur only for the uncertainty-oriented. The majority of Level 2 (conventional) should be certainty-oriented and therefore should resist principled moral thinking (Level 3).[10]

Disequilibrium and Changes in Moral Reasoning

Cognitive developmentalists assume that stage progression occurs as a result of "disequilibrium," which results because a person's moral mode of thinking proves inadequate for handling moral conflict (Piaget, 1950, p. 6). From the motivational perspective, it is only the uncertainty-oriented who are expected to be thrown into disequilibrium by a challenge to moral beliefs and to weigh alternatives. For them, the opportunity to master uncertainty provides positive rather than negative information value. Conversely, the certainty-oriented avoid disequilibrium (confusion) by clinging to a position or by cognitively restructuring the situation, in order to avoid confusion or to remove it if experienced. An interesting example of this is the study by Shaffer and Hendrick (1974). They found that closed-minded and ambiguity-intolerant subjects reported less liking for an effortful task in a dissonance condition than did open-minded and ambiguity-tolerant subjects. The latter (akin to uncertainty-oriented persons) demonstrated typical dissonance-reducing behavior. They preferred and enhanced a dissonance-producing task. The former (akin to certainty-oriented persons) showed no evidence of dissonance (see Wicklund & Brehm, 1976). Instead they chose to derogate the experiment and the experimenter. Here, paradoxically, the aversive consequences of dissonance ("disequilibrium" to the developmentalist, "confusion" to us) were greater for the open-minded than for the closed-minded. This is consistent with our notion that only uncertainty-oriented types of persons will be concerned with and attempt to resolve uncertain, inconsistent, or dissonant situations (see Sorrentino & Short, 1986). Certainty-oriented persons ignore or avoid such situations rather than becoming concerned with them.

Wonderly and Kupfersmid (1978) tested the assumption that disequilibrium explains stage progression by comparing transitional (mixed-stage) subjects with pure-stage subjects on five measures of psychological adjustment. They found that transitional subjects did not show greater "disequilibrium" than pure-stage subjects. This may have been because their subjects were primarily certainty-oriented. Had they controlled for individual differences in uncertainty orientation, they may have found evidence of disequilibrium in the uncertainty-oriented group (recall our findings on negative affect and self-discrepancy; Roney & Sorrentino, 1989a).

Moratorium and Principled Moral Thinking

Kohlberg (1973) has noted a failure to develop principled moral reasoning among those who enter the Army or the work force after high school (instead of attending college). He has suggested the importance of a college moratorium for the development of principled reasoning. In our view, both college attendance and principled thinking provide opportunities to the uncertainty-oriented to maximize positive information value by seeking clarity through mastery of uncertainty. We suggest that this "sleeper effect," which purportedly requires a moratorium experience for principled reasoning to develop, reflects the choice of the uncertainty-oriented for the challenge of uncertainty. Those who joined the Army were more likely to be certainty-oriented. Their failure to use principled reasoning would result from their certainty orientation rather than their lack of a college moratorium experience. Consistent with this view is Podd's (1972) finding that conventional students exposed to postconventional moral reasoning during college did not seriously consider this type of reasoning. Instead, they remained committed to their conventional position.

Moral Level and Familiarity

Freeman and Giebink (1979) found that the highest moral judgments were associated with the most remote moral situations and the lowest with the most familiar. In our view, the uncertainty-oriented should be attracted to remote and highly unfamiliar dilemmas, which offer greater opportunity to master uncertainty. The certainty-oriented should be attracted to the most familiar moral dilemmas, because these provide the greatest certainty.

Principled Moral Reasoning and Late Adulthood

Postconventional moral reasoning may predominate in early-stage striving, where a person considers "what might be" or "what ought to be" and weighs each possibility rationally and objectively. In late-stage striving, the cultural value of a specific moral viewpoint may predominate, limiting consideration of all sides of that moral issue. This process over time may lead the uncertainty-oriented to become dogmatic with respect to that moral viewpoint, appearing as upholding tradition, the law, or the views of "the past generation." Thus, in later life the previously "intellectual" and objective may come closer to being the passionate and biased. Conventional moral thinking has been described as a foreclosure-type process (Podd, 1972), because it involves adherence to a commitment without consideration of alternatives. Without some "nudging" or reinstatement of past values, the postconventional thinker in late-stage striving may come to display "foreclosed" moral thinking, a process of reasoning resembling that of the conventional moral thinker in early-stage striving.

Dialectical Theory of Development

The cognitive-developmental approach assumes that each successive stage of development represents a period of equilibrium. Riegel's (1976) dialectic theory places emphasis on continuous change rather than on equilibrated states. Dialectic theory stresses that both the person and the environment are constant sources of contradiction. The person continuously strives toward a goal of synchrony, though synchrony is never completely achieved. Lack of synchronization results in "crisis," the resolution of which contributes to new development or growth. The dialectic perspectives focuses on how people generate problems rather than on how they solve them. The person is viewed as inquisitive, doubtful, and "never at rest."

Dialectic Theory and Information Value

In our view, synchrony refers to "clarity" or "knowing." For dialectic psychology, the person is a seeker and a questioner. However, seeking and questioning are characteristic of the uncertainty-oriented, who value the process of finding out and anticipate that the mastery of uncertainty will provide positive information value. The certainty-oriented value the *product* of knowledge rather than the *process* of discovery or finding out. They are unlikely to seek questions to ask or problems to solve, so as not to be confused. Dialectical psychology is concerned with how individuals "succeed in overcoming tranquillity and balance" (Riegel, 1976, p. 696). From our perspective, tranquillity and balance represent clarity and the absence of confusion—states that the certainty-oriented should not wish to overcome.

Riegel proposes that the dialectical model encompasses both the "materialistic" (concrete) preference for commodity, product, and result, and the "idealistic" preference for activity, labor, and effort. In the cognitive realm, the materialistic and the idealistic represent two distinct orientations. As stated above, the certainty-oriented do value a product—knowledge. The uncertainty-oriented also value an activity—finding out. A desire to approach and to understand the unknown, to resolve inconsistencies, and to act to overcome uncertainty are characteristics of the uncertainty-oriented. Riegel's dialectical theory seems to describe only the uncertainty-oriented while neglecting the certainty-oriented, for whom a primary motivation is not to overcome contradiction, but to avoid or ignore it. The research by Gitta (1989) and Gitta and Sorrentino (1989) is consistent with this notion of two distinct orientations. These studies showed that whereas uncertainty-oriented persons were process-oriented, certainty-oriented persons were outcome-oriented. The latter were also avoidant of arousal caused by uncertainty.

The Development of Ego Identity and the Identity Statuses

Erikson's (1959, 1968) theory of psychosocial development proposes that ego development unfolds through eight stages across the life span (see Table 6.1). At each stage, the person must resolve a crisis for healthy development to take place (Ewen, 1980). The positive outcome of the crisis of identity is a firm sense of identity and commitment to an ideology and an occupation. The negative outcome of this stage is the state of identity diffusion.

The ontogeny of uncertainty orientation may be consistent with Erikson's stages. We suspect that the uncertainty-oriented person is likely to develop a basic trust early in life, leading to autonomy, which in turn leads to initiative. Hence, such a person should trust the world, seek his or her control over it, and go out in search of new and stimulating events. The certainty-oriented person, on the other hand, may go from a basic mistrust of the world, to reliance and dependence on authority and a fear of the unknown. Hence, such a person should stick to safe, or at least predictable, events.

It is our belief that individual differences in uncertainty orientation may serve as the interface among Eriksonian, Kohlbergian, and Piagetian conceptions.[11] We assume that the uncertainty-oriented person develops formal logic, principled thinking, and a positive orientation toward uncertain outcomes. We also assume that the certainty-oriented person has not reached and may not reach these levels (see Figure 6.1). Hence, we should expect these differences in uncertainty orientation to extend into various aspects of ego identity.

Based on Erikson's ideas, four identity statuses have been proposed (Marcia, 1966) that represent styles of functioning along a continuum of identity achievement. These statuses have been defined as movement from the absence of commitment ("diffusion") to crisis ("moratorium") to commitment ("achieved identity"), or alternatively, from diffusion to commitment without crisis ("foreclosure") (Munro & Adams, 1977). These now represent four possible outcomes of Erikson's stage of identity versus identity diffusion.

Identity-diffuse individuals are characterized by a lack of commitment to a self-definition. They do not have an identity and are unconcerned with establishing one. Individuals in moratorium, by definition, are in the midst of crisis; they are engaged in the process of examining alternatives and are actively seeking to establish an identity. The identity-achieved status represents the most mature resolution of the identity crisis. People in this status have actively questioned former identifications and searched among alternatives to arrive at a pronounced sense of self. They have committed themselves to an occupation and an ideology on the basis of self-derived decisions. The identity-foreclosed have established a firm identity based on identification with parents and other authorities, but have done so without examining alternatives.

Ego-Identity Status and Personality Functioning

In our view, the identity statuses deal with motivational arousal in different systems: identity diffusion in the behavioral system, moratorium in the emergent self-system, identity achievement in a psychological career, and foreclosure in the self-system (but not in a psychological career). Although so-called "identity crises" may reflect normal personality functioning, there is no inevitable need to establish or to preserve a self-identity (cf. Raynor & McFarlin, 1986; Sorrentino & Roney, 1989a; Sorrentino & Short, 1986). Adults can and do function in life without arousal in the self-system or in a psychological career (i.e., without perceived self-identities). Identity crisis is not necessary for later functioning. The manner in which perceived self-identity emerges and changes (or in which identity "crises" are resolved) is determined by opportunities to maximize positive and minimize negative affective and information value. Prior to self-system functioning, but after development of the capacity to answer the question "Who am I?", the idea of self-definition represents an opportunity to attain clarity by mastery of uncertainty. It also poses the threat of confusion and ambiguity.

IDENTITY DIFFUSION AND THE BEHAVIORAL SYSTEM   The identity-diffuse lack sufficient sources of information and affective value to be concerned about self-identity. There is no inevitable motivation to move from diffusion to other identity statuses. People can function for a lifetime without motivation in the self-system. They do so without the additional sources of positive affective and information value available to people with functioning in the self-system or a psychological career. On the other hand, they do so without the negative affective and information value (see Roney & Sorrentino, 1989a). The diffuse should be weakly motivated because they lack sources of positive value. They are characterized by relative indifference in the behavioral system and in the self-system. Their motivational arousal should be more influenced by immediate and momentary sources of value; it should be less intense and should not persist for long. The identity-diffuse have been found to base job changes on the negative aspects of the occupation, to be dissatisfied with these changes, and to be the least likely to pursue higher education or to make a vocational commitment (Waterman & Waterman, 1976).

MORATORIUM AND THE EMERGENT SELF-SYSTEM   In our view, most individuals in moratorium are uncertainty-oriented people in the process of achieving identity. A minority are certainty-oriented people in the process of becoming identity-foreclosed. Individuals in moratorium are concerned about answering the question "who am I?", but are uncertain about an answer. They derive negative information value if they are certainty-oriented and positive information value if they are uncertainty-oriented. Certainty-oriented persons in moratorium are primarily motivated to remove confusion. They should move rapidly from moratorium to foreclosure, in order to remove confusion engendered by self-questioning; they wish to adopt a clear and valued self-image without further searching for alternatives. Uncertainty-oriented persons in moratorium are primarily motivated to master uncertainty. They should move slowly through moratorium, because the process of self-discovery provides positive information value. They move to achieved status if they find a self-image with clarity that provides esteem income.

Erikson (1972) has proposed that a prolonged moratorium may result in impulsive attempts to end it with sudden choices. From our view, this would be expected only for a minority of certainty-oriented individuals in moratorium. For them, a prolonged moratorium is an extended experience of confusion. Their sudden choice is movement to foreclosed status to remove confusion without further exposure to it.

IDENTITY ACHIEVEMENT AND THE PSYCHOLOGICAL CAREER   We believe that those who have achieved identity are primarily the uncertainty-oriented who have investigated a variety of possible selves and found one by mastering uncertainty about self-definition. Research is consistent with our view of the identity-achieved as persons with a need to approach and to overcome uncertainty who place a high value on thinking (Beourne, 1978). The identity-achieved have a greater need for complexity (Matteson, 1974) and are significantly more reflective than individuals in the other statuses (Waterman & Waterman, 1974).

Successful occupational outcomes are often both clear-cut and high in positive cultural value. Hence, they are likely to become sources for self-definition (positive information value) and self-esteem (positive affective value). Self-images defined by the outcomes of action along a life path are time-linked ("who I am becoming," "who I have been," "the attributes I possess"). This is consistent with the description of identity achievement as "continuity within self" (Marcia, 1966). It reflects a synthesis of earlier identifications, and the establishment of an identity that is "unique and yet continuous" with earlier perceptions of the self (Podd, 1972). In our view, however, such continuities are not necessary for self-identity. Young people often lack a past sense of self, since valued life successes have not occurred; old people often lack a future sense of self, since valued future successes are not anticipated. In these cases, the amount of value will determine whether such a restricted self-system will provide sufficient clarity and self-esteem to sustain a psychological career.

The identity-achieved should prefer contingent and open paths, because these provide many and continued opportunities to master uncertainty with respect to the future sense of self. Waterman and Waterman (1976) found that the identity-achieved had a significantly higher level of education, such as graduate or professional training. They were also more likely to initiate career changes for self-generated reasons—an indication of active search and deliberation with regard to vocational choice.

We expect that people who have achieved an identity may explore the possibilities of new self-images because of their uncertainty orientation. However, they will also strive to maintain their perceived self-identity because they experience positive esteem income from seeing themselves clearly in a valued way. Identity-achieved individuals were found to resist self-esteem manipulations in the face of information discrepant with their self-perceptions (Marcia, 1966, 1967). We have already noted that the uncertainty-oriented are not motivated by induced confusion (i.e., discrepant information) to remove it. Their currently perceived self-image provides sufficient positive value for them to strive to maintain it. However, if the value of perceived self-images decreases, the identity-achieved are more likely to approach such discrepant information than individuals in other statuses. They do this with the goal of discovering a new self-image with greater positive value.

FORECLOSED IDENTITY STATUS   The foreclosed status should be associated with certainty orientation. Any source of value has the potential to become a means of perceived self-identity, provided that it produces clarity and self-esteem. The foreclosed arrive at an identity by adopting views of parents or other authority figures. They move rapidly away from moratorium to reduce the confusion generated by examination of alternatives, or use a clear life outcome to define a self-image. In doing so, they minimize negative information value while maximizing positive affective value. They should avoid the ambiguity involved in a struggle to achieve an identity through active questioning and search. Research has consistently shown that the foreclosed are high in authoritarianism, compared to individuals in other statuses (Marcia, 1967; Marcia & Friedman, 1970; Matteson, 1974; Schenkel & Marcia, 1972). High authoritarianism is characteristic of certainty orientation and correlates negatively with ambiguity tolerance (McBride & Moran, 1967; Millon, 1957; Zacker, 1973). This is perhaps also why our certainty-oriented subjects have smaller self-discrepancies and are less affected by them than are our uncertainty-oriented subjects (Roney & Sorrentino, 1989a; Sorrentino & Roney, 1989a).

From the stage theory perspective, a person cannot return to foreclosed identity status once he or she has left it by experiencing a crisis of self-doubt. In our view, exposure to uncertainty about a self-image should produce confusion in the certainty-oriented; they should remove this confusion by either ignoring it or suddenly changing from one foreclosed identity to another. This should depend on the value of the new relative to the old self-image. They should foreclose again and again by adopting a succession of immediately available, culturally valued self-images whenever self-doubt produces enough negative value to motivate its removal (see Rokeach's [1960] discussion of party-line thinking in closed-minded individuals).

The foreclosed should prefer a closed career path, because it provides a clear-cut future self-image that they can see themselves striving to attain. Waterman and Waterman (1976) found a lack of foreclosed subjects with graduate or professional training. The foreclosed were also found to be least likely of the four status groups to make occupational changes. High job stability would be expected of the certainty-oriented, because they may be strongly motivated to maintain clarity of self-images (images tied to the outcomes of past job performance).

Cultural value should be significant in the establishment of an identity among the foreclosed. The acceptability of the foreclosed self-image as a source of positive affective value is most easily based on valuation of parental and other authorities. Waterman and Waterman (1976) found that, among other extrinsic motivations, "family tradition" frequently determined vocational choice among the foreclosed. Certainty orientation should be related to respect for tradition, since it provides clear-cut, unambiguous, and acceptable ways of seeing oneself.[12]

Performance Difference for Identity Statuses

Marcia (1966) compared the performance of individuals in the different identity statuses on a concept attainment task. The identity-achieved performed significantly better and gave up less often than those in other statuses. This suggests a tolerance for uncertainty. The foreclosed, on the other hand, had the lowest performance and gave up more often than those in other statuses. This suggests an intolerance for uncertainty. The results for the achieved and foreclosed statuses are consistent with our expectations: The uncertainty-oriented should be more interested and the certainty-oriented should be less interested when uncertainty is great. The actual performance, again, should interact with affective value (Sorrentino & Short, 1986).

Uncertainty Orientation and Identity Status

Figure 6.2 illustrates the hypothetical relationship between uncertainty orientation and Marcia's (1966) four identity statuses. Here we have taken the data from Meilman's (1979) study of college-bound or college-educated people from age 12 to age 24 (as illustrated in Shaffer, 1979, p. 477). We have then labeled the four statuses according to the predominance of uncertainty-oriented and certainty-oriented persons in each. By age 24, we would expect most of those in the statuses of identity achievement and moratorium to be uncertainty-oriented; we would expect most of those in foreclosure and identity diffusion to be certainty-oriented. It is also important to note that the proportions here of individuals in identity achievement and moratorium would probably be much lower for a blue-collar sample. Such a sample would have much higher proportions of the foreclosed and the identity-diffuse.

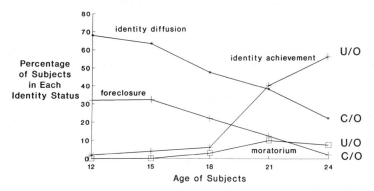

FIGURE 6.2 Hypothetical placement of uncertainty-oriented (U/O) and certainty-oriented (C/O) persons according to Meilman's (1979) data on Marcia's four identity statuses among college-bound or college-educated subjects. Adapted from Shaffer (1979).

RELATIONSHIPS AMONG OPERATIONAL THOUGHT, MORAL REASONING, AND EGO IDENTITY

Numerous studies have investigated relationships among the three developmental constructs: operational thought, moral reasoning, and ego identity (Cauble, 1976; Haan, Weiss, & Johnson, 1982; Hult, 1979; Liberman, Gaa, & Frankiewicz, 1983; Podd, 1970, 1972; Rowe & Marcia, 1980; Wagner, 1976; Walker & Richards, 1979).

Rowe and Marcia (1980) found a significant relationship between the identity-achieved status and principled moral reasoning. *Only subjects who reached at least the transition to full formal operations were at these levels of ego identity and moral development.* The foreclosed were mostly conventional moral reasoners, and some were preconventional. In an assessment of the performance of individuals in the different identity statuses on two formal operational tasks, Wagner (1976) found that a predominance of identity-achieved and moratorium subjects had reached formal operations. A greater proportion of the foreclosed and the identity-diffuse were found to employ concrete operations. Cauble (1976) found that formal thinkers used principled moral reasoning more than did concrete thinkers.

Podd (1970) found a significant use of preconventional reasoning among the foreclosed, and a substantial representation of the foreclosed at the conventional level. Similarly, Rowe and Marcia (1980) found that the foreclosed were most conventional moral reasoners, and some were preconventional. Podd (1972) found that both identity-achieved and moratorium subjects had higher mean morality scores than foreclosed and identity-diffuse subjects. Also, there were significantly fewer principled moral reasoners among the foreclosed than would be expected by chance. Similarly, Hult (1979) found that identity-achieved and moratorium subjects had significantly higher moral reasoning than the identity-diffuse, and higher moral reasoning than the foreclosed.

Kohlberg (1973) suggests that Erikson's stage progression may be a necessary part of principled reasoning. Both ego progression and moral progression may be "absent in persons permanently conventional and nonquestioning of identity" (p. 199). Liberman et al. (1983) investigated the relationship between Kohlberg's moral development stages and ego development as outlined by Loevinger's theory of personality development. They found that subjects at higher levels of ego development had significantly higher moral scores than those at lower levels of ego development.

These findings are consistent with our hypothesis that people at the highest levels of cognitive, moral, and ego-identity development may be similarly motivated to seek clarity through mastery of uncertainty with respect to logical thought, moral issues, and the self. The uncertainty-oriented are unlikely to adopt a conferred identity or a conventional moral view without examining options. Such examination involves reasoning about the possible, assuming hypothetical conditions, and making inferences about them—characteristics that define formal thinking (Kagan & Havemann, 1976). Conversely, the certainty-oriented are motivated to maintain clarity by avoiding confusion with respect to existing cognitions, moral beliefs, and the self. Hence, they are not expected to think hypothetically or to investigate alternative moral perspectives and self-definitions.

The most consistency in use of a type of moral reasoning has been found among the identity-achieved and the foreclosed (Hult, 1979). This finding is compatible with our view of these statuses as occupying the extreme positions on the uncertainty–certainty dimension.

THE CULTURAL VALUE OF KNOWING

Piaget's theory of cognitive development assumes that logical information processing—deductive reasoning—is the highest stage in cognitive development. Kohlberg places similar emphasis on the hypothetical–deductive process and contends that "each higher (moral) stage is logically, cognitively, or philosophically more adequate than the preceding stage and logically includes it" (1973, p. 199).

In our view, the claim that subsequent developmental stages are more "adequate" than previous stages is based on the cultural view of knowing. We suggest that different cultures value different modes of thinking. This cultural value of knowing provides the basis for judgments about "mature," "higher," and "more adequate" ways of thinking. In modern Western culture there is a widely shared positive cultural value associated with hypothetical–deductive thinking— that is, with knowing through the mastery of uncertainty and the unknown. Conversely, there is a negative cultural value associated with both emotionally based decision making and conforming to the status quo without examination of its origins and validity—that is, with knowing by maintaining clarity with respect to the "truth" as stated by tradition, convention, the law, the church, the family, and wisdom based on authority.[13]

A comparison of Western and Chinese cultural traditions (Shu-Fang Dien, 1982) suggests that what is considered to be the "mature" and "superior" mode of resolving moral conflict is closely associated with differences between Eastern and Western conceptions of the individual and of morality. Shu-Fang Dien points out that the Eastern value system emphasizes the subordination of the individual to the group, and the importance of "individual duties and limits." In Eastern culture the preferred mode of conflict resolution is "reconciliation and collective decision-making." Conversely, the Western value system emphasizes the "doctrine of civil liberties and individual rights" and the resolution of moral conflict through "individual choice and commitment" (p. 331). In our view, in Eastern culture there is greater positive value associated with loyalty to the group and tradition, and greater negative cultural value associated with autonomy and self-determination.[14]

Simpson (1974) has challenged Kohlberg's (1973) claim of universality, citing the failure of some individuals and cultures to reach principled thinking. We suggest that the failure to reach the "highest" moral level may be a function of the difference in positive cultural value of knowing through tradition and authority, as opposed to the positive cultural value of knowing through logical information processing.

Sullivan (1977) has criticized Kohlberg's structuralism for its separation of emotional life from intellectual life. This author suggests that "in the type of dichotomy Kohlberg presents the emotions are relegated to an epiphenomenal status in understanding and in morality" (p. 15). From Sullivan's perspective, and from ours, Kohlberg's moral stages are an "offshoot of the development of scientific understanding," and moral logic is "an extension of scientific logic" (p. 16). The scientist's value system stresses that strong affective value in the process of discovery and knowing is "bad." It is "bad" to be emotional; it is good to be "objective" by weighing all reasonable alternatives. Mature moral reasoning and cognitive functioning as defined by Kohlberg and Piaget are abstract and formal. As such, they reflect a Western bias toward reason and against feeling.

Our position emphasizes affective and information value as interacting sources of motivational impetus for arousal and functioning in terms of the personality's dual principles—to maximize positive and minimize negative (affective and information) value. The cognitive-developmentalist position emphasizes positive information value and neglects positive affective value. In our view, psychological functioning and adjustment involve maximizing both positive affective and positive information value. The most psychologically mature individuals are those who can emotionally commit themselves to a belief or a course of action that seems clear, thus maximizing both kinds of value. Thus, certainty-oriented persons, concrete thinkers, conventional moral reasoners, and foreclosed individuals are as "mature" and "advanced" in their personality functioning as are uncertainty-oriented persons, formal thinkers, principled moral reasoners, and identity-achieved individuals.

Loevinger and Wessler (1970) assert that ego progression from the lowest or impulsive stage, through opportunistic hedonism and conformity, to the highest or integrated stage of ego development represents a sequence of "coping with increasingly deeper problems" (p. 7) rather than higher levels of adjustment. However, the positive cultural value of knowing through mastery of uncertainty is evident in other formulations of ego development. The "healthy" ego is one that has achieved identity, or is at least in the process of moratorium, because these statuses are characterized by use of an investigative process—active questioning and search among alternatives. On the other hand, foreclosure, while admittedly often functional (Rowe & Marcia, 1980), is considered a less-than-ideal resolution of the "crisis" of identity because it is the result of living up to parental or societal expectations without having challenged them. But living up to such expectations is positively valued by a good many individuals in Western cultures.

Is there evidence that parental and other authority-based sources of self-esteem are less adequate for personality functioning and psychological health than those derived from self-search and struggle through uncertainty? In an application of the identity statuses to college women, Marcia and Friedman (1979) found that *both* the identity-achieved and the foreclosed chose more difficult college majors than those in other statuses. They also found that the foreclosed had the *highest* self-esteem and the *lowest* anxiety scores of the four identity status groups. In an attempt to reconcile their data with Dignan's (1965) finding that the foreclosed (assumed to be low in ego identity) scored *highest* on a measure of ego identity, Marcia and Friedman (1969) suggest that the foreclosed status may be "more adaptive" for women. In our view, the high ego-identity scores among the foreclosed, their choice of more difficult college majors, their high self-esteem, and their low anxiety are not unexpected. Positive information value results from being clear about any self-image, whatever its source. Self-esteem from it depends on its affective value. One can be equally well "adjusted" as foreclosed (and conventional) and as identity-achieved (and principled). The foreclosed in particular have large sources of positive cultural value that provide clear and valued senses of self. We find in our own data that uncertainty-oriented and certainty-oriented persons do not differ in self-esteem (Hafer, 1987), and that at least as first-year undergraduates, certainty-oriented students appear to be happier than uncertainty-oriented students (Roney & Sorrentino, 1989a).

The identity-achieved may be more vulnerable to a later change in perceived identity (e.g., a "midlife identity crisis"). On the other hand, they may also be better able to resolve it (i.e., to find new, valued self-images)—not because of their experience of previous crises, as the stage theorists assume, but rather because of their attraction to uncertain situations with the goal of working through to clarity.

SUMMARY AND CONCLUSIONS

We have shown that it is possible to reinterpret three bodies of literature in terms of the value of the outcomes of thought and action. This is done without assuming that there is an invariant sequence of change over time; that self-system functioning is inevitable or necessary; that needs such as enhancement or consistency exist; or that one way of knowing, reasoning, or self-identity is more "adequate" or "mature" than another. From this perspective, individual differences in cognitive, moral, and self-system functioning result from normal functioning of the personality's dual principles of maximizing positive and minimizing negative affective and information value. Sources and types of value depend on path characteristics that distinguish one situation from another, and personal characteristics that distinguish one person from another. In the cognitive realm of functioning, uncertainty-oriented individuals maximize positive information value by seeking clarity through mastery of uncertainty. They do so by expanding and changing their methods, moral views, and self-images as a function of changes in value resulting from this future-oriented attempt to master uncertainty. Conversely, certainty-oriented individuals maximize positive information value by maintaining clarity and minimize negative information value by avoiding or ignoring confusion with respect to established cognitions, methods, beliefs, and identity. Sources of value and expectancies of experiencing them determine motivational arousal. This, in turn, influences how individuals think, make moral decisions, and establish and change a self-definition—all in different ways, but all in the aim of feeling good or not feeling bad about themselves. We suggest that these same functions of personality can also account for motivation in life activity over time.

In closing, we wish to leave the reader with one more set of data to contemplate. Figure 6.3 shows the scores on our overall Resultant Uncertainty Measure, and their component scores (n Uncertainty; authoritarianism or F

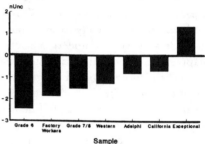

Grade 6 = grade six students from various schools near London, Canada.

Factory Workers = workers in a factory in Rhode Island.

Grade 7/8 = grade seven and eight students from a school near London, Canada.

Western = first year undergraduates from The University of Western Ontario.

Adelphi = undergraduates from Adelphi University.

California = udergraduates from The University of California at Santa Barbara.

Exceptional = grade six, seven, and eight students enrolled in a program for advanced children at a school near London, Canada.

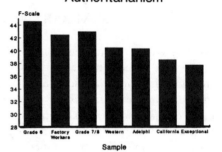

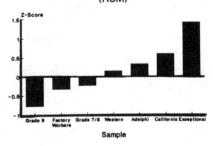

FIGURE 6.3 Scores on n Uncertainty, authoritarianism (the F Scale), and the Resultant Uncertainty Measure for various samples.

Scale), across the samples we have collected so far. *n* Uncertainty and F Scale scores are nice mirror images of each other, as we would hope. College students have higher *n* Uncertainty scores than grade school students and factory workers, as we would also hope. But the reader should pay close attention to the sample on the far right in the figure. These are students, mostly from the sixth grade, in a rural school district. Their distinguishing feature is that they are officially classified as students in an exceptional (advancement) learning program on the basis of their intelligence test scores, aptitude test scores, and teacher ratings of exceptional learning potential. This raises the question "Which came first?"

Acknowledgments

Many thanks to Kathy Denton, Tory Higgins, Patricia Raso, Chris Roney, Diane Ruble, and Lynn Zarbatany of their extremely helpful comments regarding this chapter. Research reported on uncertainty orientation was supported by various grants from the Social Sciences and Humanities Research Council (Canada) to Richard M. Sorrentino.

Notes

1. This is not to say that our theoretical approach is restricted to these levels. We do, in fact, believe that the precursors for these shifts occur very early in life. More research, however, must be conducted before we can speculate on earlier stages of development.

2. The *n* Uncertainty scoring manual provides a procedure for coding sentence leads in terms of one's concern with uncertainty (e.g., inconsistency between a thought and a behavior, two inconsistent thoughts, thoughts about the unknown) and one's desire to resolve the uncertainty. Expert scorers have interrater reliabilities above .90 with each other and the scoring manual. The measure of authoritarianism, the F Scale, is acquiescence-free and has test–retest reliabilities above .90. Uncertainty-oriented persons are those who fall in the upper tertile of *n* Uncertainty *z* scores minus authoritarian (F Scale) *z* scores. Certainty-oriented persons are those who fall in the lower tertile of these scores. Children and adult forms for each are available from Sorrentino.

3. This phenomenon cannot be explained in terms of overmotivation (see Short & Sorrentino, 1986).

4. This derivation from dynamics of action includes other elements of the theory, such as consummatory force. (See Atkinson & Birch, 1978, for the source of this derivation.)

5. A recent master's thesis by Maria Gitta (1989) gives support to many of these assumptions. For example, uncertainty-oriented persons were found to be "paratelic" or process-oriented, whereas certainty-oriented were "telic" or goal-oriented. Subscales of the Telic Dominance Scale (Murgatroyd, Rushton, Apter, & Ray, 1978) also revealed that certainty-oriented persons were arousal-avoidant (i.e., avoidant of uncertain situations), compared to uncertainty-oriented persons. Gitta found, in addition, that certainty-oriented persons had a greater preference for balanced relationships, and a lesser preference for imbalanced relationships, than did uncertainty-oriented persons.

6. We found, in the same study, that certainty-oriented persons reported fewer traits within categories than uncertainty-oriented persons, indicating less richness in their categorizations as well.

7. Sorrentino's students question his use of politics as non-achievement-oriented; but this, after all, is more related to power motivation than to achievement motivation (see Atkinson, 1958).

8. Interestingly, Kohlberg was forced to drop Stage 6, as it was difficult to find people who use this level (Colby & Kohlberg, 1987). We wonder whether there would have been more success among uncertainty-oriented samples.

9. If the notion of avoiding a situation where uncertainty can be resolved strains credulity, we invite the reader to examine the results of the Sorrentino and Hewitt (1984) study. Recall that here

certainty-oriented persons chose *not* to engage in a task that could resolve uncertainty about an important ability, even under circumstances such that the resolution would probably lead to positive affect. This is why we believe that certainty-oriented persons simply do not want to engage in the *process* of finding out.

10. Recall, also, that the certainty-oriented component of our resultant measure of uncertainty orientation is authoritarianism.

11. We also note with interest the apparent lack of continuity of infant intelligence with adult intelligence (Weinberg, 1989), except for variables that would appear to be related to uncertainty orientation. According to Weinberg (1989, pp. 99-100), "coping with novelty, a person's ability to adjust to unfamiliar tasks and life situations, appears to be dependent on certain underlying cognitive components, that is, the ability to explore and solve novel kinds of problems as well as motivational attitudes." This interface would also appear worthy of exploration.

12. Evidence that bears on this point comes from a master's thesis by Clayton (1981), where it was found that certainty-oriented persons were significantly more sex-typed, whereas uncertainty-oriented persons were significantly more androgynous.

13. Recent successes of the far right (e.g., conservatives, "the silent majority," "the moral majority") in the last two decades suggest that this value may be shifting from negative to positive in our society. We might, therefore, expect a concomitant rise in certainty orientation over the same period.

14. In her baccalaureate honors thesis, Bonita Lau (1985) found that Oriental students from Hong Kong and the Chinese mainland were significantly more certainty-oriented than Western students at the University of Western Ontario.

References

Arbuthnot, J. (1975). Modification of moral judgment through role playing. *Developmental Psychology, 11*, 319-324.

Atkinson, J. W. (Ed.). (1958). *Motives in fantasy, action, and society.* Princeton, NJ: Van Nostrand.

Atkinson, J. W., & Birch, D. (1978). *An introduction to motivation* (2nd ed.). New York: Van Nostrand.

Atkinson, J. W., & Feather, N. T. (Eds.). (1966). *A theory of achievement motivation.* New York: Wiley.

Atkinson, J. W., & Raynor, J. O. (Eds.). (1974). *Motivation and achievement.* Washington, DC: Hemisphere.

Bee, H. (1981). *The developing child.* New York: Harper & Row.

Beourne, E. (1978). The state of research on ego identity: A review and appraisal. Part II. *Journal of Youth and Adolescence, 7*, 371-392.

Berzonsky, M. D., Weiner, A. S., & Raphael, D. (1975). Interdependence of formal reasoning. *Developmental Psychology, 11*, 258.

Blatt, M. M. (1970). *The effects of classroom discussion programs upon children's level of moral judgement.* Unpublished doctoral dissertation, University of Chicago.

Byrne, D., & Lamberth, J. (1971). The effect of erotic stimuli on sexual arousal, evaluation responses, and subsequent behavior. In *Technical reports of the Commission on Obscenity and Pornography* (Vol. 8). Washington, DC: U.S. Government Printing Office.

Case, R., Hayward, S., Lewis, M., & Hurst, P. (1988). Toward a neo-piagetian theory of cognitive and emotional development. *Developmental Review, 8*, 1-51.

Cauble, M. (1976). Formal operations, ego identity, and principled morality: Are they related? *Developmental Psychology, 12*, 363-364.

Chabassol, D. J., & Thomas, D. (1975). Needs for structure, tolerance of ambiguity, and dogmatism in adolescents. *Psychological Reports, 37*, 507-510.

Clayton, J. P. (1981). *Uncertainty orientation, sex roles identity, and performance in achievement situations.* Unpublished master's thesis, University of Western Ontario.

Clayton, V., & Overton, W. F. (1976). Concrete and formal operational thought processes in young adulthood and old age. *International Journal of Aging, 7*, 237-245.

Colby, A., & Kohlberg, L. (1987). *The measurement of moral judgment: Vol. 1. Theoretical foundations and research validation.* Cambridge, MA: Harvard University Press.

Dignan, M. H. (1965). Ego identity and maternal identification. *Journal of Personality and Social Psychology, 1*, 476-483.

Edwards, C. P. (1981). The comparative study of the development of moral judgement and reasoning. In R. H. Munroe, R. L. Munroe, & B. B. Whiting (Eds.), *Handbook of cross-cultural human development* (pp. 501-528). New York: Garland Press.

Erikson, E. H. (1959). Identity and the life cycle: Selected papers. *Psychological Issues, 1*, 50-100.

Erikson, E. H. (1968). *Identity: Youth and crisis.* New York: Norton.

Erikson, E. H. (1972). Youth: Fidelity and diversity. *Humanitas, 8*, 21-35.

Ewen, R. B. (1980). *An introduction to theory of personality.* New York: Academic Press.

Feather, N. T. (Ed.). (1982). *Expectations and actions: Expectancy-value models in psychology.* Hillsdale, NJ: Erlbaum.

Fischer, L. W., & Silvern, L. (1985). Stages and individual differences in cognitive development. *Annual Review of Psychology, 36*, 613-648.

Freeman, S. J., & Giebink, J. W. (1979). Moral judgment as a function of age, sex, and stimulus. *Journal of Psychology, 102*, 43-47.

Gitta, M. Z. (1989). *Uncertainty orientation: The balance effect and other individual difference variables.* Unpublished master's thesis, University of Western Ontario.

Gitta, M. Z., & Sorrentino, R. M. (1989). *Uncertainty orientation and the balance effect: Implications for information processing models of balance.* Manuscript in preparation.

Gutkin, D. C., & Suls, J. (1979). The relation between the ethics of personal conscience-social responsibility and principled moral reasoning. *Journal of Youth and Adolescence, 8*, 433-441.

Haan, N., Weiss, R., & Johnson, V. (1982). The role of logic in moral reasoning and development. *Developmental Psychology, 18*, 245-255.

Hafer, C. L. (1987). *Personal responsibility, referent outcomes, and individual differences in relative deprivation.* Unpublished master's thesis, University of Western Ontario.

Higgins, E. T., & Eccles-Parsons, J. (1983). Social cognition and the social life of the child: Stages as subcultures. In E. T. Higgins, D. N. Ruble, & W. W. Hartup (Eds.), *Social cognition and social development: A sociocultural perspective* (pp. 15-62). New York: Cambridge University Press.

Higgins, E. T., Strauman, T., & Klein, R. (1986). Standards and the process of self-evaluation: Multiple affects from multiple stages. In R. M. Sorrentino & E. T. Higgins (Eds.), *Handbook of motivation and cognition: Foundations of social behavior* (Vol. 1, pp. 23-63). New York: Guilford Press.

Higgins, E. T., & Wells, R. S. (1986). Social construct availability and accessibility as a function of social life phase: Emphasizing the "how" versus the "can" of social cognition. *Social Cognition, 4*(2), 201-226.

Hogan, R. (1970). A dimension of moral judgment. *Journal of Consulting and Clinical Psychology, 35*, 205-212.

Holstein, C. B. (1976). Irreversible stepwise sequence in the development of moral judgment: A longitudinal study of males and females. *Child Development, 47*, 51-61.

Houston, J. P., Bee, H., Hatfield, E., & Rimm, C. (Eds.). (1979). *Invitation to psychology.* New York: Academic Press.

Hult, R. E. (1979). The relationship between ego identity status and moral reasoning in university women. *Journal of Psychology, 103*, 203-207.

Kagan, J., & Havemann, E. (Eds.). (1976). *Psychology: An introduction.* New York: Harcourt Brace Jovanovich.

Keasey, C. B. (1973). Experimentally induced changes in moral opinions and reasoning. *Journal of Personality and Social Psychology, 26*, 30-38.

Kelman, H. C., & Barclay, J. (1963). The F Scale as a measure of breadth of perspective. *Journal of Abnormal and Social Psychology, 67*, 608-615.

Kohlberg, L. (1969). Stage and sequence: The cognitive developmental approach to socialization. In D. A. Goslin (Ed.), *Handbook of socialization theory and research* (pp. 347-480). Chicago: Rand McNally.

Kohlberg, L. (1973). Continuities in childhood and adult moral development revisited. In P. Baltes & K. Schaie (Eds.), *Life-span developmental psychology: Personality and socialization* (pp. 180-204). New York: Academic Press.

Kohlberg, L., & Gilligan, C. (1971). The adolescent as a philosopher: The discovery of the self in a post-conventional world. *Daedalus, 100,* 1051-1086.

Kohlberg, L., & Hersh, R. H. (1977). Moral development: A review of the theory. *Theory into Practice, 16,* 53-59.

Kramer, D. A. (1986). Social cognition in adulthood: An overview of an emerging perspective. *Educational Gerontology, 12*(4), 273-276.

Lau, B. (1985). *Uncertainty, orientation, learned helplessness, and cross-cultural differences.* Unpublished honors thesis, University of Western Ontario.

Liberman, D., Gaa, J. P., & Frankiewicz, R. G. (1983). Ego and moral development in an adult population. *Journal of Genetic Psychology, 142,* 61-65.

Loevinger, J., & Wessler, R. (1970). *Measuring ego development* (Vol. 1). San Francisco: Jossey-Bass.

Marcia, J. E. (1966). Development and validation of ego identity status. *Journal of Personality and Social Psychology, 3,* 551-558.

Marcia, J. E. (1967). Ego identity status: Relationship to change in self-esteem, general maladjustment, and authoritarianism. *Journal of Personality, 1,* 118-134.

Marcia, J. E., & Friedman, M. L. (1970). Ego identity status in college women. *Journal of Personality, 38,* 249-261.

Matteson, R. (1974). Changes in attitudes toward authority figures with the move to college: Three experiments. *Developmental Psychology, 10,* 340-347.

McBride, L., & Moran, G. (1967). Double agreement as a function of item ambiguity and susceptibility to demand implications of the psychological situation. *Journal of Personality and Social Psychology, 6,* 115-118.

McClelland, D. C. (1961). *The achieving society.* New York: Free Press.

Meilman, P. W. (1979). Cross-sectional age changes in ego identity status during adolescence. *Developmental Psychology, 15,* 230-231.

Miller, J. G. (1984). Culture and the development of everyday social explanation. *Journal of Personality and Social Psychology, 46,* 961-978.

Millon, T. (1957). Authoritarianism, intolerance of ambiguity, and rigidity under ego- and task-involving conditions. *Journal of Abnormal and Social Psychology, 55,* 29-35.

Murgatroyd, S., Rushton, C., Apter, M. J., & Ray, C. (1978). The development of the Telic Dominance Scale. *Journal of Personality Assessment, 42,* 519-528.

Munro, G., & Adams, G. R. (1977). Ego-identity formation in college students and working youth. *Developmental Psychology, 13,* 523-524.

Piaget, J. (1950). *The psychology of intelligence.* New York: Harcourt, Brace.

Piaget, J. (1972). Intellectual evolution from adolescence to adulthood. *Human Development, 15,* 1-12.

Piaget, J., with Inhelder, B. (1969). *The psychology of the child.* New York: Basic Books.

Podd, M. H. (1970). *The relationship between ego identity status and two measures of morality.* Unpublished doctoral dissertation, State University of New York at Buffalo.

Podd, M. H. (1972). Ego identity status and morality: The relationship of two developmental constructs. *Developmental Psychology, 6,* 497-507.

Raynor, J. O. (1982). A theory of personality functioning and change. In J. O. Raynor & E. E. Entin (Eds.), *Motivation, career striving, and aging* (pp. 249-302). Washington, DC: Hemisphere.

Raynor, J. O., & Entin, E. E. (Eds.). (1982). *Motivation, career striving, and aging.* Washington, DC: Hemisphere.

Raynor, J. O., & McFarlin, D. B. (1986). Motivation and the self system. In R. M. Sorrentino & E. T.

Higgins (Eds.), *Handbook of motivation and cognition: Foundations of social behavior* (Vol. 1, pp. 315-349). New York: Guilford Press.

Riegel, K. F. (1976). The dialectics of human development. *American Psychologist, 31,* 689-700.

Rogoff, B., & Morelli, G. (1989). Perspectives on children's development from cultural psychology. *American Psychologist, 44,* 343-348.

Rokeach, M. (1960). *The open and closed mind: Investigations into the nature of belief systems and personality systems.* New York: Basic Books.

Roney, C. J. R., & Sorrentino, R. M. (1987). Uncertainty orientation and person perception: Individual differences in categorization. *Social Cognition, 5,* 369-382.

Roney, C. J. R., & Sorrentino, R. M. (1989a). *Uncertainty orientation and the self: Implications for social comparison and self-discrepancy theory.* Manuscript in preparation.

Roney, C. J. R., & Sorrentino, R. M. (1989b). *The motivating properties of self-discrepancies as a function of uncertainty orientation and achievement-related motives.* Unpublished manuscript.

Rowe, I., & Marcia, J. E. (1980). Ego identity status, formal operations, and moral development. *Journal of Youth and Adolescence, 9,* 87-99.

Schenkel, S., & Marcia, J. E. (1972). Attitudes toward premarital intercourse in determining ego identity status in college women. *Journal of Personality, 40*(3), 472.

Shaffer, D. R. (1979). *Developmental psychology: Theory, research, and applications.* Monterey, CA: Brooks/Cole.

Shaffer, D. R., & Hendrick, C. (1974). Dogmatism and tolerance for ambiguity as determinants of differential reactions to cognitive inconsistency. *Journal of Personality and Social Psychology, 29,* 601-608.

Short, J. C., & Sorrentino, R. M. (1986). Achievement, affiliation, and group incentives: A test of the overmotivation hypothesis. *Motivation and Emotion, 10*(2), 115-131.

Shu-Fang Dien, D. (1982). A Chinese perspective on Kohlberg's theory of moral development. *Developmental Review, 2,* 331-341.

Simpson, E. L. (1974). Moral development research: A case study in scientific cultural bias. *Human Development, 17,* 81-106.

Sorrentino, R. M., Bobocel, R., Gitta, M. Z., Olson, J. M., & Hewitt, E. C. (1988). Uncertainty orientation and persuasion: Individual differences in the effects of personal relevance on social judgments. *Journal of Personality and Social Psychology, 55,* 357-371.

Sorrentino, R. M., Hanna, S. E., & Roney, C. J. R. (in press). In C. P. Smith (Ed.), *Thematic content analysis for motivation and personality research.* New York: Cambridge University Press.

Sorrentino, R. M., & Hewitt, E. C. (1984). The uncertainty reducing properties of achievement tasks revisited. *Journal of Personality and Social Psychology, 47,* 884-889.

Sorrentino, R. M., & Roney, C. J. R. (1986). Uncertainty orientation, achievement-related motivation, and task diagnosticity as determinants of task performance. *Social Cognition, 4,* 420-436.

Sorrentino, R. M., & Roney, C. J. R. (1989a). Individual differences in uncertainty orientation: Implications for the self-inference process. In M. P. Zanna & J. M. Olson (Eds.), *Social influence: The Ontario Symposium* (Vol. 6, pp. 239-257). Hillsdale, NJ: Erlbaum.

Sorrentino, R. M., & Roney, C. J. R. (1989b). *The role of uncertainty orientation and state vs. trait self-discrepancies on performance.* Manuscript in preparation.

Sorrentino, R. M., & Short, J. C. (1986). Uncertainty, motivation, and cognition. In R. M. Sorrentino & E. T. Higgins (Eds.), *Handbook of motivation and cognition: Foundations of social behavior* (Vol. 1, pp. 379-403). New York: Guilford Press.

Sorrentino, R. M., Short, J. C., & Raynor, J. O. (1984). Uncertainty orientation: Implications for affective and cognitive views of achievement behavior. *Journal of Personality and Social Psychology, 46,* 189-206.

Sullivan, E. V. (1977). *Kohlberg's structuralism: A critical appraisal.* Toronto: Ontario Institute for Studies in Education.

Tomlinson-Keasey, C. (1972). Formal operations in females from eleven to fifty-four years of age. *Developmental Psychology, 6,* 364.

Tracy, J. J., & Cross, H. J. (1973). Antecedents of a shift in moral judgment. *Journal of Personality and Social Psychology, 26,* 238-244.

Trope, Y. (1975). Seeking information about one's own ability as a determinant of choice among tasks. *Journal of Personality and Social Psychology, 32,* 1004-1013.

Turiel, E. (1966). An experimental test of the sequentiality of developmental stages in the child's moral judgments. *Journal of Personality and Social Psychology, 6,* 611-618.

Wagner, J. A. (1976). *A study of the relationship between formal operations and ego identity in adolescents.* Unpublished doctoral dissertation, State University of New York at Buffalo.

Walker, L. J., & Richards, B. S. (1979). Stimulating transitions in moral reasoning as a function of stage of cognitive development. *Developmental Psychology, 15,* 95-103.

Waterman, A. S., & Waterman, C. K. (1976). Factors related to vocational identity after extensive work experience. *Journal of Applied Psychology, 61,* 336-340.

Waterman, C. K., & Waterman, A. S. (1974). Ego identity status and decision styles. *Journal of Youth and Adolescence, 3,* 1-6.

Weinberg, R. A. (1989). Intelligence and IQ: Landmark issues and great debates. *American Psychologist, 44,* 98-104.

Weiner, B. (1972). *Theories of motivation: From mechanisms to cognition.* Chicago: Markham.

Wicklund, R. A., & Brehm, J. W. (1976). *Perspectives on cognitive dissonance.* Hillsdale, NJ: Erlbaum.

Wonderly, D. M., & Kupfersmid, J. H. (1978). A test of the cognitive-developmental disequilibrium hypothesis in moral development. *Journal of Psychology, 100,* 297-304.

Zacker, J. (1973). Authoritarian avoidance of ambiguity. *Psychological Reports, 33,* 901-902.

CHAPTER 7

Activity Engagement Theory
Implications of Multiply Identifiable Input for Intrinsic Motivation

E. TORY HIGGINS
Columbia University

YAACOV TROPE
Hebrew University

What determines people's motivational responses when they are engaging an input? How do people's affective and inferential responses when they are engaging an input influence their subsequent orientation toward that input? Since the 1950s, these central issues in motivation have been addressed mostly in terms of the distinction between "intrinsic" and "extrinsic" motivation (for recent reviews, see Bandura, 1986; Deci & Ryan, 1987; Pittman & Heller, 1987). The purpose of the present chapter is to address these issues more broadly by considering the role of activity engagement in motivation generally and in intrinsic-extrinsic motivation in particular. Our model of activity engagement proposes that people's input orientations are more fluid and more numerous than traditional intrinsic-extrinsic distinctions have suggested. Given the history of the issues to be addressed, however, classic distinctions between intrinsic and extrinsic motivation provide the initial framework for our discussion.

Previous theories of social motivation have taken two basic approaches to distinguishing intrinsic from extrinsic motivation: (1) distinguishing types of needs or incentives for engaging in an activity; and (2) distinguishing types of inferences about one's engagement in an activity. Let us briefly consider each of these two approaches.

DISTINGUISHING INTRINSIC FROM EXTRINSIC MOTIVATION

Distinguishing Types of Needs or Incentives for Engagement

One basic approach to distinguishing intrinsic from extrinsic motivation has been to identify a set of needs or incentives for engaging in activities that differs from traditionally postulated drives (e.g., hunger, thirst, sex, aggression, avoidance of pain), current situational pressures (e.g., promise of reward, threat of punishment), and past reinforcements. It was proposed that animals are innately motivated to engage in activities by curiosity, a need for optimal arousal and psychological consistency, and a need to be effective and in control when dealing with their environment (see Berlyne, 1950; Festinger, 1957; Harlow, 1950; Hunt, 1965; White, 1959). Such "intrinsic" needs were postulated in order to explain why people and other animals will spontaneously engage in nonreinforced, non-drive-reducing activities, and to draw attention to properties of activities themselves that had previously received little attention (e.g., complexity, novelty, stimulation).

Delineating types of "intrinsic" needs or incentives continues to be a common approach to distinguishing intrinsic from extrinsic motivation. Deci and Ryan (1985), for example, have suggested that there is a convergence toward the view that intrinsic motivation is based on the organismic needs to be competent and in control. More recently, an additional organismic need for attachment has been proposed as a third basic intrinsic need (see Connell & Wellborn, in press). Bandura (1986) includes among intrinsic forms of motivations those types of incentives that arise from naturally occurring consequences of engaging in an activity. Pittman and Heller (1987) mention curiosity and a desire for stimulation as further intrinsic motives.

Distinguishing Types of Inferences about One's Engagement

Another basic approach to distinguishing intrinsic from extrinsic motivation has been to identify types of inferences that people make about their engagement in an activity—inferences that produce different orientations to and experiences of the activity. Based upon the earlier work of Heider (1958) and Rotter (1954), deCharms (1968), Deci (1971, 1972, 1975), Kruglanski (1975; Kruglanski, Freedman, & Zeevi, 1971), Lepper and Greene (1975; Lepper, Greene, & Nisbett, 1973), and Ross (1975; Ross, Karniol, & Rothstein, 1976) have suggested that people's motivational orientation to activities varies, depending on whether they *believe* their engagement with an activity to be intrinsically or extrinsically motivated. They suggest that whatever the true cause of their engagement, people's *inferences about themselves in relation to the activity* are what determine their motivational state.

Intrinsic and extrinsic motivation are distinguished in terms of different types of inferences about oneself in relation to the activity. For example, it has been suggested that perceptions of oneself as the locus of causality for one's own behavior (i.e., perceived self-determination) involve intrinsic motivation, whereas perceptions of one's behavior as externally controlled involve extrinsic motivation (e.g., deCharms, 1968; Deci & Ryan, 1987). Self-perceptions that one is engaging in an activity as an end in itself involve intrinsic motivation, whereas self-perceptions that one is engaging in an activity as a means to an end involve extrinsic motivation (e.g., Lepper et al., 1973; Kruglanski, 1975; Nicholls, 1975; Ross et al., 1976). Self-perceptions that one is engaging in an activity for a reward as feedback about competence and performance quality involve intrinsic motivation, but self-perceptions that one is engaging in an activity for a reward as an incentive simply to perform involve extrinsic motivation (e.g., Boggiano & Ruble, 1979; Deci, 1975; Pittman, Cooper, & Smith, 1977).

Delineating types of "intrinsic" inferences continues to be a common approach to distinguishing intrinsic from extrinsic motivation. Perceptions of self-causality, self-competence, and self-efficacy are proposed as sources of intrinsic motivation (see Bandura, 1986; Deci & Ryan, 1985; Harackiewicz, Abrahams, & Wageman, 1987; Pittman, Boggiano, & Ruble, 1983; Pittman & Heller, 1987). Bandura (1986) also suggests that the self-evaluative mechanism whereby people judge whether they have met their own standards is a form of intrinsic motivation. Morgan (1981) and Lepper, Sagotsky, Dafoe, and Greene (1982) propose that inferences based on event knowledge concerning which activities are likely to involve incentives from others to perform can determine whether an activity is experienced as intrinsically or extrinsically motivated.

Differences and Similarities in Intrinsic–Extrinsic Distinctions

These two basic approaches to distinguishing intrinsic from extrinsic motivation differ in some important respects. First, the "type-of-inference" approach considers an activity to involve intrinsic motivation as long as the actor perceives himself or herself to be intrinsically motivated, regardless of which need is actually being fulfilled. In contrast, the "type-of-need" approach considers an activity to be intrinsically motivated only when particular types of needs are fulfilled. Although the condition of having some intrinsic need fulfilled increases the likelihood of a person's inferring that he or she is intrinsically motivated, it is *not* a necessary condition. For example, regardless of which needs are actually fulfilled while actors are engaging in an activity, it should be possible after the activity to alter the actors' perceptions of their motivation during the activity (see Kruglanski, Alon, & Lewis, 1972). Second, the type-of-need approach considers an activity to involve intrinsic motivation as long as it fulfills some intrinsic need of the actor, regardless of whether the actor perceives himself or herself to be intrinsically motivated. Although making an inference that one is intrinsically motivated is likely to be associated with fulfilling an intrinsic need, such an inference is *not* a necessary condition for fulfilling intrinsic needs. Indeed, even organisms that are not capable of making inferences about their motivational state (e.g., infants) can still engage in activities that fulfill intrinsic needs.

Thus, some activities would be considered to involve intrinsic motivation according to the type-of-inference approach but would not be so considered according to the type-of-need approach, and vice versa. Activities performed to meet evaluative standards provide an important example of how these two approaches can differ in their classification of activities. According to the type-of-inference approach, if meeting evaluative standards increases people's perceived self-efficacy or perceived competence, then such activities involve intrinsic motivation (see Bandura, 1986). But according to the type-of-need approach, if people meeting evaluative standards experience pressure or concern about others' reactions, then such activities do not involve intrinsic motivation (see Deci & Ryan, 1985).

Although there are some important differences between these two approaches to distinguishing intrinsic from extrinsic motivation, a careful reading of the literature suggests that there are also important underlying similarities in the approaches. Both emphasize the classic distinction between engaging in an activity as an end in itself (intrinsic motivation) and engaging in an activity as a means to an end (extrinsic motivation). The type-of-inference approach makes this distinction in regard to people's inferred reasons for engaging in an activity, whereas the type-of-need approach makes this distinction in regard to people's orientation toward and experience of an activity.

Both approaches also distinguish between intrinsic motivation as a relatively positive state and extrinsic motivation as a relatively negative state. Intrinsic motivation has been conceptualized as interest in and enjoyment of activities (e.g., Csikszentmihalyi, 1975; Izard, 1977). Activities involving intrinsic motivation have been described as inherently desirable, satisfying, pleasurable, interesting, and enjoyable (see Deci & Ryan, 1985; Kruglanski, 1975; Lepper et al., 1973; Pittman & Heller, 1987; Ross, 1976). Pretty and Seligman (1984) have been most explicit about this distinction. They argue that people experience positive affect when they engage in intrinsically motivating activities, and that experiencing an increase in negative affect will produce a decrease in intrinsic motivation. They suggest that intrinsic motivation may be better conceived of as an internally generated need to engage in activities that make one feel good, rather than as a set of specific internal motivators.

It is interesting in this regard that when Bandura (1986) describes self-evaluation as intrinsically motivating, he refers to the enjoyment and self-satisfaction derived from meeting challenging standards, but that when Deci and Ryan (1987) describe self-evaluation as extrinsically motivating, they refer to the pressure and tension that people experience when they are ego-involved in an activity. Self-evaluation can produce both kinds of experiences (see Higgins, 1990; Higgins, Strauman, & Klein, 1986), and it is significant that conclusions about its motivational nature (i.e., intrinsic vs. extrinsic) are so closely tied to the quality of affect that is described as being associated with it.

Some Difficulties with the Intrinsic–Extrinsic Distinction

The type-of-need approach to distinguishing intrinsic from extrinsic motivation distinguishes activities in terms of whether engaging in them fulfills certain specific intrinsic needs. Typically, the need fulfillment is understood to derive from the natural or inherent properties of the activity and/or the natural or inherent consequences of engaging in the activity. But if intrinsic motivation involves responses to the natural or inherent properties of activities, why restrict it to only those responses that fulfill a particular set of needs? It is arbitrary to assert that activity engagement involves intrinsic motivation when the inherent properties of an activity fulfill a need for complexity, but not when the inherent properties of an activity fulfill a need for thirst reduction.

Let us consider these examples further. It might be argued that complexity is more inherent than thirst reduction because thirst reduction, like other tradition-ally postulated drives, varies as a function of the drive state of the person engaging in the activity rather than being just a property of the activity. But this is obviously true of other "intrinsic" needs, such as novelty and optimal stimulation. Indeed, the fulfillment of all needs necessarily involves person–activity interactions.

Another version of the type-of-need approach is that activity engagement involves intrinsic motivation when the activity is an end in itself rather than simply a means to an end. But any activity can be transformed from an end in itself to a means to an end by setting up contingency conditions, so that a person must engage in that activity in order to engage in another positive activity (see Lepper et al., 1982). Thus, the natural or inherent properties of an activity do not necessarily determine whether it will function intrinsically as an end in itself or extrinsically as a means to an end.

The emphasis of the type-of-need approach on defining intrinsic motivation in terms of need fulfillment and positive consequences is likewise problematic. Interacting with the natural or inherent properties of an activity need not fulfill needs or have only positive consequences. Why should only the positive conse-quences of activity engagement involve intrinsic motivation, when negative con-sequences can also derive from the natural or inherent properties of an activity? Again, this seems arbitrary. Indeed, if intrinsic motivation is restricted to cases of positive responses to activities, the range of applicability of models of intrinsic motivation is limited to cases of approach motivation. But people also spontane-ously avoid certain activities. Moreover, the *same* activity can involve *both* positive and negative responses to different inherent properties of the activity (e.g., it is complex but too stimulating). It seems unreasonable to consider only the positive subset of a person's responses to the inherent properties of a particular activity as intrinsically motivated.

There are also problems with the type-of-inference approach to intrinsic motivation. Like the type-of-need approach, this approach has also restricted intrinsic motivation to positive responses to an activity. Again, this restriction rules out the possibility that intrinsic motivation may be involved in the spon-taneous avoidance of activities. There are other problems as well. For example, an activity that is perceived as an end in itself can still have inherently negative properties (e.g., getting rid of the garbage). On the other hand, an activity that is perceived as a means to an end can have inherently positive properties (e.g., tasting wine to select the best vintage). Is it the affect or the perception of the means–end relation that is critical?

The self-determination and competence criteria for classifying activities in cognitive-evaluation theory (Deci & Ryan, 1985) are problematic as well. First, activities can be inherently absorbing and enjoyable but allow little self-determi-nation. People may find themselves intensely absorbed in and fascinated by a landscape, a sunset, or a street scene without necessarily experiencing a gain in self-determination during or after the activities. Second, competent performance often requires organizing complex activities according to a sequence of instrumentally related goals and subgoals. Do self-imposed planning and execution of the plan increase or decrease intrinsic motivation for the task? In fact, all problem-solving operations may be experienced as means toward the end of reaching a solution. Does this inevitable "means to an end" status of instrumental problem-solving activities necessarily detract from their intrinsic value?

Third, perceived competence is irrelevant to a wide range of activities. One can become absorbed in eating, sightseeing, watching a movie, or daydreaming without experiencing a sense of competence. In fact, assessments of competence or self-determination may interfere with and detract from the enjoyment of such activities. Within the achievement domain, failure (i.e., an absence of perceived competence) does not necessarily reduce intrinsic task attractiveness. Achievement motivation research suggests that to the extent that failures generate uncertainty about one's competence, they may increase rather than decrease the motivation to persist (Atkinson & Feather, 1966; Sorrentino & Short, 1986; Trope & Ben-Yair, 1982). Moreover, self-assessment of either success or failure would enhance motivation for a task to the extent that both success and failure are diagnostic about one's abilities (Trope, 1980, 1986a).

Another problem with the type-of-inference approach is that it restricts intrinsic motivation to activities involving higher-level inferences such as "What is the significance of this activity for my competence and self-determination?" or "Why am I doing this activity? What is my motivation for doing it?" This restriction again limits the range of applicability of intrinsic motivation. It implies that intrinsic motivation is not involved in activity engagement until and unless the activity is processed at stages beyond just attention and stimulus representation or even identification (see Higgins, 1990; Higgins et al., 1986; Trope, 1986a). It implies that people (e.g., infants) or animals that are not capable of such levels of processing or not currently utilizing their capability are not intrinsically motivated when engaging in activities. Intrinsic motivation is thereby precluded from applying to babies' fascination with faces or adults' attraction to glorious sunsets. Again, this would seem to be an unreasonable restriction.

In sum, the two basic approaches in the literature to distinguishing intrinsic from extrinsic motivation have been to delineate types of intrinsic needs and types of intrinsic inferences. These two approaches do not always agree in their classification of activities as intrinsic or extrinsic. In addition, there are difficulties in both approaches with classifying some activities, especially activities involving inherently negative properties, stimulus control, self-imposed plans, self-assessment, or self-determined failure. The major reason for these differences and difficulties in classification is the emphasis of these approaches on distinguishing activities in terms of either the types of needs or the types of inferences they involve (cf. Kruglanski, 1975).

This emphasis on differentiating activities in terms of fixed content has impeded consideration of the basic processes that underlie orientation toward activity-identified input (see also Kruglanski, 1980). The major purpose of the present chapter is to propose a preliminary model of what such processes might be. We begin with a presentation of our general theory of activity engagement. Then we propose an approach to defining intrinsic and extrinsic motivation that not only is compatible with previous classifications of basic phenomena in the area, but complements the emphasis of our activity engagement theory on motivational responses to input properties. Finally, we consider how activity engagement processes influence intrinsic and extrinsic motivation.

ACTIVITY ENGAGEMENT THEORY

As discussed earlier, previous approaches to distinguishing intrinsic from extrinsic motivation have delineated types of needs that are fulfilled and types of inferences that are made when people engage in an activity. But what exactly is the activity in which people are engaged? Is it reasonable to assume, as these approaches typically do, that there is a given experimenter-identified activity in which people initially and subsequently engage? The applicability of a construct to an input—in this case, the extent of overlap between the attributes of an identification and the attributes of an input—certainly sets constraints on how the input can be characterized (see Higgins, 1989). But even within the considerable constraints of such applicability there are still many alternative ways to identify any particular input (see Higgins & Stangor, 1988b; Trope, 1986b, 1989a).

Multiple Activity Identifications

In his classic paper "How Shall a Thing Be Called?", Roger Brown (1958) pointed out that every referent can be identified in many different ways. A dime is not only a "dime," but also "money," a "coin," and a "metal object." More recently, Wegner and Vallacher (1986) have noted that any one action identification is just one choice from among many possibilities (see also Kruglanski, 1975; Newtson, 1976). For example, "throwing a brick through a window" may also be identified as "scaring people in the building," "moving one's arm," "breaking glass," and so on. A walk in a park can be characterized as "physical exercise" as well as "sightseeing."

The literature on identification motivation has suggested that at least some aspects of the general activity event may be labeled in different ways. For example, Deci (1975) has pointed out that the rewarding of activities can decrease or increase identification motivation, depending on whether the reward is identified as "external control" or "competence feedback." Similarly, Reiss and Sushinsky (1975) suggest that the offer of a reward may be identified as a "bribe," an "aid," or a "symbol of success." More generally, Bandura (1986) states that the same incentives can have different motivational effects, depending upon the message conveyed by the rewarders.

Although the importance of alternative labeling of the circumstances surrounding an activity has been recognized in the literature on intrinsic motivation, the implications of identifying the activity itself in different ways have received little attention. When a child is given multicolored felt-tipped pens and white drawing paper, has the opportunity to draw freely, and is promised an award for helping out an adult by drawing pictures (as in a study by Lepper et al., 1973), is the child's subsequent activity "coloring," "making a picture," "learning to draw," "playing with Magic Markers," "helping out an adult," "drawing for a promised reward," or "pleasing the experimenter"? How would each of these identifications of the activity influence the way in which a child would experience the input, the child's affective and cognitive responses to the input, and the child's subsequent orientation to the input? To answer these questions, some discussion of the determinants and consequences of activity identification and its relation to input orientation is necessary.

Determinants of Activity Identification

Activity-related input should function like any input in being identifiable in multiple ways. One of the first issues, then, is what determines the identification of an input as being a particular type of activity. Brown (1958) suggests that objects are given the name that has proven most useful in the situations in which the object has most frequently appeared. Rosch (e.g., 1978) extended Brown's notion of functional utility by proposing that there are basic-level categorizations of objects that are preferred because they maximize cue validity. Wegner and Vallacher (1986; see also Vallacher & Wegner, 1985) state that people ordinarily prefer to think about an act in the most encompassing or general way possible, but will think about a detail of the act when the broader conceptualization does not facilitate performance of the act.

These proposals suggest that people have general preferences for identifying input as being particular types of objects or actions, although the preferences can be modified or disrupted by specific circumstances of usage. Such general preferences certainly constitute an important determinant of how people identify activity-related input. Like other types of judgments, however, identifications of activity-related input can also be influenced by a wide variety of chronic individual factors and momentary contextual factors. For example, people's activity identifications can be influenced by chronic individual differences in the availability and accessibility of alternative constructs, or by momentary changes in the relative accessibility of constructs resulting from contextual priming or mood and arousal effects (for reviews, see Higgins, 1989; Higgins & Stangor, 1988b; Wyer & Srull, 1986). Chronic individual differences in personal orientations and expectancies, and momentary goals and sets resulting from current needs, contextual adaptation, or experimenter instructions, can also influence how activity-related input is identified (see Higgins & Stangor, 1988a; McCann & Higgins, 1984; Trope, 1986b, 1989a; Trope & Cohen, 1989; Trope, Cohen, & Maoz, 1988).

Relevance and Significance of Input Properties as a Function of Activity Identification

Each activity construct has defining or characteristic attributes associated with it. When an activity construct is activated, these associated attributes are what underlie subsequent processing. Thus, identifying an input as being a particular type of activity makes those particular attributes associated with that activity central to subsequent processing. The centrality of the activity attributes to processing, in turn, determines the *relevance* of the different input properties. Those properties of the input that are most closely related to the attributes of the identified activity become the most relevant input properties.

The relevance of the different properties of an input, therefore, varies as a function of how the input is identified. Anderson and Pichert (1978), for example, showed that people who read a description of the inside of a house attended to and remembered different properties of the house when they pretended to be engaged in a "planning a burglary" activity than when they pretended to be engaged in a "buying a house" activity. As another example, let us consider a coffee cup made of handcrafted pottery. This object can be identified as either "a coffee cup" or "handcrafted pottery." If it is identified as a "coffee cup," the relevant properties of the object are its weight, the ease with which it can be held, the volume of liquid that it can contain, the material's ability to retain liquid and heat, and so on. If it is identified as "handcrafted pottery," the relevant properties of the object are its type of clayware and glaze, method of firing, originality of design, artistry and craftsmanship in execution, and so on.

Some properties of this object, such as retention of heat versus color design, are more relevant to one identification than the other. Other properties, such as the shape of the handle or the type of glaze used on the inside, may be equally relevant to both identifications but may still differ in how they are perceived and assessed. If the object is identified as a "coffee cup," the handle is perceived in terms of ease of holding the cup while drinking from it, and the inside glaze is perceived in terms of its effect on the taste of the coffee. If the item is identified as "handcrafted pottery," the handle is perceived in terms of its contribution to the overall structural design (e.g., composition, balance), and the inside glaze is perceived in terms of the aesthetic contribution of its color and lustre.

The primary identification assigns not only meaning to a property (e.g., "effect on taste" vs. "aesthetic quality"), but also value. For example, the inside glaze of a coffee cup may be positively valued for its aesthetic nature when the cup is identified as "handcrafted pottery," but may be negatively valued for its taste when the cup is identified as a "coffee cup." A broken window may be positively valued when one is "planning a burglary," but may be negatively valued when one is "buying a house." Thus, the primary identification of an input determines not only the relevance of the various properties of the input, but also their *significance* (i.e., their meaning and importance).

Our common experience with various types of input suggests that we often attend and respond to a mixture of the properties of the input. This is because the same input is often identified in more than one way, which can happen simultaneously (e.g., "There's a handcrafted coffee cup") or successively (e.g., "There's a coffee cup," followed by "Look at how beautifully it was crafted"). Nevertheless, it is likely that during any specific engagement with an input, one of the possible identifications will be primary and one or more of alternative identifications will be secondary. For example, a person in a store may examine either "a coffee cup that is handcrafted" or "a piece of handcrafted pottery that functions as a coffee cup"; similarly, a child in the Lepper et al. (1973) study may have been either "making a picture by playing with Magic Markers" or "playing with Magic Markers by making a picture."

Primary and Secondary Activity Identifications

We propose that when experiencing an input, people will motivationally respond (both affectively and cognitively) primarily to those properties of the input that are made relevant by their primary activity identification. For example, children in the Lepper et al. (1973) study whose primary activity identification was "playing with Magic Markers" may have responded to the picture-drawing input primarily in terms of the physical and functional properties of the Magic Markers, whereas children whose primary activity identification was "learning to draw" may have responded to the input primarily in terms of the experience of acquiring operations that facilitate drawing. A primary activity identification may also cause people to attend and respond to properties of stimuli other than the input. For example, subjects in the Lepper et al. (1973) study whose primary activity identification was "waiting for the promised award" may have responded to the picture-drawing input primarily in terms of its time-consuming properties (passing time), and may have thought mostly about the properties of the promised award.

People's motivational responses to input can also be influenced by their secondary activity identifications. Just as there are attributes central to the primary activity identification because of their association with the primary activity construct, so too there are attributes central to the secondary activity identification because of their association with the secondary activity construct. And just as the properties of the input vary in their relevance to the central attributes of the primary activity identification, they also vary in their relevance to the central attributes of the secondary activity identification. The secondary activity identification competes with the primary activity identification, and thus the input properties relevant to the secondary activity identification compete with the input properties relevant to the primary activity identification. This competition for processing attention and dominance is another factor that influences people's motivational responses to the input. These motivational responses can be both affective and cognitive. In the next two sections, we consider these responses in more detail.

Affective Responses to Input Properties

We propose that when people engage in an identified activity, they have affective responses to those properties of the input (as well as to extrainput properties) made relevant by their activity identifications. The properties to which they are most likely to respond are those made relevant by the primary identification of the activity. The affective responses to the properties can be positive or negative. Through continued responding to these properties, associations form between each property and an affective response. Over time, then, associative networks are formed that interconnect the primary identification, the identification-relevant properties of the input (as well as extrainput stimuli), and the affective responses to these properties.

As discussed earlier, people can have secondary activity identifications of an input as well, and these alternative identifications can function during the same experience with the input. Thus, associative networks can also form that interconnect a secondary identification, its identification-relevant properties, and the affective responses to these properties. What, then, distinguishes between the associations formed for the primary identification and the associations formed for the secondary identification?

The critical difference between the primary and secondary identifications is simply that the primary identification is *primary*. That is, it is first in order of time and development, as well as first in importance. It is more basic and fundamental to the engagement process. This difference has a couple of implications. First, when people are engaged in an activity, they are likely to spend more time with and pay more attention to those properties relevant to the primary identification than those properties relevant to the secondary identification. Because the properties relevant to the primary identification are more important than those relevant to the secondary identification, the affective responses are likely to be stronger to the former than to the latter properties. Thus, the affective associative network formed during engagement with the activity is likely to be stronger and more extensive for the primary identification than the secondary identification. According to this logic, input properties that are relevant neither to the primary identification nor to the secondary identification are likely to be lowest in the amount of attention they attract and in the strength of the affective associations that are formed to them.

A second implication of the primary identification's being primary is that the properties of the input that are relevant to it are the activity-relevant properties, and the responses to these properties are the activity-relevant responses. In contrast, the remaining properties of the input are activity-irrelevant, and the responses to these properties are competing, interfering responses. An activity-relevant response is more likely to be retained than an activity-interfering response. Indeed, a task-interfering response is likely to be inhibited (see Shallice, 1972). A task-interfering response is also likely to be experienced as negative. Everything else being equal, then, an activity-relevant response should produce more positive affect than an activity-interfering response. Thus, everything else being equal, responses to primary-identification-related properties should be more positive and better retained than responses to secondary-identification-related properties.

It is not only that people's affective responses to the primary-identification-related properties are different from their affective responses to the secondary-identification-related properties. In addition, people's affective responses to the primary-identification-related properties can be altered by the presence of the secondary-identification-related properties, and vice versa. The more salient the secondary-identification-related properties of an activity are, the more people will be distracted from the primary-identification-related properties. Such distraction can influence the quality of the engagement with the primary-identification-related properties, and thus can influence the affective responses to these properties. Reiss and Sushinsky (1975), for example, suggest that in the "expected award" condition of the Lepper et al. (1973) study, in which children were promised an award for engaging in the drawing activity, the expected award could have elicited many interfering responses that resulted in the children's play being more hurried, lower in quality, and thus less enjoyable. Similarly, if the primary identification of a walk in the park is "enjoying sightseeing," then a secondary identification of the walk as "physical exercise" is likely to interfere with the enjoyment of sightseeing.

The presence of the primary-identification-related properties can also influence people's affective responses to the secondary-identification-related properties. For example, under conditions in which the secondary identification competes with the primary identification for the actor's attention, the secondary-identification-related properties are likely to be experienced as interfering or distracting from the primary task. Thus, the affective responses to these secondary-identification-related properties are likely to be more negative than they would be otherwise.

It is important to note that the motivational consequences of the competition between primary- and secondary-identification-related properties can be independent of the status of the activity as a means to an end or an end in itself (Kruglanski, 1975), as well as of the extent to which the activity gratifies needs for competence and self-determination (Deci & Ryan, 1985). For example, if a walk in the park is primarily identified as physical exercise, the distraction produced by the scenery does not necessarily affect the perceived purpose of the walk or one's sense of competence and self-determination.

Inferential Responses to Input Properties

When people engage in activities they not only have affective responses to the input (and extrainput) properties; they also have inferential responses. A large body of literature suggests that people use their engagement in an identified activity as a basis for drawing inferences regarding their feelings toward the activity, their motives for undertaking it, and their more general dispositions (Bem, 1972; Deci & Ryan, 1982, 1985). The present contribution to this literature is based on the assumption that people will draw different inferences from the same activity, depending on *how it is identified*. These inferences, in turn, will affect the motivation for subsequent engagement in an activity if the inferences are applicable to the subsequent identification of the activity. Via inference, the identification of an activity thus determines the motivation for subsequent engagement in the activity. For example, a walk in the park will lead to different inferences regarding one's feelings and interests, depending on whether the walk is primarily identified as sightseeing or physical exercise. The walk is more likely to produce inferences regarding the enjoyment and interest in, say, the park scenery if it is identified as sightseeing than if it is identified as exercise. These inferences, in turn, will affect subsequent walks in the park if the walks are identified as sightseeing rather than as physical exercise.

The range of future activities affected by the immediate identification depends on the generality of the inference (see Trope, 1989b). The identification of an activity will affect a broader range of subsequent activities if the inference concerns general needs and dispositions than if it pertains to a specific property of the immediate activity. For example, the identification of a walk in the park as sightseeing will affect a broader range of subsequent activities if the actor infers from the walk that he or she enjoys nature than if the actor infers that he or she enjoys the flower gardens in the park.

Both the primary activity identification and the secondary activity identification serve as bases for inferences from experiencing an input. Because of the cognitive advantages of the primary identification described earlier, however, primary-identification-related properties will receive more attention than secondary-identification-related properties, and primary identification–inference associations are likely to be stronger and more extensive than secondary identification–inference associations. This, in turn, will produce inferences concerning the greater significance of the primary identification activity than the secondary identification activity. For example, when sightseeing is the primary identification of a walk, a person will devote more attention and thought to the scenery; in turn, this will further reinforce the person's inferences regarding his or her interest in enjoying sightseeing. Indeed, the simple fact that a particular identification *is* primary, and is recognized as such, may lead the actor to infer that he or she must be motivated to engage in activities so identified. Such an inference is less likely to occur for the secondary identification. Thus, everything else being equal, primary identifications are likely to produce stronger motivations to engage subsequently in the activity than secondary identifications.

In functioning as an alternative to the primary identification, a secondary identification can influence people's inferences regarding the primary identification. Both the competition of the secondary identification for attention and the implications for the primary identification suggested by such competition may influence a person's primary-identification-related inferences. Let us consider, first, the role of attention. To the extent that secondary-identification-related properties attract the actor's attention away from the primary-identification-related properties, the actor may infer that the activity defined by the primary identification must not be interesting. Thus, as the salience of the secondary-identification-related properties increases, the perceived motivation to engage in the primary-identification-related activity will decrease (see Ross, 1975). Indeed, to the extent that the secondary-identification-related properties attract the actor's attention away from the primary-identification-related properties, the actor may infer that the secondary-identification-related activity must be the one that is interesting or important. Thus, as the salience of the secondary-identification-related properties increases, the perceived motivation to engage in this competing activity will also increase.

Apart from its direct competition for attention, a secondary identification may affect activity engagement inferences by implying a motivational alternative to the motivation implied by the primary identification. Specifically, when the actor is experiencing an input, the feelings, motives, and dispositions implied by secondary-identification-related properties may either undermine or augment the actor's confidence in the feelings, motives, and dispositions implied by the primary-identification-related properties (Kelley, 1972; Lepper et al., 1973; Trope, 1989a). For example, the secondary identification of a walk in a park as physical exercise may lead to inferences involving properties that are related to this identification (e.g., an interest in one's physical fitness) that may undermine one's confidence in inferences involving properties that are related to the primary identification of the walk as sightseeing (e.g., an interest in scenery). On the other hand, when the properties of the secondary identification provide little or no justification for input engagement, a secondary identification may augment inferences from the primary identification. For example, if the secondary identification for a walk in the park is physical exercise but a walk in a park provides less exercise than one's usual pastimes, the inferences that derive from the properties related to the primary identification of the walk as sightseeing may be augmented, such as greater confidence that one is simply interested in the scenery.

Finally, people's inferences regarding their motivation in an identified activity also depend on its relation to available but rejected alternative activities. To the extent that an alternative activity is positive and does not overlap with the primary identified activity, people will draw strong inferences about interest in the properties of the primary identified activity. Consider, for example, someone who chooses to take a walk in the park rather than a swim in the pool and identifies the primary activity either as "sightseeing" or as "physical exercise." The inference of interest in scenery (with "sightseeing" as the primary identification) will be greater than the inference of interest in physical fitness (with "physical exercise" as the primary identification).

As before, these effects of secondary identification properties do not depend on the contribution of the activity to one's sense of self-determination or competence. The secondary identification of a walk in the park as physical exercise can undermine or augment inferences regarding interest in park scenery without influencing the perception of the sightseeing as self-determined or competent.

Traditional attributional analyses of intrinsic motivation have recognized that properties extraneous to an input can undermine or augment inferences about intrinsic motives regarding the input. However, the usefulness of these analyses is limited because they do not take into account the fact that different motives can be inferred from the same input, depending on its activity identification (see Trope, 1986b). The present approach assumes that secondary-identification-related properties will affect only those motives that are implied by primary-identification-related properties. For example, properties related to the physical exercise involved in a walk in the park will only augment or undermine inferences regarding interest in scenery if the primary identification of the walk is sightseeing and the secondary identification is physical exercise. Moreover, the inference regarding interest in the scenery will affect the motivation for subsequent walks in the park only to the extent that the primary identification of subsequent walks is also sightseeing.

Stability and Change in Activity Identifications

The preceding sections have described how affective and inferential responses become associated with primary and secondary identifications of an activity. What are the implications of these associations for subsequent engagements in the activity? To answer this question, it is necessary to consider the implications of the *relation* between initial and subsequent identifications of an activity.

Earlier, we have described various determinants of activity identification. Some of these determinants, such as the applicability (and perceived applicability) of alternative activity constructs to an input, basic-level preferences for alternative activity identifications, or the chronic accessibility of alternative activity constructs, would be expected to produce some stability in activity identifications over time. Other determinants, however, such as contextual factors and momentary goals, would be expected to produce change in activity identifications over time. There is considerable evidence, for example, that changes in context can cause changes in how people categorize events (for a review, see Higgins & Stangor, 1988b). Indeed, changes in context can even change the referential meaning of the "same" judgment over time (see Higgins & Lurie, 1983; Higgins & Stangor, 1988a). What are the implications of activity identifications' being the same or different over time?

In addressing this issue, we consider the usual case described in the literature, in which there is an initial engagement with an input under specified experimental conditions and a subsequent "free-choice" or "open" engagement. Everything else being equal, the identification of an input in a subsequent engagement is likely to be the same as the initial identification, for a number of reasons. First, the factors that caused the input to be identified initially in a particular manner, such as high applicability of the identification to the input and high chronic accessibility of the identification, should continue to increase the likelihood that the input will be identified in this manner. Second, the initial engagement should have further increased the accessibility of the identification, as well as its perceived applicability to the properties of the activity made salient by the initial identification (see Higgins, 1989). On the other hand, everything else is often *not* equal, because changes in context can change the relative accessibility of alternative identifications or the salience of alternative properties of an activity, as well as people's moods, goals, and so on. These changes increase the likelihood that the activity will not be identified in the same way (see also Wegner & Vallacher, 1986, for a discussion of other reasons why identifications change over time).

When the subsequent activity identification of an input is the same as the initial activity identification of that input, then the primary identification involved in the initial engagement will be activated prior to subsequent engagement. This, in turn, will activate the affective and inferential responses associated with the earlier primary identification. The greater the positivity of these associated responses, the greater people's motivation to engage with the input again will be. When the activity identification of an input remains the same over time, then the motivational responses that occur during the subsequent engagement with the input are likely to be basically the same as those that occurred during the initial engagement. In the case where positive motivational responses were reduced in the experimental session (e.g., because of interference from a competing identification), then the positive motivational responses are expected to remain reduced in the subsequent open session. This is the case most often assumed in the literature. No measures of subjects' initial and subsequent activity identifications of the input have been taken in these studies, however. Thus, it is possible that in some conditions a change in the context of experiencing the input between the initial and subsequent engagements produced a change in how the activity was identified. What are the implications of a change in activity identification?

There are two basic types of change in activity identification: (1) The primary identification in the subsequent engagement was a secondary identification in the initial engagement; and (2) the primary identification in the subsequent engagement was neither the primary nor a secondary identification in the initial engagement. In the first case, subsequent activity identification of the input activates the secondary identification of the initial engagement. But now this identification is primary. Activation of the secondary identification of the initial engagement, in turn, activates the affective and inferential responses associated with this earlier identification. Once again, the greater the positivity of these associated responses, the greater people's motivation to engage with the input again will be. For example, if a group of subjects in the Lepper et al. (1973) study had inferred during the initial engagement in a drawing task that they must be interested in drawing for an award because this secondary identification distracted them from their primary identification of just playing with Magic Markers, then they should have been more motivated to engage again in a drawing task identified as drawing for an award than a group of subjects who had unexpectedly received an award at the end of the initial session or who had not previously experienced the drawing task input (a "no-previous-engagement" comparison group typically missing from past studies).

The second type of change is when the primary identification in the subsequent engagement was neither the primary nor a secondary identification in the initial engagement. In this case, the identification in the subsequent engagement has no affective or inferential responses associated with it from the initial engagement with the input. Thus, when this type of change in activity identification occurs, the people involved should have the same orientation to the activity as people who currently identify the activity in the same way but have had no previous experience with the activity (again, a "no-previous-engagement" comparison group).

To illustrate more fully the motivational implications of changes in activity identification from the perspective of our model, let us consider in some detail the conditions of the classic Lepper et al. (1973) study. Subjects were assigned to three experimental conditions: no award, unexpected award, and expected award. When presenting the drawing materials to the subjects, who were preschool children ranging in age from 3 to 5 years, the experimenter told them that there was an adult stranger who had come to the nursery school to see what kinds of pictures boys and girls like to draw with Magic Markers. The subjects in the no-award and unexpected-award conditions were then asked, "Would you like to draw some pictures for him?" (p. 133). The subjects in the expected-award condition were told instead that the stranger had brought along a few awards to give to boys and girls who would help him out by drawing some pictures for him. The subjects in this condition were then asked, "Would you like to win one of these Good Player Awards?" (p. 133). Lepper et al. (1973) reported that each subject indicated assent to the question asked of him or her, typically with considerable enthusiasm.

The first experimenter left, and the stranger (another experimenter) was left alone with the subjects. The stranger sat across the subject, started a stopwatch, asked the subject what he or she would like to draw first, and attempted to show interest in the subject's performance. At the end of the drawing period, the stranger looked at the stopwatch and announced that time was up. He then said, "Thank you very much for helping me out by drawing these pictures for me. You really did a good job" (p. 133). In the unexpected-award and expected-award conditions, the stranger continued by saying, "In fact, you have been such a big help to me that I have something very special to give you . . . let me show you our special Honor Roll board where you can put your award so that everyone will know what a good player you are!" (p. 133).

The open sessions measuring spontaneous interest in the activity began 1 or 2 weeks later. The children's interest in the activity was recorded during the first hour of 3 consecutive class days, where interest was defined as either sitting down at the target activity table or handling a Magic Marker. The target activity was available to each child for an hour from the time he or she arrived in class, and "was presented by the teachers as simply another activity with which the children might choose to play" (p. 132).

A careful review of these conditions suggests that the experimental groups may have differed in their primary activity identification of the experimental input. For the no-award group, the experimental input (i.e., the drawing task) may have been identified as "helping out a stranger." For the unexpected-award group, the experimental input may have been identified as "helping out a stranger" at the beginning of the session but as "succeeding at drawing" by the end of the session. For the expected-award group, the experimental input was probably identified as "winning an award (from a stranger)." Let us assume that for each group the secondary activity identification was "playing."

At the subsequent open engagement with the input, the stranger was no longer present. Thus, it was not possible to "help out a stranger" or "win an award (from a stranger)." In the no-award and expected-award conditions, therefore, there was likely to have been a change of identification from the experimental to the open engagement with the input. In the unexpected-award condition, however, it *was* possible to "succeed at drawing" in the subsequent open engagement. Given that this identification was the last identification during the previous engagement, it may also have been more accessible than alternative identifications at the time of the open engagement. Moreover, it is likely that this identification in the previous engagement was associated with positive affective and inferential responses. Subjects in the unexpected-award condition, then, should have had an increased motivation to engage with the input. Lepper et al. (1973) reported that subjects in this group who did not have high initial interest in the activity did indeed show a substantial, significant increase in interest following the experimental engagement.

In the no-award condition, one might expect that during the experimental session subjects would have acquired positive affective and inferential associations to the primary identification, "helping out a stranger." Moreover, the secondary identification of "playing" would not have interfered or competed with "helping out a stranger" to see what kinds of pictures boys and girls like to draw. In the open engagement session, however, it was not possible for these subjects to apply the same primary identification to the input as they did in the experimental session. Therefore, the previous engagement in the activity should have had little influence on their motivation to engage with the input again. Lepper et al. (1973) reported no change in interest for subjects in this condition following the experimental engagement.

A unique prediction of our model should be noted, however. What if in the open engagement session a different stranger had been present requesting help on a different task, such as working together as a team to clean some paintbrushes and paint jars, and subjects had been asked whether they would like to help him out? In this case, subjects' identification in the experimental session, "helping out a stranger," could have been applied to the activity, and the affective and inferential responses associated with this identification would have been activated. Therefore, subjects in this group should have been more motivated to engage in the activity than subjects without previous experience with this identification. These subjects should also have been more motivated to engage in the activity than subjects in the unexpected-award condition, because the activity could not be identified as "succeeding at drawing."

In the expected-award condition, subjects identified the activity as "winning an award (from a stranger)." Given that the stranger was sitting across the table from each subject, watching and timing the subject's performance, it is likely that the subjects in this group inferred that drawing quickly was important to win one of the few awards available. If this were the case, then the quality of these subjects' drawings should have suffered. Lepper et al. (1973) reported that the quality of the pictures drawn was indeed significantly lower in this group than in the other two groups, and the production level was slightly higher (although not significantly so). In contrast to the no-award condition, the secondary identification of "playing" in this condition should have competed with the primary identification of "winning an award" and interfered with the primary-identification-related property of drawing quickly. Thus, as discussed earlier, negative affective responses (but possibly positive inferential responses) should have become associated with the "playing" identification. Given the very young age of the children and the long delay between the experimental and open engagements, it is likely that the affective associations would have predominated in this study.

No stranger was present in the open engagement session, and thus subjects in this group could not apply their identification of "winning an award (from a stranger)" to the input in this session. If they identified the input as "playing," which may have been primed by the teachers in the open engagement session, then the associations with this initially secondary but now primary identification would have been activated. Therefore, the subjects in this group should have had a decreased motivation to engage with the input. Lepper et al. (1973) reported that these subjects' interest in the input indeed decreased following the experimental engagement.

Another unique prediction of our model should be noted. In making the prediction above, we have assumed that the affective responses were more strongly associated than the inferential responses with the "playing" secondary identification from the initial experimental session, because of the age of the subjects and the intersession delay. But if older subjects had been used, the intersession delay had been shorter, and the subjects' "previous thoughts about the activity" (i.e., previous inferential responses) had been primed at the beginning of the open engagement session, then it is possible that subjects' motivation to engage with the input would have *increased* following the experimental engagement in the expected-award condition. Of course, this could only be predicted if subjects in the experimental session had been distracted from "winning an award" by the attractive "playing" properties of the activity, so that they would infer that these properties must be positive.

Summary of Activity Engagement Theory

This section has presented a general model of activity identification and input orientation. This model, "activity engagement theory," emphasizes the role of multiple and changing identifications in initial and subsequent motivational responses to input. The model makes the following proposals:
1. An input can be identified in multiple ways.
2. The primary activity identification of an input determines which proper-

ties of the input are relevant when the actor is engaged in the activity, as well as the significance of these properties.

3. Secondary activity identifications of an input can compete with the primary identification for the attention of the actor.

4. Affective responses and inferential responses become associated with both the primary-identification-related properties of an input and the secondary-identification-related properties of the input.

5. The competition between primary and secondary identifications for attention and the inferences they suggest can influence the affective and inferential responses that become associated with these identifications.

6. There can be stability or change over time in the activity identifications of an input, as a function of a variety of personal, stimulus, and contextual factors.

7. "Change of identification" can involve either a subsequent primary identification's having been a secondary identification in a previous engagement or a subsequent primary identification's having been neither a primary nor a secondary identification in a previous engagement.

8. If a current identification of an input is the same as a previous identification of the input (whether primary or secondary), then the affective and inferential responses associated with the previous identification will be activated.

9. The greater the positivity of the affective and inferential responses associated with an activated identification, the greater the motivation to engage with the input again. The greater the negativity, the less the motivation to engage with the input again.

10. Contextual factors can influence the salience, accessibility, and applicability of an activity identification and its associated affective and inferential responses.

This model has general applicability to issues regarding motivational responses and orientations to input. One issue of special interest in the present chapter is the question of how activity identification influences intrinsic (and extrinsic) motivation. To address this issue, however, we need a definition of intrinsic motivation that is compatible with both the previous literature and our general model. In the next section, we propose such a definition.

INTRINSIC–EXTRINSIC MOTIVATION AND DISPOSITIONAL INPUT PROPERTIES

Earlier in this chapter, we have described some limitations and problems with the "type-of-need" and "type-of-inference" approaches to defining intrinsic motivation as distinct from extrinsic motivation. As an alternative approach, let us begin by returning to the everyday, "naive" meaning of "intrinsic" and "extrinsic." Using a Heiderian strategy, we went to the dictionary for the everyday meaning of "intrinsic" and "extrinsic." According to *Webster's New Collegiate Dictionary* (1973), "intrinsic" means "belonging to the essential nature or constitution of a thing" (p. 606). A synonym of "intrinsic" is "inherent," which means "involved in the constitution or essential character of something; belonging by nature" (p. 593). In contrast, "extrinsic" means "not belonging to a thing; coming from or originating from outside" (p. 408). A synonym of extrinsic is "extraneous," which means "not forming an essential part; coming from the outside" (p. 407). Thus, a general definition of "intrinsic motivation" and "extrinsic motivation" consistent with these meanings would be as follows: Experiencing an input is intrinsically motivating to the extent that it involves motivational responses to the inherent, essential properties of the input. Experiencing an input is extrinsically motivating to the extent that it involves motivational responses to properties extraneous to the input.

The inherent, essential properties of an input are properties that tend to be relatively enduring and invariant over time and place. Thus, such properties are "dispositional properties," in Heider's (1958) sense of "disposition." The dispositional properties of an input, in turn, are precisely the properties that permit current and future instances of some input to be considered the same input. The question of how current experiences with an input (current activity engagement) influence subsequent responses to the input (future activity engagement) is only meaningful if the two instances of the input are basically the same. The dispositional properties of an input can (and typically do) remain the same over time and place even when the actor's identification of the input as a certain type of activity varies (e.g., the invariant properties of a dime whether identified as "a coin" or as "money"). In this way, one can avoid tautological reasoning and circularity when considering the role of activity identification in intrinsic motivation.

In this approach, then, "intrinsic motivation" involves motivational responses to the dispositional properties of the input, whereas "extrinsic motivation" involves motivational responses to properties that are extraneous to the dispositional properties of the input. One might characterize this approach as distinguishing between responses to two types of properties—motivational responses to properties that are inherent or extraneous to the input. To this extent, this approach also involves "types"—the type of property in relation to the input to which the person motivationally responds, or, briefly, the "type-of-motivating-property" approach. As described in the preceding section, however, activity engagement theory emphasizes the *relation* between activity identifications and motivational responses to input. Indeed, as we discuss later, which dispositional properties of an input are intrinsically motivating depends on which input properties have been made relevant and significant by the primary activity identification. Thus, intrinsic motivation depends on the activity identification "process" and not just the input "content."

Let us now compare this type-of-motivating-property approach to defining intrinsic motivation with the type-of-need and type-of-inference approaches. All approaches to defining intrinsic motivation recognize that neither the person alone nor the input alone is sufficient as the source of intrinsic motivation. Intrinsic motivation, like all social phenomena (see Higgins, 1990), involves a complex set of person–input relations. The type-of-motivating-property approach differs from the type-of-need and type-of-inference approaches, however, with respect to which contributing variable in the person–input relations is emphasized. The type-of-need and type-of-inference approaches both emphasize the person as the contributing variable, either in that the person fulfills certain types of needs or in that the person makes certain types of inferences or attributions. In contrast, the type-of-motivating-property approach emphasizes the input as the contributing variable, in that the motivating properties have a certain type of relation to the input.

In comparison to the type-of-need and type-of-inference approaches, the type-of-motivating-property approach has little difficulty in classifying activities involving stimulus control. When people's motivational responses to an input, such as a glorious sunset, are controlled by the dispositional properties of the input (rather than by their prior needs or inferences), intrinsic motivation is involved. When people's motivational responses to an input are controlled by properties extraneous to the dispositional properties of the input, extrinsic motivation is involved.

Another major difference between the type-of-motivating-property approach and the other two approaches concerns the treatment of negative motivational responses. As discussed earlier, both the type-of-need and type-of-inference approaches distinguish between intrinsic motivation as a relatively positive state and extrinsic motivation as a relatively negative state. Experiencing negative affect because of the inherently negative properties of an input is not treated as intrinsic motivation in these approaches. In contrast, the type-of-motivating-property approach does not distinguish intrinsic and extrinsic motivation on the basis of the affect experienced in relation to input properties. Either positive or negative affect experienced in relation to dispositional properties of the input involves intrinsic motivation. Either positive or negative affect experienced in relation to properties extraneous to dispositional properties of the input involves extrinsic motivation. By including intrinsically negative motivation as one possibility, the type-of-motivating-property approach has the potential to study intrinsically motivated avoidance responses.

For example, just as one may wish to continue walking because it is relaxing (positive intrinsic motivation), one may wish to stop walking because it is tiring (negative intrinsic motivation). Similarly, just as one may wish to stay in the concert because the music is good (positive intrinsic motivation), one may wish to leave a concert because the music is bad (negative intrinsic motivation). The same factors that determine the strength of positive intrinsic motivation should also determine the strength of negative intrinsic motivation. Thus, negative affect will become strongly associated with an activity to the extent that there is little interference with attention and affective responses to the negative properties of the input. Furthermore, the individual will make strong inferences regarding his or her dislike for the activity to the extent that he or she was induced to undertake the activity but freely chose to terminate it. The initial inducements to undertake the activity will discount self-inferences of interest in the activity, whereas the absence of inducements for avoiding the activity will enhance self-inferences of dislike for the activity.

In comparison to the type-of-need and type-of-inference approaches, the type-of-motivating-property approach also has little difficulty in classifying activities in which there is increased motivation following failure (Atkinson & Feather, 1966; Trope & Ben-Yair, 1982) or spontaneous selection of tasks in which failure in highly diagnostic (Trope, 1979, 1980). In the type-of-motivating-property approach, an activity can be intrinsically motivating even if it produces negative affect as long as the motivational responses are to the dispositional properties of the input, which would be the case for tasks selected for their inherently diagnostic properties.

The type-of-motivating-property approach has a wider range of applicability than the alternative approaches. As just mentioned, cases involving stimulus control, negative affect, and diagnostic failure are treated as intrinsic motivation possibilities. In comparison to the type-of-need approach, intrinsic motivational responses are not restricted to those involving a particular set of needs. For example, a thirsty person drinking water would be considered intrinsically motivated because the motivated response is to the inherent gratifying properties of water as input. In comparison to the type-of-inference approach, intrinsic motivational responses are not restricted to those involving a particular higher-level stage of information processing. Infants enjoying being rocked, for example, would be considered intrinsically motivated because the motivated response is to the inherent pleasurable properties of rocking as input.

Although there are some clear differences between the type-of-motivating-property approach and the type-of-need and type-of-inference approaches to classifying activities as intrinsically or extrinsically motivated, there are many cases where they would agree in their classifications. A classic distinction in the literature is that between spontaneous selection of an activity and selection of an activity in order to receive a promised reward. Traditional approaches would classify these two cases as involving intrinsic and extrinsic motivation, respectively (see Lepper & Greene, 1978). The type-of-motivating-property approach would classify these cases in the same way if one assumes that in the spontaneous selection of an activity a person is typically drawn to the dispositional properties of the input, whereas when there is a promised reward a person is likely to respond motivationally to the properties of the reward, which are extraneous to the properties of the input. Similarly, when a person selects an activity because of the threat of punishment, the person is likely to respond motivationally to the properties of the punishment, which are extraneous to the properties of the input. As would the other approaches, then, the type-of-motivating-property approach would classify such cases as involving extrinsic motivation.

Activities in which a reward has been promised have been described as involving more intrinsic motivation when the reward is not simply for engaging in the activity, but is contingent on the quality of performance during the activity (see Boggiano & Ruble, 1979; Pittman & Heller, 1987). When a person is simply waiting for an activity to end in order to receive a promised reward, one would not expect the person to pay much attention to or be motivationally responsive to the dispositional properties of the input. In comparison, a person is much more likely to pay attention to and be motivationally responsive to the dispositional properties of the input when the person is concerned about his or her performance vis-à-vis the input. Thus, the type-of-motivating-property approach would also predict more intrinsic motivation when the promised reward is contingent on the quality of performance during the activity, rather than just on engaging in the activity.

Another classic distinction in the literature is between engaging in an activity as an end in itself ("for its own sake") and engaging in an activity as a means to an end. Traditional approaches would classify these two cases as involving intrinsic and extrinsic motivation, respectively (see Kruglanski, 1975). Engaging in an activity for its own sake implies being motivated to respond to the dispositional properties of the input. In contrast, engaging in an activity as a means to an end implies that the activity is less important or central than the end, and therefore the properties of the end, which are extraneous to the input, may be motivationally responded to at least as much as the properties of the means. Therefore, the type-of-motivating-property approach would classify these two cases in the same way as traditional approaches.

The type-of-motivating-property approach is also compatible with the literature's description of the fulfillment of certain needs as being intrinsically motivating. The literature suggests, for example, that fulfilling curiosity needs and competence needs is intrinsically motivating (see Deci & Ryan, 1985; Pittman & Heller, 1987). When one is fulfilling curiosity needs, the dispositional properties of the input are likely to be extensively explored; when one is fulfilling competence needs, the dispositional properties of the input are likely to be attended to carefully and responded to repeatedly. The type-of-motivating-property approach, therefore, would consider both of these cases as involving intrinsic motivation.

The type-of-motivating-property approach, therefore, agrees with previous approaches in its classification of some classic cases. This is not surprising, since even when previous approaches have emphasized other variables in distinguishing intrinsic and extrinsic motivation, there has always been a recognition that any approach should be compatible with the "naive" distinction between "inherent" versus "extraneous" properties. What we have done is simply to propose an approach where this distinction is central and not just compatible. We believe that doing so will give the distinction between intrinsic and extrinsic motivation a broader range of applicability. The type-of-motivating-property approach also has the advantage of allowing systematic consideration of the role of activity identification in intrinsic motivation, because both this definition of intrinsic motivation and activity identification emhasize relations to input properties. Let us now turn to this issue.

ACTIVITY ENGAGEMENT AND INTRINSIC–EXTRINSIC MOTIVATION

Both activity identification and intrinsic motivation, as we define these variables, concern *relations to input properties*. When an input is characterized in terms of an activity identification, attributes associated with the activity construct are activated and determine the relevance and significance of the input properties. Experiencing an input is intrinsically motivating to the extent that it involves motivational responses to the inherent, essential properties of the input—that is, to the dispositional properties of the input. Experiencing an input is extrinsically motivating to the extent that it involves motivational responses to properties extraneous to the dispositional properties of the input. Those properties made relevant and significant by a primary activity identification can be either dispositional properties of an input or properties extraneous to the dispositional properties of the input. The properties relevant to the secondary activity identification can also be either dispositional properties of an input or properties extraneous to the dispositional properties of the input.

Because of activity identification, intrinsic motivation does not necessarily involve responses to all of the inherent or dispositional properties of an input. Instead, intrinsic motivation involves mainly the responses to those dispositional properties of an input made relevant and significant by the primary identification, although additional dispositional properties can be responded to because of their relation to secondary identifications. Similarly, extrinsic motivation does not necessarily involve responses to all of the input-extraneous properties in a situation. Primary and secondary identifications also determine which input-extraneous properties will be responded to during an input engagement.

From the joint perspective of our theory of activity engagement and our approach to intrinsic–extrinsic motivation, a purely intrinsically motivated activity involves just a primary activity identification in which the attributes of the identified activity relate solely to the dispositional properties of the input. A purely extrinsically motivated activity involves just a primary activity identification in which the attributes of the identified activity relate solely to properties extraneous to the dispositional properties of the input.

A major difference between these pure cases of intrinsically versus extrinsically motivated activities is that the affective and inferential responses experienced during interaction with the input are more likely to influence subsequent engagements with the input in the case of the intrinsically motivated activity. In this case, the affective and inferential responses are to the dispositional properties of the input. When the input is later encountered again, these dispositional properties will still be present. Thus, the activity identification of the input is likely to be the same at the subsequent encounter as at the initial encounter, which should result in the activation of the affective and inferential responses associated with the dispositional properties from the initial encounter. In the case of the extrinsically motivated activity, however, the initial affective and inferential responses are to properties extraneous to the input, and thus are not likely to be activated when the input is subsequently encountered unless all the circumstances surrounding the initial encounter with the input remain the same at the subsequent encounter. This difference between the pure cases of intrinsically versus extrinsically motivated activities is consistent with the notion in the intrinsic-extrinsic motivation literature that intrinsically motivated activities are more likely than extrinsically motivated activities to produce a prolonged orientation to engage with an input (controlling for the positivity of the initial experiences with the input).

Although cases of purely extrinsically motivated activities and, especially, purely intrinsically motivated activities do occur, it is probably more common for activities to be both intrinsically *and* extrinsically motivating. Certainly, the intrinsic–extrinsic motivation literature has been concerned mainly with activities where both intrinsic and extrinsic motivation are involved. It is also common for inputs to be encoded with both a primary identification and one or more secondary identifications. Thus, combinations of primary–secondary identifications and intrinsic–extrinsic motivation are quite common. If we consider cases where there is just a primary and one secondary identification of an input, there are four possible combinations of activity identification and intrinsic–extrinsic motivation: (1) The primary activity identification involves intrinsic motivation and the secondary activity identification involves extrinsic motivation; (2) the primary activity identification involves extrinsic motivation and the secondary activity identification involves intrinsic motivation; (3) both the primary and the secondary identifications involve intrinsic motivation; and (4) both the primary and the secondary activity identifications involve extrinsic motivation.

The first of these combinations is more likely than the second, because it is more likely that the primary activity identification will involve intrinsic than extrinsic motivation. The dispositional properties of an input are more likely to determine identification, because the significance of objects and events derives in part from the meaning of their inherent properties or "affordances" to humans in general (see Gibson, 1979; McArthur & Baron, 1983). In addition, the dispositional properties of an input are likely to be more salient than extraneous properties. By grabbing and maintaining attention, these properties should have a stronger influence on choice of identification. Extraneous, nondispositional properties are frequently context-dependent (i.e., they result from momentary situational forces) and thus tend to change over time. In contrast, the dispositional properties of an input remain part of the input across time and place. Dispositional properties of an input, therefore, tend to be identified more consistently than extraneous, nondispositional properties. The greater consistency in how dispositional properties are identified should produce associations between these properties and their identification that are stronger than the associations between the nondispositional properties and their identifications. This in turn should result in the former associations' having higher chronic accessibility than the latter associations. When exposed to an input, therefore, an identification associated with dispositional properties of the input is more likely to be activated and to function as the primary identification than an identification associated with nondispositional properties of the input.

Thus, for a variety of reasons, it is more likely that the primary identification of an input will be related to dispositional than to nondispositional properties of the input. If so, then dispositional properties of the input should be made relevant and significant. This in turn increases the likelihood that the motivational responses will be in relation to these properties. Thus, one would expect the primary activity identification to involve intrinsic motivation more often than extrinsic motivation, which make the first combination described above more likely than the second one.

There is an important theoretical implication of the relation between the primary activity identification and intrinsic motivation. Because of the primary activity identification, intrinsic motivation should not involve responses to all of the inherent or dispositional properties of an input. Instead, intrinsic motivation should involve just the responses to those dispositional properties of an input made relevant and significant by the primary identification. To this extent, our approach does *not* simply equate "intrinsic" motivation with natural responses to inherent properties. Although the content of dispositional properties sets constraints on what can be intrinsically motivating, the process of activity identification strongly influences which input properties will be experienced as intrinsically motivating. Consider the case of the handcrafted coffee cup, for example. People will have a natural response to the taste of a particular glaze on the inside of a cup that is inherent to the chemical composition of the glaze. This taste response will be intrinsic to engaging the cup if the activity identification is "drinking coffee from the cup," but it will not be intrinsic if the activity identification is "studying the cup's craftsmanship." Moreover, the intrinsic response to the property can itself vary, depending on the activity identification. For example, the response to the glaze may be either a negative taste response when the activity identification is "drinking coffee from the cup" or a positive visual response when the activity identification is "studying the cup's craftsmanship." Thus, although "content" is part of our definition of intrinsic motivation, "process" is also critical.

The combination of a primary activity identification involving intrinsic motivation and a secondary activity identification involving extrinsic motivation has motivational implications that are reflected in a variety of phenomena in the intrinsic–extrinsic motivation literature. One implication of this combination is that intrinsic motivation is likely to be experienced as more positive than extrinsic motivation is. As discussed earlier, one implication of the primary identification's being primary is that the properties of the input related to it are experienced as relevant and significant, whereas the properties related to the secondary identification are experienced as competing, interfering responses. The fact that the primary identification *is* primary, and is recognized as such, can yield the inference that one must be motivated to engage with its identification-related properties, whereas experiencing the secondary identification as interfering can yield the inference that one must not be motivated to engage with its identification-related properties. Thus, the primary identification involving intrinsic motivation is likely to be experienced as more positive than the secondary identification involving extrinsic motivation.

Another implication of this combination is that increasing the extrinsic motivation of an input engagement will *undermine* the positivity of the intrinsic motivation of the input engagement. As discussed earlier, people's affective and inferential responses to the primary-identification-related properties can be altered by the presence of the secondary-identification-related properties. The more salient the secondary-identification-related properties of an activity are, the more they will interfere with affective and inferential responses to the primary-identification-related properties. The promise of an award, for example, can make children's play more hurried, lower in quality, and less enjoyable (Reiss & Sushinsky, 1975). In addition, the fact that the secondary-identification-related properties are grabbing one's attention and orientation away from the primary-identification-related properties can yield the inference that the secondary identification is a strong motivational alternative to the primary identification; this can undermine one's confidence in the feelings, motives, and dispositions implied by the primary-identification-related properties (Kelley, 1972; Lepper et al., 1973; Trope, 1989b). Thus, a salient secondary identification involving extrinsic motivation can undermine the positivity of the intrinsic motivation associated with the primary identification.

For the reasons mentioned earlier, when the input is encountered subsequently, the identification involving intrinsic motivation (i.e., related to dispositional properties) is again likely to be the primary activity identification. When this identification is activated, the affective and inferential responses associated with it from the earlier input engagement will influence the orientation to the input. The less positive the motivational responses associated with this identification from the previous engagement, the less motivated the person will be to engage with the input again. Thus, when a salient secondary identification involving extrinsic motivation undermines the positivity of the intrinsic motivation associated with the primary identification, it is likely that the motivation to engage the input subsequently will be reduced.

The most likely combination of a primary activity identification involving intrinsic motivation and a secondary activity identification involving extrinsic motivation should, therefore, typically produce the kinds of phenomena described in the literature on intrinsic and extrinsic motivation. Other combinations, however, can also occur. There are cases, for example, where properties extraneous to the dispositional properties of an input are made so salient that the primary identification involves extrinsic motivation. Consider, for instance, a study in which children successfully avoid punishment by performing some task. The primary identification involving extrinsic motivation is thus "doing what I'm told so I won't be punished." Because the primary identification involves extrinsic motivation (i.e., relates to properties extraneous to the dispositional properties of the input), it is unlikely to function again as the primary identification when the task is subsequently encountered in an open session. If so, then the subsequent orientation of these experimental children to perform the task may not differ from the input orientation of children who have had no previous experience with the task, despite the fact that the experimental children have been reinforced (i.e., punishment avoidance) for engaging in the task. This case represents the situation where children's compliance with adult demands fails to produce spontaneous obedience on future occasions.

Another version of this combination is when children are pressured to play a game called "X" that some adult wants them to play. Again, the primary identification involving extrinsic motivation may be "doing what I'm told to avoid punishment." The secondary identification involving intrinsic motivation may be "playing game X." Because the dispositional properties of the input are related to the secondary identification, they are likely to be experienced negatively (e.g., "I must not like playing this game if I am playing it just to avoid being punished"). When the input is subsequently encountered, however, the primary identification is likely to involve intrinsic motivation (i.e., to relate to the dispositional properties of the input). If so, the negative responses associated with this (previously secondary) identification will be activated and reduce motivation to engage with the input again. This case represents the situation where pressuring children to play a "fun" game decreases rather than increases their subsequent interest in the game.

The third possible combination is a primary identification involving intrinsic motivation and a secondary identification also involving intrinsic motivation. This combination has received little attention in the literature, in part because the dispositional properties of input have received little attention. When one considers the dispositional properties of input more carefully, one realizes that an input can have different sets of dispositional properties that relate to different identifications. For instance, our earlier example of a handcrafted coffee cup is an input that has some dispositional properties related to the "coffee cup" identification (e.g., weight, ease of holding, heat retention) and other dispositional properties related to the "handcrafted pottery" identification (e.g., type of clayware and glaze, method of firing, design originality). The input of taking a walk in the park also has a set of dispositional properties related to the "physical exercise" identification and another set of dispositional properties related to the "sightseeing" identification. As another example, children's books typically contain both a written story and pictures, with different dispositional properties being related to the "storybook" than to the "picture book." When one of these identifications is primary and the other is secondary, one has the combination of a primary and a secondary identification that both involve intrinsic motivation.

Because both of the alternative identifications relate to dispositional properties of the input, they are equally likely to function as the primary identification. In either case, the responses to the input involve intrinsic motivation. But for the reasons discussed earlier, the primary-identification-related properties are likely to be experienced more positively than the secondary-identification-related properties. Thus, everything else being equal, the subsequent motivation to engage with the input will be greater if the primary identification of the input remains the same than if the previously secondary identification becomes the primary identification. Indeed, in the latter case the subsequent motivation to engage with the input may be less than if there had been no previous experience with the input, despite the fact that the previous experience involved intrinsic motivation.

Another interesting implication of this combination is that *one intrinsic motivation can undermine another intrinsic motivation.* As discussed earlier, the secondary-identification-related properties of an input can grab attention and compete with the primary-identification-related properties. This competition and interference can reduce the positivity of the affective and inferential responses to the properties of the primary identification. Thus, it is possible for the intrinsic motivation associated with the secondary identification to undermine the intrinsic motivation associated with the primary identification.

The skill-related tasks typically employed in intrinsic motivation research exemplify this possibility. It seems plausible to assume that such tasks often lead people to identify their activity as skilled performance. Competence information should therefore enhance primary-identification-related motivation and thereby subsequent interest in the task. In contrast, competence-irrelevant rewards enhance secondary-identification-related motivations—motivations that may detract from the primary-identification-related motivation. This is what past research has usually found (see Condry, 1977; Harackiewicz et al., 1987; Pittman, et al., 1983). However, it is quite possible for skilled performance to be a secondary identification of an activity. Under these circumstances, competence information may diminsh intrinsic motivation. Suppose, for example, that the primary identification of a walk in the park is "sightseeing." In this case, competence information (e.g., regarding one's physical fitness) may enhance the motivation associated with a secondary identification of the walk (physical exercise) and thus may detract from subsequent interest in simply sight seeing. Recent research by Sansone, Sachau, and Weir (in press) is consistent with the present analysis. This research investigated the effects on intrinsic motivation of giving subjects *instructions* on how to improve their performance on the task. Sansone et al. found that the instructions enhanced interest when the task was described as a "game of skill," but diminished interest when the task was described as a "fantasy game." From the present perspective, the description of the task as a game of skill made skilled performance the primary identification of the activity, whereas the description of the task as a fantasy game made skilled performance the secondary identification of the activity. As such, when the task was described as a game of skill, the instructions on how to improve performance enhanced the motivation associated with the primary identification, and thus enhanced interest in the activity. In contrast, when the task was described as a fantasy game, the instructions enhanced the motivation associated with the secondary identification, and thus undermined interest in the activity.

The present analysis suggests that when alternative identifications compete and interfere with one another, the motivational responses and orientation to an input may be *less* positive if its dispositional properties are related to multiple identifications than if they are related to only one identification, even though all identifications are intrinsically motivating. On the other hand, when alternative identifications do not interfere with one another, such as appreciating the glaze of a cup for both its aesthetic ("pottery") and heat retention ("coffee container") properties, then multiple alternative identifications involving intrinsic motivation may increase positive responses to the input. In addition, if the secondary identification involving intrinsic motivation becomes the primary identification when the input is subsequently encountered, it is possible that positive inferential responses to the properties of the secondary identification at the initial encounter may produce an augmentation effect at the subsequent encounter.

For related reasons, the combination in which both the primary and the secondary identifications involve extrinsic motivation is interesting, because there is the possibility of *one extrinsic motivation undermining another extrinsic motivation.* Of course, this combination would be unusual to begin with, because it is likely that at least one of the identifications of an input will be related to the dispositional properties of the input. However, one can imagine a boy who must eat his spinach before receiving dessert identifying his eating the spinach primarily as "getting to dessert" and secondarily as "pleasing Mother." Both identifications involve extrinsic motivation. As we have discussed earlier, to the extent that the properties related to a secondary identification attract attention away from the properties related to a primary identification, the actor may infer that the primary identified activity must be less interesting or important. If the boy, for example, begins to think about how eating the spinach will please his mother, rather than about the dessert he will receive, then the value of the dessert will be undermined.

SUMMARY AND CONCLUSIONS

The purpose of this chapter has been to address some basic issues in motivation. What determines people's motivational responses to an input? How do people's affective and inferential responses to an input influence their subsequent orientation toward that input? These issues have been addressed by considering the role of activity identification in motivation generally and in intrinsic–extrinsic motivation in particular. A general model of activity identification and motivation has been proposed, and an alternative approach to distinguishing intrinsic and extrinsic motivation has been suggested. In contrast to previous theories of intrinsic–extrinsic motivation, which have emphasized different types of needs of the actor or different types of inferences by the actor, our theory emphasizes input properties and the motivational consequences of multiple and changing relations to them.

This emphasis on input properties and the varying relations to them is reflected in the following four basic postulates of our theory:

1. *Experiencing an input involves intrinsic or extrinsic motivation, depending on the relation between the motivational responses and the properties of the input.* Experiencing an input is intrinsically motivating to the extent that it involves motivational responses to the dispositional properties (i.e., the inherent, essential properties) of the input. Experiencing an input is extrinsically motivating to the extent that it involves motivational responses to properties extraneous to the input's dispositional properties.

2. *The relevance and significance of each property of an input vary as a function of the property's relation to the primary activity identification of the input.* It is the primary activity identification of an input that determines both the

meaning and the importance of its properties. Every input can be identified in multiple ways. At any point in time there is a primary (i.e., focal or predominant) activity identification, and there can also be competing (or noncompeting) secondary activity identifications.

Because of the primary activity identification, intrinsic motivation does not necessarily involve responses to all of the inherent or dispositional properties of an input. Instead, intrinsic motivation involves mainly the responses to those dispositional properties of an input made relevant and significant by the primary identification. Primary and secondary identifications also determine which input-extraneous properties involving extrinsic motivation will be responded to during an input engagement.

For a variety of reasons, the primary identification of an input is more likely to be related to intrinsically motivating properties of the input than to extrinsically motivating properties. A purely intrinsically motivated activity involves just a primary activity identification in which the attributes of the identified activity relate solely to the dispositional properties of the input. Often, however, there are one or more secondary identifications as well. When there is a competing secondary identification, it is often related to extrinsically motivating properties. Everything else being equal, this combination of a primary identification involving intrinsic motivation and a secondary identification involving extrinsic motivation can account both for why intrinsically motivated responses are typically more positive than extrinsically motivated responses, and for why extrinsically motivated responses typically undermine the positivity of intrinsic motivation.

3. *The associations formed between input (and extrainput) properties and affective and inferential responses to those properties are the basis of the influence of initial input engagements on subsequent input engagements.* It is not just the inherent need-fulfilling nature of the properties of an input that causes initial input engagements to influence subsequent engagements. As indicated by the first postulate, the inherent or dispositional nature of a property is certainly a factor in how people respond to it. But as indicated by the second postulate, whether people even attend to a property, and which aspect of a property they assess when they do attend to it, are determined by how an input is identified in the first place. People respond affectively and inferentially to the properties of an input that are made relevant and significant by the activity identification. And these relations between the properties and the responses to them as represented in property–response associations are critical factors in motivating subsequent engagements, and not just the inherent nature of the properties.

4. *The impact of the affective and inferential responses to the properties of an input on subsequent engagements with the input depends on the relation between the subsequent and the previous activity identifications of the input.* Earlier models of input orientation have implicitly assumed that an activity will be identified in the same way in both initial and subsequent engagements. Thus, the predominant affective or inferential responses to the input during the initial engagement are assumed to determine the motivation to engage subsequently

with the input. But in our model, this would only be predicted if the activity identification of the input is the same on both occasions. If there is a change of identification over time, either subordinate affective and inferential responses to the input properties will determine the subsequent motivation to engage (when the subsequent primary identification was a secondary identification in the previous engagement), or none of the previous responses will determine the subsequent motivation to engage (when the subsequent primary identification has no relation to previous identifications).

By emphasizing both the inherent nature of input properties and basic information processes that influence relations to them, the present theory entails both an idiographic and a nomothetic perspective on motivation generally and on intrinsic–extrinsic motivation in particular. Historically, there has been some conflict between content perspectives on motivation (e.g., type-of-need models) and process perspectives on motivation (e.g., operant conditioning models). The present theory represents an initial attempt at integrating process and content perspectives, in order to capture as fully as possible the true complexity of motivational orientations to input.

References

Anderson, R. C., & Pichert, J. W. (1978). Recall of previously unrecallable information following a shift in perspective. *Journal of Verbal Learning and Verbal Behavior, 17*, 1–12.

Atkinson, J. W., & Feather, N. T. (Eds.). (1966). *Theory of achievement motivation.* New York: Wiley.

Bandura, A. (1986). *Social foundations of thought and action: A social cognitive theory.* Englewood Cliffs, NJ: Prentice-Hall.

Bem, D. J. (1972). Self-perception theory. In L. Berkowitz (Ed.), *Advances in experimental social psychology* (Vol. 6, pp. 1–62). New York: Academic Press.

Berlyne, D. E. (1950). Novelty and curiosity as determinants of exploratory behavior. *British Journal of Psychology, 41*, 68–80.

Boggiano, A. K., & Ruble, D. N. (1979). Competence and the overjustification effect: A developmental study. *Journal of Personality and Social Psychology, 37*, 1462–1468.

Brown, R. W. (1958). How shall a thing be called? *Psychological Review, 65*, 14–21.

Condry, J. (1977). Enemies of exploration: Self-initiated versus other-initiated learning. *Journal of Personality and Social Psychology, 35*, 459–477.

Connell, J. P., & Wellborn, J. G. (in press). Self-system processes from a motivational perspective. In M. R. Gunnard & L. A. Sroufe (Eds.), *Minnesota Symposium on Child Psychology: Vol. 23. Self processes in development.* Hillsdale, NJ: Erlbaum.

Csikszentmihalyi, M. (1975). *Beyond boredom and anxiety.* San Francisco: Jossey-Bass.

deCharms, R. (1968). *Personal causation.* New York: Academic Press.

Deci, E. L. (1971). Effects of externally mediated rewards on intrinsic motivation. *Journal of Personality and Social Psychology, 18*, 105–115.

Deci, E. L. (1972). Intrinsic motivation, extrinsic reinforcement, and inequity. *Journal of Personality and Social Psychology, 22*, 113–120.

Deci, E. L. (1975). *Intrinsic motivation.* New York: Plenum Press.

Deci, E. L., & Ryan, R. M. (1982). Curiosity and self-directed learning. In L. Katz (Ed.), *Current topics in early childhood education* (Vol. 4). Norwood, NJ: Ablex.

Deci, E. L., & Ryan, R. M. (1985). *Intrinsic motivation and self-determination in human behavior.* New York: Plenum.

Deci, E. L., & Ryan, R. M. (1987). The support of autonomy and the control of behavior. *Journal of Personality and Social Psychology, 53,* 1024-1037.

Festinger, L. (1957). *A theory of cognitive dissonance.* Evanston, IL: Row, Peterson.

Gibson, J. J. (1979). *The ecological approach to visual perception.* Boston: Houghton Mifflin.

Harackiewicz, J., Abrahams, S., & Wageman, R. (1987). Performance evaluation and intrinsic motivation: The effects of evaluative focus rewards, and achievement orientation. *Journal of Personality and Social Psychology, 53,* 1015-1023.

Harlow, H. F. (1950). Learning and satiation of response in intrinsically motivated complex puzzle performance by monkeys. *Journal of Comparative and Physiological Psychology, 43,* 289-294.

Heider, F. (1958). *The psychology of interpersonal relations.* New York: Wiley.

Higgins, E. T. (1989). Knowledge accessibility and activation: Subjectivity and suffering from unconscious sources. In J. S. Uleman & J. A. Bargh (Eds.), *Unintended thought* (pp. 75-123). New York: Guilford Press.

Higgins, E. T. (1990). Personality, social psychology, and person–situation relations: Standards and knowledge activation as a common language. In L. A. Pervin (Ed.), *Handbook of personality: Theory and research* (pp. 301-338). New York: Guilford Press.

Higgins, E. T., & Lurie, L. (1983). Context, categorization, and memory: The "change-of-standard" effect. *Cognitive Psychology, 15,* 525-547.

Higgins, E. T., & Stangor, C. (1988a). A "change-of-standard" perspective on the relation among context, judgment, and memory. *Journal of Personality and Social Psychology, 54,* 181-192.

Higgins, E. T., & Stangor, C. (1988b). Context-driven social judgment and memory: When "behavior engulfs the field" in reconstructive memory. In D. Bar-Tal & A. W. Kruglanski (Eds.), *The social psychology of knowledge* (pp. 262-298). New York: Cambridge University Press.

Higgins, E. T., Strauman, T., & Klein, R. (1986). Standards and the process of self-evaluation: Multiple affects from multiple stages. In R. M. Sorrentino & E. T. Higgins (Eds.), *Handbook of motivation and cognition: Foundations of social behavior* (Vol. 1, pp. 23-63). New York: Guilford Press.

Hunt, J. M. (1965). Intrinsic motivation and its role in psychological development. In D. Levine (Ed.), *Nebraska Symposium on Motivation* (Vol. 13, pp. 189-282). Lincoln: University of Nebraska Press.

Izard, C. E. (1977). *Human emotion.* New York: Holt.

Kelley, H. H. (1972). *Causal schemata and the attribution process.* Morristown, NJ: General Learning Press.

Kruglanski, A. W. (1975). The endogenous–exogenous partition in attribution theory. *Psychological Review, 82,* 387-406.

Kruglanski, A. W. (1980). Lay epistemo-logic—process and contents: Another look at attribution theory. *Psychological Review, 87,* 70-87.

Kruglanski, A. W., Alon, S., & Lewis, T. (1972). Retrospective misattribution and task enjoyment. *Journal of Experimental Social Psychology, 8,* 493-501.

Kruglanski, A. W., Friedman, I., & Zeevi, G. (1971). The effect of extrinsic incentive on some qualitative aspects of task performance. *Journal of Personality, 39,* 606-617.

Lepper, M. R., & Greene, D. (1975). Turning play into work: Effects of adult surveillance and extrinsic rewards on children's intrinsic motivation. *Journal of Personality and Social Psychology, 31,* 479-486.

Lepper, M. R., & Greene, D. (1978). *The hidden costs of rewards.* Hillsdale, NJ: Erlbaum.

Lepper, M. R., Greene, D., & Nisbett, R. E. (1973). Undermining children's intrinsic interest with extrinsic reward: A test of the overjustification hypothesis. *Journal of Personality and Social Psychology, 28,* 129-137.

Lepper, M. R., Sagotsky, G., Dafoe, J. L., & Greene, D. (1982). Consequences of superfluous social constraints: Effects on young children's social inferences and subsequent intrinsic interest. *Journal of Personality and Social Psychology, 45,* 587-597.

McArthur, L. Z., & Baron, R. M. (1983). Toward an ecological theory of social perception. *Psychological Review, 90,* 215-235.

McCann, C. D., & Higgins, E. T. (1984). Individual differences in communication: Social cognitive determinants and consequences. In H. E. Sypher & J. L. Applegate (Eds.), *Communication by children and adults* (pp. 172-210). Beverly Hills, CA: Sage.

Morgan, M. (1981). The overjustification effect: A developmental test of self-perception interpretations. *Journal of Personality and Social Psychology, 40*, 809-821.

Newtson, D. (1976). Foundations of attribution: The unit of perception of ongoing behavior. In J. Harvey, W. J. Ickes, & R. F. Kidd (Eds.), *New directions in attribution research* (pp. 223-247). Hillsdale, NJ: Erlbaum.

Nicholls, J. G. (1975). Causal attributions and other achievement-related cognitions: Effects of task outcome, attainment value and sex. *Journal of Personality and Social Psychology, 31*, 379-389.

Pittman, T. S., Cooper, E. E., Smith, T. W. (1977). Attribution of causality and the overjustification effect. *Personality and Social Psychology Bulletin, 3*, 280-283.

Pittman, T. S., Boggiano, A. K., & Ruble, D. N. (1983). Intrinsic and extrinsic motivational orientations: Limiting conditions on the undermining and enhancing effects of reward on intrinsic motivation. In J. Levine & M. Wang (Eds.), *Teacher and student perceptions: Implications for learning* (pp. 319-340). Hillsdale, NJ: Erlbaum.

Pittman, T. S., & Heller, J. F. (1987). Social motivation. *Annual Review of Psychology, 38*, 461-489.

Pretty, G. H., & Seligman, C. (1984). Affect and the overjustification effect. *Journal of Personality and Social Psychology, 46*, 1241-1253.

Reiss, S., & Sushinsky, L. W. (1975). Overjustification, competing responses, and the acquisition of intrinsic interest. *Journal of Personality and Social Psychology, 31*, 1116-1125.

Rosch, E. (1978). Principles of categorization. In E. Rosch & B. B. Lloyd (Eds.), *Cognition and categorization* (pp. 27-48). Hillsdale, NJ: Erlbaum.

Ross, M. (1975). Salience of reward and intrinsic motivation. *Journal of Personality and Social Psychology, 33*, 245-254.

Ross, M., Karniol, R., & Rothstein, M. (1976). Reward contingency and intrinsic motivation in children: A test of the delay of gratification hypothesis. *Journal of Personality and Social Psychology, 32*, 245-254.

Rotter, J. B. (1954). *Social learning and clinical psychology.* Englewood Cliffs, NJ: Prentice-Hall.

Sansone, C., Sachau, D. A., & Weir, C. (in press). Effects of instructions on intrinsic interest: The importance of context. *Journal of Personality and Social Psychology.*

Shallice, T. (1972). Dual functions of consciousness. *Psychological Review, 79*, 383-393.

Sorrentino, R. M., & Short, J. C. (1986). Uncertainty orientation, motivation, and cognition. In R. M. Sorrentino & E. T. Higgins (Eds.), *Handbook of motivation and cognition: Foundations of social behavior* (Vol. 1, pp. 379-403). New York: Guilford Press.

Trope, Y. (1979). Uncertainty reducing properties of achievement tasks. *Journal of Personality and Social Psychology, 37*, 1505-1518.

Trope, Y. (1980). Self-assessment, self-enhancement and task preference. *Journal of Experimental Social Psychology, 16*, 116-129.

Trope, Y. (1986a). Identification and inferential processes in dispositional attribution. *Psychological Review, 94*, 237-258.

Trope, Y. (1986b). Self-enhancement and self-assessment in achievement behavior. In R. M. Sorrentino & E. T. Higgins (Eds.), *Handbook of motivation and cognition: Foundations of social behavior* (Vol. 1, pp. 350-378). New York: Guilford Press.

Trope, Y. (1989a). Levels of inference in dispositional judgment. *Social Cognition, 7*, 296-314.

Trope, Y. (1989b). The multiple roles of context in dispositional judgment. In J. N. Bassili (Ed.), *Cognition and the judgments we make about other people* (pp. 123-140). Hillsdale, NJ: Erlbaum.

Trope, Y., & Ben-Yair, E. (1982). Task construction and persistence as means for self-assessment of abilities. *Journal of Personality and Social Psychology, 42*, 637-645.

Trope, Y., & Cohen, O. (1989). Perceptual and inferential determinants of behavior-correspondent attribution. *Journal of Experimental Social Psychology, 25*, 142-158.

Trope, Y., Cohen, O., & Maoz, I. (1988). The perceptual and inferential effects of situational inducements. *Journal of Personality and Social Psychology, 55,* 165–177.

Vallacher, R. R., & Wegner, D. M. (1985). *A theory of action identification.* Hillsdale, NJ: Erlbaum.

Webster's new collegiate dictionary. (1973). Springfield, MA: G. & C. Merriam.

Wegner, D. M., & Vallacher, R. R. (1986). Action identification. In R. M. Sorrentino & E. T. Higgins (Eds.), *Handbook of motivation and cognition: Foundations of social behavior* (Vol. 1, pp. 550–582). New York: Guilford Press.

White, R. W. (1959). Motivation reconsidered: The concept of competence. *Psychological Review, 66,* 297–333.

Wyer, R. S., Jr., & Srull, T. K. (1986). Human cognition in its social context. *Psychological Review, 93,* 322–359.

CHAPTER 8

Happiness, Sadness, and Helping

A Motivational Integration

MARK SCHALLER
University of Texas at Arlington
ROBERT B. CIALDINI
Arizona State University

In recent years, reviews documenting the effects of induced happiness and sadness on helping have sprung up in the social-psychological literature like mushrooms after a summer rain (e.g., Carlson, Charlin, & Miller, 1987; Carlson & Miller, 1987; Clark & Isen, 1984; Isen, 1984; Rosenhan, Karylowski, Salovey, & Hargis, 1981; Salovey & Rosenhan, 1989; Shaffer, 1985/1986). This surge may be representative of the fecund conceptual soil that over the last 20 years has spawned a veritable thicket of empirical reports. Less encouragingly, the number of recent reviews may betray the inevitable conceptual disagreement that has burgeoned alongside the empirical research.

Twenty years of research on mood and helping might well be expected to lead to a clear, perhaps even definitive, explanation of exactly how and why temporary positive and negative moods affect altruistic behavior. Unfortunately, this has not been the case; in addition to the vast empirical literature, there exists no shortage of possible explanatory accounts for the effects of sadness and elation on helping. Hypotheses concerning the effects of these affective states on helping have been derived from models stressing such processes as mood management (e.g., Cialdini, Baumann, & Kenrick, 1981; Cialdini, Kenrick, & Baumann, 1982; Clark & Isen, 1982), equity and focus of attention (e.g., Rosenhan et al., 1982), objective self-awareness and locus of responsibility (e.g., Rogers, Miller, Mayer, & Duval, 1982), perceptions of the social community (Hornstein, 1982; Hornstein, LaKind, Frankel, & Manne, 1975), and differential access to cognitions (Clark & Isen, 1982; Isen, Shalker, Clark, & Karp, 1978). However, these explanatory accounts cannot be considered fully developed theories of helping behavior, as each has focused exclusively upon a constrained set of moderator variables or mediating processes of particular theoretical interest. As a result, with few exceptions (see Carlson & Miller, 1987), these accounts have for the most part not attempted to explain the results of experiments conducted as tests of other accounts of mood effects on helping. The reviews have not integrated the vast literature or reconciled differing accounts. Most have drawn conclusions about the basic effects: The experience of a positive mood and—although somewhat less consistently—the experience of a negative mood both lead to enhanced helping. Moderators of the effects of mood on helping, as well as attentional and cognitive processes that may mediate the relationship, have been reviewed in commendable detail, but only passing attention has been given to the mechanisms that drive social actions. In other words, motivation has been largely ignored.

We believe that it is imperative to address explicitly questions of motivation. Why is it that happiness consistently leads to greater helping? Why is it that sadness also enhances helping, but less consistently? Is it the same motivation underlying both, or are the two effects due to entirely different motivational processes? The framework we advance in this chapter focuses explicitly upon the motivation that underlies the effects of happiness and sadness on helping. In attending to the role of motivation in directing the effects of mood on helping, we hope to expand the scope of explanation for these effects. However, we cannot understand the role of motivation in the mood–helping relationship without also attending to the processes so thoroughly discussed by other researchers in the area. In particular, we discuss the role of attentional and cognitive processes that interact with motivational processes in directing the effects of mood on helping.

HAPPINESS AND SADNESS: DEFINITIONAL ISSUES

Before we proceed further, it is crucial that the reader understand the boundaries of the present perspective on mood. Our framework is specific to the experience of happiness and sadness; we do not extend the model to all types of positive and negative affect. Therefore, we distinguish temporary happiness ("elation," "joy") from other positive mood states, such as pride.[1] And we distinguish sadness ("sorrow") from other commonly researched negative states, such as anger, frustration, and guilt.

We must also make it clear that in discussing happiness and sadness, we refer to *temporary* mood states. We do not extend this perspective to account for behavior associated with more chronic affective states. For instance, although at times we highlight commonalities between clinical depression and temporarily induced sadness, our model should not be taken as an account of the cognitive or motivational processes associated with chronic depression. We speak only of the processes engaged by relatively short affective episodes of the sort that most people experience frequently in the course of their daily lives.

OVERVIEW OF THE THEORETICAL FRAMEWORK

There are five different levels to our analysis. Our primary goal is to arrive at a conceptualization of mood-induced motivation to help others. As a means toward developing a coherent and empirically consistent motivational perspective, we review four other processes that we believe are important in understanding the effects of mood on helping behavior. Before we discuss each in detail, it may be useful to introduce each level briefly.

First, we discuss the effect of mood states on cognitive processes. A number of researchers (e.g., Bower, 1981; Isen et al., 1978) have suggested that material may be stored in memory according to its affective tone. Therefore, different mood states may temporarily enhance retrieval of mood-congruent material from memory. This differential access to affect-related information can have an impact on resulting cognitions, perceptions, and behavior.

As a second level of analysis, we propose that happiness and sadness are associated with different attentional processes and different orientations toward the environment. When sad, people tend for the most part to avoid interaction with the environment, because they will probably see it as harsh and punishing. When happy, however, people tend to seek such interaction, because they are likely to view the environment as rich and rewarding. One consequence is that the experience of sadness will lead attention away from the surround and toward a different area of concern—the self. In contrast, elated persons, who are more trusting of the environment, will be less concerned with the self and may redirect or even expand their focus of attention.

Third, we discuss support for the assertion that happiness and sadness are associated with different levels of physiological and physical activity. Temporary elation is associated with enhanced arousal and activity, whereas sadness is often associated with reduced physiological arousal and physical activity. This we take as evidence that the mechanisms for action associated with happiness and sadness are quite different.

Fourth, we review evidence to suggest that saddened individuals will make decisions and emit social responses only after careful consideration; those feeling happy will offer responses that are much less considered. Therefore, the helping responses offered by saddened persons will be dependent upon consideration of factors that affect the hedonic consequences of helping. The helping responses offered by elated persons will be less dependent upon carefully considered hedonic considerations, and instead will be offered in a more unthinking, impulsive manner.

Finally, in light of the processes we have outlined above and of the amassed data from the helping literature, we expand upon the proposal offered by Cunningham and his colleagues (e.g., Cunningham, Shaffer, Barbee, Wolff, & Kelley, 1990; Cunningham, Steinberg, & Grev, 1980; Shaffer, 1985/1986) that happiness and sadness are associated with two distinctly different sets of motivational concerns. These distinct motives can nonetheless lead to the same behavioral outcome: increased helping. How might we characterize these two different motives? On a general level, we propose that the motivation instigated by the onset of a negative mood is one of homeostasis—a drive to restore mood to a prior, non-negative equilibrium state. In contrast, we propose that the motivation attendant upon the feeling of happiness is not homeostatic, but instead is marked by a striving away from equilibrium. More specifically, we suggest that that the experience of sadness leads to an enhanced drive to restore the disrupted mood state to its prior level. The experience of happiness, we suggest, leads not to concern over restoration of a prior state, but to a less focused motive to move toward greater personal attainment.

Although we discuss these five assertions in the order just outlined, we do not suggest that this outline represents the temporal order of processes engaged by temporary shifts in mood. For instance, in locating our discussion of motivation after our presentation of cognitive and attentional processes, we do not mean to imply that the structure and form of the motives are purely consequences of cognition or attention. In fact, we would argue that the motivational concerns are conceptually independent of the processes of cognition and attention. It is likely that each is affected independently by changes in mood, and yet that the processes are conceptually consistent and may under many circumstances be self-perpetuating.

We now address each of our assertions in detail.

MOOD, MEMORY, AND EVALUATION OF THE ENVIRONMENT

Interest in the relation between mood and cognition has existed as long as the study of psychology itself (see Wundt, 1897, p. 26). This interest has flowered over the last 15 years with the conceptualization of mood as an important component in the human memory system (e.g., Bower, 1981; Isen et al., 1978; Teasdale & Fogarty, 1979). In his influential "network theory of affect," Bower (1981; Bower & Cohen, 1982) proposed that mood may be a node within an associative network of memory. Affectively toned material encoded into memory may therefore be accessed by activation of the relevant affective node. The onset of a certain mood may be sufficient to activate the particular affective node, and thus may automatically facilitate recall of mood-congruent cognitive material from memory.

A considerable body of literature has emerged that examines the relation between mood state and recall; others have reviewed this literature in considerable depth (e.g., Blaney, 1986; Clark & Isen, 1982; Isen, 1984; Singer & Salovey, 1988). Although there are exceptions, a number of studies provide compelling evidence that temporary positive affect does indeed faciliate the recall of positively toned material (e.g., Laird, Wagener, Halal, & Szegda, 1982; Teasdale & Fogarty, 1979; Teasdale & Russell, 1983; see Singer & Salovey, 1988, for a comprehensive review). Other studies have shown that induced sadness may facilitate recall of negatively toned material (e.g., Teasdale & Russell, 1983; see Singer & Salovey, 1988, for a review). However, most reviewers of this literature (Blaney, 1986; Clark & Isen, 1982; Isen, 1984; Singer & Salovey, 1988) have noted some asymmetry in these effects. Specifically, the effects of positive mood-congruent recall are generally stronger and more consistent than the effects of negative mood-congruent recall.

Mood, Memory, and Perception of the Social Environment

Happiness apparently makes happy memories more accessible; in a more qualified way, sadness makes sad memories more accessible. Research in a number of domains suggests that mood-congruent recall may affect a considerable body of perceptual phenomena, any or all of which may be linked to helping behavior. A number of studies have shown that happy individuals register greater liking for others or view others more positively than do sad individuals (e.g., Forgas & Bower, 1987; Gouaux, 1971; Griffitt, 1970; Mayer, Mamberg, & Volanth, 1988; Mayer & Volanth, 1985; Veitch & Griffitt, 1976). Others have found that ambiguous stimuli are rated more positively by happy subjects than by sad subjects (e.g., Forest, Clark, Mills, & Isen, 1979; Isen & Shalker, 1982; Schiffenbaur, 1974). Personal possessions (Isen et al., 1978) and social interactions (Forgas, Bower, & Krantz, 1984) are also rated more positively by happy subjects than by controls.

Other studies have examined perceptions of particular situations. A number of researchers have found that, compared to controls, temporarily elated subjects are more optimistic about future events (Feather, 1966; Forgas & Moylan, 1987; Masters & Furman, 1976). In a similar vein, compared to negative affect, positive affect decreases the judged likelihood of a number of unpleasant events (Johnson & Tversky, 1983; Mayer et al., 1988). This suggests that happy individuals perceive the world in general to be a less risky place than do those in sad moods. Other research has corroborated this interpretation in demonstrating that induced positive affect enhances the likelihood of taking moderate risks in a specific situation (Isen, Means, Patrick, & Nowicky, 1982). Perceptions of control are also influenced by affect. Chronic negative affect is associated with the perception of reduced control over one's environment (Alloy & Abramson, 1979). Similarly, Alloy, Abramson, and Viscusi (1981) found that temporarily induced sadness eliminates the "illusion of control" commonly experienced by nondepressed individuals.

These studies all suggest that people, inanimate objects, and a wide variety of situations are likely to be judged more positively by temporarily elated individuals than by those in either a sad or a neutral mood. These perceptual effects are consistent with the thesis that affect facilitates the retrieval of mood-congruent cognitions from memory, and that these cognitions in turn influence judgments of a variety of stimuli.

Note that a number of the judgmental effects of mood are found on social stimuli. This is consistent with our assertion that sadness is less likely than happiness to induce an outward focus upon the external environment. More direct evidence for the impact of positive mood upon cognitions about the social environment has been obtained by Isen, Herren, and Geva (1986). These researchers found that temporarily elated subjects recalled a greater number of words with socially oriented (but affectively neutral) content than did subjects in a neutral mood. This same effect was not found on recall for intellectually oriented words.

Helping

How might these automatic cognitive consequences of mood be related to helping behavior? Clark and Isen (1982) have suggested that a "helping node" may exist in an associative memory network, and may be activated whenever one perceives the opportunity to help another. Activation of this helping node may activate other memory nodes associated with various concequences of helping. If one is in a happy mood, those nodes that are associated with helping and also associated with happy moods are more likely to be activated than nodes that are associated with helping and also associated with negative moods. Therefore, positive consequences of helping are likely to be conjured up in the mind of the potential helper. The same helping situation may therefore be viewed more positively by the elated individual than by someone in a neutral mood. Indeed, Clark and Waddell (1983) found that in response to a hypothetical helping situation, elated subjects generated thoughts that were more positive in content than were those generated by control subjects. Although to our knowledge no one has coded the semantic content of such thoughts, it seems likely that the elated individual may see the helping situation as less risky, may expect greater control over the outcome, and may simply expect better outcomes than a nonelated person may. Furthermore, compared to someone in a neutral mood, the elated individual may perceive the needy other as more deserving of aid. Finally, the happy helper may view the needy other as particularly pleasant and attractive, and therefore may perceive the helping situation as having additional positive social benefits for the self. Indeed, evidence from several studies support the hypothesis that more help is offered to those who are more interpersonally attractive (e.g., Carlsmith, Lepper, & Landauer, 1974; Daniels & Berkowitz, 1963; Staub & Sherk, 1970).

If happiness generates positive cognitions about the helping situation, does this mean that sadness will inevitably lead to negative thoughts about the helping situation? There may be such a natural tendency, but for several reasons it seems fair to argue that this tendency does not fully determine helping behavior. First, as noted above, mood-congruent recall effects tend to be stronger for positive mood than for negative mood. The perceptual effects may also lack full symmetry. For instance, although Masters and Furman (1976) found happy subjects to be more optimistic than those in a neutral mood, their results did not show temporarily saddened subjects to be more pessimistic. Furthermore, there is evidence that negative material is not interconnected in memory to the same elaborate degree as is positive material (Isen et al., 1978). Therefore, sadness may be a less efficient memory cue than happiness.

Finally, let us not overlook the most obvious reason to discard the notion that negative mood leads only to negative thoughts about helping: Sadness often leads to enhanced helping. This well-demonstrated effect is fully incompatible with the notion that saddened individuals view helping situations particularly unfavorably. Instead, it is likely that the automatic cognitive consequences of sadness are superseded by the motivational concern to reachieve affective homeostasis. We concur with others (e.g., Clark & Isen, 1982; Fiske & Taylor, 1984; Isen, 1984) who have suggested that individuals concerned with their moods will rebel against the automatic self-perpetuating processes associated with negative moods, and will instead adopt controlled mechanisms to manage their moods. Or, as Fiske and Taylor (1984) put it, "People often take charge of their minds' propensity to jump from gloomy thought to gloomy thought" (p. 328). Salovey (1988) has suggested that immediately following the induction of negative moods, there may be an initial period of automatically accessed mood-congruent thoughts. This may then give way to controlled processing as the individual attempts to reachieve a more desirable mood state. We argue later that saddened individuals may therefore actively assess the potential positive aspects of helping—particularly when helping may serve as an instrument toward mood repair.

MOOD, ATTENTION, AND ORIENTATION TO THE ENVIRONMENT

We suggest that temporary mood states influence the manner in which people approach their social environment. This approach to the environment is manifested in either the withdrawal of attention from the environment (as in sadness) or the expansion or redirection of attention to the environment (as in happiness). We are hardly the first to suggest this distinction. Almost three decades ago, Tomkins (1962) proposed that negative affect produces "sociophobia" and positive affect produces "sociophilia." Cunningham and his associates have for several years incorporated similar reasoning into their "separate-processes" approach to positive and negative moods (Cunningham, 1988a, 1988b; Cunningham et al., 1980, 1990). Following the lead of these authors, we wish to propose a mechanism whereby differential attention to the environment results from the onset of positive and negative mood. Specifically, we propose that this shift in attention may be an automatic process, and a process that is adaptive to the living organism. We therefore must address two assumptions. The first is that shifts in moods are typically based upon changes in a person's immediate environment (although this is not invariably the case; e.g., Strauman & Higgins, 1987). The second assumption is that the valence of the shift in the environment will result in an automatic tendency either to approach or to avoid the environment.

Although rarely articulated, the first assumption is implicit in the operations psychologists have traditionally used in mood research: success or failure at a task (Weyent, 1978); committing or witnessing a transgression (Cialdini, Darby, & Vincent, 1973; Cunningham et al., 1980); and receiving an unexpected gift (Isen, Clark, & Schwartz, 1976) or finding a dime (Isen & Levin, 1972). Other manipulations involve nonaction procedures, such as the Velten Mood Induction Procedure (Velten, 1968) or reflective thinking (Cialdini & Kenrick, 1976; Moore, Underwood, & Rosenhan, 1973), but these too invariably retain the suggestion that the subjects imagine changes in their environment. Even further illustrating the almost invariant nature of this relation are studies in which mood has been operationalized according to changes in the physical environment itself—the weather (Cunningham, 1979).

Our second assumption is that negative shifts in the environment are associated with withdrawal of attention from the environment, and positive shifts are associated with an expansion or redirection of attention to the environment.[2] We suggest that this shift in attention may be automatic. Several lines of research offer evidence in support of this notion.

An Ethological Perspective

An organism is more likely to survive and successfully reproduce if it withdraws from an immediately harmful environment. Similarly, an organism is more likely to reproduce if it remains open to further rewards from a currently rewarding environment. Studies of nonhuman species offer a compelling portrait of organisms withdrawing attention from a harsh environment but responding to a pleasant one. As indicated above, the equation of happiness with sunshine and sadness with rain is not simply metaphorical, but empirically valid. Therefore, it is worth noting that nonhuman primates respond in a revealing manner to rain and sun. For instance, in his monograph on the mountain gorilla, G. B. Schaller (1963) noted that "gorillas seemingly enjoy the sun when it appears. . . . [T]hey roll onto their backs, spread their arms above the head or to the side, and expose their chests to the rays. . . . I have not made a single observation in which a gorilla avoided the sun" (pp. 294-295). However, during days of rain, "they sit hunched over, head held low, with the chin sometimes resting against the chest or on the folded arms. . . . At such times the gorillas are not very excitable. I once walked inadvertently through a group of huddled animals and only one raised its head" (p. 295). The weather affects the responses of the mountain gorilla not only to the physical environment, but also to the social environment. For instance, in his description of gorilla play behavior, Schaller reported, "Frequently several days went by without my observing a single instance of this behavior, especially when the clouds hung low in the saddle and the vegetation was wet" (p. 249). Surely these descriptions of mountain gorillas resonate with our own experiences under similar conditions.

The adaptability of withdrawal responses has also been noted by a number of researchers who adopt a sociobiological perspective on human social behavior (e.g., Averill, 1973; Cunningham, 1985/1986; Kenrick, Montello, & MacFarlane, 1985; Schmale, 1970). For instance, Schmale (1970) has argued that a "conservation–withdrawal response" may facilitate recuperation among physically or emotionally depleted animals. Both Schmale and Kenrick et al. (1985) applied this notion to the experience of depression, suggesting that the withdrawal associated with depression is an adaptive strategy for responding to a nonrewarding environment. In contrast, happiness typically accompanies situations that are ecologically adaptive (Cunningham, 1985/1986). Cunningham suggests that positive mood may enhance the likelihood of performing somewhat risky but potentially rewarding behaviors as a result of a more direct influence on "external perceptions." In fact, Cunningham offers the intriguing suggestion that happiness "may have evolved in part to facilitate the expression of helping behavior" (1985/1986, p. 57).

Social-Psychological Evidence

This ethological perspective suggests that positive and negative shifts in the environment elicit different orientations to that environment. Given the highly persuasive evidence that positive and negative shifts in the environment elicit different moods as well, it is possible that onsets of positive and negative mood may also be accompanied by attentional shifts. Recent social-psychological evidence has been amassed in support of the hypothesis that the onset of different mood states leads to differential shifts of attention to the self and to others. For instance, both chronic depression (e.g., Pyszczynski & Greenberg, 1987) and temporary sadness (Rogers et al., 1982; Salovey, 1988) have been shown to lead to a greater degree of self-directed attention.

Extrapolations to other-directed attention have primarily remained speculative and involve the implicit assumption that there is a hydraulic relation between attention focused upon the self and attention focused outside the self. Furthermore, there is little demonstrated evidence that happiness leads to reduced self-focus. In fact, some recent evidence (Salovey, 1988) suggests that the experience of happiness may also redirect attention to the self, at least initially. This should not be viewed as inconsistent with our reasoning, however, as it is likely that any unexpected or personally relevant event will lead to self-focus initially, but that attention will shift again shortly thereafter (e.g., Pyszczynski & Greenberg, 1987).

Our reasoning about mood-based attentional shifts is supported by studies that examine the effects of mood on social behaviors other than helping. For instance, Archer, Hormuth, and Berg (1982) found that the experience of negative events resulted in both self-reflection and reduced confidence in social behavior. Crandall (1978) reported two studies to show that personal threat increases self-concern and reduces social concerns. In two recent studies Cunningham (1988b) found that relative to subjects in a neutral mood, temporarily depressed subjects reported a reduced interest in a number of social activities. Conversely, temporarily elated subjects reported an increased interest in these activities. Researchers have also found happy subjects to be more willing to initiate conversations (Batson, Coke, Chard, Smith, & Taliaferro, 1979) and to demonstrate higher levels of self-disclosive behavior (Cunningham, 1988a). It is worth noting that in this latter study, happy subjects did not simply appear to talk more in general; the effects were specific to behaviors high in self-disclosive content.

These studies offer evidence that happiness does enhance the focus upon the environment, and decreases focus upon the self. However, one might also argue that the effect of mood is not to change the direction of attentional focus so much as to change the specificity of attentional focus. By removing focus from the self, happiness may lead to a less specified focus of attention. It is likely that the attentional focus of elated individuals is simply less "fixed" than that of sad individuals, and that the elated person may focus upon any number of self- or other-oriented stimuli in quick succession. Most of us have experienced moments of joy marked by the energy and desire to obtain many goals at once, but the inability to concentrate on any single goal before another occupies our giddy attention. We argue that after an initial stage of reorientation and reflection, elated individuals will approach the environment in this open and playful manner.

Helping

We have argued that sad individuals will withdraw attention from the environment and focus upon the self, whereas happy individuals will be more likely to focus upon the environment. How does focus of attention affect helping behavior? Several researchers have examined this issue. Gibbons and Wicklund (1982), for instance, found in two studies that self-focused attention does in fact lead to reduced prosocial behavior. However, these authors found in an additional study that, under conditions in which helping-relevant values are salient, self-focus may increase helping. Duval, Duval, and Neely (1979) also found that self-focus may increase helping when the distress of the helping target is salient. These results suggest that withdrawal of attention from the environment may reduce responsiveness to cues associated with helping situations, and that focus upon the environment may increase responsiveness to these cues. For example, McMillen, Sanders, and Solomon (1977) found that saddened subjects were generally less responsive to environmental stimuli and were less likely than control subjects to respond to an opportunity to help unless their attention was "accidentally" drawn to it, in which case they became more likely to help than controls. Mayer, Duval, Holtz, and Bowman (1985) offered corroborating evidence in a study showing that increasing focus upon the self enhanced helping *only* under conditions in which the helping opportunity was salient.

These studies indicate that there are at least two conceptually distinct effects of self-focus: (1) reduced attention to the social environment; and (2) increased attention to self-based motivational states, including self-discrepancies (cf. Carver, 1979; Higgins, 1987) and an unsatisfactory mood state. This distinction makes clear the hypothesis that individuals who have withdrawn attention from the environment are likely to help more only under certain circumstances. In particular, the environment may need to be structured in a manner to bring the need of the helping target (and its attendant potential for self-reward) to the attention of the withdrawn individual. Furthermore, the results of Gibbons and Wicklund (1982) indicate that self-focus may enhance helping only under circumstances in which the evaluative consequences of helping are salient.

It should be noted that the studies just reviewed conceptualized and operationalized attentional focus according to the theory of "objective self-awareness" (Duval & Wicklund, 1972), in which self-focused attention is caused by events that induce the individual to examine the self as an object of perception. The state of heightened self-awareness is hypothesized to induce the drive to bring one's behavior in line with an ideal or behavioral standard. In terms of helping behavior, this state is suggested to enhance adherence to altruistic values (Gibbons & Wicklund, 1982) and helping-related norms of responsibility (Duval et al., 1979; Mayer et al., 1985). Other researchers have examined the interaction of mood and focus of attention, but have employed very different conceptualizations of attentional focus. For instance, Rogers et al. (1982) discussed this construct in terms of attribution of responsibility for the negative mood—that is, whether the onset of the negative mood is internally or externally attributed. A third conceptualization of attentional focus has been advanced in the work of Rosenhan and his colleagues (Rosenhan, Salovey, & Hargis, 1981; Thompson, Cowan, & Rosenhan, 1980). These researchers operationalized focus of attention according to the recipient of a positive or negative event—that is, whether the happiness or sadness is felt for oneself or experienced empathically for another.

The reader should recognize that these three conceptualizations of attentional focus are different in their relationship to helping from what we have discussed in our theoretical framework. Perhaps the most notable distinction in its relevance to helping behavior is the distinction between mediators and moderators of the mood–helping relationship (see Baron & Kenny, 1986). Most researchers have discussed attentional focus as a *moderator* of the relationship between transient mood and helping behavior, and have generally attempted to manipulate attentional focus independently of mood manipulations (e.g., Berkowitz, 1987; Rosenhan et al., 1981; Thompson et al., 1980). In contrast, we have advanced the notion that differences in attentional focus (defined according to our environmental orientation perspective) may *mediate* the relationship between mood and helping behavior: Changes in mood may lead to attendant shifts in attentional focus. In offering this distinction, we do not mean to invalidate the moderator approach offered by others. In fact, as indicated in the preceding discussion, the results offered by others are taken to be generally consistent with our theoretical framework. As yet, there exist no data that explicitly examine the predicted role of attentional focus in mediating the mood–helping relationship. However, the results from one study that manipulated mood and attentional focus independently (Rogers et al., 1982) did indicate that attentional focus may mediate the relation between sadness and helping. Specifically, these researchers found that a manipulation of locus of responsibility had similar effects on both focus of attention and helping.

In all these studies, the operations were designed to enhance self-concern, and consequently to reduce the orientation to the environment. The results just reviewed may then be more clearly relevant to sadness-based helping than to helping resulting from positive moods. There has been scarce attention to variables that directly affect focus on the social environment. Enhanced orientation to the social environment may, however, be related to other constructs such as empathy or role taking, both of which have been persuasively documented to enhance helping behavior (for reviews, see Eisenberg & Miller, 1987; Underwood & Moore, 1982). To our knowledge, a recent study by Cunningham and his colleagues (Cunningham, Barbee, Wolff, & Kelley, 1989) provides the only attempt to enhance orientation to the environment directly and measure the subsequent effects on helping. Using a variant of the Velten Mood Induction Procedure (Velten, 1968), Cunningham and his colleagues induced both externally and internally oriented positive and negative moods in their subjects. They found that an external orientation facilitated helping on a group activity, but that an internal orientation facilitated helping on a solitary activity.

MOOD, AROUSAL, AND PHYSICAL ACTIVITY

The Arousal–Mood Association

Arousal has been an integral part of the social-psychological study of emotional experience (e.g., Schachter & Singer, 1962) and of helping behavior (e.g., Piliavin, Dovidio, Gaertner, & Clark, 1981, 1982). The perspective we adopt is somewhat different from these prominent perspectives, but it is not incompatible with them. We propose that happiness and sadness are differentially related to arousal. In particular, the experience of elation is associated with an increase in both physiological arousal and activity level, whereas the experience of sadness is associated with no such increase. In fact, sadness is associated with reduced activity.

There is growing evidence that these different mood states are associated with different levels of arousal. This evidence is clear for positive moods, with a number of researchers reporting that the experience of induced positive affect is associated with enhanced arousal (e.g., Averill, 1969; Schwartz, Fair, Salt, Mandel, & Klerman, 1976; Schwartz, Weinberger, & Singer, 1981). However, the evidence has been less clear that sadness is not associated with enhanced arousal. For instance, Averill (1969) and Schwartz et al. (1981) obtained evidence to suggest that sadness might be associated with an increase in arousal as well. These results may be misleading, however, as the experience of sadness is closely related to other, more clearly arousing negative states, such as personal distress (see Fultz, Schaller, & Cialdini, 1988; Russell, 1980). Negative mood inductions that do not specifically control for this high affective overlap may not accurately reflect the level of arousal associated specifically with sadness. Recent research attending to this concern has found that induced sadness and sorrow do not lead to increases in arousal, but are, in fact, associated with *decreases* in physiological arousal (Eisenberg, Fabes, et al., 1988; Eisenberg, Schaller, et al., 1988; Ridgeway & Waters, 1987). Recent results from other lines of research also offer evidence of the reduced arousal associated with sadness. For instance, Strauman and Higgins (1987) found that the cognitive activation of a certain type of self-discrepancy was associated both with greater sadness and with reduced physiological arousal.

The Activity–Mood Association

Not only are happiness and sadness associated with different levels of physiological arousal; they are associated with different levels of physical activity as well.

Among the primary symptoms of chronic depression are lethargy and inactivity (cf. Seligman, 1975; Seligman, Klein, & Miller, 1976). Temporarily induced moods have much the same effect on activity level, as sadness is associated with slower responses and less activity than is elation. For instance, recent tests of Higgins's (1987) self-discrepancy theory demonstrate that sadness is associated with reduced activity on both written tasks (Higgins, Bond, Klein, & Strauman, 1986) and verbal tasks (Strauman & Higgins, 1987). Indeed, it is notable that a number of researchers interested in sadness and elation have employed as a mood manipulation check the speed at which subjects perform a task (e.g., Mayer et al., 1985).

The evidence pertaining to arousal and activity differences associated with happiness and sadness is consistent with other aspects of our framework. For instance, we have suggested that when people are elated, their attentional orientation may be less focused than when they are sad. This unhinged focus of attention would be consistent with an increase in physiological arousal and heightened physical activity. Also consistent with an increase in arousal is the evidence that happiness leads to more rapid responses (Isen & Means, 1983) and, as we discuss shortly, to more heuristic responding (Worth & Mackie, 1987). Thus, elated individuals may well show enhanced arousal relative to nonelated individuals.

Helping

The relationship between arousal and helping has not been examined extensively, except in regard to the relationship between personal distress and helping. Within this domain, it has been found that the drive to reduce arousal may predict helping in bystander intervention situations (e.g., Gaertner & Dovidio, 1977; Sterling & Gaertner, 1984). However, it is unlikely that the aversive arousal examined by these authors is comparable to the arousal associated with positive affect. This distinction suggests that arousal reduction motives bear little relevance to our discussion of happiness-based helping.

In fact, this distinction underscores the necessity of differentiating between different mood states on dimensions other than arousal. This is crucial not only for a consideration of happiness, but for sadness as well. As noted above, sadness is an unusual negative mood, in that it is not associated with an increase in arousal. Much other research has examined the prosocial consequences of other negative states that do have an arousal component. For instance, a number of studies have shown that helping behavior was increased following an unintentional transgression, a result often interpreted as driven by guilt (e.g., Carlsmith & Gross, 1969; Darlington & Macker, 1966; Freedman, Wallington, & Bless, 1967; Konecni, 1972; D. T. Regan, Williams, & Sparling, 1972; J. W. Regan, 1971; Wallace & Sadalla, 1966). Although others have offered alternative interpretations of these results (e.g., Brock, 1969; Cialdini et al., 1973; McMillen, 1971), it would seem reasonable to allow that the experience of guilt will increase helping behavior. Other studies have found that experiences of embarrassment (Apsler, 1975) and cognitive dissonance (Kidd & Berkowitz, 1976) also may enhance helping behavior. Other arousal-based negative states, however, may have very different effects on helping. For example, De Nicholas (1987) tested Cialdini et al.'s (1973) prediction that the negative emotional state of anger would lead to diminished helping, because refusal to help would serve as an aggression-like response that would reduce the anger-based negative arousal. In a pair of studies, she found (1) that anger increased subjects' tendencies to refuse to help, and (2) that refusing to help significantly reduced angered subjects' negative arousal (as measured by systolic blood pressure).

Results such as these highlight the importance of recognizing that, when considered alone, arousal is not a good predictor of helping behavior. Although the positive experience of happiness, as well as such negative states as guilt, embarrassment, dissonance, and anger, may be rooted in arousal, it is likely that the attentional and cognitive effects of these arousal-based states differ in important ways. Regardless of the accompanying mood, arousal may itself have effects on memory (Clark, Milberg, & Erber, 1988), attentional focus (Easterbrook, 1959), and the use of cognitive short cuts in the judgment process (Kim & Baron, 1988), as well as on behavior (Hull, 1943, 1952; Spence, 1960). As a result, a number of additional contextual and psychological factors are likely to interact with arousal in determining one's behavioral reaction to a helping situation. Furthermore, general affective state is not a good predictor of helping when examined apart from other factors. Although both sadness and anger are classified as negative states, they differ in their psychological effects and in their consequent effects upon helping. That is, sadness is likely to increase helping because helping reduces the negative state (as we discuss more fully later in this chapter), whereas anger is likely to increase *refusal* to help for precisely the same reason—it reduces the relevant negative state.

These considerations further underscore our thesis that for a full understanding of why helping behavior is facilitated by both happiness and sadness—states that differ in affective valence and in arousal—it is necessary to consider a multiplicity of psychological and motivational concomitants of these moods. The difference in arousal level represents only one of several important distinctions that provide the clues to understanding and motivational processes by which happiness and sadness affect helping behavior.

MOOD, MINDLESSNESS, AND THE DECISION PROCESS

The differential effects of mood may also be manifested in the decision process. We propose that temporarily elated and temporary saddened individuals arrive at their decision to help through processes that are dramatically different. The helping decision arrived at in a state of temporary sadness is likely to be carefully considered, with particular attention to the personal consequences of the helping act. In contrast, the helping decision made while one is elated is likely to be less carefully considered, and may even be characterized as impulsive or "mindless" (Langer, Blank, & Chanowitz, 1978).

The Link between Mood and Level of Scrutiny

A number of researchers have examined the influence of mood states on the processes by which judgments and decisions are made (e.g., Bless, Bohner, Schwarz, & Strack, 1988; Isen et al., 1982; Mackie & Worth, 1989; Worth & Mackie, 1987). The resulting evidence strongly indicates that positive and negative affective states lead to different levels of scrutiny of relevant information. In Chapter 15 of this volume, Schwarz (see also Schwarz, 1988; Schwarz & Clore, 1988) argues that in making decisions or judgments, people may employ a "How do I feel about it?" heuristic. Positive affective states offer the indication that the world is a positive place, and therefore that there is little need to engage in effortful cognitive processing or further scrutiny. In contrast, and consistent with our earlier reasoning, negative affective states indicate some threat or possible negative outcome. As a consequence, negative mood will elicit greater cognitive appraisal, a higher level of scrutiny of the situation, and considerable attention to relevant information

This perspective on affect-induced processing has received compelling empirical support. Isen and her colleagues have demonstrated over a number of studies that the onset of positive mood results in more rapid and less effortful decision strategies. Relative to those in a neutral mood, happy individuals use broader and more inclusive categories in classification tasks (Isen & Daubman, 1984), and are more likely to employ judgmental heuristics or simple, intuitive solutions to problems (Isen et al., 1982). Also indicating differential scrutiny is evidence that happy subjects reach decisions more quickly than do neutral subjects (Isen & Means, 1983).

Several recent studies in the persuasion literature offer a similar interpretation of the processing differences introduced by mood states. Bless et al. (1988) showed that subjects in negative moods were more likely to be persuaded by strong than weak arguments, but that subjects in positive moods were equally persuaded by strong and weak arguments. Worth and Mackie (1987) found that relative to controls, happy subjects were less influenced by the quality of the persuasion message and were more susceptible to the presence of a simple persuasion cue. Additional measures from these investigations have indicated that happy subjects demonstrate less cognitive elaboration of the persuasion messages. In fact, Bless et al. (1988) found that happy subjects paid attention to the quality of the arguments only when explicitly instructed to do so. Recent research by Mackie and Worth (1989) examined the processes underlying the tendency for elated subjects to respond less analytically and more heuristically to persuasive appeals; their study specifically tested the question of whether the effect is due to reduced cognitive capacity or to a motivated tendency to maintain a positive mood. They obtained evidence consistent with the hypothesis that heuristic responding results from arousal-based reductions in cognitive processing capacity. More importantly, as we discuss shortly, their data offer no evidence for the alternative based upon the motivation to maintain positive mood.

Helping

Research within the mood–helping literature is consistent with the results from the persuasion studies reviewed above in suggesting that saddened subjects take a more considered approach to helping opportunities, whereas elated subjects take a less considered approach. Several experiments (e.g., Manucia, Baumann, & Cialdini, 1984; Switzer, 1989; Weyent, 1978) obtained results indicating that helping responses under happy moods are relatively unaffected by changes in the perceived costs and benefits of helping, whereas changes in these factors do influence helping under sad moods. This reasoning is consistent with the general finding that happiness enhances helping over a broader range of situations that does sadness. These studies suggest that sad individuals will be more likely to consider the features of the helping situation carefully, to weigh the potential costs and benefits, and only then to decide whether to offer help. Happy individuals may respond in a more impulsive manner; their decision may be swayed only by a few salient cues, such as their present elation.

MOOD AND MOTIVATION

In the preceding pages, we have reviewed evidence to suggest that the experience of sadness will result in the following: (1) enhanced access to negative thoughts and nonoptimistic (if not actually pessimistic) cognitions about the self and the environment; (2) an avoidance of the external environment and heightened attentional focus on the self; (3) reduced levels of arousal and activity; and (4) careful consideration of and scrutiny of external stimuli prior to response decisions. We have also reviewed evidence to suggest that the experience of happiness will result in contrasting reactions along the same dimensions: (1) enhanced access to positive thoughts and optimistic perceptions about the self and the environment; (2) an approach to the external environment and a more diffuse, wide-ranging focus of attention; (3) enhanced levels of arousal and activity; and (4) a rather mindless and cavalier orientation to the decisions one encounters in the environment. These processes have been documented outside the helping literature, and have generally received support within the helping literature as well.

On the basis of this evidence, we may sketch a broader picture in which the experience of a negative or positive mood normally flows from the receipt of punishments or rewards from the environment. All else being equal, the ratio and recency of the rewards and punishments should predict the likelihood of future such events in the immediate setting. Consequently, sadness should result in a reluctance to interact further with the environment in all but clearly rewarding ways, whereas elation should result in a less restrictive, more active, more wide-ranging approach to the environment. Therefore, sadness should result in a behavioral orientation that is carefully considered and goal-specific, whereas elation should result in a behavioral orientation that, although perhaps goal-oriented, is more encompassing and more impulsive.

What conclusions, then, may we draw about motivation? First, we are compelled to assert that the motives underlying sadness-based helping and happiness-based helping are not the same. Helping offered by sad individuals is motivated out of concern for managing their own mood; helping offered by happy individuals is not. Although this distinction is intuitively appealing and broadly consistent with the mood research we have just reviewed, other researchers in mood and helping have proposed different motivational frameworks. Most notably, several researchers (e.g., Clark & Isen, 1982) have offered the possibility that both sadness and happiness spur helping as an instrumental means of meeting mood-based concerns: Sad individuals are concerned with repairing their negative moods, and happy individuals are concerned with maintaining their positive moods. Others have argued that no instrumental motive is necessary to explain the effect of sadness on helping (Carlson & Miller, 1987). In light of these other perspectives, our motivational perspective might be considered somewhat controversial. Therefore, we now turn to an examination of motivational theory and empirical evidence bearing on these issues.

Sadness and the Mood Management Hypothesis

We suggest that the experience of sadness induces a focused motivational drive to restore one's mood to the previous state of equilibrium. The drive to regulate one's mood may be a rather basic human motive in maintaining general welfare. Within the context of human motivation, one set of primary motives includes those drives toward homeostatic regulation evoked by some change of psysiological or psychological condition. Thus, if you are hungry, you eat; if you are thirsty, you drink. Although mood regulation certainly cannot be viewed as quite so primary as regulation of physiological needs, the desire to maintain a reasonably positive mood state nonetheless would seem to fall within the realm of homeostatic regulation. Therefore, just as hunger instigates the drive to eat, we propose that when one experiences a negative mood, it may dominate attention until the mood deficit is eliminated and a normal mood state is restored. The motivational energy derived from sadness is directed toward achieving affective homeostasis.

For almost two decades, research from our own and others' laboratories has demonstrated a tendency for saddened individuals to help as a function of the reward value of helping. Weiss and his colleagues (Weiss, Boyer, Lombardo, & Stitch, 1973; Weiss, Buchanan, Alstatt, & Lombardo, 1971) have provided compelling evidence of the self-reinforcing function of helping. This function may be of particular interest to temporarily saddened individuals, who, we hypothesize, have a greater need for self-gratification so as to restore affective homeostasis. Baumann, Cialdini, and Kenrick (1981) provided evidence that sad subjects were less likely to engage in self-gratification as a means of mood management if they had recently helped another; this evidence suggests that helping and self-gratifying behaviors are perceived as equivalent means of alleviating sadness. In addition, a number of studies have demonstrated that the effects of sadness on helping are moderated by the availability of other avenues toward mood repair. Several studies have shown that if a rewarding event occurs between the onset of the negative mood and the helping opportunity, subjects are no more likely to offer help than subjects in a neutral mood (Cialdini et al., 1973; Cunningham et al., 1980). In another study, results indicated that saddened subjects are likely to help more than neutral-mood subjects only if they believe that the act of helping will actually alter their moods (Manucia et al., 1984). Finally, recent evidence has been obtained that sad subjects will not show enhanced helping if they anticipate a low-cost mood-elevating experience to occur immediately following the helping opportunity (Batson et al., 1989; Switzer, 1989).

The studies just reviewed have obtained support for a sadness-induced mood management motive through such "traditional" mood induction methods as transgression manipulations and reminiscence procedures. It is interesting to note that we have obtained equivalent results in several recent studies in which sadness was induced through procedures intended to directly manipulate empathic concern for the person in need (Cialdini et al., 1987; Schaller & Cialdini, 1988). These results offer a further indication of the generality of the sadness-based mood management motive.[3] Together with the results reviewed in the preceding paragraph, these studies offer strong support for the hypothesis that saddened individuals are concerned with their moods and use helping in an instrumental manner to reachieve affective homeostasis.

Happiness and the Mood Management Hypothesis

In contrast to sadness, the experience of happiness is not based upon an affective deficit. Therefore, there is no corresponding drive to focus attention and motivational energy upon the affective state. If one has satisfied one's hunger, one no longer searches for food to eat. Similarly, if one is no longer sad, one no longer searches for ways of managing or maintaining one's mood.

Supporting this view, we note that evidence is scarce that happy subjects help as a means to maintain positive moods. Several studies have offered experimental tests of the mood maintenance hypothesis. Baumann et al. (1981) tested whether helping and self-gratification were equivalent responses among happy subjects. Results indicated that, in contrast to the results found among sad subjects, happy subjects did not treat the two as equivalent. The tendency of elated subjects to gratify themselves was not moderated by the intervention of a prior helping act. To test the instrumental hypothesis directly, three studies (to our knowledge) have manipulated the utility of helping as a means of maintaining a positive mood. In the study by Manucia et al. (1984) discussed earlier, results showed that unlike sad subjects, elated subjects helped at equally high levels, regardless of the perceived likelihood that helping could influence the positive mood. In contrast, a recent study (Yinon & Landau, 1987) found that elated subjects offered less help if they expected an unrelated positive experience to occur immediately after the helping opportunity than if no such experience was expected. Although these data do not fit well with the implications of the findings of Manucia et al. (1984), a potential confound in the expectancy manipulation renders the mood maintenance interpretation ambiguous. Specifically, in this experiment, subjects who did not expect an upcoming positive experience presumed that the experiment was over, whereas those who did expect the positive experience had no such presumption. It is plausible that those who felt that their experimental task was done would be more likely to leave their seats to come to aid the experimenter (the helping opportunity) than those who felt bound by experimental constraints. This alternative explanation seems all the more plausible in light of recent results from the Arizona State laboratory (Switzer, 1989) indicating that elated individuals help at equally high levels whether they expect an unrelated positive experience to occur immediately thereafter or a week hence; this suggests that the helping act is not used tactically to maintain affective positivity.

In less direct tests of the mood maintenance hypothesis, several other studies have examined the notion that temporarily elated subjects will be more likely to help on pleasant tasks than on unpleasant tasks. Three studies have obtained results showing that subjects made to feel happy helped more on a pleasant than an unpleasant task (Forest et al., 1979; Isen & Simmonds, 1978; Shaffer & Graziano, 1983). On the surface, these results seem to suggest that the mood-related reward value of the helping opportunity is important in elated subjects' decisions to help. However, this may not be the case. It should be noted that in each of these three studies, the helping task involved the reading of Velten Mood Induction Procedure statements (either pleasant or unpleasant ones), and the dependent variable was the number of statements read. In contrast to the mood maintenance interpretation, an equally plausible explanation for these results is that subjects reading the negative mood induction statements (the unpleasant task) found their earlier positive mood quickly reduced to neutral levels, and that this made them less likely to help further by reading additional statements. In fact, research has shown that reading mood-inconsistent Velten statements is an effective way in which to remove the earlier induction (Frost & Green, 1982). Why, then, did happy subjects in the unpleasant task condition help less? Because, as a result of reading negative statements, they were no longer happy.

Supporting this reasoning is further evidence from the Shaffer and Graziano (1983) study that the pleasantness of the task did not moderate happy subjects' initial decisions to help or not. Whether they were to help on an unpleasant task or a pleasant task, elated subjects volunteered at equally high rates; this indicates that before the task itself reduced their moods, the happy subjects did not decide to help on the basis of the hedonic features of the task. Additional studies have cast further doubt on the mood maintenance explanation. O'Malley and Andrews (1983) found that happy subjects showed increased helping on even a particularly unpleasant task, such as donating blood. Weyent (1978) found that elated subjects helped at equally high levels, regardless of whether the personal costs of helping were high or low. Finally, a recent study by Cunningham et al. (1990) found that, regardless of whether the helping task was presented as boring or engaging, happy subjects helped at higher levels than did those in neutral moods.

Finally, a recent study by Mayer and Gaschke (1988) provides additional data indicating that sadness and happiness engender different motives. In their research on the metaexperience of mood, these researchers provide correlational evidence for the relations between affective dimensions and metaexperiences. Most relevant to our discussion is the result that pleasant mood is strongly correlated with typicality and stability. In short, subjects in a pleasant mood report that they commonly experience this mood and expect that it will persist indefinitely. These metaexperience results suggest that concern over maintaining one's happy mood may be remote in the elated individual's mind. On the basis of these results and those of the other studies reviewed above, our view is compatible with that of Shaffer (1985/1986), who concludes that "altruism inspired by negative moods might well be interpreted as an instrumental strategy for brightening one's spirits, whereas benevolence associated with positive moods seems much less self-serving or hedonic in character" (p. 208).

Happiness and the "Elan to Maximize"

In light of the preceding discussion, we conclude that happiness does not enhance helping as a result of a mood management motive. But if happy individuals are not practicing affective self-regulation, why do they help more than nonelated individuals? Two distinct alternative hypotheses may be advanced that are largely consistent with the literature we have reviewed.

First, we may propose that positive mood leads to enhanced helping via the more positive outlook and enhanced activity that appear to spring automatically from the experience of happiness. Because the arousal level of happy people inclines them to interact more with the environment, and because they see themselves and that environment more favorably—for instance, they feel more competent (Alloy et al., 1981) and optimistic (Masters & Furman, 1976), and they have access to more positive thoughts about the people (Forgas & Bower, 1987), things (Isen et al., 1978), and opportunities (Clark & Waddell, 1983), they encounter—it makes sense that elated individuals are more willing to give up resources to others. Although this hypothesis is consistent with the bulk of the helping research we have reviewed (see Cialdini et al., 1982, for further elaboration of how such natural cognitive and perceptual concomitants of happiness can account for enhanced benevolence), we wish to focus our discussion upon a second alternative that has not yet been addressed explicitly by helping theorists.

The second alternative is rooted in a hierarchy of motives that is enunciated explicitly by some motivation theorists (e.g., Buck, 1985; Maslow, 1954) and discussed implicitly by most (see Mook, 1987). It follows, too, from the observations of Weiner (1986) that "the greater part of human behavior cannot be subsumed within the concept of homeostasis" (p. 282). We argue that the effects of positive mood may be subsumed within this greater part of human behavior. Specifically, we argue that happiness is associated with a motivation toward disequilibrium—toward the possible attainment of additional personal rewards that transcend the basic concern over one's mood. That is, with the basic goals satisfied (including the goal of eliminating a negative mood), one may pursue additional, less basic goals. Let us return to the analogy of hunger—or, in this case, the converse of hunger. If one has not only satisfied one's hunger and thirst, but has indeed enjoyed the gustatory delight of a gourmet dinner, the motivation that results is very different from that of the unsatisfied state. There is no basic physiological deficit to attend to; instead, with the satisfaction of basic needs, an organism may pursue higher needs.[4] Similarly, the experience of elation offers not a mood deficit, but a surfeit. As a result, the motivational energy is not directed at reachieving homeostasis. Instead, this surfeit brings with it the luxury of basic need fulfillment, and the motivation to disrupt homeostasis in other areas of importance to the self. In his theory of invested self-expression, McCall (1963) states:

> Behind and sustaining all or virtually all particular human motives there is an *elan to maximize*; not merely to maintain life—though that of course is basic to the enterprise of maximization—but to live it as fully as possible, to develop one's capacities, extend and deepen experience, exercise one's powers in the highest; in a word to achieve for one's self *the greatest possible self-enrichment psychologically speaking.* (p. 302; emphasis in original)

We concur, and assert that the experience of happiness brings with it the "elan to maximize."

This self-enrichment is expected to be manifested in complex social motives. What might these motives be? Motivation theorists have identified a number of social motives that may be served by helping behavior, including motives of attachment and affiliation (e.g., Bowlby, 1969; Maslow, 1954), achievement (e.g., McClelland, 1961, 1964; Weiner, 1974), competence (White, 1959), and esteem (Maslow, 1954). Our intention is not to describe these motives in detail, nor to specify any one in particular that may be specifically activated by temporary elation. Instead, we wish simply to identify these as higher-order, nonhomeostatic goals that may be satisfied by helping.

This latter notion is intuitively compelling and consistent with general theories of human motivation; furthermore, it is consistent with the helping literature we have reviewed. And yet we are aware of no direct tests of this hypothesis. Nonetheless, there are certain studies outside the literature on helping behavior that are perhaps more consistent with this alternative than with the purely concomitant alternative. For instance, recall that Cunningham (1988a) found that elation led to an increase in self-disclosing communications, but that it was not associated with an increase in less self-disclosing communications. This may be an indication that happiness activates an affiliative or attachment motive.

There are also previous studies within the helping literature that are consistent with this reasoning. For example, Carlsmith et al. (1974) found that happy children were more likely to accede to the helping request of an adult who was likeable rather than one who was punitive. Aderman (1972) found that happy adults offered more help on a task when it was presented as a favor rather than as a requirement. More persuasive evidence was obtained by Isen and Levin (1972), who found that happy subjects helped more than neutral-mood subjects only when the helping task was presented as a creativity task, but not when it involved distracting others from this task. All these studies might indicate a sensitivity to needs for affiliation, esteem, competence, or achievement—needs that may be satisfied through prosocial behavior. Finally, Cunningham et al. (1980) found that happiness enhanced helping responses only when the helping task was presented in a manner that highlighted the positive achievement of helping ("Help keep the children smiling") rather than obligation ("You owe it to the children"). We should note that each of these studies has been interpreted according to the "separate-processes" model, which suggests that elated individuals emphasize social concerns and saddened individuals emphasize personal concerns (Cunningham et al., 1990). We do not disagree with this interpretation; indeed, it is entirely consistent with the motivational perspective we have outlined.

We offer these results as consistent with the hypothesis that temporary elation induces a motivation to disrupt homeostasis—the elan to maximize. However, the results cannot definitively rule out the first (less purposive, more automatic) alternative. It would seem that testing these alternatives constitutes the next important conceptual hurdle to clear in understanding the relationship between mood and helping.

IMPLICATIONS FOR FUTURE RESEARCH

Implicit Hypotheses

In reviewing past research on sadness, happiness, and helping behavior, our intent has been to offer an integration consistent with the wealth of results describing the effects of mood on attention, cognition, and motivation. A by-product of this integration is the realization that, despite the vast empirical literature in this area, many of the hypotheses implicit in our framework have yet to be subjected to direct disconfirmation.

For instance, as yet there is no direct evidence supporting the notion that increased access to positive cognitions mediates the relationship between happiness and helping. Methodologies are needed that allow measurement of the cognitive concomitants of mood as well as prosocial behavior. Within such designs, one could also test the implicit hypothesis that mood-consistent cognitions should play a more prominent role in the relationship between happiness and helping than they should in the relationship between sadness and helping. Furthermore, there is little research that has directly examined the effect of mood on attentional focus, and the few studies that have examined this relationship (Rogers et al., 1982; Salovey, 1988) employed very different measures of attentional focus. It is necessary not only to determine the relative differences in self-versus non-self-focus, but also the stability or "fixity" of attentional focus under sad versus happy moods. Future research should also explore the role of attentional focus as an unconstrained mediator of the mood–helping relationship.

Moreover, research must examine more explicitly the hypothesis that happiness leads to poorly considered, heuristic-based decisions to help, whereas sadness leads to highly scrutinized and carefully considered decisions to help. The methodologies employed in recent research on affect and persuasion (Bless et al., 1988; Mackie & Worth, 1989; Worth & Mackie, 1987) might well be adapted to helping situations. Finally, the motivational hypotheses we have outlined should be subjected to direct empirical tests. In particular, there have been no studies directly testing the hypothesis that positive mood induces a motivation to seek greater social rewards. This hypothesis might be tested as an important alternative to the mood maintenance hypothesis offered by others (e.g., Carlson et al., 1988; Isen & Simmonds, 1978). Researchers might take particular care in the manipulation of helping measures that might discriminate between these two alternatives.

Broader Implications

In addition to the specific hypotheses extracted from our model, the framework we have advanced also offers some broader implications for the study of mood and social behavior. One implication bears on a current debate over the existence of a truly altruistic motive to help others (cf. Batson, 1987). Although in a different theoretical context we have argued against the possibility of an altruistic motive (Cialdini et al., 1987; Schaller & Cialdini, 1988), our present perspective suggests that happiness may elicit helping without consideration of the personal costs and benefits of this act. Does this suggest that helping elicited by elation is altruistic? We do not think so. Although the available evidence strongly indicates that elated individuals help without carefully considering the costs or benefits to the self, the evidence does not indicate that these individuals help purely out of concern for others. Furthermore, we have suggested that elation-based helping may satisfy unspecified higher-order social goals. Nonetheless, it is worth considering the possibility that happiness may elicit helping that, by nature of its impulsiveness, may come closer to true altruism than any other human behavior.

An additional consequence of writing the present review is that it has allowed us to come to see the plausibility of a broader view of the nature of mood. It seems possible that moods may be conceived of as affective indices of the state of the environment, serving to cue internal responses that are congenial with the contemporary aspects of the external world. It may be that certain rewarding or nonrewarding environments produce moods (e.g., happiness or sadness) that have within them (or trigger) arousal levels that are adaptive for those environments. For example, the heightened arousal associated with elation may lead naturally to the energization of general activity and to the cognitive-capacity-based inhibition of controlled information processing and analytical decision making. This view of mood as an internal representation of the external experience that automatically directs and shapes responding to that environment is speculative. However, it does resonate with a theory of emotion and motivation that has recently been articulated by Buck (1985), in which emotion is viewed as a readout mechanism associated with self-regulatory and environmentally adaptive functioning. Clearly, this conceptualization of mood warrants future study.

SUMMARY AND CONCLUSIONS

In order to understand the differential effects of happy and sad mood states on helping, we have felt it necessary to examine how the states differ more generally in their character and consequences. In our investigation of relevant literatures, we have identified five dimensions that, taken together, allow an improved understanding of when and why elated and saddened individuals will help. Specifically, it appears that such individuals are likely to differ in the following ways:

1. *Access to affect-related memories and thoughts*, with positive recollections, attributions, and cognitions more accessible to elated than to saddened persons.
2. *Attention/orientation to the environment*, with elated individuals showing a greater tendency to attend to and make contact with external stimuli in a broad, encompassing fashion, and saddened individuals showing a greater tendency to attend to the self and to make contact with the environment only in a most selective manner.
3. *Level of arousal and physical activity*, with happy persons demonstrating greater than normal levels of physiological arousal and behavioral activity, and saddened persons demonstrating reduced arousal and activity.
4. *Process of decision making*, with elation leading to a less controlled, more heuristic decisional style, and sadness leading to a more controlled, highly considered approach.
5. *General motivational drive*, with elated individuals striving for a counterhomeostatic enhancement of higher-order goals (e.g., affiliation, attachment, competence, achievement) and saddened individuals striving primarily for the homeostatic restoration of affective equilibrium.

Our general orientation to the relationship between happy–sad mood and behavior, especially helping, is a functional/adaptive one. We view happy versus sad moods as the characteristic affective states of individuals who have recently experienced a rewarding versus a punishing environment. Furthermore, we view each of the five identified differences between elated and saddened persons as an adaptive reaction to those environmental circumstances. The cognitive, attentional, and motivational tendencies of an elated individual are likely to be functional in an environment that has given evidence of being rich and yielding. The cognitive, attentional, and motivational tendencies of a saddened individual are likely to be adaptive in an environment that has recently given evidence that it is potentially dangerous. Thus, a saddened person would be well advised to be receptive to opportunities for reward (and consequent mood shifts), but not to engage actively in diffuse attempts to generate them. The elated person may be best served by impulsive exploration of the environment and its apparently rich opportunities for higher rewards. These differing response patterns of elated and saddened persons account very well for the behaviors of such persons in the helping research we have reviewed.

This review has led us to conclude that the motives arising from sadness and happiness are different. The motivational perspective we have adopted is consistent not only with the bulk of evidence within the helping literature, but also with the findings in other literatures and with a larger motivational framework. Some readers may find it inelegant that the helping arising from sadness and happiness cannot be explained with a single motivational construct. However, we are conceptually bound by the inelegant asymmetry of the empirical results. The more complex perspective we have presented may lack the explanatory simplicity that psychologists so often seek. We believe that what it lacks in utter simplicity, however, it makes up for in self-consistency. Furthermore, we believe that this perspective may further enrich a conceptual soil that promises to yield another two decades of provocative research on mood and helping.

Acknowledgment

We are grateful to Michael Cunningham for his helpful comments on an earlier draft of this chapter.

Notes

1. It may be worth mentioning a special case of positive affect that has received some attention, and to which our framework may not apply. Rosenhan, Salovey, and Hargis (1981) found that joy experienced for the self enhanced helping, but when joy resulted from another's good fortune, subjects offered less help than controls. The happiness we discuss here is that which is experienced for the self—happiness resulting from a positive change in the personal environment. The joy derived from the success of another is likely to be qualitatively different, and is probably compounded by the experience of social comparison jealousy (Salovey & Rodin, 1984).

2. We recognize that not all negative events will lead to behavioral withdrawal. For instance, certain persons may be motivated by an initial failure at a task to approach the same or another task. In such cases, it is likely that the person perceives the environment as potentially rewarding, and therefore these occurrences are consistent with our present analysis. Conversely, success at a task—and the resulting positive affect—may lead to withdrawal from the task. However, this by no means indicates withdrawal from the environment as a whole. In fact, success at one task may typically lead to engagement in an unrelated activity, such as helping.

3. Although we have explicitly resisted the temptation to extend our framework to account for arousal-based negative affective states, we have not been so conservative in our interpretation of the prosocial consequences of sympathy. This is controversial, as Batson and his colleagues (see Batson,

1987, for a review) have argued that sympathy (or "empathy," as it has often been labeled in the recent helping literature) may lead to an altruistic rather than a self-serving motivation to help. Recent data from our own laboratories have indicated that the results of Batson and his colleagues may be interpreted according to the motive of egoistic mood management that apparently underlies sadness-based helping (Cialdini et al., 1987; Fultz & Cialdini, 1986; Schaller & Cialdini, 1988). Although our results have compelled us to extend our framework to sympathy-based helping, other researchers have obtained differing results (Batson et al., 1989; Schroeder, Dovidio, Sibicky, Matthews, & Allen, 1988), and as yet there is no definitive resolution concerning the motivation of sympathetic helping.

4. This may also occur at a sociological level. Note the difference between a starving culture and an affluent culture: Where there is a deficit of food, one finds primarily activities that revolve around agriculture and production; in a nation where everything exists at a surplus, one finds such nonessential activities as video games, dog shows, and social psychology.

References

Aderman, D. (1972). Elation, depression and helping behavior. *Journal of Personality and Social Psychology, 24,* 91-101.

Alloy, L. B., & Abramson, L. Y. (1979). Judgment of contingency in depressed and nondepressed students: Sadder but wiser? *Journal of Experimental Psychology: General, 108,* 441-485.

Alloy, L. B., Abramson, L. Y., & Viscusi, D. (1981). Induced mood and the illusion of control. *Journal of Personality and Social Psychology, 41,* 1129-1140.

Apsler, R. (1975). Effects of embarrassment on behavior toward others. *Journal of Personality and Social Psychology, 32,* 145-153.

Archer, R. L., Hormuth, S. E., & Berg, J. H. (1982). Avoidance of self-disclosure: An experiment under conditions of self-awareness. *Personality and Social Psychology Bulletin, 8,* 122-128.

Averill, J. R. (1969). Autonomic response patterns during sadness and mirth. *Psychophysiology, 5,* 399-414.

Averill, J. R. (1973). Personal control over aversive stimuli and its relationship to stress. *Psychological Bulletin, 80,* 286-303.

Baron, R. M., & Kenny, D. A. (1986). The moderator-mediator variable distinction in social psychological research: Conceptual, strategic, and statistical considerations. *Journal of Personality and Social Psychology, 51,* 1173-1182.

Batson, C. D. (1987). Prosocial motivation: Is it ever truly altruistic? In L. Berkowitz (Ed.), *Advances in experimental social psychology* (Vol. 20, pp. 65-122). New York: Academic Press.

Batson, C. D., Batson, J. G., Griffitt, C. A., Barrientos, S., Brandt, J. R., Sprengelmeyer, P., & Bayly, M. J. (1989). Negative-state relief and the empathy-altruism hypothesis. *Journal of Personality and Social Psychology, 56,* 922-933.

Batson, C. D., Coke, J. S., Chard, F., Smith, D., & Taliaferro, A. (1979). Generality of the "glow of goodwill": Effects of mood on helping and information acquisition. *Social Psychology Quarterly, 42,* 176-179.

Baumann, D. J., Cialdini, R. B., & Kenrick, D. T. (1981). Altruism as hedonism: Helping and self-gratification as equivalent responses. *Journal of Personality and Social Psychology, 40,* 1039-1046.

Berkowitz, L. (1987). Mood, self-awareness, and willingness to help. *Journal of Personality and Social Psychology, 52,* 721-729.

Blaney, P. H. (1986). Affect and memory: A review. *Psychological Bulletin, 99,* 229-246.

Bless, H., Bohner, G., Schwarz, N., & Strack, F. (1988). *Happy and mindless? Moods and the processing of persuasive communications.* Unpublished manuscript, Zentrum für Umfragen, Methoden und Analysen, Mannheim, Federal Republic of Germany.

Bower, G. H. (1981). Mood and memory. *American Psychologist, 36,* 129-148.

Bower, G. H., & Cohen, P. R. (1982). Emotional influences in memory and thinking: Data and theory. In M. S. Clark & S. T. Fiske (Eds.), *Affect and cognition: The 17th Annual Carnegie Symposium on Cognition* (pp. 291-331). Hillsdale, NJ: Erlbaum.

Bowlby, J. (1969). *Attachment and loss: Vol. 1. Attachment.* New York: Basic Books.

Brock, T. C. (1969). On interpreting the effects of transgression upon compliance. *Psychological Bulletin, 72,* 138-145.

Buck, R. (1985). Prime theory: An integrated view of motivation and emotion. *Psychological Review, 92,* 389-413.

Carlsmith, J. M., & Gross, A. (1969). Some effects of guilt on compliance. *Journal of Personality and Social Psychology, 11,* 240-244.

Carlsmith, J. M., Lepper, M. R., & Landauer, T. (1974). Children's obedience to adult requests: Interactive effects of anxiety arousal and apparent punitiveness of the adult. *Journal of Personality and Social Psychology, 30,* 823-828.

Carlson, M., Charlin, V., & Miller, N. (1988). Positive mood and helping behavior: A test of six hypotheses. *Journal of Personality and Social Psychology, 55,* 211-229.

Carlson, M., & Miller, N. (1987). Explanation of the relationship between negative mood and helping. *Psychological Bulletin, 102,* 91-108.

Carver, C. S. (1979). A cybernetic model of self-attention processes. *Journal of Personality and Social Psychology, 37,* 1251-1281.

Cialdini, R. B., Baumann, D. J., & Kenrick, D. T. (1981). Insights from sadness: A three step model of the development of altruism as hedonism. *Developmental Review, 1,* 207-223.

Cialdini, R. B., Darby, B., & Vincent, J. (1973). Transgression and altruism: A case for hedonism. *Journal of Experimental Social Psychology, 9,* 502-516.

Cialdini, R. B., & Kenrick, D. T. (1976). Altruism as hedonism: A social developmental perspective on the relationship of negative mood state and helping. *Journal of Personality and Social Psychology, 34,* 907-914.

Cialdini, R. B., Kenrick, D. T., & Baumann, D. J. (1982). Effects of mood on prosocial behavior in children and adults. In N. Eisenberg (Ed.), *The development of prosocial behavior* (pp. 339-359). New York: Academic Press.

Cialdini, R. B., Schaller, M., Houlihan, D., Arps, K., Fultz, J., & Beaman, A. L. (1987). Empathy-based helping: Is it selflessly or selfishly motivated. *Journal of Personality and Social Psychology, 52,* 749-758.

Clark, M. S., & Isen, A. M. (1982). Toward understanding the relationship between feeling states and social behavior. In A. H. Hastorf & A. M. Isen (Eds.), *Cognitive social psychology* (pp. 73-108). New York: Elsevier.

Clark, M. S., Milberg, S., & Erber, R. (1988). Arousal-state-dependent memory: Evidence and implications for understanding social judgments and social behavior. In K. Fiedler & J. P. Forgas (Eds.), *Affect, cognition, and social behavior* (pp. 63-83). Toronto: Hogrefe International.

Clark, M. S., & Waddell, B. A. (1983). Effects of moods on thoughts about helping, attraction and information acquisition. *Social Psychology Quarterly, 46,* 31-35.

Crandall, J. E. (1978). Effects of threat and failure on concern for others. *Journal of Research in Personality, 12,* 35-360.

Cunningham, M. R. (1979). Weather, mood, and helping behavior: Quasi-experiments with the sunshine Samaritan. *Journal of Personality and Social Psychology, 37,* 1947-1956.

Cunningham, M. R. (1985/1986). Levites and brother's keepers: A sociobiological perspective on prosocial behavior. *Humboldt Journal of Social Relations, 13,* 35-67.

Cunningham, M. R. (1988a). Does happiness mean friendliness? Induced mood and heterosexual self-disclosure. *Personality and Social Psychology Bulletin, 14,* 283-297.

Cunningham, M. R. (1988b). What do you do when you're happy or blue? Mood, expectancies, and behavioral interest. *Motivation and Emotion, 12,* 309-331.

Cunningham, M. R., Barbee, A. P., Wolff, P. L., & Kelley, D. J. (1989). *Mood, focus of attention, social and hedonic motives in helping.* Paper presented at the 97th annual convention of the American Psychological Association, New Orleans.

Cunningham, M. R., Shaffer, D. R., Barbee, A. P., Wolff, P. L., & Kelley, D. J. (1990). Separate processes in the relation of elation and depression to altruism: Social and personal concerns. *Journal of Experimental Social Psychology, 26,* 13-33.

Cunningham, M. R., Steinberg, J., & Grev, R. (1980). Wanting to and having to help: Separate motivations for positive mood and guilt-induced helping. *Journal of Personality and Social Psychology, 38,* 181-194.

Daniels, L., & Berkowitz, L. (1963). Liking and response to dependency relationships. *Human Relations, 16,* 141-148.

Darlington, R. B., & Macker, C. E. (1966). Displacement of guilt-produced altruistic behavior. *Journal of Personality and Social Psychology, 4,* 442-443.

De Nicholas, M. E. (1987). *Refusal to help under conditions of anger: Rejection as hedonism.* Unpublished doctoral dissertation, Arizona State University.

Duval, S., Duval, V. H., & Neely, R. (1979). Self-focus, felt responsibility, and helping behavior. *Journal of Personality and Social Psychology, 37,* 1769-1778.

Duval, S., & Wicklund, R. A. (1972). *A theory of objective self-awareness.* New York: Academic Press.

Easterbrook, J. A. (1959). The effect of emotional on cue utilization and the organization of behavior. *Psychological Review, 66,* 183-200.

Eisenberg, N., Fabes, R. A., Bustamante, D., Mathy, R. M., Miller, P. A., & Lindholm, E. (1988). Differentiation of vicariously induced emotional reaction in children. *Developmental Psychology, 24,* 237-246.

Eisenberg, N., & Miller, P. A. (1987). The relation of empathy to prosocial and related behaviors. *Psychological Bulletin, 101,* 91-119.

Eisenberg, N., Schaller, S., Fabes, R. A., Bustamante, D., Mathy, R. M., Shell, R., & Rhodes, K. (1988). Differentiation of personal distress and sympathy in children and adults. *Developmental Psychology, 24,* 766-775.

Feather, N. T. (1966). Effects of prior success and failure on expectations of success and subsequent performance. *Journal of Personality and Social Psychology, 3,* 287-298.

Fiske, S. T., & Taylor, S. E. (1984). *Social cognition.* Reading, MA: Addison-Wesley.

Forest, D., Clark, M., Mills, J., & Isen, A. M. (1979). Helping as a function of feeling state and nature of the helping behavior. *Motivation and Emotion, 3,* 161-169.

Forgas, J. P., & Bower, G. H. (1987). Mood effects on person-perception judgments. *Journal of Personality and Social Psychology, 53,* 53-60.

Forgas, J. P., Bower, G. H., & Krantz, S. E. (1984). The influence of mood on perceptions of social interactions. *Journal of Experimental Social Psychology, 20,* 497-513.

Forgas, J. P., & Moylan, S. (1987). After the movies: The effects of mood on social judgments. *Personality and Social Psychology Bulletin, 13,* 467-477.

Freedman, J. L., Wallington, S. A., & Bless, E. (1967). Compliance without pressure: The effects of guilt. *Journal of Personality and Social Psychology, 7,* 117-124.

Frost, R. O., & Green, M. L. (1982). Duration and post-experimental removal of Velten Mood Induction procedure effect. *Personality and Social Psychology Bulletin, 8,* 341-342.

Fultz, J., & Cialdini, R. B. (1986). *Focus of attention, sadness, and the empathy-helping relationship.* Paper presented at the 94th annual convention of the American Psychological Association, Washington, DC.

Fultz, J., Schaller, M., & Cialdini, R. B. (1988). Empathy, sadness, and distress: Three related but distinct vicarious affective responses to another's suffering. *Personality and Social Psychology Bulletin, 14,* 312-325.

Gaertner, S. L., & Dovidio, J. F. (1977). The subtlety of white racism, arousal, and helping. *Journal of Personality and Social Psychology, 35,* 691-707.

Gibbons, F. X., & Wicklund, R. A. (1982). Self-focused attention and helping behavior. *Journal of Personality and Social Psychology, 43,* 462-474.

Gouaux, C. (1971). Induced affective states and interpersonal attraction. *Journal of Personality and Social Psychology, 20,* 37-43.

Griffitt, W. B. (1970). Environmental effects on interpersonal affective behavior: Ambient effective temperature and attraction. *Journal of Personality and Social Psychology, 15,* 240-244.

Higgins, E. T. (1987). Self-discrepancy: A theory relating self and affect. *Psychological Review, 94,* 319-340.

Higgins, E. T., Bond, R. N., Klein, R., & Strauman, T. (1986). Self-discrepancies and emotional vulnerability: How magnitude, accessibility, and type of discrepancy influence affect. *Journal of Personality and Social Psychology, 51*, 5-15.

Hornstein, H. A. (1982). Promotive tension: Theory and research. In V. J. Derlega & J. Grzelak (Eds.), *Cooperation and helping behavior: Theories and research* (pp. 229-248). New York: Academic Press.

Hornstein, H. A., LaKind, E., Frankel, G., & Manne, S. (1975). Effects of knowledge about remote social events on prosocial behavior, social conception, and mood. *Journal of Personality and Social Psychology, 32*, 1038-1046.

Hull, C. L. (1943). *Principles of behavior*. New York: Appleton-Century-Crofts.

Hull, C. L. (1952). *A behavior system: An introduction to behavior theory concerning the individual organism*. New Haven, CT: Yale University Press.

Isen, A. M. (1984). Toward understanding the role of affect in cognition. In R. S. Wyer & T. K. Srull (Eds.), *Handbook of social cognition* (Vol. 3, pp. 179-235). Hillsdale, NJ: Erlbaum.

Isen, A. M., Clark, M., & Schwartz, M. F. (1976). Duration of the effect of good mood on helping: "Footprints on the sands of time." *Journal of Personality and Social Psychology, 34*, 385-393.

Isen, A. M., & Daubman, K. A. (1984). The influence of affect on categorization. *Journal of Personality and Social Psychology, 47*, 1206-1217.

Isen, A. M., Herren, L. T., & Geva, N. (1986). *The effect of positive affect on recall of social information*. Paper presented at the 94th annual convention of the American Psychological Association, Washington, DC.

Isen, A. M., & Levin, P. F. (1972). The effect of feeling good on helping: Cookies and kindness. *Journal of Personality and Social Psychology, 21*, 384-388.

Isen, A. M., & Means, B. (1983). The influence of positive affect on decision-making strategy. *Social Cognition 2*, 18-31.

Isen, A. M., Means, B., Patrick, R., & Nowicky, G. (1982). Some factors influencing decision-making strategy and risk-taking. In M. S. Clark & S. T. Fiske (Eds.), *Affect and cognition: The 17th Annual Carnegie Symposium on Cognition* (pp. 243-261). Hillsdale, NJ: Erlbaum.

Isen, A. M., & Shalker, T. E. (1982). The influence of mood state on evaluation of positive, neutral and negative stimuli: when you "accentuate the positive," do you "eliminate the negative"? *Social Psychology Quarterly, 45*, 58-63.

Isen, A. M., Shalker, T., Clark, M., & Karp, L. (1978). Affect, accessibility of material in memory and behavior: A cognitive loop? *Journal of Personality and Social Psychology, 36*, 1-12.

Isen, A. M., & Simmonds, S. F. (1978). The effect of feeling good on a helping task that is incompatible with good mood. *Social Psychology, 41*, 345-349.

Johnson, E., & Tversky, A. (1983). Affect, generalization, and the perception of risk. *Journal of Personality and Social Psychology, 45*, 20-31.

Kenrick, D. T., Montello, D. R., & MacFarlane, S. (1985). Personality: Social learning, social cognition, or sociobiology? In R. Hogan & W. Jones (Eds.), *Perspectives in personality* (Vol. 1, pp. 201-234). Greenwich, CT: JAI Press.

Kidd, R. F., & Berkowitz, L. (1976). Dissonance, self-concept, and helpfulness. *Journal of Personality and Social Psychology, 33*, 613-622.

Kim, H., & Baron, R. S. (1988). Exercise and the illusory correlation: Does arousal heighten stereotypic processing? *Journal of Experimental Social Psychology, 24*, 366-380.

Konecni, V. J. (1972). Some effects of guilt on compliance: A field replication. *Journal of Personality and Social psychology, 23*, 30-32.

Laird, J. D., Wagener, J. J., Halal, M., & Szegda, M. (1982). Remembering what you feel: The effects of emotion on memory. *Journal of Personality and Social Psychology, 42*, 646-657.

Langer, E. J., Blank, A., & Chanowitz, B. (1978). The mindlessness of ostensibly thoughtful action: The role of "placebic" information on interpersonal interaction. *Journal of Personality and Social Psychology, 36*, 635-642.

Mackie, D. M., & Worth, L. T. (1989). Processing deficits and the mediation of positive affect in persuasion. *Journal of Personality and Social Psychology, 57*, 27-40.

Manucia, G. K., Baumann, D. J., & Cialdini, R. B. (1984). Mood influences on helping: Direct effects or side effects? *Journal of Personality and Social Psychology, 46*, 357-364.

Maslow, A. H. (1954). *Motivation and personality.* New York: Harper.

Masters, J. C., & Furman, W. (1976). Effects of affect states on noncontingent outcome expectancies and beliefs in internal or external control. *Developmental Psychology, 12*, 481-482.

Mayer, F. S., Duval, S., Holtz, R., & Bowman, C. (1985). Self-focus, helping request salience, felt responsibility, and helping behavior. *Personality and Social Psychology Bulletin, 1985*, 133-144.

Mayer, J. D., & Gaschke, Y. N. (1988). The experience and meta-experience of mood. *Journal of Personality and Social Psychology, 55*, 102-111.

Mayer, J. D., Mamberg, M. H., & Volanth, A. J. (1988). Cognitive domains of the mood system. *Journal of Personality, 56*, 453-486.

Mayer, J. D., & Volanth, A. J. (1985). Cognitive involvement in the emotional response system. *Motivation and Emotion, 9*, 261-275.

McCall, R. J. (1963). Invested self-expression: A principle of human motivation. *Psychological Review, 70*, 289-303.

McClelland, D. C. (1961). *The achieving society.* Princeton, NJ: Van Nostrand.

McClelland, D. C. (1964). *The roots of conciousness.* Princeton, NJ: Van Nostrand.

McMillen, D. L. (1971). Transgression, self-image, and compliant behavior. *Journal of Personality and Social Psychology, 20*, 176-179.

McMillen, D. L., Sanders, D. Y., & Solomon, G. S. (1977). Self-esteem, attentiveness, and helping behavior. *Personality and Social Psychology Bulletin, 3*, 257-261.

Mook, D. G. (1987). *Motivation: The organization of action.* New York: Norton.

Moore, B. S., Underwood, B., & Rosenhan, D. L. (1973). Affect and altruism. *Developmental Psychology, 8*, 99-104.

O'Malley, M. N., & Andrews, L. (1983). The effect of mood and incentives on helping: Are there some things money can't buy? *Motivation and Emotion, 7*, 179-189.

Piliavin, J. A., Dovidio, J. F., Gaertner, S. L., & Clark, R. D., III. (1981). *Emergency intervention.* New York: Academic Press.

Piliavin, J. A., Dovidio, J. F., Gaertner, S. L., & Clark, R. D., III. (1982). Responsive bystanders: The process of intervention. In V. J. Derlega & J. Grzelak (Eds.), *Cooperation of helping behavior* (pp. 279-304). New York: Academic Press.

Pyszczynski, T., & Greenberg, J. (1987). Self-regulatory perseveration and the depressive self-focusing style: A self-awareness theory of reactive depression. *Psychological Bulletin, 102*, 122-138.

Regan, D. T., Williams, M., & Sparling, S. (1972). Voluntary expiation of guilt: A field experiment. *Journal of Personality and Social Psychology, 24*, 42-45.

Regan, J. W. (1971). Guilt, perceived injustice, and altruistic behavior. *Journal of Personality and Social Psychology, 18*, 124-132.

Ridgeway, D., & Waters, E. (1987). Induced mood and preschoolers' behavior: Isolating the effects of hedonic tone and degree of arousal. *Journal of Personality and Social Psychology, 52*, 620-625.

Rogers, M., Miller, N., Mayer, F. S., & Duval, S. (1982). Personal responsibility and salience of the request for help: Determinants of the relations between engative affect and helping behavior. *Journal of Personality and Social Psychology, 43*, 956-970.

Rosenhan, D. L., Karylowski, J., Salovey, P., & Hargis, K. (1981). Emotion and eltruism. In J. P. Rushton & R. M. Sorrentino (Eds.), *Altruism and helping behavior* (pp. 233-248). Hillsdale, NJ: Erlbaum.

Rosenhan, D. L., Salovey, P., & Hargis, K. (1981). The joys of helping. *Journal of Personality and Social Psychology, 40*, 899-905.

Russell, J. A. (1980). A circumplex model of affect. *Journal of Personality and Social Psychology, 39*, 1161-1178.

Salovey, P. (1988). *Mood, attention, and self-relevant thought.* Unpublished manuscript, Yale University.

Salovey, P., & Rodin, J. (1984). Some antecedents and consequences of social-comparison jealousy. *Journal of Personality and Social Psychology, 47*, 780-792.

Salovey, P., & Rosenhan, D. L. (1989). Mood states and prosocial behavior. In H. L. Wagner & A. S. R. Manstead (Eds.), *Handbook of psychophysiology: Emotion and social behavior* (pp. 371-391). Chichester, England: Wiley.

Schachter, S., & Singer, J. L. (1962). Cognitive, social, and physiological determinants of emotional state. *Psychological Review, 69,* 379-399.

Schaller, G. B. (1963). *The mountain gorilla.* Chicago: University of Chicago Press.

Schaller, M., & Cialdini, R. B. (1988). The economics of empathic helping: Support for a mood management motive. *Journal of Experimental Social Psychology, 24,* 163-181.

Schiffenbauer, A. (1974). Effect of observer's emotional state on judgements of the emotional state of others. *Journal of Personality and Social Psychology, 30,* 31-35.

Schmale, A. H. (1970). Adaptive role of depression in health and disease. In J. P. Scott & E. C. Senay (Eds.), *Separation and depression* (pp. 187-214). Washington, DC: American Association for the Advancement of Science.

Schroeder, D. A., Dovidio, J. F., Sibicky, M. E., Matthews, L. L., & Allen, J. L. (1988). Empathic concern and helping behavior: Egoism or altruism? *Journal of Experimental Social Psychology, 24,* 333-353.

Schwartz, G. E., Fair, P. L., Salt, P. S., Mandell, M. R., & Klerman, J. L. (1976). Facial muscle patterning to affective imagery in depressed and nondepressed subjects. *Science, 192,* 489-491.

Schwartz, G. E., Weinberger, D. A., & Singer, J. A. (1981). Cardiovascular differentiation of happiness, sadness, anger, and fear following imagery and exercise. *Psychosomatic Medicine, 43,* 343-364.

Schwarz, N. (1988). *Happy but mindless? Mood effect on problem solving and persuasion.* Paper presented at the 24th International Congress of Psychology, Sydney, Australia.

Schwarz, N., & Clore, G. L. (1988). How do I feel about it? The informative function of affective states. In K. Fiedler & J. Forgas (Eds.), *Affect, cognition, and social behavior* (pp. 44-63). Toronto: Hogrefe International.

Seligman, M. E. P. (1975). *Helplessness: On depression, development, and death.* San Francisco: W. H. Freeman.

Seligman, M. E. P., Klein, D. C., & Miller, W. (1976). Depression. In H. Leitenberg (Ed.), *Handbook of behavior modification and behavior therapy* (pp. 168-210). Englewood Cliffs, NJ: Prentice-Hall.

Shaffer, D. R. (1985/1986). Is mood induced altruism a form of hedonism? *Humboldt Journal of Social Relations, 13,* 195-216.

Shaffer, D. R., & Graziano, W. G. (1983). Effects of positive and negative moods on helping tasks having pleasant or unpleasant consequences. *Motivation and Emotion, 7,* 269-278.

Singer, J. A., & Salovey, P. (1988). Mood and memory: Evaluating the network theory of affect. *Clinical Psychology Review, 8,* 211-251.

Spence, K. W. (1960). *Behavior theory and conditioning.* New Haven, CT: Yale University Press.

Staub, E., & Sherk, L. (1970). Need for approval, children's sharing behavior, and reciprocity in sharing. *Child Development, 41,* 243-252.

Sterling, B., & Gaertner, S. L. (1984). The attribution of arousal and emergency helping: A bidirectional process. *Journal of Experimental Social Psychology, 20,* 586-596.

Strauman, T. J., & Higgins, E. T. (1987). Automatic activation of self-discrepancies and emotional syndromes: When cognitive structures influence affect. *Journal of Personality and Social Psychology, 53,* 1004-1014.

Switzer, G. E. (1989). *Altruism and mood: Limits of an instrumental model.* Unpublished master's thesis, Arizona State University.

Teasdale, J. D., & Fogarty, S. J. (1979). Differential effects of induced mood on retrieval of pleasant and unpleasant events from episodic memory. *Journal of Abnormal Psychology, 88,* 248-257.

Teasdale, J. D., & Russell, M. C. (1983). Differential effects of induced mood on the recall of positive, negative, and neutral words. *British Journal of Clinical Psychology, 22,* 163-171.

Thompson, W. C., Cowan, C. L., & Rosenhan, D. L. (1980). Focus of attention mediates the impact of negative affect on altruism. *Journal of Personality and Social Psychology, 38,* 291-300.

Tomkins, S. S. (1962). *Affect, imagery, and consciousness: Vol. 1. The positive affects.* New York: Springer.

Underwood, B., & Moore, B. (1982). Perspective-taking and altruism. *Psychological Bulletin, 91*, 143–173.

Veitch, R., & Griffitt, W. (1976). Good news—bad news: Affective and interpersonal effects. *Journal of Applied Social Psychology, 6*, 69–75.

Velten, E. (1968). A laboratory task for induction of mood states. *Behaviour Research and Therapy, 6*, 473–482.

Wallace, J., & Sadalla, E. (1966). Behavioral consequences of transgression: I. The effects of social recognition. *Journal of Experimental Research in Personality, 1*, 187–194.

Weiner, B. (1974). *Achievement motivation and attribution theory.* Morristown, NJ: General Learning Press.

Weiner, B. (1986). Attribution, emotion, and action. In R. M. Sorrentino & E. T. Higgins (Eds.), *Handbook of motivation and cognition: Foundations of social behavior* (Vol. 1, pp. 281–312). New York: Guilford Press.

Weiss, R. F., Boyer, J. L., Lombardo, J. P., & Stitch, M. H. (1973). Altruistic drive and altruistic reinforcement. *Journal of Personality and Social Psychology, 25*, 390–400.

Weiss, R. F., Buchanan, W., Alstatt, L., & Lombardo, J. P. (1971). Altruism is rewarding. *Science, 171*, 1262–1263.

Weyent, J. M. (1978). Effects of mood states, costs, and benefits of helping. *Journal of Personality and Social Psychology 36*, 1169–1176.

White, R. W. (1959). Motivation reconsidered: The concept of competence. *Psychological Review, 66*, 297–333.

Worth, L. T., & Mackie, D. M. (1987). Cognitive mediation of positive affect in persuasion. *Social Cognition, 5*, 76–94.

Wundt, W. (1897). *Outlines of psychology.* New York: Stechert.

Yinon, Y., & Landau, M. O. (1987). On the reinforcing value of helping behavior in a positive mood. *Motivation and Emotion, 11*, 83–93.

CHAPTER 9

Political Motivation and Political Cognition

RICHARD R. LAU

Rutgers University

Unlike psychology, political science has not staked out theories of individual behavior that are "unabashedly cognitive" or "unabashedly motivational." The great philosophers, upon whose political ideas most of modern political science is based, all had theories of individual behavior, of course.[1] But most of political science gets by quite nicely with only passing reference to any theory of individual behavior, because institutions, governments, and the relations between them are the basis of the field. One subarea of political science, however—political behavior research—explicitly studies individuals' political actions, and the study of individual political behavior must be based, at least implicitly, on some underlying psychological theory of human behavior.

Even when turning to psychology for a theory of individual behavior, however, political scientists have tended to be eclectic, borrowing here and there for ideas that help explain phenomena of interest without worrying too much about being "true" to the original theory. Nevertheless, as psychology was dominated by motivational theories, so did political behavior research come to have mostly motivational theories underlying it, and as psychology has become much more cognitive, so has political behavior research.

Thus, through the 1960s, most research in the field had an underlying motivational basis. In the first half of the century, research in political behavior was largely psychodynamic in flavor, exploring the conscious and unconscious motives that guided individual political actors. With a few notable exceptions, this research focused on political elites. The development of sophisticated survey research techniques after World War II changed the focus of political behavior research from elites to the masses. By the 1960s the field was dominated by the "Michigan" or social-psychological approach. Motivation for cognitive consistency became supreme. The decisions of most voters are chiefly based, according to the Michigan approach, on the early-learned, long-standing "decision" of party identification that "colors" any and all new political information that voters acquire and "brings it into line" with the prior predispositions. Thus perception, along with motivation, is also an integral part of the Michigan approach, and no sharp distinction is ever made between motivation and cognition.

At the same time that the social-psychological approach was in its heyday, economic/rational-choice models of political behavior were becoming more and more popular in political science, and they became the chief rival of the Michigan approach. Although these models are based on the idea that people are motivated by self-interest, at least as much emphasis is on the thoughtful, "rational" calculation of, rather than the motivation by, self-interest. Monroe (1983) makes the interesting distinction between economics as methodology and economics as motive. The rational-choice theory to be outlined below is economics as methodology; it supposes some value-maximizing way of achieving one's goals, whatever they are. Economic motives are those goals that are essentially financial or material in nature. Tangible, material, financial self-interest is often the goal that decision makers are assumed to attempt to maximize rationally, and therefore economics as motives and economic methodology are closely intertwined. This is another way in which cognition and motivation have been closely linked in models of political behavior.

These powerful rational-choice theories have been used to explain the behavior of both political elites and the general public. The early work concentrated on model building rather than theory testing, but with increasing frequency the advocates of these theories began testing them empirically, first at the aggregate level and then at the individual level. As many social scientists began to realize, however, rational-choice theories of political behavior make assumptions about human cognitive abilities that are psychologically unrealistic. Thus, in the 1980s, the field began to utilize information-processing theories of political behavior that are explicitly based on "boundedly rational" views of human cognitive functioning.

This chapter focuses on these two most recent, and radically different, approaches to political behavior. For historical perspective, I begin with a brief discussion of the early uses of psychodynamic theory in political behavior research. Then the once-dominant social-psychological or Michigan model is reviewed in somewhat greater detail. After this background material has been presented, the economic/rational-choice model is discussed as it has been applied to political behavior. The data supporting this model's major contribution to the political behavior literature—the effect of macroeconomic conditions on political support for incumbents—are discussed. Then two alternatives to this simple economic approach are presented. The symbolic politics model challenges the economic model on empirical grounds, arguing that simple calculations of self-interest—the basic motivation underlying the economic approach—rarely have important effects in politics. Information-processing theories challenge the cognitive requirements of the rational-choice model. Although there is as yet no dominant political cognition theory, the various perspectives are discussed in some detail. The final section summarizes what has been said and suggests further ways in which motivational and cognitive concerns may be integrated in the study of political behavior.

MOTIVATIONAL APPROACHES

Unconscious Motivations: Psychodynamic Theory and Political Behavior

Some of Freud's writings during the later years of his life addressed the political or societal consequences of intrapsychic conflicts (e.g. *Civilization and Its Discontents*; Freud, 1930/1961), but it was the political scientist Harold Lasswell who brought psychodynamic theory to bear most directly on political questions. Relying on the theorizing of both Freud and Adler, Lasswell (1930) posited that political behavior is often a displacement of intrapsychic needs that have little or nothing to do with politics. Lasswell stressed the Adlerian notion of a "pathogenic importance of insufficient self-respect" that often leads to a compensatory "power motivation" that can be realized through political power (see also Lasswell, 1948). Thus the majority of Lasswell's examples are of politicians, judges, and other people with political power. More recent "psychobiographies" of prominent political leaders also tend to be psychodynamic in nature (see Barber, 1985; George & George, 1956; Mazlish, 1972), although they draw on the work of many theorists in addition to Freud and consider motives other than a need for power. The basic idea is the same, however: People are driven to seek political power and to use it in certain ways because of aspects of their lives that have little or nothing to do with politics.

The best-known application of psychoanalytic theory to the political behavior of the general public is *The Authoritarian Personality* (Adorno, Frenkel-Brunswik, Levinson, & Sanford, 1950). Based on the psychoanalytic theorizing of Reich (1933/1946), Fromm (1941), Erikson (1942), and Maslow (1943), *The Authoritarian Personality* was an attempt to describe the underlying personality dynamics that would lead people to adopt fascist, anti-Semitic, and generally ethnocentric political attitudes. A strict superego leads authoritarians to be highly conventional, submissive to authority, and aggressive toward violators of social norms, according to this theory. A weak ego leads authoritarians to be anti-intraceptive (i.e., afraid of self-awareness and of expressing strong emotion), highly superstitious, and strongly stereotypic (thinking in black-and-white terms, with "rigid, oversimplified categories"; Sanford, 1973). The origins of authoritarianism, like the origins of personality, are in early childhood experiences in the family. Later research has questioned the methodological soundness of the original authoritarianism scale (see Christie & Jahoda, 1954), but not the underlying motivational theory.

Political scientists who take a psychoanalytic perspective on political behavior attempt to address the reasons that underlie and motivate political attitudes and behavior. Researchers more closely tied to Freud (Adorno et al., 1950; Lasswell, 1930, 1948) look to early childhood experience; those adopting a broader functional approach (Lane, 1962, 1969; Smith, Bruner, & White, 1956) look to contemporary needs as well as historical ones. For example, Lane (1962) concluded that his working-class respondents preferred an *in*egalitarian society because they feared the threats to their self-esteem and motivation for self-improvement that greater income equality would bring. In most cases, the hypothesized underlying motivations are far removed from politics, and therefore have often been considered "irrational" and unthinking.

This approach is, by necessity, a relatively individual, personalized one. It is methodologically better suited for in-depth interviews than for mass surveys. When applied to political leaders, it is usually based on official biographies and public speeches and appearances, with the analyst attempting to "see around" any self-presentational biases that must be present in such data. As in all research using psychodynamic theories, the strength of the approach is in explanation, not prediction. Perhaps for this reason, the early motivational approaches to political behavior never had more than a few practitioners, and their influence on the field as a whole has been somewhat limited. However, if it were possible to get reliable measures of motivational concepts such as "uncertainty orientation" (Sorrentino, Bobocel, Gitta, Olson, & Hewitt, 1988) or "cognitive style" (Tetlock, 1983, 1984) from a broad cross-section of voters early in a campaign, it might be possible to predict voters' reactions to different styles of political arguments or advertisements during the course of the campaign, and thus their candidate evaluations and vote choice. Recent advances in psychology in measuring motivational constructs make their application to political behavior much more feasible, but so far few such applications exist.

The Michigan Social-Psychological Approach

The American Voter (Campbell, Converse, Miller, & Stokes, 1960), and all the research that derives from that seminal work, begins with a "funnel of causality" that describes metaphorically what has become known as the social-psychological or Michigan approach. A time dimension runs through the funnel, with the relevant political decision (e.g., a vote choice) at the narrow end of the funnel. Basic demographic characteristics (e.g., race) and prior historical events (e.g., one's father being unemployed during the Great Depression) may have many different types of effects, including some that are political, and these factors are represented further back in the funnel. Despite the widespread popularity of "explaining" electoral outcomes from historical events and basic demographic characteristics, however, it is in fact quite difficult to predict a priori exactly what effect such distant events will have; the same event can have very different effects on different people. The funnel narrows as prior events that no longer have political effects are excluded. According to the Michigan approach, such distant events will have political repercussions only to the extent they have been translated into an attitude (e.g., distrust of Republican economic policies) that is part of a voter's psychological field at the time of the vote decision. Only these attitudes remain at the narrow end of the funnel.

The political attitudes fall into three main categories: party identification, issue orientations, and candidate perceptions. Each of these can be considered a vector, with a certain force (strength) and a certain valence (direction). Some vectors point toward (or motivate) a Democratic vote, others toward a Republican vote. The sum of the vectors in a voter's psychological field at the time of the vote decision determines that decision.

It is clear from this brief sketch that Lewin's (1939, 1951) field theory underlies *The American Voter* (and its predecessor, *The Voter Decides*; Campbell, Gurin, & Miller, 1954). Thus political scientists from the "social-psychological school" search for attitudes or beliefs or values that motivate political behavior. These motivations include both long-term factors (summarized by party identification) and short-term factors (specific to the major presidential candidates or the nature of the times surrounding a particular election). One of the most important findings to come from the Michigan school was the predominance of party identification in the vote choice—a "standing decision," learned at one's mother's knee[2]—with almost as much surety as one learns religion. Perceptions of current political actors and events are "colored" by party identification. For example, people project their own issue stands onto their party's candidates, thus "perceiving" a great deal of agreement with those candidates on the issues (Brent & Granberg, 1982; Kinder, 1978). Thus party identification is important not only because of its direct effect on the vote decision, but also because it indirectly affects the vote choice through its influence on perceptions of candidates and perceptions of candidates' issue stands. Thus the Michigan model integrates both motivational concerns and more cognitive, perceptual processes in the same basic model.

The predominance of (very stable) party identification led to a theory of a "normal" vote—the percentage of votes the two parties *should* get in any election, in the absence of an imbalance of short-term factors. The normal-vote theory, in turn, allows the Michigan theorists to have much to say about macro-level political outcomes. To give only one illustration, consider the familiar pattern of a president's party gaining seats in Congress during the presidential election but losing seats during the off-year elections. According to the Michigan model, this "surge and decline" can be explained by the fact that short-term factors generally favor the winning presidential candidate, and he can usually pull many of his party's Congressional candidates to victory on his "coattails." In 1980, for example, the Republican Ronald Reagan won the election, even though there were more Democrats than Republicans in the general public, because the short-term forces—the hostages in Iran, high inflation, the growing perception that Jimmy Carter was a very ineffective president—were overwhelmingly in Reagan's favor. The Republicans picked up 33 seats in the House and 12 seats in the Senate that year. In a case like this, however, the president is *not* running 2 years later, and those short-term factors will therefore be absent. A return to "normal" voting patterns will almost always reduce the support for the president's party in Congress (Campbell, 1962). In the 1982 election, for example, the Democrats regained 26 of their lost seats in the House of Representatives.[3]

The predominance of party identification at the individual level comes at the expense of more thoughtful, rational concerns, such as the issue stands of the candidates. Indeed, *The American Voter* concluded that very few people (in the neighborhood of 20%, on any given issue) are even *capable* of voting on an issue, if in order to do so they must hold an opinion on an issue, know the stands of the competing candidates on that issue, and perceive some difference between the candidates' stands. This finding has important implications for the association between public opinion and government policy, or the very nature of how our "democratic" government actually functions. If voters depend chiefly on party identification, then the issue stands of the candidates (indeed, virtually the entire election campaign) are mostly irrelevant. For that matter, what candidates do in office (within limits) is mostly irrelevant, as long as citizens continue to vote their party identification.

Converse (1964, 1970) has gone on to argue that the mass public is for the most part "ideologically innocent." Less than 12% of the American public in 1956 showed any evidence of being able to use the abstractions "liberal" or "conservative" in their descriptions of the parties and candidates of the day. Nor was there any evidence that the political beliefs of the general public were at all organized into tightly constrained wholes. That is, knowing a person's stand on one issue tells us little about the person's stand on any other issue. Most damning of all were Converse's data showing that even individual issue stands seem to have little substance for most people, in that they have little or no stability over time. For many people, expressions of opinions on many political issues are more "nonattitudes" than attitudes.

Thus *The American Voter* and the research stemming from it painted a somewhat discouraging picture of the American voter. Although unconscious, irrational motives had disappeared, the view of the average voter that came out of this literature was hardly flattering. Ill-informed and generally uncaring about politics, the typical American simply pulls the lever of party identification whenever he or she enters a voting booth. The general public is not very sophisticated politically, and is mostly incapable of performing (or at least unwilling to perform) the type of careful monitoring of our elected representatives that good citizenship in a democracy requires.

The Michigan model does have the advantage of being cognitively realistic. It makes few demands on human cognitive abilities. Nevertheless, its view of the general public was too stark to go unchallenged, and soon the field saw a wealth of studies designed to show that "voters are not fools" (e.g., Key, 1966). The literature on issue voting has become rich and varied (see Boyd, 1972; Miller, Miller, Raine, & Brown, 1976; Nie, Verba, & Petrocik, 1976; Pomper, 1972; Shapiro, 1969). Most of these studies (or at least those parts of them dealing with issue voting) were inspired by a more economic approach to political behavior. Rational considerations of self-interest guide the economic person, and they are assumed by economic theories of political behavior to guide the political person as well. The next section provides a more complete review of the economic or rational-choice approach to political behavior.

Economic Motives: Self-Interest and Rational Choice

There are nearly as many definitions of "rationality" in political science, economics, and philosophy as there are definitions of "attitudes" in social psychology.

Nonetheless, most definitions assume that rational decision makers have a coherent set of known and fixed preferences, and a consistent set of beliefs about the world. Rational behavior is behavior that, in some value-maximizing way, applies those beliefs to achieve goals that are associated with the individual's preferences. The most rational goal, according to economists, and the one we can safely assume everyone shares, is self-interest.

The economic/rational-choice model assumes that politicians are essentially amoral vote maximizers who have no strong policy preferences or ideologies of their own, desiring only to win elections by as large a margin as possible (e.g., Davis, Hinich, & Ordeshook, 1979; Downs, 1957; Riker & Ordeshook, 1968; see Weatherford, 1988, for a recent review). To do this, they adopt any issue positions that will attract the largest coalition of supporters; they are constrained into moderate consistency only by fears of losing all credibility with voters. Campaigns are the crucial events in the economic model, not only because they involve all the interesting strategic maneuvering between candidates (or parties), each trying to adopt issue positions that are closest to those held by the median voter, but also because the actual governing between elections is mostly irrelevant. Politicians must strive to live up to their campaign promises or they will be voted out of office in the next election. (Indeed, actually having to govern is an inconvenience, for governing establishes a record, which makes it more difficult to maneuver and manipulate one's issue stands at the next election.) Thus the important policy choices are made during campaigns.

Citizens are essentially self-interested and short-sighted, according to the economic/rational-choice model.[4] They are concerned with what the government can do for *them*; they worry about how the government's actions affect their own (and their families') welfare. They are, in the terminology popularized by Downs (1957), "pocketbook" voters. Citizens are assumed to have clear and fixed issue positions that reflect rational calculations of their own self-interest. They are assumed to pay attention to politics and the platforms offered by the different candidates, and to vote for the candidate or party that, on balance, takes the stands closest to their own (and therefore for the candidate or party that will, on balance, be most beneficial to their self-interest).

The rational-choice model makes its clearest predictions and has had its biggest successes with economic matters. If voters are self-interested, then they should support those policies that would clearly benefit them, and they should vote for candidates whose policies have benefited them. There are two main lines of evidence for this basic claim of the rational-choice model. First, there is a very sophisticated econometric literature linking macroeconomic conditions to political outcomes. These econometric analyses, although usually at the aggregate level, either explicitly or implicitly assume the rational, self-interested economic person sketched out above. The seminal work in the field is Kramer's (1971) study linking aggregate changes in real disposable income and unemployment to support for the president's party in Congress. Kramer's theory holds that people's personal economic well-being is their most important concern; that they view past economic performance as the best indicator of future economic performance;

and that they view Congressional candidates as essentially party members who share the president's economic policies. Thus if voters are better off now than they were 2 years ago, they will vote for Congressional candidates of the incumbent president's party, whereas if voters are worse off now than they were 2 years ago, they will vote for Congressional candidates of the opposite party. Although there are a few dissenters (Stigler, 1973, is the most notable), most subsequent research with aggregate data (e.g., Arcelus & Meltzer, 1975; Bloom & Price, 1975; Goodman & Kramer, 1975; Tufte, 1973, 1975; see Monroe, 1979, for a review of this literature) has supported Kramer's general conclusion; researchers differ only in which economic indicators are believed to be the most important (e.g., inflation rates, changes in real disposable income), how to measure them (e.g., what time lags are appropriate), and how to best specify the dependent variable (e.g., how to treat votes for minor-party candidates). Other investigators (e.g., Kernell, 1978) have extended the analysis to predicting changes in the public's support for the president (as indicated by the proportion of the public "approving" of the president's job performance in periodic Gallup polls). There are now several prominent models (each slightly different), based mostly on economic indicators and presidential popularity, that do very good jobs of predicting how many seats the incumbent president's party will gain in Congress each election (Abramowitz & Segal, 1986; Campbell, 1985; Lewis-Beck & Rice, 1984, 1985; Tufte, 1975).

The second line of evidence for the self-interest hypothesis comes from group differences in political beliefs: Women support the Equal Rights Amendment (ERA) more than men do; blacks support busing to a greater extent than do whites; retired people oppose Social Security cuts more than young people do; and so on. These examples, like the econometric data presented above, are all at the aggregate level, illustrating mean differences across groups in some political response. But the underlying individual-level theory is obvious: Those voters who have been hurt economically are the ones who vote against the incumbent president's party; those women who would benefit most from the ERA are its strongest supporters; and so on. When Ronald Reagan urged voters during his 1980 debate with Jimmy Carter to ask themselves whether they were better off now than they were 4 years ago, the answer for the great majority of voters must have been "No," and Reagan won a big electoral victory.

The Symbolic Politics Alternative

There is one major flaw in the self-interest hypothesis: When the underlying theory is tested at the individual level, self-interest in fact appears to have very little to do with most political responses! White parents whose children are being bused are no more opposed to busing than are white parents whose children are not threatened with busing, or whites without school-age children (Gatlin, Giles, & Cataldo, 1978; Kinder & Rhodebeck, 1982; Kinder & Sears, 1981; McConahay, 1982; Sears, Hensler, & Speer, 1979; Sears, Lau, Tyler, & Allen, 1980); people without health insurance or people who believe their health insurance is inadequate for present needs are no more supportive of national health insurance than are people with good health insurance coverage (Sears et al., 1980); people who have served in Vietnam, or people with children or spouses or close friends who have served in Vietnam (or who were serving in Vietnam at the time of the survey), held no different opinions toward the war than people without such personal associations (Lau, Brown, & Sears, 1978); victims of crime or people living in high-crime neighborhoods are no more opposed to ensuring the rights of those accused of crimes than are people who have not been victimized by crimes (Sears et al., 1980); people greatly inconvenienced by the energy crisis of the mid-1970s were no more supportive of greater energy conservation policies than were people who suffered few such inconveniences (Sears, Tyler, Citrin, & Kinder, 1978).

Even when it comes to economics and pocketbooks, there seems to be little individual-level evidence for the self-interest hypothesis: People who are unemployed or underemployed, people who have suffered from inflation, and people who claim to be worse off financially now than they were a few years ago are no more opposed to the incumbent president or his party, and are no more supportive of government policies to guarantee jobs and income, than are people who have not suffered such financial setbacks (Kinder, 1981; Kinder & Kiewiet, 1979, 1981; Lewis-Beck, 1986; Sears et al., 1980). This general lack of support for self-interest holds whether the indicators of self-interest are objective (e.g., unemployment) or subjective ("Would you say it is safe to go out walking around here alone at night?"), retrospective ("Would you say that you are better off or worse off financially than you were a year ago?") or prospective ("Do you think that a year from now you will be better off financially, or worse off, or just about the same as now?"). Only when the consequences of a political policy are particularly clear, tangible, and large do voters show any evidence of self-interested political behavior (Sears & Citrin, 1985), and even here (proposed property tax cuts that could save home owners hundreds or even thousands of dollars, and cost many government employees their jobs), the political ramifications are very limited and narrowly focused.

What can explain the macroeconomic results reported above? One possibility is that people are motivated by collective economic (or "sociotropic") concerns more than by personal economic concerns. In a series of intriguing studies, Kinder (1981; Kinder & Kiewiet, 1979, 1981) has shown that political behavior (approval of the president's job performance; Congressional and presidential voting) is much more strongly a function of collective or sociotropic judgments (e.g., evaluations of how the economy as a whole is doing) than it is of personal economic judgments. Moreover, these collective judgments do not appear to be rationalizations of personal economic well-being. They do have their partisan components, to be sure (i.e., Democrats are more likely to say that the economy is going down the tubes when there is a Republican president than when there is a Democratic president, and vice versa), but they have substantial elements that are independent of partisanship. The macro-level results are produced not because more individuals suffer financial setbacks during times of high inflation or high unemployment and vote against the incumbent president and his party, but because more people believe that the country is suffering because the economy is being mismanaged during such times (regardless of their personal economic situation) and vote accordingly.

More generally, the limited or nonexistent support for self-interest effects on political behavior is consistent with Sears's "symbolic politics" theory (Sears et al., 1979, 1980). Sears and his colleagues argue that political attitudes and behavior are most frequently "unthinking, reflexive, affective responses to remote attitude objects" (Sears et al., 1980, p. 681). Thus Sears would not expect rational calculations of self-interest to have much of an effect on policy attitudes. As an alternative, Sears hypothesizes that children acquire stable affective responses to political objects on the basis of simple conditioning and social learning from their parents, with little or no calculation of costs and benefits associated with those attitudes. These early learned "symbolic attitudes" include party identification, liberalism–conservatism,[5] racism, and nationalism. Later in life, if some new political object evokes one of these early learned symbolic attitudes (through stimulus similarity), attitudes toward the new political object will be based largely on the early learned symbolic attitude. Thus one need not have developed simple affective responses to buses (say) as a child for adult policy attitudes toward busing to be influenced primarily by symbolic attitudes; if some new attitude object evokes symbols (blacks) toward which one has a symbolic attitude (racism), the later policy attitude can be guided by the symbolic attitude by simple stimulus generalization. Indeed, in all of the studies cited above that found little or no effect of self-interest, one or more of the symbolic attitudes were found to have very strong effects on the policy attitude of interest.

Thus, symbolic politics theory challenges one of the basic underlying assumptions of the rational-choice model. Self-interest motivations appear not to be very important determinants of political attitudes and behavior. There is another prominent attack on rational-choice theories, however—one that challenges the reasonableness of the cognitive requirements of the model. It is to this challenge that I now turn.

COGNITIVE APPROACHES

Cognitive Requirements of Rational-Choice Models

Recall that the rational-choice model assumes that people vote for the candidate or party that takes the stands closest to their own. Figuring out which party or candidate takes positions that are closest to one's own issue stands is no mean task. The difficulty can be demonstrated by illustrating how this task is usually represented in the rational-choice literature.

There is a vector I of a person's stand on all relevant political issues during an election campaign. Most voters will not have stands on all of those issues, of course, and therefore many of the individual issue stands i_j will be missing. There is also a vector W of weights attached to each of these issues, reflecting how important each issue is to the voter. D represents the stands taken by the Democratic party or candidate on those issues, whereas R represents the stands taken by the Republican party or candidate. Both of these party or candidate vectors are weighted by credibility factors (c_d and c_r, respectively), reflecting how much the voter trusts the candidates or parties to actually do what they pledge to do during a campaign. The voter's task, then, is to calculate the "distance" between his or her own stands on the issues and those of the candidates or parties, or

$$| W(I - c_d D)| - | W(I - c_r R)|$$

The voter will presumably vote for the Republicans if this difference is greater than 0 (i.e., the voter is closer to the Republicans on the issues than to the Democrats), and for the Democrats if this difference is less than 0. This is a "prospective" decision, based on calculations of what is likely to happen in the future.

The task becomes even more difficult if we realize that the credibility factor is likely to be low, and information about where the candidates or parties stand on the issues is generally going to be difficult to obtain.[6] Instead, what the candidates or parties have actually done while in office (P_d and P_r) must also be figured into the calculation, balanced perhaps by other beliefs (b_d and b_r) about how reliably the parties can be counted on to continue doing in the future what they have done in the past. Then the voter's task looks more like this: Calculate

$$| W[I - (b_d P_d + c_d D)]| - | W[I - (b_r P_r + c_r R)]|$$

and vote as above.

It is *conceivable* that "single-issue" voters could make the calculation above and vote "rationally." Once voters are allowed to care about more than one or two issues, however, the cognitive requirements of this type of calculation become psychologically unrealistic. The litany of cognitive limitations need not be repeated for this audience (see Fiske & Taylor, 1984, or Lau & Sears, 1986, for recent summaries). But it is these very limitations that have led some political psychologists to seek alternative models of political cognition—models that are psychologically more realistic in what is demanded of the voter. I turn now to examining some of the different models of political cognition.

The Content of Political Schemata

Virtually all political cognition research assumes that cognition is structured, and most researchers adopt the term "schema" to describe these structures. A fairly generic definition of "schema" will suffice: It may include a category label, general descriptions of the stimulus domain, specific instances of it, and interconnections between these. Schema content is based on experience, and schemata are usually assumed to be hierarchically organized within any domain (Rumelhart & Ortony, 1977; Taylor & Crocker, 1981). They serve two important purposes: They guide the processing and storage of incoming information, and they guide recall and interpretation of information in memory.

Whereas all researchers in political cognition would be comfortable accepting this basic definition, they differ greatly in which function of schemata they have explored, the level of specificity or abstraction they are concerned with, and how they have operationalized the schemata they have chosen to study. As the following review indicates, whereas most cognitive and social-cognitive researchers have been concerned with the effects of consensually held schemata, researchers in political cognition have more typically been concerned with individual differences in political schemata. This difference may be due to the fact that politics is more on the periphery of day-to-day life (at least in the United States) than furniture or basic personality types are, and therefore one would expect people to differ in how much and what type of experience they have had with the stimuli in question. In any case, the following discussion begins by presenting research at the most general level of overall political expertise and then proceeds to research on more specific types of political schemata.

Expertise

Several researchers have looked at general political expertise, operationalized in terms of interest in political campaigns, following politics through the media, political activity (voting, campaigning, contributing money, etc.), awareness of the candidates and issues of the day, and basic political knowledge (e.g., which party controls the House of Representatives, how long a senator's term is). The cognitive literature suggests not only that experts (by definition) should know more about their domain of expertise, but that their knowledge should be more tightly structured, with more links between concepts. Knowledge tends to be "chunked" or grouped together, and the knowledge chunks of experts also tend to contain more information than the chunks of novices (Chase & Simon, 1973). The tighter structure means that experts' knowledge can be more quickly and efficiently "brought to mind" (Chi & Koeske, 1983), and the large chunks means that experts can contemplate and manipulate more information in active memory (Larkin, McDermott, Simon, & Simon, 1980; McKeithen, Reitman, Rueter, & Hirtle, 1981).

Fiske, Kinder, and Larter (1983) hypothesized that everyone has schemata for democratic and communist countries, and that information that is consistent with a schema will be more easily processed. Because the schemata of political experts are more coherently and tightly structured, however, they will have sufficient remaining cognitive capacity in active memory to also process information that is *in*consistent with the schema. Thus novices should process chiefly schema-consistent information, whereas experts should process both schema-consistent and schema-inconsistent information. To test this hypothesis, Fiske et al. (1983) created a description of an obscure country on an island in the Indian

Ocean that included some information that was stereotypic of a democratic country (e.g., elections occur regularly) and other information that was stereotypic of a communist country (e.g., the economy is state-owned and controlled). The first sentence of the description labeled the country as either democratic or communistic, thereby determining what information was consistent and what information was inconsistent. Results showed the hypothesized expert–novice differences in recall: Experts recalled more information that was inconsistent with the label than novices, whereas novices recalled more information that was consistent with the label than did experts.[7]

Ralph Erber and I explored expert–novice differences in responses to political surveys (Lau & Erber, 1985). We hypothesized first that experts, with more highly developed and cohesive political schemata, would be more likely to assimilate new information into a schema without drastic changes, whereas novices, with more rudimentary political schemata, would be more likely to revise a schema to accommodate the new information (see Piaget & Inhelder, 1973). Therefore, the political attitudes of experts were hypothesized to be more stable across a political campaign. Using data from a nationally representative survey of voters interviewed in February and September 1980, we found that party identification, ideological self-placement (on a liberal–conservative scale), affective evaluations of the three major candidates (Jimmy Carter, Ronald Reagan, and Edward Kennedy), and competence ratings of Carter and Reagan (but not Kennedy) were significantly more stable for experts than for novices.[8] Second, we hypothesized that the efficiency of larger knowledge chunks would allow experts to bring more information to bear on their evaluations of the candidates. Indeed, experts' evaluations of the three candidates correlated significantly with three or four of their issue stands, whereas novices' candidate evaluations correlated significantly with only one or two issue stands.

Probably the most elaborate exploration of political expertise is provided in a later study (Fiske, Lau, & Smith, 1990). We collected a wide variety of different types of political expertise measures from a sample of registered voters in Pittsburgh. These measures made up a fairly comprehensive list of the different measures of political expertise being used by researchers in the field. Factor analyses revealed five different types of political expertise: Political Knowledge, Political Activity, Electronic Media Use (TV), Print Media Use (newspapers and magazines), and Political Self-Schematicity (e.g., the importance of thinking of oneself as a liberal or conservative). These factors were then linked to various measures of information processing of (printed) political stimuli, including reading time, cognitive responses, and recall. A general (second-order) Political Expertise factor, measured by Political Knowledge, Political Activity, and Print Media Use, predicted 20% of the variance in a general Political Information Processing factor, comprised of reading time and recall. Electronic Media Use and Political Self-Schematicity had no effects on the processing of printed political material. Thus political expertise is multidimensional, and the various dimensions have distinct effects on the processing of different types of political information.

More Specific Schemata

Conover and Feldman (1984) have studied the contents of people's political "belief systems." They were concerned with three different levels of specificity. At a superordinate level, they explored people's beliefs about human nature and social interaction; at an intermedite level, they explored more classic "ideological" principles about preferences for government intervention in society; and at a more specific level, they explored the nature of people's beliefs in four general areas of politics: foreign affairs, economics, racial policy, and social policy. (Stimuli at this last level were not at the most subordinate level of specific policy proposals, however.) Conover and Feldman utilized a methodology that is particularly well suited for studying the contents of the mind, but one that, surprisingly, has been utilized by few other cognition researchers: Q-sort methodology (see also Bolland, 1985; Brown, 1980).

With Q-sort methodology, subjects sort a list of statements according to some criteria. For each of their six domains of interest, Conover and Feldman had subjects sort a list of 40–50 items according to how much they agreed with each statement. "Forced-distribution" instructions were employed to require subjects to place a specified number of statements at each level of agreement. A Q-sort is essentially a factor analysis that simplifies the rows rather than the columns of a data matrix. That is, rather than illustrating how all subjects group a set of items, thus forming subsets of items (as in a traditional factor analysis), a Q-sort illustrates how the entire set of items are structured by different groups of subjects, thus forming subsets of the subjects.[9]

For present purposes, the individual results of each of the six Q-sorts are not important (but see Conover & Feldman's [1984] Table 1, pp. 106–107). More important are several summary conclusions that can be drawn about the results across the various domains and levels of abstraction. First, each Q-sort revealed from two to four distinct ways of grouping the same political information (or two to four distinct schemata). That is, there was no single dimension along which everyone grouped the various statements. Furthermore, these ways of grouping the information were by no means totally idiosyncratic: Each one of them involved at least 10% of the subjects. Second, with only one exception (for economic beliefs), the groupings were essentially orthogonal to each other, even though an oblique rotation was employed. Third, and again with only one exception, the factors were not bipolar; that is, they did not involve a group of subjects who held one set of beliefs and another group of subjects who held the opposite set of beliefs. This finding casts serious doubt on any analysis of political belief systems that relies on a single (typically, liberal–conservative) bipolar dimension. And finally, within each domain a reasonable number of subjects (10–20%) were totally *a*schematic—they did not think about these items in an identifiable manner. However, this tendency was not a general one: Only 12% of the subjects were aschematic in more than one domain.

In contrast to Conover and Feldman (1984), who looked for individual differences in the ways people structure political information, Miller, Wattenberg, and Malanchuk (1986) explored the consensual ways in which people view presidential candidates. Employing a set of open-ended questions that have been asked in nationally representative surveys about the major candidates in every presidential contest from 1952 to 1984,[10] Miller et al. identified five common dimensions of candidate evaluations: competence (including comments about political experience, statesmanship, and intelligence), integrity (including comments about trustworthiness and corruption in government), reliability (comments about dependability, strength vs. weakness, decisiveness, aggressiveness vs. passivity, etc.), charisma (leadership, dignity, humility, patriotism, ability to inspire), and a purely personal factor (including comments about easily observable features, such as a candidate's appearance, age, previous employment or military background, religion, social class, etc.). Miller et al. found these same five dimensions in every election year from 1952 to 1984, which they took as evidence that "people share common expectations across time about what presidential candidates should be like" (Miller et al., 1986, p. 528), and thus as evidence for schematic as opposed to piecemeal processing of candidate information.

Somewhat surprisingly, Miller and colleagues found that the use of person-related information (as opposed to party or policy information) was *positively* associated with education, interest in politics, and media exposure to politics. This was particularly true of the competence, reliability, and integrity dimensions. This general finding is surprising because, for a long time, evaluating candidates on the basis of personal (and personality) factors was considered irrational, emotional, and mostly uninformed. It is clear, however, that this conventional view should be revised. Dimensions of candidate evaluation concentrate more on factors (such as competence, integrity, and reliability) that are instrumental to how a president will perform in office than on factors (here, the purely personal dimension) that carry little performance information.

No one has been more careful in measuring and validating an operationalization of political schema than Milton Lodge and his colleagues at the State University of New York at Stony Brook (Hamill & Lodge, 1986; Hamill, Lodge, & Blake, 1985; Lodge & Hamill, 1986; Lodge, McGraw, & Stroh, 1989; Sharp & Lodge, 1985). Lodge views schemata primarily as declarative knowledge structures in a particular domain, and he operationalizes them by asking subjects to categorize politicians, issues, and social groups as liberal or conservative, as Democratic or Republican, and as favored by rich people or favored by poor people. Thus Lodge and his colleagues have looked at partisan, ideological, and class schemata.

A measure of "schema usage" is created by calculating the proportion of issues, people, and groups that are correctly categorized as Democratic or Republican, say. "Correct" is defined as the consensual response of the subjects studied. That is, if "favor more defense spending" is categorized by most subjects as a Republican issue stance, then all subjects who categorize it as Republican are scored correct, whereas those who categorize it as Democratic are categorized as incorrect.

In a series of careful studies using this knowledge-based measure of different types of political schemata, Lodge and his colleagues have documented some of the information-processing differences between schematics and aschematics. For example, Hamill and Lodge (1986) have shown that ideology schematics are better able to recognize ideological issue stands when they are presented for very brief periods of time (50 milliseconds); they are more accurate, and faster, at verifying the truth of simple sentences about liberals and conservatives (e.g., "Conservatives favor more defense spending"). Greater recognition, accuracy, and speed are three advantages of schematic processing, and Lodge has shown that these familiar effects extend to political schemata.

Some of Lodge's most ingenious work comes from experiments about a hypothetical "Congressman Williams from upstate New York." Congressman Williams is labeled as a Democrat or a Republican, and his stands on 40 different political issues are described. Thirty of his issue positions are consistent with his ideological label (e.g., a Democrat favoring a higher minimum wage), whereas 10 issue positions are inconsistent with the label. After reading this description of Williams and then performing a distractor task, subjects receive an unexpected recognition task. Forty policy stands are presented, and subjects are asked to recall whether Congressman Williams took that stand. Of the 40 test stimuli, 20 are old (Williams actually took that stand) and 20 are new (Williams said nothing about that issue); 20 are stereotypically Democratic positions (and therefore either consistent or inconsistent with Williams's partisan label), and 20 are stereotypically Republican positions. Lodge and Hamill (1986) predicted that schematics, relative to aschematics, would be better able to correctly recognize old statements that were consistent with the partisan label and to correctly reject new statements that were inconsistent with the partisan label; they predicted no such advantage for schematics for old items that were inconsistent with the partisan label, however, or for new statements that were consistent with the label. The observed results supported this hypothesis. Moreover, Lodge and Hamill showed that their schematic effects were independent of verbal ability (as measured by the Civil Service Commission's vocabulary test), for when verbal ability was entered as another factor in the analyses of variance, a main effect for schematicity was still observed.

Chronicities

All of Lodge's results are consistent with the position that schematic knowledge is more accessible than aschematic knowledge. In a similar vein, I have looked for individual differences in the generic *type* of political information that voters chronically notice and/or seek out, and that they have available for subsequent recall about a variety of different political stimuli (Lau, 1986, 1989). Such cognitive constructs should be relatively stable, and should guide the processing of information about a variety of different political objects in a variety of different situations. One could call these hypothesized cognitive structures "schemata," for they clearly perform many of the functions ascribed to schemata. Following Higgins (Higgins & King, 1981; Higgins, King, & Mavin, 1982) and Bargh (Bargh & Pratto, 1986; Bargh & Thein, 1985), however, I refer to these constructs as "chronically accessible political constructs," or more simply as "political chronicities."

I operationalized political chronicities from responses to open-ended questions of nationally representative surveys. Using some of the same questions employed by Miller et al. (1986; see present note 10), I hypothesized the existence of four basic types of political chronicities: persons, issues, groups, and parties. Responses to the open-ended questions were classified as relevant to one of these four categories, and a weighted count of the number of responses falling into each category was calculated. This counting algorithm gives more weight to the first responses to any open-ended question than it does to later responses, under the assumption that the first things that "come to mind" are more indicative of the type of information in memory.[11] I have shown that political chronicities are, as hypothesized, fairly stable over time (stability coefficients ranging from .27 to .78 over 4-year periods). Moreover, they guide the processing of information about a variety of different political objects in a variety of different contexts. For example, people with a strong political person chronicity in 1956 gave more person-related reasons for their vote in 1960; knew more about the social class, religion, and family backgrounds of the candidates that year; and most impressively, recalled more person-related information from the Kennedy–Nixon debates than did people without a strong person chronicity. Similar validity information is presented for the other political chronicities.

The Structure of Political Schemata

Some political cognition research provides evidence for the presumed hierarchical structure of schemata. Recall that Conover and Feldman (1984) had subjects perform six different Q-sorts of information at three different levels of generality, varying from beliefs about human nature (the most general level) to beliefs about basic ideological principles to beliefs about four policy areas (the most subordinate level). Correlating individuals' factor loadings across factors (and across Q-sorts) provides an indication of the relationship between schemata, and thus of the structure of political schemata. The Q-sort of information at the most general level revealed four distinct schemata ("altruistic–positive," "Hobbesian–Freudian," "individualistic," and "altruistic–complex"), each of which was associated with one of the three schemata pertaining to ideological principles ("neoconservatism," "free-market conservatism," and "democratic socialism"). Each of these higher-level schemata was related to various lower-level schemata concerning economic, racial, social, and foreign affairs beliefs. The results revealed two fairly simple conservative ideologies, one fairly simple liberal ideology, and one very complex ideology. The three simpler patterns are shown in Figures 9.1 through 9.3. One very simple conservative structure (shown in Figure 9.1) links a Hobbesian–Freudian view of human nature with a free-market conservative view of ideological principles, with pro-free enterprise economic beliefs, and with two distinct sets of foreign affairs beliefs. There are no racial or social beliefs associated with this structure. A second conservative structure (shown in Figure 9.2) links an individualistic view of human nature with neoconservative ideological principles and with a variety of economic, racial, social, and foreign affairs beliefs.

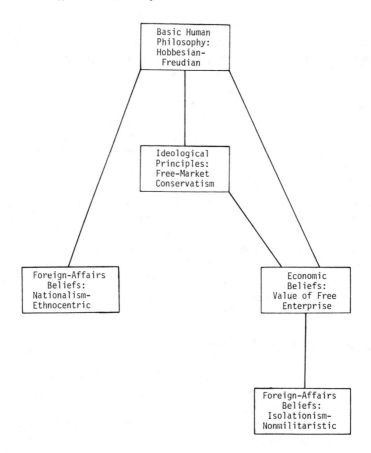

FIGURE 9.1 The simple conservative structure based on a Hobbesian–Freudian view of human nature. Data from Conover and Feldman (1984).

The one clearly liberal perspective (Figure 9.3) links an altruistic–complex view of human nature with a democratic-socialist ideology and corresponding economic and racial beliefs, and with two sets of social and foreign affairs beliefs.

These different cognitive structures or "belief systems" are important because they suggest that Converse's (1964, 1970) conclusions about the ideological innocence of the American public were overstated. It is true that very few members of the general public structure their political beliefs in terms of an overarching liberalism or conservatism in the way that members of political elites do. But most people have more limited ideologies that do help them structure and make sense of political affairs. For example, people make schema-based inferences about candidates' issue stands, as discussed below, and evaluate them in terms of information that is relevant to strong political chronicities.

Models of Political Cognition

Inference

One question that political cognition research is particularly useful in addressing concerns inference. In political campaigns, one of the most important questions is that of how voters attribute issue stands to different candidates. Rarely do candidates actually commit themselves to specific policies; everyone favors peace and a strong economy. Yet voters do make more specific inferences about candidates' issue stands, and even apparently vote on the basis of those inferences (see the literature on issue voting, cited above). How, then, are these inferences made? How do voters cope with a very ambiguous political world? One answer is given by balance theory: People "project" their own issue stands to liked

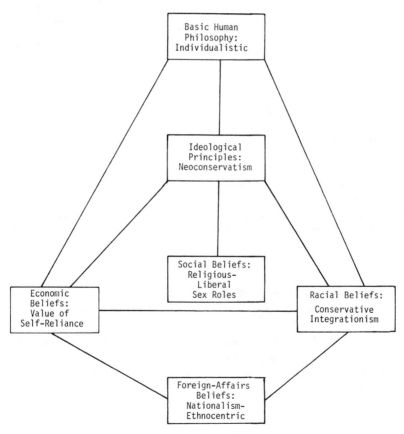

FIGURE 9.2 The fairly simple conservative structure based on an individualistic view of human nature. Data from Conover and Feldman (1984).

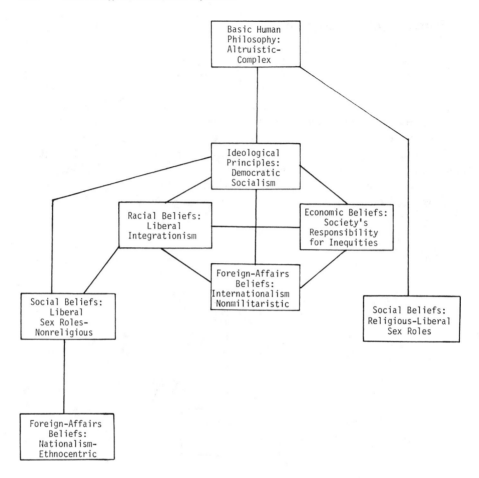

FIGURE 9.3 The fairly simple liberal ideology on an altruistic–complex view of human nature. Data from Conover and Feldman (1984).

candidates (Brent & Granberg, 1982; Kinder, 1978), and perhaps "contrast" their own stands with their perceptions of the stands of disliked candidates. Indeed, there is much evidence that such projection does go on, in that some voters will attribute the most liberal issue stands to the most conservative politicians and others will attribute the most conservative issue stands to the most liberal politicians, depending on the extent of their liking for the candidates and their own stands on these issues.

But there is another process by which such inferences can be made, and this one generally produces more accurate results. Because there is some generic information associated with most schemata, schematics often infer that the generic information is present even when no such information was actually presented. Certainly there are issue stands that are prototypically associated with Democrats and Republicans, liberals and conservatives. One of the first things one learns about any candidate is his or her party, and without too much additional difficulty one can learn whether a candidate is generally liberal or conservative. These generic labels can be the basis for inferring issue stands, at least for people who have a partisan and/or an ideological schema.

To illustrate this inference process, Hamill et al. (1985) correlated measures of partisan, ideology, and class schematicity with correct placement of Ronald Reagan on the issues. The partisan schema was the most useful, correlating .83 with correct knowledge of Reagan's policy stands. An ideological schema was somewhat less useful ($r = .68$), and a class schema was only useful for correctly inferring Reagan's economic policies ($r = .60$, vs. $r = .21$ for noneconomic issues).

Conover and Feldman (1986, 1989) explored the inference process in even greater detail. They utilized a panel study in which respondents were interviewed several times during the 1976 presidential campaign. At the beginning of the campaign, voters were mostly ignorant of the issue stands of a little-known former governor of Georgia who was running for president. By the time of the election, however, most people felt that they knew Jimmy Carter's stands on most of the important issues of the campaign. Among the bases on which people made these inferences were their perceptions of the stands of Democrats on those same issues. Moreover, as the campaign progressed and Carter became more closely identified as a Democrat, these inferences became stronger.

Candidate Evaluation and Vote Choice

I posited a simple model of candidate evaluation and the vote decision based on political chronicities (Lau, 1986, 1989). I hypothesized that not only should voters notice and have available for recall political information that is related to their political chronicities, but they should evaluate candidates disproportionately on the basis of those chronicities. That is, people with a party chronicity should be chiefly party voters, those with an issues chronicity should be disproportionately issues voters, and so on. To test this model, I regressed measures of differential candidate evaluation (liking one candidate more than the other) on standard affective orientations that are used by political scientists to explain the vote (e.g., party identification, closeness to the candidates on the issues, trait evaluations of the candidates), my chronicity measures, and interactions between the two. The model predicts that the interactions should be significant: The standard affective measures should predict candidate preference disproportionately for those with an appropriate chronicity. As hypothesized, the interaction terms were generally significant (eight of nine at the .05 level) and were substantively large (see Lau, 1989, Tables 1 and 2). This model is an important improvement over more standard models of the vote decision because it predicts what *type* of information will be important to *which* voters. Thus it has the real potential to explain the success or failure of different campaign strategies and political advertisements on the basis of the political chronicities of the audience.

Herstein (1981) presented subjects with three different "elections" involving pairs of hypothetical candidates. Different pieces of information about each candidate were written on index cards placed on an "information board." These cards had a brief description of the information contained on one side (e.g., "position on the Middle East"), but subjects had to turn the card over to read the information. This allowed Herstein to trace the order in which information was accessed—a far more detailed record than is possible with any post hoc report from a voter. He also asked subjects to "think aloud" while they went about making their vote choice so that a verbal record of the thought processes could be recorded. Because exactly comparable information was available about each candidate, Herstein could determine whether information search was mostly intraitem (i.e., the same information was accessed about each candidate) or intracandidate (i.e., a variety of different information was assessed about one candidate, then information was gathered about the other candidate). His results showed much more intraitem searching than intracandidate searching, which led him to prefer a memory-based "moment-of-decision" model rather than an on-line "running-evaluation" model of the vote choice. Evidence from the verbal protocols further supported the moment-of-decision model: There were few (less than one, on the average) overall evaluative statements per protocol (which one would expect from a running-evaluation model), but many particular evaluative statements (e.g., "I like that stand"—an average of 9.5 per protocol).

This led Herstein to propose the following model. People gather information about candidates without necessarily forming evaluations of the candidates as they go. At some unspecified "choice point," overall evaluations of both candidates are formed. If one evaluation is negative and the other is positive or neutral, the voter chooses the non-negatively evaluated candidate. If neither candidate is negatively evaluated, the person compares the candidates on a few salient bits of information and votes for the candidate preferred on these items. If both candidates are negatively evaluated, the model predicts abstention.

Lodge et al. (1989) used a variant on their Congressman Williams experiments to explore the same question, which they pose as a distinction between a "memory-based" and an "impression-based" strategy for candidate evaluation. A memory-based strategy suggests that when people make an evaluation (of a political candidate, for instance), they recall as much information as is possible about that person and then base their evaluation on the recalled information. This is Herstein's moment-of-decision model. If this strategy is employed, one should observe a correlation between the valence of the information recalled and the evaluation of the person in question. An impression-based strategy, on the other hand, suggests that people keep a "running total" or "running evaluation" of a person that is constantly updated as new information is gathered. Thus evaluation occurs naturally, almost inevitably. This running total is entered into long-term memory, and when one is asked for an evaluation of the person in question, it is a simple matter to retrieve the total score. Any additional information recalled about the person would not be a particularly good indicator of that summary evaluation, however, because memory of specific bits of information may be based on factors (e.g., salience) that have little to do with evaluation. Thus the impression-based strategy predicts no correlation between valence of the information recalled and overall evaluation (see also Hastie & Park, 1986).

I do not have the space to go into all the details of this experiment, but the crucial manipulation involved instructions to subjects telling them what to do while reading about Congressman Williams. A quarter of the subjects were asked to rate each policy statement made by Williams in terms of its "readability." These instructions were designed to discourage subjects from making an evaluation of Williams while they were learning about him, thus forcing them to use a memory-based strategy when later they were asked to evaluate Williams. The remaining subjects were in one of three impression-based conditions. The initial description of Williams in this experiment contained a one-sentence evaluation by the "Troy Civic Association" designed to create an initial positive, neutral, or negative impression of Williams. Then subjects read the 40 policy statements, but evaluated them in terms of how much they personally liked the statements. These instructions were designed to encourage the use of an "on-line operator" to keep a running total of the current evaluation of Williams.

As predicted, subjects' evaluations of the policy statements they could remember Congressman Williams making correlated with their evaluation of him only in the memory-based condition. Because the memory-based condition was artificially designed to prevent the formation of an on-line evaluation, we must conclude that normal candidate evaluation processes would involve such on-line evaluation, and thus voters' reports of why they preferred one candidate over another would not be a very good indicator of the actual reasons for candidate evaluation. Thus Lodge et al. (1989) reach conclusions that are directly at odds with those of Herstein (1981). One way to reconcile this discrepancy is to assume that the short biography of Congressman Williams and the initial description of him provided by the Troy Civic Association made the stimulus object in Lodge et al.'s experiment more familiar than the candidates in Herstein's experiment. Ostrom, Prior, and Simpson (1981) found that social information is more likely to be organized in memory in terms of persons when those persons are familiar than when they are unfamiliar. Thus differences in familiarity could account for the differences between Herstein's findings and Lodge et al.'s results.

SUMMARY: RECONCILING MOTIVATION AND COGNITION

This chapter has argued that the two dominant paradigms of political behavior research must both be revised in light of advances in political cognition research. There is nothing inherently wrong or unrealistic about the Michigan approach. It presents a reasonable model of political behavior, although it could now be greatly expanded in light of new theories of social cognition. Party identification is probably still the most important influence on the vote decision (even if it has declined in importance since the time *The American Voter* was written—see Beck, 1977, or Wattenberg, 1981; see also Miller, 1986, for a schematic interpretation of this decline), but it is important in ways that the Michigan model does not delineate very well. Party identification is not so much a standing decision as it is a very valuable heuristic that summarizes much important political information and allows people to make reasonable inferences in a very ambiguous political environment. Similarly, as Converse (1964, 1970) has argued, the average citizen does not have the well-defined, tightly constrained liberal or conservative ideology that political elites have. But citizens do have political belief systems that are not totally idiosyncratic (i.e., similar belief systems are held by large groups of people); they may contain only a subset of the information and structure of an elite's ideology, but they nonetheless serve the purpose of a political belief system—to help make sense of politics.

I cannot be as sanguine in my view of the economic/rational-choice model. The basic self-interest motivation underlying it seems not to be very important for most political behavior, and its cognitive requirements for rational decision making are clearly unrealistic. It continues to have many advocates, however, and it continues to make reasonable predictions, although in most cases those predictions are based on "auxiliary assumptions" (e.g., about actors' goals) that have nothing to do with rationality per se (Simon, 1985). The political cognition models that have been reviewed here are much more cognitively realistic than even those rational-choice models that are most aware of "information costs" and other cognitive limitations (e.g., Fiorina, 1981). But none of the political cognition models have anywhere near the mathematical precision that is necessary for extensive deductive reasoning and theory building, a major advantage of the rational-choice model.

If the organization of this chapter has created the impression in the casual reader that motivation and cognition in political behavior research are distinct, again let me correct that impression. Both the Michigan approach and the economic/rational-choice approach combine features that are clearly cognitive and clearly motivational. Indeed, both are necessary for a full understanding of any phenomenon as complicated as politics, and frequently the explicit combination of the two answers questions that cannot be addressed by ignoring either one.

Recall the classic "surge and decline" interpretation of the incumbent president's party losing seats in Congress at midterm elections (Campbell, 1962). Kernell (1977) has offered an alternative explanation for this phenomenon, one based on negative voting rather than coattail effects. According to Kernell, public opinion punishes presidents for their failures but does not comparably reward them for their successes. Using Gallup poll data from 1948 to 1970, Kernell has shown that people who disapprove of the president's job performance are more likely to turn out and vote in off-year elections than are those who approve of his job performance. And those who do vote are more likely to be negative voters. For example, members of the president's party who disapprove of his job performance are more likely to defect and vote for a Congressional candidate of the opposite party than are members of the opposite party who approve of the president's job performance. Similarly, Congressional candidates from the president's party typically receive less support from members of their own party who approve of the president's job performance, compared to the support that Congressional candidates from the other party get from members of that party who disapprove of the job the president is doing. I (Lau, 1982) extended Kernell's theory to the perception of presidential candidates, using the amount of positive and negative information respondents offered as to why they might vote for and against each candidate as the independent variables and affective "feeling thermometer" evaluations of the candidates as the dependent variables. As hypothesized, negative information had a much stronger effect on predicting evaluations of presidential candidates than positive information.

Of more concern to us here are possible explanations for negative voting. I offer two: one based on a motivational "cost orientation," an almost biological or genetic tendency to be more concerned about possible losses than possible gains; the other based on more perceptual, figure–ground processes that make negative information stand out against a generally positive background (Lau, 1985b). Cost orientation is measured by a single question about whether respondents "care" about the outcome of the election (clearly a motivational concept), whereas the perceptual process (the "ground") is determined by a five-item "trust-in-government" scale that measures how strongly a respondent believes that people in Washington "know what they are doing" and "can be trusted to do what is right." I hypothesize that perceptual processes will best explain negative voting in Congressional elections, when potential costs and gains are relatively low (after all, each member of the House has only 1/435th of the votes), but that motivational processes will better explain negativity in perceptions of presidential candidates during presidential campaigns, because presidents can affect people's lives much more dramatically than can Congressmen (and thus potential costs and benefits resulting from the outcome of the election are much higher). I have found clear support for these hypotheses in survey data from the elections of 1968 through 1980. Specifically, the effect of negative information on the evaluation of presidential candidates was much greater than the effect of positive information among those who cared about the outcome of the election than among those who did not care about the outcome of the election, whereas no differences were found for turnout and vote choice in congressional elections. On the other hand, the difference in the size of the effect of turnout and vote preference in congressional elections between those who disapproved rather than approved of the job the president was doing was much greater among those with a diffuse trust in government than among those who generally distrusted those in government. This same perceptual process influenced the effect of positive and negative information on evaluations of presidential candidates, although the effect was notably weaker compared to the motivational process described above.

Let us also consider the surprising conclusion that self-interest rarely has important political consequences. Are there special conditions or circumstances under which people's political behavior is motivated by self-interest? Research (Brody & Sniderman, 1977; Lau & Sears, 1981) suggests one such circumstance: People who attribute responsibility to the president for changes in their financial status do appear to be self-interested voters. Such attributions are relatively rare, given the American ethic of self-reliance (Sniderman & Brody, 1977); when they are made, however, there is clear evidence of greater self-interested voting. Making attributions involves a cognitive, thoughtful, reasoned process, so here is another case in which combining cognitive and motivational concerns increases our understanding of political questions.

Neither of these examples involve the application of more recent information-processing theories to political behavior. It is true that research in political cognition, like much research in social cognition, tends to ignore motivation. Lane (1986) clearly notes the absence of motivation (or "purpose") in political cognition, and finds it lamentable. As he puts it,

> People are doing more than trying "to organize their political world"; . . . they are making their thoughts more comfortable to themselves; they are watching with a sports fan's eye and passion, impressing others, evaluating a process that, in the end, they cherish; and they are trying to understand and achieve something beyond the election that requires them to enlist their theories, interpret government boundaries and capabilities, and decide who should get what, themselves included. Each of these purposes will give color and tone, transience or durability, shape and content to their political schemata. (Lane, 1986, pp. 316–317)

The Lodge et al. (1989) article is the one example of political cognition research in which different goals clearly lead to different information-processing strategies. However, this only captures a little of what Lane means by "purpose." I doubt that any information-processing theory will ever be able to model the broader meaning of "purpose" that Lane has in mind. But I join him in calling for more progress in this direction.

Let me conclude with one final point about political cognition research. On one level, politics are a very important part of all of our lives. They do determine "who gets what, when, and where"; they help determine the very structure of society. But on another level—a very immediate, day-to-day level—they are at the periphery. In general, psychologists study the more immediate, the day-to-day phenomena. And politics is much more complicated, more ambiguous, more difficult to understand than is most of what psychologists (and certainly cognitive psychologists) study. Political behavior researchers must be careful in borrowing the methods of cognitive psychologists and applying them to politics, because the "fit" may be poor.

An inappropriate methodology may explain the discrepancy in the results of Herstein (1981) and Lodge et al. (1989). Any experiment has some artificiality built into it, but Herstein's paradigm is particularly vulnerable to this criticism. With all information about candidates displayed on information boards, not only is the total sum of the available information easily seen before any of it is processed in detail, and not only is the *same* information available about both candidates, but all information is equally difficult (or easy) to obtain.

None of these conditions is ever true in a real campaign, and it is therefore unclear how generalizable Herstein's results are to an actual political campaign. For example, a reasonable strategy for subjects in his experiment to follow is to look at all the available information and plot out a strategy for accessing the type of information they care about, holding off making evaluations until all relevant information is obtained. Such a strategy is only feasible when one can see all the information that might be obtained, but it is unlikely to be followed in the information environment of a typical political campaign. Likewise, schema-based inferences are made about candidates' issue stands because information is ambiguous or difficult to obtain, but there is no need for such inferences within Herstein's paradigm.

This is not to say that one cannot learn anything from the information search methodologies that have been developed by cognitive psychologists and behavioral decision theorists.[12] But one must either revise the basic research strategies so that they better fit the realities of politics and political campaigns, or be very careful in the inferences drawn from the results.

Notes

1. Some of these theories were basically motivational (e.g., Bentham, Mill), whereas others were much more cognitive (e.g., Descartes, Kant, Leibniz, Spinoza). See Lau (1985a) for a brief review.

2. When parents differ in their party identification, there is some evidence that the children are more likely to adopt their mother's party identification than their father's party identification. As Sears (1975) put it, while the fathers are out proselytizing the world, the mothers are home subverting the children.

3. The Democrats regained none of their lost Senate seats in 1982. The odds were stacked in the Republicans' favor in the Senate that year, however, because only 13 of the 33 Senate seats up for re-election were held by Republicans. Hence the Democrats had relatively few targets to try to defeat. (In fact, one Republican and one Democratic incumbent were defeated, so there was no net change.) In subsequent elections the odds shifted the other way, and by 1986—the second off-year election of the Reagan administration—the Democrats recaptured the Senate.

4. People are assumed to be short-sighted mainly because the future is very difficult to predict with any certainty. However, "self-interested" goals must be defined in such a tangible, material, short-term manner, or the term becomes nonfalsifiable and therefore mostly useless. It can be argued, for example, that bashing one's head against the wall is in the basher's self-interest, or else why would he or she be doing it? This all-encompassing usage of the term is much too broad. Tangible short-term self-interest is not limited solely to financial considerations, however. One's health, one's safety, and one's children's well-being are all clearly part of self-interest as the term is used here.

5. Treating liberalism–conservatism as a symbolic attitude is clearly inconsistent with any definition of liberalism–conservatism that defines it as a tightly constrained, policy-based ideology (e.g., Converse, 1964). Symbolic politics theory treats liberalism–conservatism as a simple affective response ("Liberals are bad," "Conservatives are good," etc.). As such, the meaning is most consistent with Conover and Feldman's (1981) results.

6. Indeed, the rational-choice literature has sketched out the reasons why politicians should actively refrain from taking clear issue stands (see, e.g., Page, 1978; Shepsle, 1972).

7. A closer look at the means raises some questions, however. The biggest difference *should* have come from experts' recalling more inconsistent information than novices; the actual difference, although in the hypothesized direction, was moderate in size (.62). There should have been relatively small differences between experts and novices in the recall of consistent information, but in fact the observed differences were larger (.85). To view the results in another light, there was a slight tendency for experts to recall more inconsistent information than consistent information (.28), but a much larger tendency for novices to recall more consistent information than inconsistent information (1.19). These data are more compatible with an input orientation model (Higgins & Bargh, 1987),

which states that whereas experts are interested in forming an impression, novices are more interested in confirming a prior impression.

8. We (Lau & Erber, 1985) also reported an expert–novice difference between the stability of respondents' opinions on only one of four political issues, and no differences on their integrity ratings of the three candidates. With the exception of the question of greater defense spending (one of the issues for which no expert–novice differences on stability were found, and one of Ronald Reagan's major campaign issues), there was no new information provided during the campaign on these issues or on the candidates' integrity, and therefore there was no reason for either experts or novices to be tempted to revise their schemas.

9. See Brown (1980) for an elaborate discussion of *Q*-sort methodology.

10. The questions read: "Is there anything in particular about [Democratic candidate] that might make you want to vote *for* him? Is there anything about [Democratic candidate] that might make you want to vote *against* him?" These same questions are repeated about the Republican candidate (and in a few years—e.g., 1968, 1980—about a major third-party candidate). Typically, these questions have been preceded by an analogous set of questions asking respondents what they like and dislike about the two major parties. I have utilized these same open-ended questions in my work on political chronicities (Lau, 1986, 1989), to be discussed below.

11. This "inversely-weighted-proportion" method controls for verbosity by dividing the weighted counts by similarly weighted counts of the total number of responses to the open-ended questions, regardless of the content of the response. I (Lau, 1989) have also employed a straight count of the number of responses falling into each of the four hypothesized categories, without any inverse weighting and without any control for verbosity. The disadvantages of the inversely-weighted-proportion method are two: First, there is some "built-in" negative correlation between the measures of the different categories because the higher the proportion of responses that fall into one category, the lower *ceteris paribus* the proportions of responses that can fall into the other categories. (The negative correlation is not perfect, because all responses do not fall into one of the four categories.) Second, the inversely-weighted-proportion method equates one out of one response falling into a particular category with six out of six responses falling into that category, when in fact we might believe that the latter respondent has a "stronger" or more accessible chronicity. As it turns out, however, both the inversely-weighted-proportion method and a straight counting method produce equivalent results. In subsequent work (Fiske et al., 1990; Lau, Smith, & Fiske, 1988), I have continued to employ the inversely-weighted-proportion method because a straight count does not control for verbosity, and the effect of education and political experience on the constructs measured by the straight counting method is substantial (explaining between 10% and 60% of the variance of the chronicity measures); in addition, the inversely-weighted-proportion method produces a summary measure with more variance, which is an advantage with smaller samples.

12. Herstein has been very considerate in sharing his materials with me, and I have already begun to explore information search strategies during political campaigns.

References

Abramowitz, A. I., & Segal, J. A. (1986). Determinants of the outcomes of U.S. Senate elections. *Journal of Politics, 48,* 433–439.

Adorno, T. W., Frenkel-Brunswik, E., Levinson, D. J., & Sanford, R. N. (1950). *The authoritarian personality.* New York: Harper & Row.

Arcelus, F., & Meltzer, A. H. (1975). The effect of aggregate economic conditions on Congressional elections. *American Political Science Review, 69,* 1232–1239.

Barber, J. D. (1985). *The presidential character: Predicting performance in the White House.* Englewood Cliffs, NJ: Prentice-Hall.

Bargh, J. A., & Pratto, F. (1986). Individual construct accessibility and perceptual selection. *Journal of Experimental Social Psychology, 22,* 293–311.

Bargh, J. A., & Thein, R. D. (1985). Individual construct accessibility, person memory, and the recall–

judgment link: The case of information overload. *Journal of Personality and Social Psychology, 49*, 1129–1146.

Beck, P. (1977). Partisan realignment in the postwar South. *American Political Science Review, 71*, 477–496.

Bloom, H. S., & Price, H. D. (1975). Comment. *American Political Science Review, 64*, 1240–1254.

Bolland, J. M. (1985). The structure of political cognition: A new approach to its meaning and measurement. *Political Behavior, 7*, 248–265.

Boyd, R. W. (1972). Popular control of public policy: A normal vote analysis of the 1968 election. *American Political Science Review, 66*, 429–449.

Brent, E., & Granberg, D. (1982). Subjective agreement with the presidential candidates of 1976 and 1980. *Journal of Personality and Social Psychology, 42*, 393–403.

Brody, R., & Sniderman, P. (1977). From life space to polling place: The relevance of personal concerns for voting behavior. *British Journal of Political Science, 7*, 337–360.

Brown, S. R. (1980). *Political subjectivity: Applications of Q methodology in political science*. New Haven, CT: Yale University Press.

Campbell, A. (1962). Surge and decline: A study of electoral change. In A. Campbell, P. S. Converse, W. S. Miller, & D. E. Stokes (Eds.), *Elections and the political order* (pp. 40–62). New York: Wiley.

Campbell, A., Converse, P. S., Miller, W. S., & Stokes, D. E. (1960). *The American voter*. New York: Wiley.

Campbell, A., Gurin, G., & Miller, W. S. (1954). *The voter decides*. Evanston, IL: Row, Peterson.

Campbell, J. E. (1985). Explaining presidential losses in midterm Congressional elections. *Journal of Politics, 47*, 1140–1157.

Chase, W. G., & Simon, H. A. (1973). Perception in chess. *Cognitive Psychology, 4*, 55–81.

Chi, M. T. H., & Koeske, R. (1983). Network representation of a child's dinosaur knowledge. *Developmental Psychology, 19*, 29–39.

Christie, R., & Jahoda, M. (Eds.). (1954). *Studies in the scope and method of "The authoritarian personality."* New York: Free Press.

Conover, P. J., & Feldman, S. (1981). The origins and meaning of liberal/conservative self-identifications. *American Journal of Political Science, 25*, 617–645.

Conover, P. J., & Feldman, S. (1984). How people organize the political world: A schematic model. *American Journal of Political Science, 28*, 95–126.

Conover, P. J., & Feldman, S. (1986). The role of inference in the perception of political candidates. In R. R. Lau & D. O. Sears (Eds.), *Political cognition: The 19th annual Carnegie Symposium on Cognition* (pp. 127–155). Hillsdale, NJ: Erlbaum.

Conover, P. J., & Feldman, S. (1989). Candidate perception in an ambiguous world: Campaigns, cues, and inference processes. *American Journal of Political Science, 33*, 912–940.

Converse, P. E. (1964). The nature of belief systems in mass publics. In D. E. Apter (Ed.), *Ideology and discontent* (pp. 206–261). London: Collier-Macmillan.

Converse, P. E. (1970). Attitudes and non-attitudes: Continuation of a dialogue. In E. R. Tufte (Ed.), *The quantitative analysis of social problems* (pp. 168–189). Reading, MA: Addison-Wesley.

Davis, O., Hinch, M., & Ordeshook, P. (1970). An expository development of a mathematical model of the electoral process. *American Political Science Review, 64*, 426–448.

Downs, A. (1957). *An economic theory of democracy*. New York: Harper & Row.

Erikson, E. H. (1942). Hitler's imagery and German youth. *Psychiatry, 5*, 475–493.

Fiorina, M. (1981). *Retrospective voting in American national elections*. New Haven, CT: Yale University Press.

Fiske, S. T., Kinder, D. R., & Larter, W. M. (1983). The novice and the expert: Knowledge-based strategies in political cognition. *Journal of Experimental Social Psychology, 19*, 381–400.

Fiske, S. T., Lau, R. R., & Smith, R. A. (1990). On the variety and utility of political knowledge structures. *Social Cognition, 8*, 31–48.

Fiske, S. T., & Taylor, S. E. (1984). *Social cognition*. Reading, MA: Addison-Wesley.

Freud, S. (1961). *Civilization and its discontents* (J. Strachey, Trans.). New York: Norton. (Original work published 1930)

Fromm, E. (1941). *Escape from freedom*. New York: Holt, Rinehart & Winston.

Gatlin, D. S., Giles, M. W., & Cataldo, E. F. (1978). Policy support within a target group: The case of school desegregation. *American Political Science Review, 72*, 985-995.

George, A. L., & George, J. L. (1956). *Woodrow Wilson and Colonel House: A personality study*. New York: Day.

Goodman S., & Kramer, G. H. (1975). Comment on Arcelus and Meltzer, "The effect of aggregate economic conditions on Congressional elections." *American Political Science Review, 69*, 1255-1265.

Hamill, R., & Lodge, M. (1986). Cognitive consequences of political sophistication. In R. R. Lau & D. O. Sears (Eds.), *Political cognition: The 19th annual Carnegie Symposium on Cognition* (pp. 69-93). Hillsdale, NJ: Erlbaum.

Hamill, R., Lodge, M., & Blake, F. (1985). The breadth, depth, and utility of class, partisan, and ideological schemata. *American Journal of Political Science, 29*, 850-870.

Hastie, R., & Park, B. (1986). The relationship between memory and judgment depends on whether the task is memory-based or on-line. *Psychological Review, 93*, 258-268.

Herstein, J. A. (1981). Keeping the voter's limits in mind: A cognitive process analysis of decision making in voting. *Journal of Personality and Social Psychology, 40*, 843-861.

Higgins, E. T., & Bargh, J. A. (1987). Social cognition and social perception. *Annual Review of Psychology, 38*, 369-425.

Higgins, E. T., & King, G. A. (1981). Accessibility of social constructs: Information-processing consequences of individual and contextual variability. In N. Cantor & J. F. Kihlstrom (Eds.), *Personality, cognition, and social interaction* (pp. 69-121). Hillsdale, NJ: Erlbaum.

Higgins, E. T., King, G. A., & Mavin, G. H. (1982). Individual construct accessibility and subjective impression and recall. *Journal of Personality and Social Psychology, 42*, 35-47.

Kernell, S. (1977). Presidential popularity and negative voting: An alternative explanation of the midterm Congressional decline of the president's party. *American Political Science Review, 71*, 44-65.

Kernell, S. (1978). Explaining presidential popularity. *American Political Science Review, 72*, 506-522.

Key, V. O., Jr. (with the assistance of M. Cummings, Jr.). (1966). *The responsible electorate: Rationality in presidential voting, 1936-1960*. Cambridge, MA: Belknap Press.

Kinder, D. R. (1978). Political person perception: The asymmetrical influences of sentiment and choice on perceptions of presidential candidates. *Journal of Personality and Social Psychology, 36*, 859-871.

Kinder, D. R. (1981). Presidents, prosperity, and public opinion. *Public Opinion Quarterly, 45*, 1-21.

Kinder, D. R., & Kiewiet, D. R. (1979). Economic discontent and political behavior: The role of personal grievances and collective economic judgments in Congressional voting. *American Journal of Political Science, 23*, 495-527.

Kinder, D. R., & Kiewiet, D. R. (1981). Sociotropic politics. *British Journal of Political Science, 11*, 129-161.

Kinder, D. R., & Rhodebeck, L. A. (1982). Continuities in support for racial equality, 1972-1976. *Public Opinion Quarterly, 46*, 195-215.

Kinder, D. R., & Sears, D. O. (1981). Prejudice and politics: Symbolic racism versus racial threats to the good life. *Journal of Personality and Social Psychology, 40*, 414-431.

Kramer, G. (1971). Short-term fluctuations in U.S. voting behavior, 1896-1964. *American Political Science Review, 65*, 131-143.

Lane, R. E. (1962). *Political ideology: Why the American common man believes what he does*. New York: Free Press.

Lane, R. E. (1969). *Political thinking and consciousness*. Chicago: Markham.

Lane, R. E. (1986). What are people trying to do with their schemata: The question of purpose. In R. R. Lau & D. O. Sears (Eds.), *Political cognition: The 19th annual Carnegie Symposium on Cognition* (pp. 303-317). Hillsdale, NJ: Erlbaum.

Larkin, J. H., McDermott, H., Simon, D. P., & Simon, H. A. (1980). Models of competence in solving physics problems. *Science, 208,* 1335–1342.

Lasswell, H. D. (1930). *Psychopathology and politics.* New York: Norton.

Lasswell, H. D. (1948). *Power and personality.* New York: Norton.

Lau, R. R. (1982). Negativity in political perception. *Political Behavior, 4,* 353–378.

Lau, R. R. (1985a). *Changing perspectives on political thinking.* Paper presented at the annual meeting of the American Political Science Association, New Orleans.

Lau, R. R. (1985b). Two explanations for negativity effects in political behavior. *American Journal of Political Science, 29,* 119–138.

Lau, R. R. (1986). Political schemata, candidate evaluations and voting behavior. In R. R. Lau & D. O. Sears (Eds.), *Political cognition: The 19th annual Carnegie Symposium on Cognition* (pp. 95–126). Hillsdale, NJ: Erlbaum.

Lau, R. R. (1989). Construct accessibility and electoral choice. *Political Behavior, 11,* 5–32.

Lau, R. R., Brown, T. A., & Sears, D. O. (1978). Self-interest and civilians' attitudes toward the Vietnam war. *Public Opinion Quarterly, 42,* 464–483.

Lau, R. R., & Erber, R. (1985). Political sophistication: An information-processing perspective. In S. Kraus & R. M. Perloff (Eds.), *Mass media and political thought: An information-processing approach* (pp. 37–64). Beverly Hills, CA: Sage.

Lau, R. R., & Sears, D. O. (1981). Cognitive links between economic grievances and political response. *Political Behavior, 3,* 279–302.

Lau, R. R., & Sears, D. O. (1986). Social cognition and political cognition: The past, the present, and the future. In R. R. Lau & D. O. Sears (Eds.), *Political cognition: The 19th annual Carnegie Symposium on Cognition* (pp. 347–366). Hillsdale, NJ: Erlbaum.

Lau, R. R., Smith, R. A., & Fiske, S. T. (1988). *Political beliefs, policy interpretations, and political persuasion.* Paper presented at the annual meeting of the American Political Science Association, Washington, DC.

Lewin, K. (1939). Field theory and experiments in social psychology: Concepts and methods. *American Journal of Sociology, 44,* 868–896.

Lewin, K. (1951). *Field theory in social science.* New York: Harper & Row.

Lewis-Beck, M. S. (1986). Comparative economic voting: Britain, France, Germany, Italy. *American Journal of Political Science, 30,* 315–346.

Lewis-Beck, M. S., & Rice, T. W. (1984). Forecasting U.S. House elections. *Legislative Studies Quarterly, 9,* 475–486.

Lewis-Beck, M. S., & Rice, T. W. (1985). Are Senate election outcomes predictable? *PS, 18,* 746–754.

Lodge, M., & Hamill, R. (1986). A partisan schema for political information processing. *American Political Science Review, 80,* 505–519.

Lodge, M., McGraw, K., & Stroh, P. (1989). An impression-driven model of candidate evaluation. *American Political Science Review, 83,* 399–419.

Maslow, A. H. (1943). Authoritarian character structure. *Journal of Social Psychology, 18,* 401–411.

Mazlish, B. (1972). *In search of Nixon: A psychohistorical inquiry.* New York: Basic Books.

McConahay, J. B. (1982). Self-interest versus racial attitudes as correlates of anti-busing attitudes in Louisville. *Journal of Politics, 44,* 692–720.

McKeithen, K. B., Reitman, J. S., Rueter, H. H., & Hirtle, S. C. (1981). Knowledge organization and skill differences in computer programmers. *Cognitive Psychology, 13,* 307–325.

Miller, A. H. (1986). Partisan cognitions in transition. In R. R. Lau & D. O. Sears (Eds.), *Political cognition: The 19th annual Carnegie Symposium on Cognition* (pp. 203–231). Hillsdale, NJ: Erlbaum.

Miller, A. H., Miller, W. E., Raine, A. S., & Brown, T. A. (1976). A majority party in disarray: Policy polarization in the 1972 election. *American Political Science Review, 70,* 753–778.

Miller, A. H., Wattenberg, M. P., & Malanchuk, O. (1986). Schematic assessments of presidential candidates. *American Political Science Review, 80,* 521–540.

Monroe, K. R. (1979). Econometric analyses of electoral behavior: A critical review. *Political Behavior, 1,* 137–173.

Monroe, K. R. (1983). *The blinding light of rationality and the dark areas of political economy: The need for theoretical clarification.* Paper presented at the annual meeting of the Midwest Political Science Association, Chicago.

Nie, N. H., Verba, S., & Petrocik, J. R. (1976). *The changing American voter.* Cambridge, MA: Harvard University Press.

Ostrom, T. M., Pryor, J. B., & Simpson, D. D. (1981). The organization of social information. In E. T. Higgins, C. P. Herman, & M. P. Zanna (Eds.), *Social cognition: The Ontario Symposium* (Vol. 1, pp. 3–38). Hillsdale, NJ: Erlbaum.

Page, B. I. (1978). *Choices and echoes in presidential elections.* Chicago: University of Chicago Press.

Piaget, J., & Inhelder, B. (1973). *Memory and intelligence.* New York: Basic Books.

Pomper, G. M. (1972). From confusion to clarity: Issues and American voters. *American Political Science Review, 66,* 415–428.

Reich, W. (1946). *The mass psychology of fascism* (3rd ed.). New York: Orgone Press. (Original work published 1933)

Riker, W., & Ordeshook, P. C. (1968). A theory of the calculus of voting. *American Political Science Review, 62,* 25–42.

Rumelhart, D. E., & Ortony, A. (1977). The representation of knowledge in memory. In R. C. Anderson et al. (Eds.), *Schooling and the acquisition of knowledge* (pp. 99–135). Hillsdale, NJ: Erlbaum.

Sanford, N. (1973). Authoritarian personality in contemporary perspective. In J. N. Knudson (Ed.), *Handbook of political psychology* (pp. 139–170). San Francisco: Jossey-Bass.

Sears, D. O. (1975). Political socialization. In F. I Greenstein & N. W. Polsby (Eds.), *Handbook of political science* (Vol. 2, pp. 93–153). Reading, MA: Addison-Wesley.

Sears, D. O., & Citrin, J. (1985). *Tax revolt: Something for nothing in California* (enlarged ed.). Cambridge, MA: Harvard University Press.

Sears, D. O., Hensler, C. P., & Speer, L. K. (1979). Whites' opposition to "busing": Self-interest or symbolic politics? *American Political Science Review, 73,* 369–384.

Sears, D. O., Lau, R. R., Tyler, T. R., & Allen, H. M. (1980). Self-interest vs. symbolic politics in policy attitudes and presidential voting. *American Political Science Review, 74,* 670–684.

Sears, D. O., Tyler, T. R., Citrin, J., & Kinder, D. R. (1978). Political system support and public response to the energy crisis. *American Journal of Political Science, 22,* 56–82.

Shapiro, M. J. (1969). Rational political man: A synthesis of economic and social-psychological perspectives. *American Political Science Review, 63,* 1106–1119.

Sharp, C., & Lodge, M. (1985). Partisan and ideological belief systems: Do they differ? *Political Behavior, 7,* 147–166.

Shepsle, K. (1972). The strategy of ambiguity: Uncertainty and electoral competition. *American Political Science Review, 66,* 555–568.

Simon, H. A. (1985). Human nature in politics: The dialogue of psychology with political science. *American Political Science Review, 79,* 293–304.

Smith, M. B., Bruner, J. S., & White, R. W. (1956). *Opinions and personality.* New York: Wiley.

Sniderman, P. M., & Brody, R. A. (1977). Coping: The ethic of self-reliance. *American Journal of Political Science, 21,* 501–521.

Sorrentino, R. M., Bobocel, R., Gitta, M. Z., Olson, J. M., & Hewitt, E. C. (1988). Uncertainty orientation and persuasion: Individual differences in the effects of personal relevance on social judgments. *Journal of Personality and Social Psychology, 55,* 357–371.

Stigler, G. (1973). General economic conditions and national elections. *American Economic Review, 63,* 160–167.

Taylor, S. E., & Crocker, J. (1981). Schematic bases of social information processing. In E. T. Higgins, C. P. Herman, & M. P. Zanna (Eds.), *Social cognition: The Ontario Symposium* (Vol. 1, pp. 89–134). Hillsdale, NJ: Erlbaum.

Tetlock, P. E. (1983). Cognitive style and political ideology. *Journal of Personality and Social Psychology, 45,* 118–126.

Tetlock, P. E. (1984). Cognitive style and political belief systems in the British House of Commons. *Journal of Personality and Social Psychology, 46*, 365–375.

Tufte, E. R. (1973). The relationship between seats and votes in two-party systems. *American Political Science Review, 67*, 540–554.

Tufte, E. R. (1975). Determinants of the outcomes of midterm Congressional elections. *American Political Science Review, 69*, 812–826.

Wattenberg, M. P. (1981). The decline of political partisanship in the United States: Negativity or neutrality? *American Political Science Review, 75*, 941–950.

Weatherford, M. S. (1988). *Self-interest, commitment, and economic policy choice.* Paper presented at the annual meeting of the American Political Science Association, Washington, DC.

PART III

Motivation and Cognition in Understanding Self and Others

CHAPTER 10

Motivations for Judging and Knowing
Implications for Causal Attribution

ARIE W. KRUGLANSKI
University of Maryland–College Park

The historical relation between motivational and informational factors in social-cognitive theory has been one of uneasy tension (Tetlock & Levi, 1982). Early on, motivation was portrayed as an irrational influence on judgment, often responsible for serious biases and misrepresentations. Thus, the predominantly "motivational" models of cognitive consistency (such as dissonance or balance) were assumed to reflect an image of an irrational person, whose cognitive process is distorted by powerful wishes and desires (Festinger, 1957; Heider, 1958). By contrast, information was typically regarded as a rational influence, one that enhances judgmental accuracy or veridicality. Thus, in attribution theory (e.g., Kelley, 1967), laypersons are thought to examine various informational patterns in semiscientific ways, and to reach largely rational judgments about causal relationships.

Such disparate models of the human cognitive process naturally raise the question of their relative validity. In the late 1960s and early 1970s, this issue inspired a heated dispute between dissonance theorists (representing the motivational perspective) and proponents of Bem's self-perception theory (representing the informational perspective; see Bem, 1972, for a discussion of this particular controversy). Alternatively, it is possible to ask under what conditions the motivational or the informational influence would prevail. A notable attempt to delineate the boundary conditions for motivational and informational effects was undertaken by Zanna and Cooper (1976). These authors proposed that under intense arousal, motivational, dissonance-like processes are likely to take effect, whereas in the absence of arousal, judgments are often mediated by the dispassionate information processing depicted in self-perception theory. Thus, an intertheoretic "truce" was proposed, based on a separation of the domains to which motivational versus informational processes were assumed to apply.

The disjunction between motivational and informational influences has had *intra-* as well as *inter*theoretic implications. A particularly interesting case is attribution theory, where no satisfactory integration of motivational and informational influences has been achieved this far. As already noted, attribution theory has been initially considered an informational approach in which motivation plays no major part. However, though the informational (or cognitive) turn in the

Zeitgeist may have relegated motivational notions to the status of "ground" rather than "figure" in attribution theory, they were nonetheless contained in leading attributional analyses. (Prominent examples are Jones & Davis's [1965, p. 237] concept of "hedonic relevance," and Kelley's [1967, p. 193; 1971, p. 22] notions of "ego-protective tendencies" and of "control motivation.")

Following those early formulations, considerable motivational research in attribution has been carried out. Thus, vigorous work on ego-protective or enhancing attributions has continued under the label of "self-serving" biases, amidst a controversy as to whether these are essentially motivational or informational (Ajzen & Fishbein, 1975; Miller & Ross, 1975; Tetlock & Levi, 1982; Zuckerman, 1979). Further studies have explored the attributional effects of outcome dependency (Berscheid, Graziano, Monson, & Dermer, 1976; Erber & Fiske, 1984; Fiske & Pavelchak, 1986) or of subjects' involvement in an attributional issue (Harvey, Yarkin, Lightner, & Town, 1980; Heller, 1972; Pittman, Schemrer, & Wright, 1977).

Other motivationally relevant lines of attribution research included work on attribute ambiguity (Snyder & Wicklund, 1981), self-handicapping (Arkin & Baumgardner, 1985; Berglas & Jones, 1978; Jones & Pittman, 1982), the effects of control deprivation (Pittman & D'Agostino, 1985), and spontaneously initiated attributional activity (Smith & Miller, 1983; Weiner, 1985).

The foregoing research notwithstanding, the motivational dimension *as such* has not been systematically incorporated with the more informational aspects of attribution. Thus, it has not been made clear whether motivational influences signify a separate route to attributions, juxtaposed to the informational route, or whether motivational and informational factors are parameters of the same process whereby all attributions are rendered. Similarly, it has not been made clear whether the motives typically studied in reference to attributions (viz., needs for control, mastery, esteem, or social approval) are to be considered special, or whether any motive may be potentially relevant to attribution.

The purpose of the present chapter is twofold. The primary objective is to present an integrated model of judgmental activity in which essential roles are assigned to *both* motivational and informational components. The model is based on my theory of lay epistemics (Kruglanski, 1980, 1989; Kruglanski & Ajzen, 1983), which is concerned with the process whereby people form and change their knowledge on different topics. The secondary objective is to apply the model toward a reinterpretation and integration of several motivationally relevant lines of research on causal attributions. The chapter concludes by noting some general implications of the present analysis for further social-cognitive issues.

THE LAY EPISTEMIC PROCESS

The Epistemic Sequence

According to the theory of lay epistemics (see, e.g., Bar-Tal & Bar-Tal, 1988; Kruglanski, 1989; Kruglanski & Ajzen, 1983; Kruglanski & Klar, 1987), knowl-

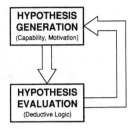

FIGURE 10.1 Schematic representation of the epistemic process.

edge is formed in the course of a two-phase sequence in which hypotheses are generated and evaluated. The epistemic process and the major categories of factors assumed to affect it are schematically depicted in Figure 10.1.

The hypothesis evaluation stage is assumed to be accomplished deductively.[1] The individual departs from a premise linking (in an "if–then" fashion) a given category of evidence with a given hypothesis, and proceeds to infer the hypothesis upon affirming the evidence. However, the deductive evaluation of hypotheses has no unique or natural point of termination. In principle, it should be always possible to generate further alternate hypotheses compatible with the same body of evidence (cf. Campbell, 1969; Weimer, 1979).

Because at most times we possess definite knowledge on various topics, *the epistemic sequence must come to a halt somehow*. Hence, we need to identify the mechanisms that effect the cessation (or, conversely, the initiation or continuation) of the epistemic sequence. The lay epistemic model recognizes two broad categories of such mechanisms, respectively related to notions of cognitive capability and epistemic motivation.

Capability Notions: Availability and Accessibility

Two broad types of capability, long-term and momentary, are sometimes discerned in the social-cognitive literature. Long-term capability to generate hypotheses on a given topic has to do with the concept of "availability" (Higgins, King, & Mavin, 1982). This refers to the individual's general repertory of social knowledge stored in long-term memory. Short-term capability to generate hypotheses on a given topic has to do with the concept of "accessibility" (Bruner, 1957; Higgins, Bargh, & Lombardi, 1985; Higgins & King, 1981; Higgins, Rholes, & Jones, 1977).

Epistemic Motivations: The Closure-Seeking and Specificity Dimensions

The second category of mechanisms related to the initiation, continuation, or cessation of the epistemic sequence has to do with the person's epistemic motivation, defined as motivation toward knowledge as object. Two general issues are addressed from this perspective: whether in a given case knowledge is desired or avoided, and what the characteristics of such knowledge are. Accordingly, epistemic motivations are presently classified on two orthogonal dimensions: "closure seeking versus avoidance," and "specificity versus nonspecificity." The first dimension bears on the issue of whether cognitive closure on an issue is deemed desirable or undesirable. The second dimension has to do with the distinction between motivating features of specific closures versus motivating properties of closure in general. Together, the two distinctions give rise to the 2×2 matrix depicted in Table 10.1, which yields a typology of four motivational orientations: needs *for* nonspecific and specific closure, and needs to *avoid* nonspecific and specific closure. Let us first consider the aspects that the epistemic motivations share in common, and subsequently those on which they differ.

Common Features

All epistemic motivations are assumed to arise from the individual's cost–benefit analysis of given epistemic end states. The perceived costs and benefits are assumed to vary as a function of the situation as well as of the person. For instance, cognitive closure may be perceived as advantageous if a person is under time pressure to reach a decision; in addition, some persons may generally value closure more than others. Furthermore, the perceived costs and benefits may originate from diverse motives. For instance, the costs of lacking closure may relate to the inability to satisfy one's desire for control, or to the lowering of self-esteem when one feels confused on a topic where easy familiarity is commonly assumed (e.g., in matters of etiquette). Such diverse motivational origins of the need for closure are assumed to be functionally equivalent as far as the epistemic process is concerned. For instance, regardless of whether the need for closure originates from considerations of control or self-esteem, its information-processing try to bring uping to avoid double-effects are presumed to be the same.

The epistemic system can be "at rest" or "in motion." From a motivational standpoint, a state of rest may occur in cases of a "match" (i.e., an absence of discrepancy) between actual and desired epistemic states. In such circumstances, the epistemic process is "frozen," hypothesis generation is arrested, and the individual is generally insensitive to further relevant stimulus information on a topic. The system is "unfrozen" or set in motion by a "discrepancy" between actual and desired epistemic states (e.g., a lack of a desired closure). This stimu-

TABLE 10.1   A Two-Dimensional Classification of Epistemic Motivations

Type of motivating closure	Disposition toward closure	
	Avoidance	Seeking
Nonspecific	Need to avoid nonspecific closure	Need for nonspecific closure
Specific	Need to avoid a specific closure	Need for a specific closure

lates hypothesis generation and sharpens the knower's sensitivity to relevant stimulus information (see also Kruglanski & Freund, 1983).

Unique Features

The nonspecific epistemic motivations are unbiased with respect to particular types of knowledge. By contrast, specific epistemic motivations represent particular preferences among knowledge types, and in this sense are biased. Both types of motivation are now described.

NEEDS TO SEEK AND TO AVOID NONSPECIFIC CLOSURE   By "nonspecific closure," I mean *an* answer on a given topic, *any* answer, as compared to confusion or ambiguity. As with all epistemic motivations, the need for nonspecific closure is assumed to be proportionate to the perceived benefits of having such closure and/ or the perceived cost of lacking it. For instance, a potential benefit of nonspecific closure is that it affords predictability and a base for action. Thus, in situations where the importance of predictability and action looms large, need for nonspecific closure is likely to be high. A very different benefit of nonspecific closure derives from the social esteem and prestige accorded the possessors of knowledge. In contexts where such social rewards are salient to the individual (e.g., where he or she is *expected* to have expertise on a topic), a strong need for this type of closure may exist.

A potential cost of lacking nonspecific closure is failing to act or decide on an issue in time to meet an important deadline. Thus, need for nonspecific closure is assumed to be heightened in situations involving time pressure. Alternative costs of lacking nonspecific closure may relate to the perceived effortfulness of information processing (which the possession of closure would have spared the person), reluctance to expend the required effort (e.g., because of a state of fatigue), or the unpleasantness of information processing where the task is dreary and boring.

In addition to situational costs and benefits associated with lacking or having nonspecific closure, respectively, a need for this type of closure may also represent a stable feature of certain personality types. "Authoritarianism" (Adorno, Frenkel-Brunswik, Levinson, & Sanford, 1950) and "dogmatism" (Rokeach, 1960) are individual-difference variables akin to the need for nonspecific closure in their postulated effects on the intolerance for ambiguity (Frenkel-Brunswik, 1949). However, whereas need for nonspecific closure is assumed to be content-free, authoritarianism and dogmatism are typically tied to right-wing and to bipolar (leftist or rightist) political extremism, respectively. Furthermore, whereas authoritarianism or dogmatism is generally assumed to undermine rational decision making, need for nonspecific closure has no such pejorative connotations; in fact, it is considered capable of improving decision quality by occasionally promoting freezing on the correct option.

A more recently identified individual-difference dimension akin to the need for nonspecific closure is "uncertainty orientation" (Sorrentino & Hewitt, 1984; Sorrentino & Short, 1986). A certainty-oriented person is inclined to *maintain* "present clarity about the self or the environment" (Sorrentino & Short, 1986, p. 382), whereas an uncertainty-oriented person seeks to *attain* such clarity through careful processing of relevant information. That is, an uncertainty-oriented person is sensitive to new stimulus information concerning a problem, presumably in order to attain the most valid knowledge possible. By contrast, a certainty-oriented individual is insensitive to new information, because his or her dominant tendency is to maintain current beliefs. In present terms, then, it seems that the certainty-oriented person is primarily motivated to seek nonspecific cognitive closure, whereas the uncertainty-oriented person occupies a more balanced position in which the need for closure is tempered by validity concerns motivating a (temporary) suspension of closure. Thus, an uncertainty-oriented person may exhibit a tension between the desire for nonspecific closure and the need to avoid such closure.

Whether it is aroused situationally or represents a stable personality disposition, the need for nonspecific closure is assumed to affect the epistemic process by facilitating the attainment of such closure. Specifically, a heightened need for nonspecific closure is likely to foster an unfreezing of the epistemic activity, where no initial knowledge existed. However, the same need is assumed to promote freezing (i.e., cessation of epistemic activity once a plausible hypothesis has been advanced and supported by extant evidence; (see Freund, Kruglanski, & Schpitzajzen, 1985; Kruglanski & Ajzen, 1983; Kruglanski & Freund, 1983).

Opposite to the need *for* nonspecific closure is the need to *avoid* nonspecific closure. In fact, those two needs are thought of as opposite poles of a continuum. The need to avoid nonspecific closure is assumed to be proportionate to the perceived benefits of lacking such closure and/or the perceived costs of such closure. The potential benefits of lacking this type of closure may include avoidance of a premature commitment to an invalid opinion, especially where invalidity may bring heavy penalties upon the knower. Furthermore, any judgmental commitment may be perceived as costly because of the unwanted restriction of potential it entails. Snyder and Wicklund (1981) furnish an illuminating discussion of cases in which definite self-knowledge may connote unattractive predictability and dullness; in such instances, persons may prefer to maintain an open mind and eschew closure. In other cases discussed by Snyder and Wicklund, "mystery" may be compatible with a cherished, romantic world view. On those occasions, too, sanguine ambiguity (i.e., lack of closure) may be preferred over somber closure. Wisconsin's Senator William Proxmire articulated such a sentiment clearly. In critically commenting on social-psychological investigations of romantic love, he said: " . . . I believe that 200 million . . . Americans want to leave some things in life a mystery, and right at the top of things we don't want to know is why a man falls in love with a woman and vice versa" (cited in *Wisconsin State Journal*, March 20, 1975).

Thus, the need to avoid nonspecific closure may arise in a variety of situational circumstances; it may also represent a stable personality inclination to shun definite judgment (see, e.g., Hofstede, 1980). Regardless of its particular origin, the need to avoid nonspecific closure is assumed to exert the same effect on the epistemic process—namely, to retard the formation of such closure. Thus, with an absence of this type of closure to begin with (i.e., "ignorance" on a topic), high need to avoid closure would effect a freezing of the epistemic activity, whereas in the presence of early nonspecific closure, high need to avoid closure would promote unfreezing (Kruglanski & Freund, 1983).

NEEDS TO SEEK AND TO AVOID SPECIFIC CLOSURE   Often persons may desire particular answers to their questions; these desires represent needs for specific closure. A need for specific closure is assumed to be proportionate to the perceived benefits of holding a particular belief and/or the perceived costs of failing to hold it. Those costs and benefits may relate to any of the belief's properties— for instance, to its particular contents, which may be flattering or otherwise desirable (Kruglanski & Ajzen, 1983; Kunda, 1987); to its novelty (Berlyne, 1960; Klar, Bar-Tal, & Kruglanski, 1988); or to its apparent creativity. In short, they may relate to any content-related, structural, or formal feature that may appear desirable in given circumstances.[2]

A need for specific closure is assumed to facilitate the attainment of such closure and to retard its modification or dissolution. This means a facilitation of freezing when the desired closure has been formed, and of unfreezing when it has not. For example, a person who surmises that he or she is about to receive a desirable job offer or did well on an exam may be refractory to contrary information, and quick to dismiss alternative, less optimistic interpretations of available evidence. By contrast, someone who entertains the possibility that he or she has contracted a dangerous illness or is about to lose an attractive position may seek out new information that (the person hopes) will be contrary to such undesirable conclusions, and/or may be ready to accept alternative, less negative interpretations of existing evidence.

Often, persons may be motivated to *avoid* specific closures because of the perceived costs of such closures or the perceived benefits of their absence. The need to avoid a specific closure may occasionally represent the need *for* the opposite closure; this may not always be the case, however. Thus, on some occasions individuals may focus on the closure to be avoided and may not be particularly concerned about its positive opposite. In other cases, persons may focus on the closure to be sought and may not be particularly concerned with its negative counterpart. Somewhat similarly, investigators of achievement motivation (e.g., Atkinson & Birch, 1970) have distinguished between individuals who are motivated to avoid failure and those who strive to attain success. In present terms, "failure avoiders" may be persons who shy away from specific closures, asserting that they have failed on some task, whereas "success approachers" may be individuals who seek out specific closures, asserting that they have succeeded. The need to avoid a specific closure is assumed to promote unfreezing when that particular closure exists or is about to form, and freezing when it does not exist.

Perceived benefits or costs of specific closures may vary as a function of the situation. For instance, the perceived benefit of knowing that one has done well on a test, or the cost of knowing that one has failed, is likely to vary according to whether the test is a minor quiz or a major exam. It is also possible that stable individual differences exist with respect to the tendency to discriminate between positively valenced beliefs and neutral or negative beliefs, or between negatively valenced beliefs and neutral or positive beliefs; the former tendency may represent stable individual differences in needs to seek specific closure, and the latter, such differences in needs to avoid specific closure. Those notions are at present speculative and in need of further empirical probing for their substantiation.[3]

Compatibility among the Epistemic Motivations

It is of interest to consider whether the four motivational states just described are mutually compatible or incompatible. Clearly, the desired end states of the various epistemic needs are often incompatible. Thus, one cannot simultaneously seek and avoid closure. Furthermore, the goals of nonspecific and specific closure may occasionally conflict. For instance, a need for nonspecific closure is equally gratified by success or failure information, as either makes a performance outcome unambiguous. By contrast, a need for specific closure may be gratified only by success information, and may be frustrated by failure information.

Although the various epistemic ends are often at odds, they may nonetheless coexist in the same individual's mind. In this sense, then, there is "compatibility." One may simultaneously desire nonspecific closure and the absence of closure, or wish for a specific closure as well as for nonspecific closure—in short, strive to "have one's cake and eat it too." For example, a scientist may desire nonspecific cognitive closure on a problem of interest, yet may concomitantly experience high fear of invalidity stemming from an anticipated criticism of the work by his or her colleagues (inducing a need to avoid nonspecific closure).[4] A request for feedback on a manuscript may be motivated by the writer's genuine interest in a colleague's opinion (representing a need for nonspecific closure), as well as by a strong wish for an approving reaction (representing a need for a specific closure). And so on.

The simultaneous existence of incompatible epistemic goals may create conflict and tension, which presumably are resolved in the direction of the stronger of the opposing forces (cf. Lewin, 1938, 1951). In fact, in natural settings persons may only rarely have a single epistemic goal; more typically, they may experience a *mix* of epistemic motivations (e.g., they may ultimately crave closure while temporarily avoiding it). In such cases, the relative magnitudes of the epistemic forces may affect the extent, direction, and outcome of information gathering. Thus, it is important to understand the effects of each epistemic motivation separately, even if in natural circumstances it often comes blended with other epistemic motivations.

Summary: The Epistemic Motivations Compared and Contrasted

The four motivations described above are assumed to fulfill the same general function of initiating and/or terminating the epistemic activity. In this sense, motivation may fulfill a similar epistemic role to that of cognitive capability (related to the "availability" and "accessibility" factors discussed earlier). Both motivation and capability may affect the individual's tendency to "freeze" on a given knowledge structure, or, conversely, to "unfreeze" and seriously entertain alternate plausible hypotheses or "possible worlds."

Beyond similarity of general function, the epistemic motivations are assumed to vary in their desired end states. The need for nonspecific closure is gratified when *any* closure on a topic is attained; the need for specific closure is gratified when *some* preferred closure is achieved; the need to avoid nonspecific closure is gratified when, generally, *no* one closure seems warranted; and the need to avoid a specific closure is gratified when the formation of a particular belief is averted.

The desired ends of the motivations for closure are illustrated in Figure 10.2, and those of the motivations to avoid closure are depicted in Figure 10.3. In Figure 10.2, the left circle represents a set of closures with property A and the right circle a set of closures with property B. As indicated by the arrows, the need for nonspecific closure is gratified by closures in either set (i.e., A *or* B). By contrast, the need for a specific closure (say, with property A or B) is gratified exclusively via a closure in the corresponding set (A or B, respectively).

In Figure 10.3, absence of closure is represented either by X, the hatched area of overlap between the circles (where closures of types A and B are in competition), or by Y, the stippled area around the circle, signifying the total lack of cognitive structures (hypotheses) on a topic. As shown, a need to avoid nonspecific closure is gratified where either X or Y obtains. By contrast, a need to avoid a specific closure such as A is gratified either by a closure of another type (e.g., B) or by the absence of any closure (X or Y).

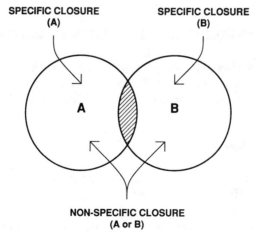

FIGURE 10.2 Desired ends of the needs for specific and nonspecific closure.

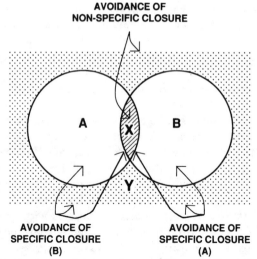

FIGURE 10.3   Desired ends of the needs to avoid nonspecific and specific closure.

All epistemic motivations are assumed to arise from the individual's cost-benefit analysis of given epistemic end states. The perceived costs and benefits may vary as a function of the situation, as well as of stable personality dispositions.[5] A match between actual and desired epistemic states is assumed to "freeze" the epistemic process, whereas a mismatch or a discrepancy is assumed to "unfreeze" it. Finally, although the various epistemic goals are often incompatible, they may be simultaneously entertained by an individual. Such a mix of epistemic motivations may give rise to temporary tension, the particular resolution of which will affect the extent, direction, and outcome of the informational search.

EXPERIMENTAL STUDIES OF EPISTEMIC MOTIVATIONS

In several recent studies, my colleagues and I have tested various implications of the foregoing motivational analysis. The studies differed in the judgmental tasks employed and in the specific predictions tested. This research is briefly described in what follows.

Subjective Confidence

We (Mayseless & Kruglanski, 1987) investigated the phenomenon of subjective confidence as it is affected by the need for nonspecific closure and the need to avoid such closure. In previous analyses, subjective confidence was assumed to depend on the degree of consistency between one's hypothesis and one's evidence: Confidence was assumed to be high when available evidence was consistent with the hypothesis, and to be low when it was inconsistent (see Edwards, 1982; Kelley, 1967; Kruglanski, 1980).

According to the present analysis, however, the individual's cognitive openness to inconsistent data or hypotheses is dynamic rather than static. In particular, it may be affected by the various motivational forces impinging on the individual. Thus, under high fear of invalidity a person may be (temporarily) disposed to avoid cognitive closure[6] and to consider numerous competing interpretations for every received item of information. Such a tendency to ponder multiple competing (and hence inconsistent) hypotheses may well cause the person's confidence in any given hypothesis to wane (cf. Kelley, 1971; Kruglanski, 1980, 1989a). By contrast, with a high need for nonspecific closure, persons' tendency to consider numerous alternate hypotheses may be low, and their confidence in the hypotheses may be correspondingly high. It follows that subjective confidence should be negatively affected by persons' need to avoid nonspecific closure, induced by a fear of invalidity, and positively affected by the need for nonspecific closure.

To test these predictions, we (Mayseless & Kruglanski, 1987, Study 2) had subjects perform a tachistoscopic recognition task of identifying barely visible digits flashed on a screen. In the need-to-avoid-closure condition, subjects were promised extra experimental credits for correctly identifying 9 out of the 10 digits. Theoretically, this was expected to increase the tolerance for ambiguity, and to prompt subjects to entertain numerous possible hypotheses concerning a digit's identity.

In the need-for-closure condition, subjects were given verbal instructions stressing the importance of forming *unambiguous, clear-cut* opinions, an ability said to correlate with "high mental concentration and intelligence" (p. 172). Thus, in the need-for-closure condition, instructions stressed the definiteness and clarity of an opinion and made no reference to the issue of correctness. In addition, a neutral control condition was included, in which no motivational induction was attempted.

Subjects were allowed to operate the tachistoscope an unlimited number of times. Following each presentation, they ventured a hypothesis concerning the digit's identity and rated their confidence in that hypothesis. As shown in Figure 10.4, subjects' confidence in their initial hypothesis, as well as the magnitude of confidence shifts (upward or downward) occasioned by each successive stimulus presentation, was significantly lower in the need-to-avoid-closure condition than in the need-for-closure condition ($p < .05$), with the neutral control condition falling between the two. Finally, subjects' extent of informational search (the number of times they operated the tachistoscope) was higher in the need-to-avoid-closure condition than in the need-for-closure condition ($p < .05$), with the control condition again in the middle.

Hypothesis Generation

Lowered magnitude of initial confidence and of confidence shifts in the need-to-avoid-closure condition of the study described above might have been mediated by

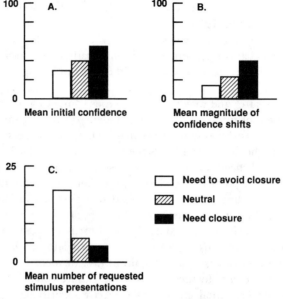

FIGURE 10.4   Effects of epistemic motivations on subjective confidence. From "What Makes You So Sure?: Effects of Epistemic Motivations on Judgmental Confidence" by O. Mayseless and A. W. Kruglanski, 1987, *Organizational Behavior and Human Decision Processes, 39,* 162–183. Copyright 1987 by Academic Press, Inc. Reprinted by permission.

subjects' increased tendency to consider alternative interpretations of the information provided. This process was tapped directly in an additional experiment (Study 3) contained in the same report (Mayseless & Kruglanski, 1987).

Subjects were shown enlarged photographs of parts of common objects; the photos were taken from unusual angles, so the objects were not readily recognizable. Subjects first listed down all conceivable hypotheses concerning an object's identity, then noted their final judgment and their confidence in it. The need-for-closure condition was instituted as in the preceding experiment. The need-to-avoid-closure instructions stated that the "capacity for correct visual recognition has considerable functional significance, and constitutes a component of general intelligence" (p. 176). A neutral control condition was also included.

As shown in Figure 10.5, subjects in the need-to-avoid-closure condition generated more hypotheses on the average than subjects in the neutral condition ($p < .05$), who, in turn, generated more hypotheses than subjects in the need-for-closure condition. These findings accord with the present predictions.

Primacy Effects

"Primacy effects" in impression formation (Asch, 1946) refer to the tendency to base one's impressions of a target more on early than on late information. Such effects may be conceived of as an instance of epistemic "freezing," because they represent early closure and relative insensitivity to subsequent information. If so, primacy effects should be augmented by a heightened need for nonspecific closure, and reduced by a heightened need to avoid nonspecific closure. Those predictions were tested in an experiment (Kruglanski & Freund, 1983, Study 1).

Subjects were presented with serial information about a target, and rated that person's attractiveness as a job candidate. In some cases, positive target information was given first, followed by negative information; in the remaining cases, the order was reversed. Primacy effects were indexed by the degree to which subjects' overall judgments were influenced more by the early as opposed to the late information.

The need for nonspecific closure was manipulated via degrees of time pressure. As suggested earlier, we assumed that under time pressure individuals would experience a heightened need for closure because of the potential costs involved in missing the deadline. The need to avoid nonspecific closure was instituted via evaluation apprehension. In the high-need-to-avoid-closure condition, subjects expected their judgments to be compared with those of professional psychologists. In the low-need-to-avoid-closure condition, subjects were told that the evaluation method was at a pilot stage and its validity was unknown.

The relevant results are shown in Figure 10.6. As predicted, primacy effects were significantly ($p < .01$) higher under high (vs. low) need for nonspecific closure and significantly ($p < .01$) lower under high (vs. low) need to avoid such closure.

In later experiments, we (Freund et al., 1985) replicated the effects of epistemic motivations on impressional primacy with different operational defini-

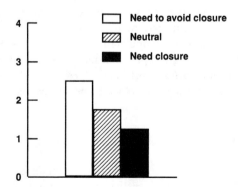

FIGURE 10.5 Mean number of hypotheses generated under various motivational conditions. From "What Makes You So Sure?: Effects of Epistemic Motivations on Judgmental Confidence" by O. Mayseless and A. W. Kruglanski, 1987, *Organizational Behavior and Human Decision Processes*, 39, 162–183. Copyright 1987 by Academic Press, Inc. Reprinted by permission.

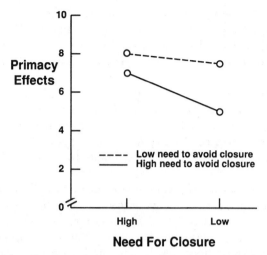

FIGURE 10.6 Primacy effects as a function of need for closure and need to avoid closure. From "The Freezing and Unfreezing of Lay Inference: Effects on Impressional Primacy, Ethnic Stereotyping, and Numerical Anchoring" by A. W. Kruglanski and T. Freund, 1983, *Journal of Experimental Social Psychology, 19,* 448–468. Copyright 1983 by Academic Press, Inc. Reprinted by permission.

tions of the need for nonspecific closure and the need to avoid such closure. In one replication, the need for closure was operationalized via demands for undimensional (hence, global and undifferentiated) versus multidimensional judgments, and the need to avoid closure was operationalized via potential costs *to the target person* of the subject's judgmental mistake. In the second replication, the need to avoid closure was manipulated as in the first experiment, and the need for closure was manipulated via degrees of time pressure. In the third replication, the need for closure was manipulated as in the first experiment, and the need to avoid closure was manipulated via degrees of evaluation apprehension. All three designs strongly replicated our original findings (Kruglanski & Freund, 1983). Specifically, primacy effects were consistently more pronounced in conditions of high (vs. low) need for closure and of low (vs. high) need to avoid closure.

Anchoring Effects

Tversky and Kahneman (1974) identified persons' tendency to anchor numerical estimates in initial values without sufficient adjustments made in the light of subsequent information. According to the present analysis, the anchoring phenomenon may represent an instance of epistemic "freezing," in which information processing comes to a halt after an initial estimate has been generated and slightly adjusted. If so, anchoring tendencies should be strengthened by a heightened need for nonspecific closure, and weakened by a heightened need to avoid such closure. Those predictions were tested (Kruglanski & Freund, 1983, Study 3).

For reasons discussed elsewhere (e.g., Bar-Hillel, 1973; Kruglanski & Freund, 1983, pp. 458–459), the anchoring tendency may lead persons to *overestimate* the probabilities of conjunctive events (e.g., coming up with a red marble on every single draw from an urn containing the proportion q of red marbles), and to *underestimate* the probabilities of disjunctive events (e.g., coming up at least once in n draws with a red marble). Following the procedure developed by Bar-Hillel (1973), we (Kruglanski & Freund, 1983) asked subjects to choose within pairs of events the one more likely to occur. Some pairs contrasted conjunctive events with simple events, whereas other contrasted disjunctive events with simple ones. Need for closure was manipulated via degrees of time pressure, and need to avoid closure was manipulated via evaluation apprehension. As shown in Figure 10.7, subjects' tendencies to overestimate the likelihood of conjunctive events and to underestimate the likelihood of disjunctive events (both indicative of anchoring) increased, as predicted, under high (vs. low) need for closure and decreased under high (vs. low) need to avoid closure.

Stereotypic Judgments

The research paradigms described thus far examined the effects of epistemic motivations on the formation of new knowledge structures. But the same motivations may also affect persons' tendency to base judgments on pre-existing knowledge or to be "theory-driven" rather than "data-driven." A pre-existing knowledge structure affords a ready base for launching a judgment. Thus, in conditions of high (vs. low) need for nonspecific closure, individuals may be more disposed to base their judgments on pre-existing structures. Conversely, in conditions of high (vs. low) need to avoid nonspecific closure, subjects may be less inclined to base judgments on pre-existing structures, and instead may assign greater weight to situational information.

To investigate those notions, we (Kruglanski & Freund, 1983, Study 2) made use of prevalent ethnic stereotypes of various Jewish subgroups in Israel. The Sephardi Jews originate predominantly in the Middle East and North Africa, and their stereotype in the domains of academic performance and achievement is generally negative. By contrast, the Ashkenazi Jews originate mostly in Europe and/or North America, and their corresponding stereotype in academic domains is generally positive.

Students in the senior class of an Israeli teachers' college assigned a grade to a literary composition ostensibly written by an eighth-grader. All subjects responded to exactly the same composition; the only difference was in the alleged writer's surname. In one condition, the name (Blumenthal) suggested an Ashkenazi origin, whereas in the other condition the name (Abutbull) suggested a Sephardi origin. The need for closure was manipulated via degrees of time pressure, and the need to avoid closure was manipulated via degrees of evaluation apprehension. The main findings of this study are summarized in Figure 10.8.

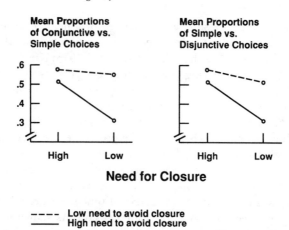

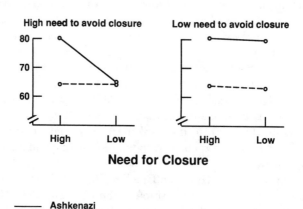

FIGURE 10.7   Anchoring effects as a function of need for closure and need to avoid closure. From "The Freezing and Unfreezing of Lay Inference: Effects on Impressional Primacy, Ethnic Stereotyping, and Numerical Anchoring" by A. W. Kruglanski and T. Freund, 1983, *Journal of Experimental Social Psychology, 19,* 448–468. Copyright 1983 by Academic Press, Inc. Reprinted by permission.

FIGURE 10.8   Stereotypic judgments as a function of need for closure and need to avoid closure. From "The Freezing and Unfreezing of Lay Inference: Effects on Impressional Primacy, Ethnic Stereotyping, and Numerical Anchoring" by A. W. Kruglanski and T. Freund, 1983, *Journal of Experimental Social Psychology, 19,* 448–468. Copyright 1983 by Academic Press, Inc. Reprinted by permission.

As may be seen, ethnic stereotypes exerted substantial effects on grading. In all but one condition, the grades assigned to the Ashkenazi writer were considerably higher on the average than those assigned to the Sephardi writer ($p < .01$). The stereotype effect disappeared almost entirely, however, in the cell that combined an absence of time pressure with a high degree of evaluation apprehension (i.e., the condition of high need to avoid closure). Thus, it appears that individuals' tendency to base judgments on pre-existing knowledge may depend on their epistemic motivations. In particular, stereotype-driven judgments may be more likely when a high need for nonspecific closure exists and less likely when a high need to avoid such closure exists.

Presumably, the tendency of persons experiencing a high need for closure to base their judgments on pre-existing stereotypes is due to the economy such stereotypes afford, by removing the necessity for laborious information processing. Similar economy may be afforded by the use of simplistic inference rules or "heuristics" (Chaiken, 1980). Indeed, Sorrentino, Bobocel, Gitta, Olson, and Hewitt (1988) found that certainty-oriented individuals (assumed to have a high need for nonspecific closure) utilized such heuristics to a greater degree than did uncertainty-oriented individuals.

Interactive Effects of Epistemic Motivations and Initial Confidence

In the research described thus far, the need for nonspecific closure appeared to inhibit epistemic activity, and the need to avoid such closure appeared to facilitate such activity. However, those effects may be moderated by the degree to which the individual departs from a fairly crystallized knowledge structure versus a relative ambiguity: To the extent that the person has a high (vs. low) need for nonspecific closure *and* starts out with crystallized knowledge, a match exists between what the person has and what he or she desires; this may foster epistemic freezing and suppress the tendency to search for further information. Indeed, in the studies previously described, the observed curtailment of epistemic activity typically occurred *after* some preliminary knowledge (e.g., an ethnic stereotype, an early impression, or an initial estimate) had been formed.

The outcome may be very different, however, in cases where the epistemic departure point is characterized by relative ambiguity. In these circumstances, a person with a high (vs. low) need for nonspecific closure should experience a discrepancy between actual and desired epistemic states. This may induce an unfreezing of the epistemic search, which (the person hopes) will lead to the coveted state of knowledge. Opposite effects may be expected if the individual has a need to avoid closure: Specifically, in cases where the individual has fairly crystallized knowledge to begin with, but what he or she prefers (if only temporarily) is lack of closure, unfreezing may be expected to occur. However, if the same person *begins* with a lack of closure, he or she may be unmotivated to "jeopardize" it via additional search, inducing freezing. These notions were investigated in a pair of recent studies (Peri, Kruglanski, & Zakai, 1986), described next.

Experiment 1: Need-for-Closure Effects

Subjects were presented with five series of drawings. Each series contained either two or four standard drawings on a given topic ("man," "woman," or "tree"), each drawn by a different person, and a criterion drawing on a different topic (invariably, "house"), drawn by *one* of the persons who had prepared the standard drawings. Subjects' task was to identify for each series the particular standard drawing by the individual responsible for the criterion drawing. The time allotted was 3 minutes. Subjects stated their interim judgment after 1 minute, and during the remaining 2 minutes were given the opportunity for social comparison with previous subjects in the same experiment. This was accomplished by having subjects turn over some (or all) of the standard drawings, which bore on their backs the percentages of previous subjects choosing them as correct answers.

The design of the study was a 2×2 factorial with these independent variables: (1) need for closure (high vs. low) and (2) initial confidence in the hypothesis (high vs. low). According to our earlier logic, in the high-initial-confidence condition subjects with a high (vs. low) need for closure were expected to engage less in social comparison. By contrast, in the low-initial-confidence condition subjects with a high (vs. low) need for closure were expected to engage more in social comparison.

Need for closure was manipulated via varying task clarity. In the low-need-for-closure condition, subjects were informed of four criteria for assessing the drawings' similarity. These, based on pilot work, were as follows: linear quality of the drawing (thick or thin, strong or weak, and continuous or discontinuous lines); the drawing's size and location on the page (big or small, centered or off center); its degree of elaboration (detailed and elaborate or simplistic and unadorned); and perspective (containing depth or flat). Subjects in the high-need-for-closure condition received no comparable criteria for assessing the drawings' similarity. We assumed that in the absence (vs. presence) of criteria subjects would be unpleasantly confused, and hence would feel a need for nonspecific closure regarding the nature of their task.

Initial confidence was manipulated via the number of choice alternatives presented to subjects. In the high-initial-confidence condition, subjects were choosing from among two standard drawings, whereas those in the low-initial-confidence condition were choosing from among four standard drawings. There were two dependent variables, both designed to tap subjects' tendency to engage in informational search via social comparison: (1) the number of standard drawings subjects turned over to ascertain the percentages of other people choosing them as correct answers; and (2) the latency (in seconds) of their turning over the first standard drawing. The relevant results are displayed in Table 10.2.

As may be seen, our predictions were supported. In the high-initial-confidence condition, the average number of standard drawings turned over by subjects with a high need for closure was lower than the corresponding number turned over by subjects with a low need for closure. This trend was reversed in the low-initial-confidence condition, and the appropriate two-way interaction was signif-

TABLE 10.2   Mean Extent of Social Comparison and Latency of First Comparison as Functions of Initial Confidence and Need for Closure

Dependent variable	Initial confidence	
	High	*Low*
Extent of social comparison[a]		
High need for closure	2.60	3.52
Low need for closure	4.37	2.82
Latency to first comparison[b]		
High need for closure	60.39	33.67
Low need for closure	19.47	49.01

Note. Adapted from *Interactive Effects of Initial Confidence and Epistemic Motivations on the Extent of Informational Search* by N. Peri, A. W. Kruglanski, and D. Zakai, 1986, unpublished manuscript, Tel-Aviv University. Adapted by permission of the authors.

[a]Extent of social comparison was based on number of drawings turned over, corrected for the available number of drawings. To obtain a uniform index, that number was divided by a factor of 2 in the high-confidence condition and by a factor of 4 in the low-confidence condition.

[b]In seconds.

icant ($p < .01$). Furthermore, in the high-initial-confidence condition the latency of turning over the first standard drawing was longer for subjects with a high (vs. low) need for closure; this trend was again reversed in the low-initial-confidence condition, and the appropriate two-way interaction was again significant ($p < .01$). Finally, a multivariate analysis of variance (MANOVA) that took into account both our dependent variables also yielded a significant interaction ($p < .02$).

Experiment 2: Need-to-Avoid-Closure Effects

The procedure of our next experiment was essentially identical to that of the preceding study, as were our manipulation of initial confidence and measurement of the dependent variables. The only significant departure from the preceding procedure concerned the way in which subjects stated their final choice. Specifically, they did so now by distributing 10 coins (of equal value) across some (or all) of the standard drawings, in proportion to the perceived likelihood of their representing the correct choice.

The experimental design was a 2 × 2 factorial in which two levels of initial confidence (high vs. low) were manipulated orthogonally to two levels of the need to avoid closure. Our basic predictions stated that in the high-initial-confidence condition, subjects with a high (vs. low) need to avoid closure would tend to engage more in informational search. By contrast, in the low-initial-confidence condition, we expected subjects with a high (vs. low) need to avoid closure to engage less in informational search.

Need to avoid closure was manipulated via different degrees of the fear of invalidity. In the high-need-to-avoid-closure condition, subjects expected their overall performance to be evaluated against that of other subjects. This was to be accomplished via computing each subject's score in accordance with the number of coins he or she placed on the correct drawings across the five series. In principle, a subject's score could range from 0 (if he or she did not place any "bets" on the correct drawings in any of the five series) to 50 (if he or she placed 10 coins on the correct drawings in all five series).

In addition, subjects in the high-need-to-avoid-closure condition were constrained in the number of coins they could "safely" bet on any one drawing. To the extent that they placed more than 5 coins (in the low-confidence condition) or more than 7 coins (in the high-confidence conditions) on the wrong drawings, they would lose all of their points for that particular series. Thus, subjects in the high-need-to-avoid-closure condition were discouraged from making a definite commitment to any particular judgment: Such commitment might result in a loss of valuable points, lowering their total score. Subjects in the low-need-to-avoid-closure condition, by contrast, were not informed of an evaluative scoring system, and were not constrained in distributing their bets across different standard drawings.

TABLE 10.3   Mean Extent of Social Comparison and Latency of First Comparison as Functions of Initial Confidence and Need to Avoid Closure

	Initial confidence	
Dependent variable	*High*	*Low*
Extent of social comparison[a]		
High need to avoid closure	3.94	3.00
Low need to avoid closure	2.62	3.60
Latency to first comparison[b]		
High need to avoid closure	37.01	47.84
Low need to avoid closure	65.11	39.79

Note. Adapted from *Interactive Effects of Initial Confidence and Epistemic Motivations on the Extent of Informational Search* by N. Peri, A. W. Kruglanski, and D. Zakai, 1986, unpublished manuscript, Tel-Aviv University. Adapted by permission of the authors.

[a]Extent of social comparison was based on number of drawings turned over, corrected for the available number of drawings. To obtain a uniform index, that number was divided by a factor of 2 in the high-confidence condition and by a factor of 4 in the low-confidence condition.

[b]In seconds.

The main experimental results are displayed in Table 10.3. As may be seen, those data generally support our predictions. In the high-initial-confidence condition, subjects with a high (vs. low) need to avoid closure turned over more drawings on the average. This trend was reversed (albeit not significantly) in the low-initial-confidence condition. The appropriate two-way analysis of variance (ANOVA) was statistically significant ($p < .02$). Furthermore, in the high-initial-confidence condition, subjects with a high (vs. low) need to avoid closure manifested shorter information search latencies, whereas the reverse trend was evident in the low-initial-confidence condition. Although the appropriate two-way ANOVA was not significant, a MANOVA taking into account both our dependent variables did yield a significant interaction ($p < .05$).

Summary: Empirical Evidence for the Epistemic Motivations

The studies reported above are generally consistent with implications of the present theoretical model concerning the effects of epistemic motivations. Typically, subjects with a high (vs. low) need for nonspecific closure tended to generate fewer hypotheses concerning a problem of interest, and exhibited higher confidence concerning the hypothesis generated. Furthermore, subjects with a high (vs. low) need for nonspecific closure tended more to form impressions on the basis of early information, to anchor their estimates in initial values, and to render stereotype-based rather than data-based judgments.

The opposite effects typically obtained where high (vs. low) fear of invalidity could be assumed to heighten subjects' need to avoid closure. Under those conditions, subjects tended to generate more hypotheses and to exhibit lower confidence in the hypotheses generated. Furthermore, they tended less to base impressions on early information, to anchor their estimates in initial values, and to render stereotype-based rather than data-based judgments.

Finally, when subjects' initial confidence in a judgment was high, high (vs. low) need for nonspecific closure decreased the tendency for informational search, and high (vs. low) need to avoid such closure increased this tendency. By contrast, where the initial confidence was low, high (vs. low) need for nonspecific closure increased the tendency for informational search, whereas high (vs. low) need to avoid such closure decreased this tendency. It is noteworthy that the present studies employed a wide variety of judgmental tasks, and operationalized the epistemic needs in a variety of ways. Thus, although each individual experiment may be open to alternative interpretations, the collective body of data described above provides a measure of support for the present epistemic model.

The various motivational orientations featured in the present chapter are assumed to apply to all possible judgments, irrespective of content. If so, they ought to apply also to causal judgments (cf. Kruglanski, 1980, 1989a). The following review of motivationally relevant research on causal attributions explores whether this is the case.

MOTIVATIONAL EFFECTS ON ATTRIBUTIONS: REVIEW AND REANALYSIS

Effects of the Need for Nonspecfic Closure

The attributional literature often mentions persons' need to clearly comprehend their environment as a powerful motivating force behind causal assignments. For instance, Kelley (1967, p. 193) has stressed the individual's motivation "to attain cognitive mastery of the causal structure of the environment" as a pervasive motive base for attributions. Kelley and others allude to an unbiased or non-preferential need for causal closure concerning one's environment, rather than a selective preference for specific causal structures.

According to the lay epistemic analysis, individuals' need for nonspecific closure regarding causality is likely to be limited to topics of particular significance. This suggests that attributional activity is likely where causal knowledge is of special interest or use to the individual. Accordingly, Berscheid et al. (1976) found in a dating study that females who expected to be highly outcome-dependent on a target person (i.e., expected this person's conduct in a forthcoming interaction to determine whether the interaction would be pleasant or unpleasant) paid more attention to him, evidenced better memory of his characteristics and behavior, and evaluated him more extremely and confidently.

Outcome dependency may induce a need for nonspecific cognitive closure about the other's properties, to serve as a base for one's own behavioral decisions in the interaction. This much is implied by Berscheid et al. (1976, p. 978), who view those effects as "manifestations of an underlying motivation to predict and control the social environment." Such motivation may prompt intensive cognitive work aimed at the attainment of clarifying closure. Consistent with this reasoning, Erber and Fiske (1984) found that outcome dependence on another increased subjects' tendency to attend to inconsistent (vs. consistent) information about that individual and to generate more dispositional attributions for the inconsistent information.

Note that outcome dependency studies (e.g., Berscheid et al., 1976; Erber & Fiske, 1984) typically create a situation characterized by initial ambiguity (e.g., meeting an unknown individual) combined with a need to attain cognitive closure (getting to know the person on whom one is dependent). The intense epistemic activity manifested in those conditions is thus consistent with implications of the present model, and with our findings (Peri et al., 1986) described earlier.

It is also noteworthy that outcome dependency studies do not typically contain a "pure" manipulation of the need for nonspecific closure. Although outcome-dependent subjects may well experience higher motivation for closure than their nondependent counterparts, they probably experience also a higher "fear of invalidity" that temporarily induces a greater need to avoid closure, and this is manifested in special attention to inconsistent information. Indeed, Erber and Fiske (1984) noted outcome-dependent subjects' predictive *accuracy* needs, alongside their desire to maintain "the *unity* of their *impressions*" (pp. 710–711; emphasis mine).[7]

A need for cognitive closure may be induced by an explicit experimental requirement to answer a specific attributional question (e.g., McArthur, 1972; Orvis, Cunningham, & Kelley, 1975). Alternatively, it may be aroused under conditions where prior knowledge has proved inadequate, as where an expectancy has been disconfirmed (Pyszczynski & Greenberg, 1981) or failure has been encountered. Spontaneous attributional activity in both types of circumstances (Weiner, 1985) is thus compatible with the present notion of need for nonspecific closure.

Effects of Needs for Specific Closure and the Avoidance of Specific Closure

Most motivational research in attribution represents the effects of needs for specific closure or the avoidance of specific closure. This is research investigating how the desirability of given attributional conclusions (e.g., whether they are flattering or damaging to one's ego) may affect the process and outcomes of attributional activity. Heider (1958, pp. 120–121) seemed to have just such directional effects in mind when he mentioned "subjective forces of needs and wishes" possibly swaying attributions. Similarly, the notion of "hedonic relevance" introduced by Jones and Davis (1965, p. 237) refers to individuals' preference for specific attributions that may fulfill rather than obstruct a purpose. Kelley (1967) alludes to specific closure effects in his discussions of ego-protective or ego-enhancing biases, and of the motivation to control one's environment (see Kelley, 1971, p. 22). Kelley suggests that environmental control involves the balance between controlling the "controllable" and the "important." In this sense, perceived controllability or importance may represent specific preferential features that attract attributions to the appropriate causal factor.

Self-Serving Biases

A clear example of research on needs for specific closure is work on "self-serving biases." Despite early reservations (Ajzen & Fishbein, 1975; Miller & Ross, 1975), a series of later reviews (Harvey & Weary, 1984; Kelley & Michela, 1980; Zuckerman, 1979) uniformly concluded that such biases are easily interpretable in motivational terms.

In a typical study of self-serving biases (e.g., Johnson, Feigenbaum, & Weiby, 1964), subjects attribute positive outcome (success) to themselves and negative outcome (failure) to external circumstances. However, more recent research has identified conditions that can reverse the pattern. For example, Arkin, Appleman, and Burger (1980) found that subjects accepted less credit for success than for failure when they expected their behavior to be evaluated by a group of experts. Tetlock (1980) provided subjects with descriptions of a teacher who had either succeeded or failed and had made either self-serving or counterdefensive attributions. Subjects evaluated the counterdefensive teacher more highly than the self-serving teacher, which shows that counterdefensive attributions may function to gain social approval.

According to the present analysis, both self-serving and social approval concerns represent needs for specific closure. In some instances, the two needs may conflict; when this happens, attributions will probably be biased in a direction of the stronger motivation. In the research by Arkin et al. (1980), approval motivation presumably prevailed over esteem motivations, resulting in a preponderance of counterdefensive attributions. In other instances, however, the relative magnitudes of these motivations may be reversed, with corresponding effects on attributions.

Self-Handicapping

Another line of research interpretable in terms of needs for specific closure is work on "self-handicapping" (Berglass & Jones, 1978; see also Jones & Berglass, 1978; Jones & Pittman, 1982), defined as behavior whose consequences are likely to lower one's performance on a subsequent task (e.g., ingestion of a debilitating drug). Such actions may be regarded as subjects attempts to manufacture evidence that may elicit the desired attributions (for reviews, see Arkin & Baumgardner, 1985; Berglas, 1985).

General Comments

To conclude, diverse concepts and findings in the attribution literature are compatible with the notion that needs for specific closure often exert biasing effects on causal ascriptions. Although most of the research to date has examined specific effects due to esteem or approval motivations, the present analysis implies that such effects may be expected to emerge with numerous alternative motivations as well. Some causal explanations may be preferred over others because they appear "controllable" or "important" (Kelley, 1971). It is further possible to imagine situations where preferred explanations are based on needs for physical safety or comfort, needs for novelty, or needs for complexity—in fact, needs for any conceivable property or attribute. In this sense, Jones and Davis's (1965) concept of "hedonic relevance" comes closest to capturing the broad flavor of the "need-for-specific-closure" notion, as it refers to the degree to which an attribution gratifies or obstructs a perceiver's purpose of whatever kind.

Effects of the Need to Avoid Nonspecific Closure

A third type of motivational force occasionally implicit in attributional analyses is the need to avoid nonspecific closure. In its pure form, a heightened degree of such a need defines a lack of nonspecific closure as the desired goal state. Often, however, the need to avoid this type of closure may coexist with a need *for* such closure; in those conditions, a temporary avoidance of closure may be induced and extend the duration of the attributional search until some judgment is ultimately reached. Both types of situations have been captured by attributional researchers.

Attribute Ambiguity

Situations in which lack of nonspecific closure represents the preferred state of affairs have been dealt with by Snyder and Wicklund (1981) in an essay on "attribute ambiguity," referred to earlier. According to the present analysis, with lack of nonspecific closure as the desired goal, individuals will engage in considerable attributional search *if* they intially possess cognitive closure. Under such conditions, they are likely to generate competing hypotheses to a current attribution and/or to seek out (or actively manufacture) evidence inconsistent with this attribution. In so doing, attributors may be guided by the deductive logic of hypothesis evaluation, and in particular by the notion that cognitive inconsistency undermines confidence in a proposition (cf. Kruglanski, 1980; Mayseless & Kruglanski, 1987), thus undermining closure. Snyder and Wicklund (1981, p. 211) describe such tendencies as instances of "using the traditional attribution logic" to attain desired ambiguity. However, with lack of nonspecific closure as the desired end state, individuals should refrain from attributional activity if they possess ambiguity to start with. Snyder and Wicklund (1981, pp. 205–207) discuss research findings demonstrating such tendencies, and label them as the "leaving-the-field" mode of securing ambiguity.

Control Deprivation

Research by Pittman and colleagues (for a review, see Pittman & D'Agostino, 1985) on the effects of control deprivation may represent a case in which fear of invalidity (Freund et al., 1985; Kruglanski & Freund, 1983; Kruglanski & Mayseless, 1988; Mayseless & Kruglanski, 1987) may induce a temporary avoidance of nonspecific closure. In a typical experiment, subjects in the high-control-deprivation condition receive failure feedback on a concept formation task. As compared with baseline or low-deprivation controls, they generally tend more to utilize relevant information on a subsequent attributional task, to process such information more cautiously, and to take more time before reaching a judgment. According to the present interpretation, subjects in the high-deprivation condition who believe that they have already failed once may be particularly concerned about the possibility of a repeat failure and its consequences for their self-esteem. Such fear of invalidity may well enhance subjects' motivation to avoid premature closure and prompt their in-depth consideration of extensive information that is apparently relevant to the judgment at hand.

Motivational Research in Attribution Theory: Implications of the Epistemic Analysis

As the foregoing review indicates, extant motivational findings in attribution may be ordered in terms of the present epistemic categories. In this sense, a considerable body of attributional data seems compatible with the predictions of the epistemic model concerning the effects of needs for nonspecific and specific closure and the need to avoid nonspecific closure. Furthermore, the present interpretation has several conceptual and empirical implications of interest. Those relate to the proposed (1) integration of motivational and informational aspects of attribution; (2) emphasis on the aspects of attributional activity that are not unique; and (3) emphasis on the targeted epistemic ends (vs. origins) of such activity. Let us consider these in turn.

Integrating Informational and Motivational Aspects of Attribution

Previous motivational research on attribution has not been clearly integrated with the informational aspects of the process. For instance, the various ego-enhancing or ego-protective tendencies were typically considered "less rational" than the informational principles assumed to guide attributions (e.g., informational criteria of "consistency," "consensus," and "distinctiveness," or rules such as "covariation," "discounting," or "augmentation"). Similarly, motivational and informational accounts of self-serving biases were sometimes juxtaposed to each other (Ajzen & Fishbein, 1975; Miller & Ross, 1975; Zuckerman, 1979). All of this implies a disjunctive model with two distinct routes to attribution: an informational route (typically regarded as more rational) and a motivational route (regarded as less rational).

By contrast, the present epistemic model suggests that the motivational dimension constitutes an inseparable part of all attributional (in fact, all judgmental) activity. According to this approach, an essential function of motivation in attribution is to stimulate or arrest the sequence of hypothesis generation and evaluation, whereby all knowledge (including causal knowledge) forms. The tendencies described above are assumed to be coextensive with the application of various "informational" principles identified by attribution theorists. For instance, the generation of alternate hypotheses driven by the need to avoid closure may result in confidence decrements, in accordance with "discounting" logic (Kelley, 1971). Similarly, a need for nonspecific closure may increase the knower's sensitivity to evidence *against* competing alternatives to one's hypotheses, resulting in "augmentation" effects (Kelley, 1971). Needs for specific closures or the need to avoid specific closures may lead to increased or decreased sensitivity to information (e.g., on the "consensus" or "distinctiveness" type), depending on its apparent congruency with the desired attribution.

Thus, motivational forces are assumed to affect the *extent, direction,* and *outcome* of attributional information processing. However, such processing may still be governed by various informational principles, so a disjunction between motivational and informational modes of attribution may not be warranted.

The proposed integration of the informational and motivational aspects of attribution has empirically testable consequences. For instance, motivational conditions assumed to facilitate hypothesis generation (viz., a high need to avoid nonspecific closure, given initial closure) should strengthen the "discounting" tendency (Kelley, 1971), which depends on the individual's sensitivity to competing causal hypotheses. By the same token, conditions assumed to inhibit hypothesis generation (e.g., a high need for closure given initial closure) should weaken "discounting."

Motivation as a Nonunique Aspect of Attribution

The present analysis suggests that the same motivational orientations that affect judgments in general affect attributions. Attributions are thus regarded as a special subcategory of judgments, whose contents are causal. According to this view, attributions are mediated by the same general process whereby all judgments are acquired and modified (see Kruglanski, 1980, 1989a; Kruglanski, Hamel, Maides, & Schwartz, 1978). The epistemic motivations exemplify parameters of that general process. For instance, arousal of the need for closure via a disconfirmed expectancy (Weiner, 1985) should prompt an informational search concerning noncausal matters as well as causal ones. Suppose that in a cab en route to the airport, one notes a discrepancy between one's own watch and the driver's. This unexpected occurrence may give rise to a frantic informational search that is not necessarily aimed at causally explaining the discrepancy, but rather at finding out which of the two contradictory bits of information is correct.

A motivation to avoid closure may exert similar effects, regardless of the judgmental contents involved. For example, if the "control deprivation" manipulation in Pittman's research (see Pittman & D'Agostino, 1985) indeed arouses subjects' fear of invalidity, the intense information-processing activity on a subsequent task should be replicated with noncausal assignments as well. Intensified information processing under heightened fear of invalidity was manifested in our studies (Mayseless & Kruglanski, 1987) described earlier, where the tasks involved tachistoscopic recognition rather than causal assignment.

Needs for specific closure should affect noncausal judgments just as they do causal ones. For instance, self-serving needs may lead to an interpretation of an ambiguous remark as a compliment rather than a criticism, to an overestimation of one's popularity or physical attractiveness, or to optimistic expectations regarding the outcome of a job interview. None of these judgments qualifies as causal, yet they may all be biased toward a positive view of oneself, just as causal judgments may be (cf. Miller, 1976; Ross & Sicoly, 1979).

Epistemic Ends versus Origins of Attributional Activity

Previous motivational research in attribution often stressed the *origins* of attributional tendencies (e.g., in esteem concerns, in the need for control, or in the need for social approval). By contrast, the present analysis emphasizes the epistemic *ends* (of nonspecific or specific closure, or the avoidance of either kind of closure) desired in each particular instance. This shift of focus rests on the assumption that different possible origins of the same epistemic motivation are *functionally equivalent* as far as the attributional (or judgmental) process is concerned. For instance, the motivation for nonspecific closure may variously arise from esteem needs, the need for "control," or the need for social approval. In all those cases, individuals' epistemic activities (e.g., information gathering, hypothesis generation, or sensitivity to inconsistent evidence) may be affected identically, regardless of the particular basis of the need for nonspecific closure. Similar examples could be cited in reference to needs for specific closure or the needs to avoid nonspecific or specific closure.

Just as different possible origins may give rise to the same epistemic motivation, different epistemic motivations may often emanate from the same origin. As Kelley (1971, p. 22) implied, the need to exercise control may occasionally serve as the origin for strivings toward specific closures, notably toward causal structures appearing "controllable" or "important," whereas on alternate occasions it may motivate striving toward nonspecific closure—toward causal structures of whatever kind. Similarly, esteem concerns may at times arouse a need for nonspecific closure (as in the case of an expert whose reputation depends on having *an* answer to a problem); in other instances they may serve as the origin of the need for a specific closure (e.g., for a conclusion with a self-serving content); and in yet others they may serve as the origin of the need to avoid nonspecific or specific closure (cf. Snyder & Wicklund, 1981). In sum, as far as the attribution *process* is concerned, the ultimate epistemic end may be of greater consequence than its origin in particular motives.

The foregoing discussion suggests the possible interchangeability of dependent variables related to the different motivational constructs. For instance, in past research, effects of needs for specific closures (e.g., of self-serving contents) were demonstrated primarily via attributional *products*—that is, via the contents of ultimate causal ascriptions. By contrast, effects of the need for nonspecific closure or the need to avoid such closure were typically demonstrated via such *process* variables as the initiation and/or the extent of attributional activity (Pittman & D'Agostino, 1985; Weiner, 1985). However, the same process measures might well be employed also with needs for specific closures, the basic prediction being that the extent of subsequent attributional activity would vary negatively with the desirability of an initial attribution.

Similarly, attributional products may often be affected by the essentially unbiased motivations for nonspecific closure or for the avoidance of such closure. For instance, to the extent that a given causal category (say, the "person" category) is readily accessible (cf. Higgins & King, 1981) and the individual has a high need for nonspecific closure, such a category may well be assigned as the cause of the event. By contrast, the likelihood that a less accessible category will be ultimately assigned as the cause should increase under conditions where the need to avoid nonspecific closure is aroused (e.g., via a fear of invalidity).

GENERAL DISCUSSION AND CONCLUSIONS

Beyond Causal Attribution: Implications for the Motivation–Cognition Interface

The debate whether purely cognitive or motivational analyses are more fit to account for judgmental phenomena is probably unresolvable (Tetlock & Levi, 1982). Instead of prolonging the dispute, the present approach sets out to specify complementary judgmental functions for motivational and cognitive factors. According to this proposal, any judgment is at once motivated and informationally based. In this sense, the lay epistemic theory represents an interface approach to motivation and cognition, of the type advocated recently by Sorrentino and Higgins (1986). As the foregoing review indicates, such an approach is capable of generating novel empirical predictions as well as integrating large bodies of previous data.

Furthermore, the present epistemic model attempts a systematic typology of judgmentally relevant needs, represented in the fourfold classification of Table 10.1. This *general* typology is offered as an alternative to a roster of *specific* motivations (e.g., needs for esteem, self-presentation, control) with possible judgmental effects. Depending on the specific context, each of these specific motivations is assumed capable of giving rise to any one of the general epistemic needs, and hence of affecting the judgmental process in different ways. In addition, the present analysis refines those motivational constructs that have been recently linked with increased cognitive effort or extent of information processing, such as "personal involvement" (Chaiken & Stangor, 1987), "outcome dependency" (Neuberg & Fiske, 1986), "decision importance," or "accountability" (Tetlock, 1985; Tetlock & Kim, 1986). For instance, "personal involvement" may variously denote arousal of a need for specific closure on an issue (implying defensiveness and bias) or a need to avoid nonspecific closure (stemming from a fear of invalidity). Similarly, "outcome dependency" on another may conceal divergent epistemic needs (Neuberg & Fiske, 1986)—for example, the need to judge that person as friendly (Berscheid et al., 1976), the need to accurately assess his or her characteristics (Erber & Fiske, 1984), and the need for orienting closure about that individual. Those epistemic needs may often affect judgments in opposite ways; thus, their relative magnitudes in different "outcome-dependent" situations may give rise to seemingly inconsistent findings. In sum, the present choice of motivational constructs has been dictated by their relatively unambiguous linkage to the epistemic process (its intensity, duration, and directionality). By contrast, previously identified judgmental motivations have been often ambiguous in their postulated effects, and hence less capable of yielding clear-cut judgmental predictions.

Further Research Implications of the Epistemic Paradigm

Debiasing

The present analysis has implications for understanding the conditions under which the various biases assumed to characterize lay judgments (see Nisbett & Ross, 1980) may be reduced, eliminated, or reversed. The prevalent conception of the layperson has been that of a cognitive miser (e.g., Fiske & Taylor, 1984) who often relies on oversimplified judgmental heuristics, and whose failure to systematically process the available information may result in serious bias and error. However, recent theorizing and research (e.g., see Lord, Lepper, & Preston, 1984; Neuberg & Fiske, 1986; Pittman & D'Agostino, 1985; Tetlock & Kim, 1986) suggest that under some conditions the various biases may be overcome and persons may be induced to process information in more extensive, effortful, or attentive ways.

According to the present approach, all human judgment is, in a sense, biased (Kruglanski, 1989a, 1989b; Kruglanski & Ajzen, 1983). The reason is that the process of hypothesis generation and evaluation has no natural or "objective" point of termination. Thus, the formation of a given judgment depends critically on various psychological or "subjective" forces that may prompt different persons (e.g., the subject and the experimenter) to render vastly different judgments of seemingly the same situation. From this perspective, "debiasing" may consist of inducing psychological forces that foster "unfreezing" of a given judgment, processing of further pertinent information, and "refreezing" on a different (more "appropriate") judgment.

More specifically, the lay epistemic model implies that debiasing requires the joint operation of informational and motivational factors. Alternatives to the "frozen" judgment need to be made accessible, and the appropriate epistemic motivation has to be aroused, for those alternatives to be considered seriously. Thus, neither information nor motivation alone is likely to accomplish debiasing. Indeed, studies of impression formation (Asch, 1946) or belief perseverance (Ross, Lepper, & Hubbard, 1975) demonstrate that persons may often ignore extant information and persist with previous judgments and impressions. Other research (see Neuberg & Fiske, 1986, for a review) suggests that motivation alone is also insufficient for debiasing. Furthermore, research in which debiasing did occur may have involved the joint combination of appropriate informational and motivational factors. For instance, Lord et al. (1984) found that merely admonishing subjects to be as objective and unbiased as possible (motivational factor) was unsuccessful in eliminating bias. However, asking them in addition to "consider the opposite"—that is, to entertain a competing or inconsistent hypothesis (informational factor)—totally abolished bias. Further debiasing research that jointly manipulates informational and motivational factors seems clearly to be in order.

The epistemic model also has implication for the *timing* of specific motivational inductions aimed at debiasing. Arousal of a fear of invalidity *prior* to a judgmental commitment may induce a need to avoid nonspecific closure, and hence may lessen the tendency to neglect relevant information. On the other hand, arousal of the same fear following an irrevocable commitment may induce a need for specific closure—namely, for the belief that one's judgment has been correct. This may promote defensiveness and induce biased attention to supportive versus refuting information (cf. Frey, 1986; Lord et al., 1984). Consistent with this reasoning, we (Mayseless & Kruglanski, 1987) found that although fear of invalidity reduced subjects' *initial* confidence, and the magnitude of confidence shifts occasioned by new information, it actually increased subjects' *final* confidence. Possibly, after a final judgment has been reached, fear of invalidity instills defensiveness (i.e., a need for specific closure) that may bolster confidence. Somewhat similarly, Tetlock and his associates (e.g., Tetlock & Kim, 1986) have repeatedly found that manipulation of *accountability* (the need to justify one's judgments to others) affects information processing only when it occurs *before* exposure to the relevant evidence, and not after exposure. Those findings may mean that in the postfreezing period, fear of invalidity occasionally instills a need for specific closure (i.e., defensiveness), rather than the need to avoid nonspecific closure.

Epistemic Motivations and Social Interaction

Finally, the present motivational constructs may yield testable implications for affect and behavior in interpersonal contexts: On numerous occasions, individuals may be "informationally interdependent" (cf. Kelley & Thibaut, 1969). This means that persons' interpersonal reactions may vary in accordance with their epistemic motivations, and with the ways in which those are affected (e.g., gratified or frustrated) by information provided by the other.

For example, criticism of one's work by another (suggesting a need to revise it extensively) may be attended to more when the criticized individual has a high need to avoid nonspecific closure, and less when he or she has the need for such closure. Similarly, the group's tendency to reject a deviate may be greater when the predominant motivation among group members is a high need for nonspecific closure, and lesser when it is a high need to avoid such closure. A dyad (say, a married couple) in which one member has a high need for nonspecific closure (affecting early "freezing" on a judgment), whereas the other has a high need to avoid such closure, may experience greater difficulties in effecting coordination and "group locomotion" (cf. Festinger, 1954) than a dyad in which both members share similar epistemic motivations. The foregoing conceptual and empirical implications of the present motivational analysis may render it a useful framework for the future study of diverse social cognitive problems.

Acknowledgments

I am indebted to Reuben Baron, Lou Boudreau, Susan Fiske, Tory Higgins, John Holmes, Dick Sorrentino, and Phil Tetlock for comments on an earlier draft.

Notes

1. This is not meant to imply that laypersons are skillful deductive logicians or that they do not err on a variety of logical tasks (cf. Wason & Johnson-Laird, 1972). Rather, it is suggested that the form of the validation process is deductive in the general sense of inferring conclusions *from* evidence, which implies a prior premise whereby *if* the evidence were affirmed, the conclusion would be warranted. For further discussion, see Kruglanski (1989a, Ch. 2).

2. The present construct of "need for specific closure" replaces that of the "need for conclusional contents" mentioned in previous versions of the lay epistemic theory (Kruglanski & Ajzen, 1983; Kruglanski & Freund, 1983), in recognition that a preference for a cognitive closure may occasionally be based on noncontentual properties of knowledge structures (such as novelty or complexity).

3. Conceivably, individuals may reliably differ in the disposition toward "wishful thinking" across different dimensions of preference among knowledge structures (e.g., their contents or novelty). Such tendencies, if found, may signify stable individual differences in needs for specific closure.

4. As noted subsequently, fear of invalidity need not invariably induce a need to avoid nonspecific closure. For example, in situations where one is irrevocably committed to a judgment or a

decision, the higher the perceived costs of a mistake (inducing high fear of invalidity), the higher the wish to perceive one's own judgment as correct may be. This may induce a need for specific closure, rather than a need to avoid nonspecific closure.

5. Individuals may reliably differ in their *general* tendency to avoid closure—for example, as a function of their desire for freedom and unpredictability.

6. In all studies reported here, the need to avoid closure was manipulated via a fear-of-invalidity induction. The reason is that in previous statements of the lay epistemic theory (e.g., Kruglanski & Ajzen, 1983; Kruglanski & Freund, 1983) serving as background for this research, fear of invalidity was conceived as the major motivational factor effecting judgmental "unfreezing." In the present formulation, "unfreezing" is linked instead to the need to avoid closure, which under some conditions only, rather than generally, may arise out of a fear of invalidity (see footnote 4).

7. As noted subsequently, the case may be even more complex than that. Specifically, beyond the need for nonspecific closure and the need to avoid such closure, outcome dependency on another may also induce a need for a specific closure (a hope that this person will be positively disposed, so that good outcomes will be forthcoming). Consistent with this analysis, Berscheid et al. (1976) found that the target person was perceived as more likeable by outcome-dependent than by nondependent subjects, attesting to possible need-for-specific-closure effects.

References

Adorno, T. W., Frenkel-Brunswick, E., Levinson, D. J., & Sanford, R. N. (1950). *The authoritarian personality.* New York: Harper & Row.

Ajzen, I., & Fishbein, M. (1975). A Bayesian analysis of attribution processes. *Psychological Bulletin, 82,* 261-277.

Arkin, R. M., Appleman, A. J., & Burger, J. M. (1980). Social anxiety, self-presentation, and the self-serving bias in causal attribution. *Journal of Personality and Social Psychology, 38,* 23-25.

Arkin, R. M., & Baumgardner, A. H. (1985). Self-handicapping. In J. H. Harvey & G. Weary (Eds.), *Attribution: Basic issues and applications* (pp. 169-202). New York: Academic Press.

Asch, S. E. (1946). Forming impressions of personality. *Journal of Abnormal and Social Psychology, 41,* 258-290.

Atkinson, J. W., & Birch, D. (1970). *The dynamics of action.* New York: Wiley.

Bar-Hillel, M. (1973). On the subjective probability of compound events. *Organizational Behavior and Human Performance, 9,* 396-406.

Bar-Tal, D. & Bar-Tal, Y. (1988). A new framework for social psychology. In D. Bar-Tal & A. W. Kruglanski (Eds.), *The social psychology of knowledge.* Cambridge, England: Cambridge University Press.

Bem, D. J. (1972). Self-perception theory. In L. Berkowitz (Ed.), *Advances in experimental social psychology* (Vol. 6, pp. 1-62). New York: Academic Press.

Berglas, S. (1985). Self-handicapping and self-handicappers: A cognitive/attributional model of interpersonal self-protective behavior. *Perspectives in Personality, 1,* 235-270.

Berglas, S., & Jones, E. E. (1978). Drug choice as a self-handicapping strategy in response to noncontingent success. *Journal of Personality and Social Psychology, 36,* 405-517.

Berlyne, D. E. (1960). *Conflict, arousal, and curiosity.* New York: McGraw-Hill.

Berscheid, E., Graziano, W., Monson, T., & Dermer, M. (1976). Outcome dependency: Attention, attribution, and attraction. *Journal of Personality and Social Psychology, 34,* 978-989.

Bruner, J. S. (1957). On perceptual readiness. *Psychological Review, 64,* 123-152.

Campbell, D. T. (1969). Perspective: Artifact and control. In R. Rosenthal & R. L. Rosnow (Eds.), *Artifact in behavioral research* (pp. 351-383). New York: Academic Press.

Chaiken, S. (1980). Heuristic versus systematic information processing and the use of source versus message cues in persuasion. *Journal of Personality and Social Psychology, 39,* 752-766.

Chaiken, S., & Stangor, C. (1987). Attitudes and attitude change. *Annual Review of Psychology, 38,* 575-630.

Edwards, W. (1982). Conservatism in human information processing. In D. Kahneman, P. Slovic, & A. Tversky (Eds.), *Judgment under uncertainty: Heuristics and biases.* Cambridge, MA: Harvard University Press.

Erber, R., & Fiske, S. T. (1984). Outcome dependency and attention to inconsistent information. *Journal of Personality and Social Psychology, 47,* 709-726.

Festinger, L. (1954). A theory of social comparison processes. *Human Relations, 7,* 117-140.

Festinger, L. (1957). *A theory of cognitive dissonance.* Stanford, CA: Stanford University Press.

Fiske, S. T., & Pavelchak, M. A. (1986). Category-based versus piecemeal-based affective responses: Developments in schema-triggered affect. In R. M. Sorrentino & E. T. Higgins (Eds.), *Handbook of motivation and cognition: Foundations of social behavior* (Vol. 1, pp. 167-203). New York: Guilford Press.

Frenkel-Brunswik, E. (1949). Intolerance of ambiguity as an emotional and perceptual personality variable. *Journal of Personality, 18,* 108-143.

Freund, T., Kruglanski, A. W., & Schpitzajzen, A. (1985). The freezing and unfreezing of impressional primacy: Effects of the need for structure and the fear of invalidity. *Personality and Social Psychology Bulletin, 11,* 479-487.

Frey, D. (1986). Selective exposure to information: A review of recent research. In L. Berkowitz (Ed.), *Advances in experimental social psychology* (Vol. 19, pp. 41-81). New York: Academic Press.

Harvey, J. H., & Weary, G. (1984). Current issues in attribution theory and research. *Annual Review of Psychology, 35,* 427-459.

Harvey, J. H., Yarkin, K. L., Lightner, J. M., & Town, J. P. (1980). Unsolicited attributions and recall of interpersonal events. *Journal of Personality and Social Psychology, 38,* 551-568.

Heider, F. (1958). *The psychology of interpersonal relations.* New York: Wiley.

Heller, J. F. (1972). *Attribution theory: Self and other attributions as a determinant of attitude change.* Unpublished doctoral dissertation, University of Iowa.

Higgins, E. T., Bargh, J. A., & Lombardi, W. (1985). The nature of priming effects on categorization. *Journal of Experimental Psychology: Learning, Memory, and Cognition, 11,* 99-69.

Higgins, E. T., & King, G. A. (1981). Accessibility of social constructs: Information processing consequences of individual and contextual variability. In N. Cantor & J. Kihlstrom (Eds.), *Personality, cognition, and social interaction* (pp. 69-121). Hillsdale, NJ: Erlbaum.

Higgins, E. T., King, G. A., & Mavin, G. H. (1982). Individual construct accessibility and subjective impressions and recall. *Journal of Personality and Social Psychology, 43,* 35-47.

Higgins, E. T., Rholes, W. S., & Jones, C. R. (1977). Category accessibility and impression formation. *Journal of Experimental Social Psychology, 13,* 141-154.

Hofstede, G. (1980). *Culture's consequences: International differences in work-related values.* Beverly Hills, CA: Sage.

Johnson, T. J., Feigenbaum, R., & Weiby, M. (1964). Some determinants and consequences of the teacher's perception of causation. *Journal of Educational Psychology, 55,* 237-246.

Jones, E. E., & Berglas, S. (1978). Control of attributions about the self through self-handicapping strategies: The appeal of alcohol and the role of under-achievement. *Personality and Social Psychology Bulletin, 4,* 200-206.

Jones, E. E., & Davis, K. E. (1965). From acts to dispositions: The attribution process in person perception. In L. Berkowitz (Ed.), *Advances in experimental social psychology* (Vol. 2, pp. 220-267). New York: Academic Press.

Jones, E. E., & Pittman, T. S. (1982). Toward a general theory of strategic self-presentation. In J. Suls (Ed.), *Psychological perspectives on the self* (pp. 231-262). Hillsdale, NJ: Erlbaum.

Kelley, H. H. (1967). Attribution theory in social psychology. In D. Levine (Ed.), *Nebraska Symposium on Motivation* (pp. 192-241). Lincoln: University of Nebraska Press.

Kelley, H. H. (1971). Attribution in social interaction. In E. J. Jones, D. E. Kanouse, H. H. Kelley,

R. E. Nisbett , S. Valins, & B. Weiner (Eds.), *Attribution: Perceiving the causes of behavior* (pp. 1–27). Morristown, NJ: General Learning Press.

Kelley, H. H., & Michela, J. L. (1980). Attribution theory and research. *Annual Review of Psychology, 31*, 457–501.

Kelley, H. H., & Thibaut, J. W. (1969). Group problem solving. In G. Lindzey & E. Aronson (Eds.), *Handbook of social psychology* (2nd ed., Vol. 4, pp. 1–102). Reading, MA: Addison-Wesley.

Klar, Y., Bar-Tal, D., & Kruglanski, A. W. (1988). Conflict as a cognitive schema: An epistemological approach. In W. Stroebe, A. W. Kruglanski, D. Bar-Tal, & M. Hewstone (Eds.), *Social psychology of intergroup and international conflict* (pp. 73–89). New York: Springer.

Kruglanski, A. W. (1980). Lay epistemo-logic—process and contents: Another look at attribution theory. *Psychological Review, 87*, 70–87.

Kruglanski, A. W. (1989a). *Lay epistemics and human knowledge: Cognitive and motivational bases.* New York: Plenum.

Kruglanski, A. W. (1989b). The psychology of being "right": On the problem of accuracy in social perception and cognition. *Psychological Bulletin, 106*, 395–409.

Kruglanski, A. W., & Ajzen, J. (1983). Bias and error in human judgment. *European Journal of Social Psychology, 13*, 1–44.

Kruglanski, A. W., & Freund, T. (1983). The freezing and unfreezing of lay inferences: Effects on impressional primacy, ethnic stereotyping, and numerical anchoring. *Journal of Experimental Social Psychology, 19*, 448–468.

Kruglanski, A. W., Hamel, J. A., Maides, S. A., & Schwartz, J. M. (1978). Attribution theory as a special case of lay epistemology. In J. H. Harvey, W. J. Ickes, & R. F. Kidd (Eds.), *New directions in attribution research* (Vol. 2, pp. 299–335). Hillsdale, NJ: Erlbaum.

Kruglanski, A. W., & Klar, Y. (1987). A view from a bridge: Synthesizing the consistency and attribution paradigms from a lay epistemic perspective. *European Journal of Social Psychology, 17*, 211–241.

Kruglanski, A. W., & Mayseless, O. (1988). Contextual effects in hypothesis testing: The role of competing alternatives and epistemic motivations. *Social Cognition, 6*, 1–21.

Kunda, Z. (1987). Motivated inference: Self-serving generation and evaluation of causal theories. *Journal of Personality and Social Psychology, 53*, 637–654.

Lewin, K. (1938). *The conceptual representation and measurement of psychological forces.* Durham, NC: Duke University Press.

Lewin, K. (1951). *Field theory in social science.* New York: Harper.

Lord, C. G., Lepper, M. R., & Preston, E. (1984). Considering he opposite: A corrective strategy for social judgment. *Journal of Personality and Social Psychology, 47*, 1231–1243.

Mayseless, O., & Kruglanski, A. W. (1987). What makes you so sure?: Effects of epistemic motivations on judgmental confidence. *Organizational Behavior and Human Decision Processes, 39*, 162–183.

McArthur, L. Z. (1972). The how and what of why: Some determinants and consequences of causal attributions. *Journal of Personality and Social Psychology, 22*, 171–193.

Miller, D. T. (1976). Ego involvement and attributions for success and failure. *Journal of Personality and Social Psychology, 34*, 901–906.

Miller, D. T., & Ross, M. (1975). Self-serving biases in the attribution of causality: Fact or fiction? *Psychological Bulletin, 82*, 213–225.

Neuberg, S. L., & Fiske, S. T. (1986). *Motivational influences on impression formation: Outcome dependency, accuracy-driven attention and individuating process.* Unpublished manuscript, University of Massachusetts–Amherst.

Nisbett, R. E., & Ross, L. (1980). *Human inference: Strategies and shortcomings of social judgment.* New York: Prentice-Hall.

Orvis, B. R., Cunningham, J. D., & Kelley, H. H. (1975). A closer examination of causal inference: The roles of consensus, distinctiveness, and consistency information. *Journal of Personality and Social Psychology, 32*, 605–616.

Peri, N., Kruglanski, A. W., & Zakai, D. (1986). *Interactive effects of initial confidence and epistemic motivations on the extent of informational search.* Unpublished manuscript, Tel-Aviv University.

Pittman, T. S., & D'Agostino, P. R. (1985). Motivation and attribution: The effects of control deprivation on subsequent information processing. In J. H. Harvey & G. R. Weary (Eds.), *Attribution: Basic issues and applications* (pp. 117-143). New York: Academic Press.

Pittman, T. S., Schemrer, F. W., & Wright, J. B. (1977). The effect of commitment on information utilization in the attribution process. *Personality and Social Psychology Bulletin, 3,* 276-279.

Pyszczynski, T. A., & Greenberg, J. (1981). Role of disconfirmed expectancies in the instigation of attributional processing. *Journal of Personality and Social Psychology, 40,* 31-38.

Rokeach, M. (1960). *The open and closed mind: Investigations into the nature of belief systems and personality systems.* New York: Basic Books.

Ross, L., Lepper, M. R., & Hubbard, M. (1975). Perseverance in self-perception and social perception: Biased attributional processes in the debriefing paradigm. *Journal of Personality and Social Psychology, 32,* 880-892.

Ross, M., & Sicoly, F. (1979). Egocentric biases in availability and attribution. *Journal of Personality and Social Psychology, 37,* 332-336.

Smith, E. R., & Miller, F. (1983). Mediation among attributional inferences and comprehension processes: Initial findings and a general method. *Journal of Personality and Social Psychology, 44,* 492-506.

Snyder, M. L., & Wicklund, R. A. (1981). Attribute ambiguity. In J. H. Harvey et al. (Eds.), *New directions in attribution research* (Vol. 3, pp. 199-225). Hillsdale, NJ: Erlbaum.

Sorrentino, R. M., Bobocel, R., Gitta, M. Z., Olson, J. M., & Hewitt, E. C. (1988). Uncertainty orientation and persuasion: Individual differences in the effects of personal relevance on social judgments. *Journal of Personality and Social Psychology, 55,* 357-371.

Sorrentino, R. M., & Hewitt, E. (1984). Uncertainty-related properties of achievement tasks as a function of uncertainty orientation and achievement-related motives. *Journal of Personality and Social Psychology, 47,* 884-899.

Sorrentino, R. M., & Higgins, E. T. (1986). Motivation and cognition: Warming up to synergism. In R. M. Sorrentino & E. T. Higgins (Eds.), *Handbook of motivation and cognition: Foundations of social behavior* (Vol. 1, pp. 3-19). New York: Guilford Press.

Sorrentino, R. M., & Short, J. C. (1986). Uncertainty orientation motivation and cognition. In R. M. Sorrentino & E. T. Higgins (Eds.), *Handbook of motivation and cognition: Foundations of social behavior* (Vol. 1, pp. 379-403). New York: Guilford Press.

Tetlock, P. E. (1980). Explaining teacher explanations of pupil performance: A self-presentation interpretation. *Social Psychology Quarterly, 43,* 283-290.

Tetlock, P. E. (1985). Accountability: The neglected social context of judgment and choice. *Research in Organizational Behavior, 7,* 297-332.

Tetlock, P. E., & Kim, J. I. (1986). *Accountability and judgment processes in a personality prediction task.* Unpublished manuscript, University of California-Berkeley.

Tetlock, P. E., & Levi, A. (1982). Attribution bias: On the inconclusiveness of the cognition-motivation debate. *Journal of Experimental Social Psychology, 18,* 68-88.

Tversky, A., & Kahneman, D. (1974). Judgment under uncertainty: Heuristics and biases. *Science, 185,* 1124-1131.

Wason, P. C., & Johnson-Laird, P. N. (1972). *Psychology of reasoning: Structure and content.* Cambridge, England: Cambridge University Press.

Weimer, W. B. (1979). *Psychology and the conceptual foundations of science.* Hillsdale, NJ: Erlbaum.

Weiner, B. (1985). "Spontaneous" causal thinking. *Psychological Bulletin, 97,* 74-84.

Zanna, M. P., & Cooper, J. (1976). Dissonance and the attribution process. In J. H. Harvey, W. J. Ickes,

& R. F. Kidd (Eds.), *New directions in attribution research* (Vol. 1, pp. 199–219). Hillsdale, NJ: Erlbaum.

Zuckerman, M. (1979). Attribution of success and failure revisited, or: The motivational bias is alive and well in attribution theory. *Journal of Personality*, 47, 245–287.

CHAPTER 11

Understanding Self and Other

Developmental and Motivational Aspects of Perceiving Persons in Terms of Invariant Dispositions

WILLIAM S. RHOLES
Texas A&M University
LEONARD S. NEWMAN
DIANE N. RUBLE
New York University

The attribution of dispositional characteristics, such as personality traits and abilities, to ourselves and others is among the most basic elements of social perception (Heider, 1958; Kelley, 1972). In this chapter, we discuss developmental changes in children's understanding of dispositions and the impact of such changes on motivational processes. Two basic theses are addressed: first, that during the early and middle childhood years children gradually come to understand dispositions to be invariant structures—that is, to be abiding, constant aspects of persons that exert a consistent influence on behavior across situations and time; and, second, that following this development some social experiences and information acquire new dimensions or meanings for children, which at least partially transform earlier motivational processes.

The chapter is divided into two major sections. The first deals with research on children's understanding of dispositional invariance. By way of outline, we begin with a discussion of adult conceptions of dispositions and a brief review of the findings of the "free-description" person perception literature, which provided the first indication of developmental changes in the way dispositions are understood (e.g., Livesley & Bromley, 1973). The largest part of this section of the chapter, however, is devoted to a group of recent studies that have followed up on issues initially raised in the free-description literature. We argue that this more recent research, in conjunction with the free-description literature, strongly implies that there are fundamental differences between younger children (e.g., 5- to 6-year-olds) and older children in their understanding of dispositional invariance. In reviewing this literature, our goal is first to illustrate those changes in the dispositional concept that we think are relevant to motivation, and then to discuss the limitations of the work done to date in this area. Finally, we conclude the first section of the chapter with a summary of cognitive and social–environmental factors that may produce developmental changes in the way dispositions are understood.

In the second section of the chapter, we address three related topics. First, we review studies dealing with a number of motivational issues—achievement motivation and self-evaluation; interpersonal interactions; and the internalization of prosocial values—as they relate to developmental changes in the dispositional concept. Second, we attempt to point out parallels between research on the dispositional concept and a related form of social invariance, gender constancy (Kohlberg, 1966). Finally, drawing on the findings in these two areas, we attempt to outline a set of principles concerning the relationship between developmental changes in social cognition and related changes in social motivation and behavior.

THE DISPOSITIONAL CONCEPT

The Concept of Dispositions among Adults

One informal indication of the importance of dispositions is their frequency of appearance within the language. In a survey by Allport and Odbert (1936) over 4,500 terms referring to stable individual differences were located in a standard English dictionary. Such terms typically dominate adults' descriptions of other persons (e.g., Fiske & Cox, 1979), and even severe critics of the scientific value of broad trait constructs (e.g., Mischel, 1973) recognize the role played by traits in the layperson's perceptions of the social environment. Gordon and Wyer (1987) reported that when adults are asked to form impressions of people, they organize behaviors in memory in terms of trait concepts even if such categories have not been provided for them explicitly; this indicates these concepts' pervasive impact on cognition. Moreover, Uleman (1987) has further argued that adults extract trait meanings from behavior even in the absence of an impression formation goal. In fact, his work seems to indicate that traits are often inferred without either intention of conscious awareness.

Despite their importance, the meaning of dispositional terms remains elusive. As constructs in a formal psychology of personality, dispositions have been defined in a variety of ways (Alston, 1975; Buss & Craik, 1983; see also Zuroff, 1986), but most discussions of definition center on three principal issues: the stability of dispositions over time; the degree and nature of cross-situational consistency in disposition-related behaviors; and the causal influence of dispositions. Similarly, investigations of lay conceptions of dispositions have focused on these same three issues. With regard to the first one, temporal stability, studies have confirmed that the person-descriptive concepts that adults classify as dispositions are viewed as being stable over time (Chaplin, John, & Goldberg, 1988; Rholes & Walters, 1982; Wimer & Kelley, 1982). In fact, adults often try to interpret new behavior that is inconsistent with a previous trait impression in such a way as to confirm their original impressions (Crocker, Hannah, & Weber, 1983; Hayden & Mischel, 1976).

In connection with the second issue, research has shown that adults base predictions for future behavior in new situations on prior disposition-related behavior, and this seems to imply a belief in cross-situational consistency (Reeder & Spores, 1983; Rholes & Ruble, 1984, Study 2). The third issue, that of dispositions as causal constructs, is potentially the most complex of the three and unfortunately has received the least attention. Although it would be difficult to explain adult beliefs in cross-situational consistency without the corresponding belief that dispositions are causal structures or are closely affiliated with causal structures, it is nevertheless the case that invoking dispositions as causes sometimes leads to circular reasoning (e.g., "He acted aggressively because he is aggressive").

Fletcher (1984) and Alston (1975) address this problem by dividing dispositions into (1) patterns of similar or conceptually related behaviors and (2) underlying motivational and/or capacity-related constructs, such as values, needs, beliefs, attitudes, and skills, that motivate or otherwise account for such patterns. Extrapolating this distinction to lay conceptions, one can argue that dispositional terms are used at times simply to characterize trends in behavior and at other times both to characterize trends and invoke stable underlying factors that produce behavior. This distinction is intuitively compelling, but has yet to inspire much empirical work, developmental or otherwise. Nevertheless, we wish to emphasize it because it highlights some of the complexities of the dispositional concept. In acquiring this concept, children must first grasp the conceptual relationships among behaviors that constitute dispositional categories. For instance, to understand aggression and be able to notice patterns of aggression in behavior, a child must first understand the conceptual similarities among behaviors that may be as diverse as hitting, lying, and "tattling." This is a difficult task in and of itself, and one that links the acquisition of the dispositional construct with the acquisition of other natural language categories. However, according to the distinction mentioned earlier, children must also come to understand the psychological forces (i.e., the needs, capacities, values, etc.) that underlie such patterns if they are to achieve a full understanding of dispositions.

In the sections that follow, we examine research on children's understanding of dispositions. We begin with research on the use of dispositional constructs in descriptions of others and of the self, and then turn to studies concerned with their use in forming expectations for patterns of behavior over time and across situations (e.g., Rholes & Ruble, 1984) and their stability and constancy within the person's psychological constitution (Rotenberg, 1982).

Description Studies

A number of studies have investigated children's use of dispositional constructs by analyzing the descriptions of others made by children of different ages (e.g., Barenboim, 1977, 1981; Bigner, 1974; Gollin, 1958; Livesley & Bromley, 1973; Peevers & Secord, 1973; Scarlett, Press, & Crockett, 1971; Wood, 1978; Yarrow & Campbell, 1963). Similarly, other studies have investigated children's use of dispositional constructs in the self-concept by analyzing self-descriptions and analyses (e.g., Livesley & Bromley, 1973; Mohr, 1978; Rholes, Jones, & Wade, 1988). The description method has both advantages and disadvantages. One of its strengths is that it permits one to investigate children's perceptions of familiar persons with whom they have a significant "real-world" interaction history. Another is that it does not unduly canalize responses. The major disadvantage, or criticism, of the method centers on its output requirements. It imposes stringent demands on children's verbal capacities and consequently could lead one to underestimate younger children's conceptual level, if they are unable to verbalize their ideas and perceptions adequately. Other potential problems concern children's motivation to provide complete accounts of their perceptions, and potential age differences in children's understanding of the goals of the description task.

In spite of the potential problems, studies using this method obtain data that make an intuitively compelling case in favor of important age-related changes in self- and other-perceptions. Consider the following self-descriptions reported by Livesley and Bromley (1973). The first is that of a girl aged 7, and the second is that of a boy aged 9.

> I am 7 years old. I have one sister. Next year I will be eight. I like colouring. The game I like is hide the thimble. I go riding every Wednesday. I have lots of toys. My flowers is a rose, and a buttercup and a daisy. I like milk to drink and lemon. I like meat to eat and potatoes as well as meat. Sometimes I like jelly and soup as well. (p. 237)

> I have dark brown hair, brown eyes, and a fair face. I am a quick worker, but am often lazy. I am good but often cheeky and naughty. My character is sometimes funny and sometimes serious. My behavior is sometimes silly and stupid and often good. It is often funny my daddy thinks. (p. 238)

Livesley and Bromley's principal analysis of descriptions involved coding statements like those above into two major categories: "peripheral" statements, which refer to appearance, identity information (such as name or age), routine activities or habits, possessions, details of life events, likes and dislikes, social roles, and kinship relations; and "central" statements, which include personality traits, general trends in behavior (such as "always hits people"), motives, needs, values, and finally attitudinal orientation (e.g., "very religious").[1] Consistent with the self-descriptions of the younger child and the older child above, Livesley and Bromley found a clear increase with age in the use of central statements to describe the self and other persons. Moreover, the most pronounced change occurred between the ages of 7 and 8; there was little further increase in the proportion of central statements after 8 years. Finally, the descriptions of self and other were found to be "strikingly similar" (p. 236) in terms of age-related changes in content.

Livesley and Bromley's (1973) main results have been replicated in many free-description studies (see references above). In fact, it is one of the most widely replicated findings in the social development literature. But what does the finding mean in connection with our present concerns? If we set aside potential methodological problems for the moment, the findings first seem to indicate that younger children are less likely to extract dispositional categorizations of persons from the behavior that they observe. This is particularly interesting, in light of the fact that younger children have a reasonably well-developed personality trait vocabulary. When asked to characterize a behavior in trait terms, they often can do so appropriately (e.g., Rholes & Ruble, 1984). Livesley and Bromley have interpreted their findings in terms of cognitive maturation. In essence, their argument is that the young child is cognitively ill equipped to perceive general themes that link behaviors together into dispositional patterns (1973, pp. 211–220). Consequently, younger children may be able to label behaviors with trait terms when asked to do so, but such terms function principally as descriptions of individual behaviors, rather than as more general characterizations of the person (Rholes & Ruble, 1984). Thus, dispositional terms appear more often in the descriptions of older children because they mean something different to them.

Prediction Studies

As mentioned above, serious questions have been raised about the free-description method. Partially in response to these, a number of studies have been conducted recently using a different method. In these studies, children typically observe behavior that is intended to reveal a personality trait or ability level, and are asked to predict how the actor would behave in a new situation that is relevant to the trait or ability. In other words, questions are asked that assess expectations for cross-situational consistency. This has the distinct advantage over the free-description method of not requiring extensive verbalization by respondents.

The fundamental concern of the studies reviewed below is whether there are developmental differences in the expectations children form when they observe behaviors that can potentially be related to dispositions. If, as Livesley and Bromley (1973) and others suggest, younger children do not understand dispositions to be invariant characteristics of persons, they should be less likely to expect cross-situationally consistent patterns of behavior. The cross-situational component of dispositions is the primary concern of these studies, because (1) it is one of the critical defining features of dispositions in most theoretical accounts, and (2) attributional theories (e.g., Abramson, Seligman, & Teasdale, 1978; Weiner, 1985) suggest that events attributed to causal entities perceived to have an abiding, cross-situational presence have very different effects on behavior and emotions than do events attributed to other types of causal factors. Consequently, if developmental differences in expectations for cross-situational stability are found, the apparent implication is that both children's basic understanding of dispositions and the range of potential effects of at least some experiences (e.g., task failure, social rejection) may change with age as well.

To illustrate, in one set of studies (Rholes & Ruble, 1984), children aged 5–6 and 9–10 observed videotaped vignettes that were designed to reveal either an actor's personality traits or the actor's level of ability. Prior to making predictions, half of the subjects were asked to label the actor in terms of his or her personality traits or abilities, and half were not asked to do so. The children made predictions after stories were read to them that depicted behaviors either consistent with the observed behavior (e.g., a new instance of generosity), inconsistent with it (e.g., an instance of stinginess when generous behavior had been observed), or unrelated to the observed behavior. The primary measure of interest was the degree to which children expected new instances of consistent behavior.

The results showed that all age groups were able to label the actors' behavior with appropriate trait-related or ability-related terms, but that the 5- to 6-year-olds did not predict substantial degrees of cross-situationally consistent behavior. The 9- to 10-year-olds, on the other hand, did form expectations for cross-situationally consistent patterns of behavior. The results were essentially the same for abilities and personality traits, and among children who had and had not labeled the actors prior to making predictions. The latter finding suggests that younger children did not fail to make cross-situationally consistent predictions simply because they did not relate the observed behaviors to dispositional categories.

In a second study, we (Rholes & Ruble, 1984) replicated these findings using different stimuli and response measures. Children and adults heard stories and were also provided covariation information—specifically, high- or low-consistency information (Kelley, 1972)—that would encourage or discourage a person attribution for the actor's behavior. The prediction measure, however, differed from the one described above. Respondents were asked to rate in how many other situations, from just a few to many, they would expect the actor to behave as he or she had in the story. The purpose of this more global measure was to circumvent concerns that situations targeted for predictions may be viewed differently by children at different ages. Persons in all age groups made stronger person attributions for behaviors described as temporally consistent, as would be expected from attribution theory and other attribution studies (e.g., DiVitto & McArthur, 1978). The prediction results, however, did not parallel the attributional patterns. Children aged 5-6 did not form stronger expectations for cross-situational consistency in the behavior of actors whose observed behaviors elicited stronger person attributions. Adults and children aged 9-10, in contrast, did expect greater consistency from such actors, and children aged 7-8 showed a mixed pattern of results. These results led us (Rholes & Ruble, 1984) to argue that younger children can label behaviors in dispositional terms, but that they use dispositions primarily to describe behavior without making reference to an underlying quality of the person.

Several other studies have obtained results that are consistent with this conclusion, but, as we discuss later, not all studies have. Ferguson, van Roozendaal, and Rule (1986) presented children with stories in which an actor consistently behaved either helpfully or aggressively toward other children. Five-year-olds appropriately labeled the actors as mean or helpful, but did not hold strong expectations that the actors so labeled would continue to exhibit consistent behavior in new situations. Children aged 8 and 11, in contrast, both attributed dispositions *and* predicted new behaviors that were congruent with the observed behavior. The results of this study are very similar to ours (Rholes & Ruble,

1984), and further suggest that young children differ from older ones in their conception of dispositions.

MacLennan and Jackson (1985) used a very different version of the prediction method, but nevertheless obtained similar results. They began with modal trait profiles obtained from adult personality trait self-reports on the Personality Research Form (Jackson, 1974). Two hypothetical child actors were shown behaving in ways congruent with four different traits that were most characteristic of two different trait profiles. One was shown engaging in behavior indicative of high levels of nurturance, play, affiliation, and exhibition; the other was shown engaging in behaviors representative of autonomy, dominance, thrill-seeking, and aggression. Children then made predictions about the occurrence of new behaviors related to the same traits, as well as new traits that the profile data showed to be correlated with the four traits depicted in the actors' behavior. The key procedural differences were that children observed the actors engaging in several behaviors relevant to four empirically intercorrelated traits, and that the dependent measure was the degree to which the children's predictions correlated with empirically derived trait–behavior profiles. In spite of the differences, the results were quite consistent with those of the previously described studies. The youngest children, 6-year-olds, made predictions that showed very modest (though in some cases significant) correlations with the profiles. The older children, 9- and 12-year-olds and college students, showed substantial correlation between the profiles and their expectations. The correlations increased with each age level, but the greatest gain occurred between the ages of 6 and 9. Thus, these results show age trends consistent with those found in the previous studies.

The basic developmental differences described in the studies above have also appeared in a number of other studies (Calveric, 1979; Dix & Grusec, 1983; Eisenberg, Cialdini, McCreath, & Shell, 1987; Josephson, 1977; Rholes & Ruble, 1983; Rotenberg, 1980, 1982; Ruble & Flett, 1988). Moreover, Gnepp and Chilamkurti (1988) have found similar age differences in children's use of information related to dispositions to predict emotional responses as well as behavior. In fact, in this study the age differences in predictions of emotions were more pronounced than those found in the prediction of behavior, which, though present, were comparatively weak.

Over and above the description of developmental differences themselves, a number of interesting issues are raised by the studies listed above. For example, in a study influenced by the literature on gender constancy, Rotenberg (1982) examined children's beliefs about the temporal stability of personality traits and their constancy across superficial changes in the person. He found that kindergartners and first-graders were less likely than second- and third-graders to believe that an actor would have the same traits at different points in time, and that they were less likely to believe that traits would remain unchanged when changes occurred either in attire or in the facial expressions of actors. Moreover, he found a stage-like sequence in which expectations for for temporal stability emerged before expectations for constancy across superficial changes in clothing and expression.

In a second study, Rotenberg (1982) examined beliefs about the stability and constancy of the self and found parallel trends. Younger children were less likely than older ones to believe in the temporal stability of their own self-attributed characteristics and in their constancy, given changes related to dress and facial expression. Again, a stage-like developmental pattern emerged, with temporal stability being attained before constancy over superficial changes. Finally, Rotenberg reported that beliefs about constancy and stability of the other were correlated with the use of prior behavior to predict new behavior, and that beliefs about stability and constancy of the self were correlated with the use of traits in a free description of the self; this latter finding was significant only among the oldest children, third-graders. The significance of these findings is that they show a correspondence between the stability and constancy of beliefs on the one hand, and both the cross-situational prediction measure used in many of the previously described studies (e.g., Rholes & Ruble, 1984) and the dispositional content measure employed in the free-description literature (e.g., Livesley & Bromley, 1973) on the other.

Rotenberg's research is important because it focuses attention on three key questions: the relationship between beliefs about the self and the other; the difference between expectations for temporal stability and other forms of dispositional invariance; and the interrelationship of the prediction measure and other conceptually related measures. Some of these topics have been addressed in other research as well. In connection with temporal stability, we (Rholes & Ruble, 1983) found that even 5- to 6-year-olds expect future behavior to be consistent with past behavior, provided that the situation is the same. Similarly, we (Rholes & Ruble, 1984, Study 2) found that 5- to 6-year-olds are more likely to expect temporal consistency of behavior that has been attributed to person causes than they are to expect cross-situational consistency. Regarding the convergence of conceptually related measures, two studies (Ferguson, Olthof, Luiten, & Rule, 1984; Rholes, Jones, & Wade, 1988) found as Rotenberg (1982) did that the prediction measure correlates with use of dispositional constructs in free descriptions: Persons who expect greater cross-situational consistency use more dispositional material in descriptions. The final issue raised by Rotenberg's research (1982), conceptions of one's own dispositions versus those of other persons, is a difficult issue to address using the prediction method, because predictions regarding the self may involve self-presentation and defensive motives that do not complicate predictions of the behavior of others. Aside from Rotenberg's study, this topic has received little investigation. However, in support of Rotenberg's assertion that the two develop in parallel, research has shown that self- and other-descriptions appear to change developmentally in parallel (Livesley & Bromley, 1973). This is a topic that warrants further study, however, because many of the implications of change in the dispositional concept for motivation and behavior derive from the perception of invariant characteristics in the self.

In light of the developmental trends discussed so far, it is interesting that adults have been shown to overattribute causality to personal factors (Ross, 1977) and have been characterized as rigid "trait theorists" (Nisbett, 1980). With the development of the concept of invariant dispositions, one might anticipate an eventual overreliance on the predictive capacity of dispositions. A study by Josephson (1977), however, suggests that this may not be completely accurate. Josephson examined children's use of both prior trait-relevant behavior and information about the current situation to make predictions for behavior. Consistent with the results of the studies above, the youngest children (5-year-olds) made little use of the trait-relevant information, but they did use the situational information. Older children (8- to 11-year-olds), in contrast, made predictions that were strongly in line with the trait-relevant behaviors of the actors. Finally, adolescents and young adults (15- and 20-year-olds) made predictions that were sensitive to both the trait information and the situation; their predictions were more interactionist in nature. These results indicate a U-shaped developmental trend in the tendency to generalize from traits to behavior. In middle childhood, the perceived relationship between dispositions and behaviors seems to peak and be at its most inflexible. A similar U-shaped developmental trend has been reported by Newman (1990).

In addition to Josephson (1977), several other studies also indicate that adults' social judgments are not rigidly based on dispositions (Allen & Smith, 1980; Epstein & Teraspulsky, 1986; Zuroff, 1982). Moreover, a recent study by Allen, Walker, Schroder, and Johnson (1987) links at least one form of flexibility to advances in cognitive development. They found that college students in the concrete operational stage of development, relative to those in the formal operational stage, showed a bias toward explanations of behavior in person terms and failed to make optimal use of covariation information to infer other potential causes. Interestingly, recent work linking cognitive development to personality, specifically to authoritarianism (see Sorrentino, Raynor, Zubek, & Short, Chapter 6, this volume), suggests that patterns of attribution similar to those found by Allen et al. (1987) may emerge from a comparison of authoritarian and nonauthoritarian persons.

Although there is substantial evidence of developmental differences in perceptions of invariant traits, some studies using the prediction method have failed to find age effects (Heller & Berndt, 1981; Smetana, 1985), and another, while finding some age effects, also found considerable cross-situational consistency in the predictions of younger children (Ruble, Newman, Rholes, & Altshuler, 1988). The procedure of Heller and Berndt's study was very similar to that of the prediction studies described above. Children heard stories about generous and ungenerous actors, and then predicted their behavior in a variety of new situations. The basic result was that even kindergartners predicted new behaviors that were consistent with the observed generous or ungenerous behavior of the actor. Smetana's research similarly failed to find developmental differences congruent with the findings of the studies described above. One possible explanation of the inconsistency in results is simply that by using small samples of younger children (usually fewer than 20), the different studies may have tapped into groups at different developmental levels, and in fact suggestions of sample effects resulting from socioeconomic differences can be found in the literature (Newman, 1990; Ruble et al., 1988). A second possibility is that differences may have resulted from the particular traits used in the studies. There is some evidence that children's most mature use of trait concepts occurs in studies focusing on the generosity–stinginess dimension (Feldman & Ruble, 1988, Study 2; Heller & Berndt, 1981; Ruble et al., 1988). It seems likely that, at least in its earliest manifestations, the concept of invariance would appear in connection with some traits but not others. A third possibility, however, is that differences in procedures may account for the different results. Our findings (Ruble et al., 1988) show that even seemingly minor variations in methods can influence the predictions that children make.

In this study, kindergarten and third-grade children heard stories about actors who behaved generously or ungenerously or who displayed high or low athletic ability. They then predicted the future behavior of these target children. In the first experiment, pictures of the actors engaging in the target behaviors were left in view during the procedure to serve as a memory aid. Older subjects, as expected, overwhelmingly made predictions of trait-consistent behavior (44 out of 48 predictions). Younger children, on the other hand, clearly predicted consistency only for athletic ability. This discrepancy across type of trait was puzzling, and in a second experiment, involving only kindergarten children, the presence or absence of the pictures was included as a factor in the design. The results of the first experiment were replicated in the "with-pictures" condition, but actually reversed themselves in the "without-pictures" condition: Ability predictions now seemed random, whereas predictions of trait-consistent behavior were made for generosity and selfishness. Thus, the pictures affected predictions in opposite ways for the two types of behavior.

This curious pattern of findings raises a number of intriguing issues. It indicates that under some conditions young children will use past behavior as a cue to future behavior, as do the findings of Heller and Berndt (1981) and Smetana (1985), but it suggests that even quite subtle variations in conditions can have dramatic consequences. Specifically, it seems clear that the pictures highlighted information that sometimes worked in favor of and sometimes worked against cross-situational predictions. In spite of their odd pattern, however, these variations apparently did not operate randomly. The results of the "with-pictures" conditions in the two studies were identical. Moreover, using stimulus materials and a procedure quite similar to that of the "without-pictures" condition, Heller and Berndt (1981) found comparable results—namely, that kindergarten subjects predicted behavioral consistency for selfish and generous targets. The reversal of results in the Ruble et al. (1988) study raises interesting questions about how younger children make predictions, and leads us to think that cross-situationally consistent predictions may not always be based on a dispositional logic. (This issue is discussed below in more detail, when we describe several different prediction "rules" that can lead to predictions of cross-situational stability.)

Summary and Interpretation of the Research

In summary, the results of most of the studies reviewed above, but not all, indicate that younger children (5-6 years of age) are less likely to make cross-situationally consistent predictions than are older children and adults. Studies have also shown that, when age is controlled for, children who use dispositional constructs in free descriptions are more likely to make cross-situationally consistent predictions (e.g., Ferguson et al., 1984; Rholes et al., 1988), and that children who believe traits are stable over time and across superficial changes in persons (Rotenberg, 1982) are also more likely to make cross-situationally consistent predictions. These convergent findings suggest that the prediction measure can in fact be regarded as a valid index of the dispositional construct. (However, as mentioned above, it is important in using the method to be sensitive to the possibility that nondispositional information may cue cross-situational predictions in some cases.) Finally, studies have shown that parallel trends exist for development of ideas about the dispositional characteristics of the self and the other (Rotenberg, 1982), and that expectations for temporally stable and consistent traits (Rotenberg, 1982) and behaviors (Rholes & Ruble, 1983, 1984) precede expectations for cross-situational consistency. Taken as a whole, the evidence suggests that there are important developmental differences in children's understanding of dispositions, but that it would be incorrect to conclude that younger children never use past behavior as a cue to predict future behavior (e.g., Heller & Berndt, 1981; Ruble et al., 1988).

In spite of what we view as overall support for the hypothesis that younger and older children understand dispositions differently, the studies described earlier showing cross-situationally consistent predictions by younger children raise questions and suggest that important issues about the way younger children form expectations for behavior remain to be resolved. These findings clearly suggest the need for more detailed studies of the expectancy formation process. We discuss four "rules" that children might use to form expectations in the following paragraphs. The first two of these rules are not dispositional in nature, and their use could lead to a mistaken conclusion that younger children have a more sophisticated conception of dispositions than is actually the case. The third and fourth rules are more closely related to the dispositional concept, but emphasize different components of it. The third rule emphasizes the categorical/conceptual relationships that bind behaviors together into dispositional groupings, whereas the fourth rule emphasizes the psychological forces that underlie and produce coherent groupings of behavior.

One way in which children may sometimes form expectations is by matching the situation in which behavior is observed to the situational context of the to-be-predicted behavior. If they are sufficiently similar, the child may expect the same behavior to appear in both. This may occur either because the child engages in an unsophisticated, "mechanical" matching process in which similarities in situations imply similarities in behavior, or because the child views the situation as the primary cause of behavior and thus expects similar situations to produce similar behavior. With this in mind, it is interesting that Ruble, Feldman, Higgins, and

Karlovac (1979) found that younger children are biased toward explanations for behavior that center on nondispositional, contextual factors. This tentatively suggests that younger children's predictions may indeed be substantially influenced by the perceived similarity or dissimilarity of situations, with little or no consideration or understanding of the actor's dispositions. Moreover, if this is an important element of the expectancy formation process among younger chlidren, one would expect cross-situational predictions sometimes (when situations match closely enough) and situation-specific predictions at other times (when the match is not sufficiently close). Unfortunately, the prediction research described earlier has in most cases not been attentive to this process; consequently, it is not clear whether the discrepant findings of some studies can be explained in these terms.

An alternative to situation matching is matching the observed behavior to the to-be-predicted behavior in terms of valence. According to this rule, if the valence of a new behavior matches that of the observed behavior, the new behavior is predicted to occur. This process could take place either because of the same "mechanical" matching described above (i.e., any cue implying similarity is taken as a basis for predicting similarities in behavior across situations), or because the child's earliest sense of dispositional categories is dominated by considerations of valence. Research relevant to the valence-matching process has yielded mixed findings. Some studies have found evidence that appears consistent with a valence-matching rule. For example, Stipek and Daniels (1987) found that younger children made predictions that crossed dispositional boundaries in such a way as to suggest a valence-based rule. They predicted, for instance, that intelligent persons would be successful at tasks far removed from intelligence, such as hurdle jumping, and that unintelligent persons would be unsuccessful. Although this finding is not conclusive, it is consistent with a valence-matching process. Other studies, however, have not found evidence of this process (Rholes & Ruble, 1983). Additional research is thus needed to determine when and how valence might enter into the expectancy formation process.

In the material above, we have suggested that the young child's sense of dispositional categories may be dominated by valence based considerations. An examination of how such a situation might arise suggests a variant of the basic valence rule. We assume that even very young children (e.g., 3-year-olds) are inclined to categorize behaviors, but that they do not have available to them anything like the highly differentiated category systems of adults. If these assumptions are correct, they raise questions about what the earliest categories of behavior may be like. We think that a reasonable working hypothesis is that behaviors first are categorized in terms of the impact of a behavior on the child's sense of well-being. In other words, the earliest categorizations may simply group all behaviors that have a positive impact on the child and all that have a negative one. Such a category system would be valence-based and egocentric, in that categorization would be determined by the impact of the behavior on the child. Such categories may become progressively less egocentric as the child grows older, but continue to be based on liked versus disliked behaviors. Correspondent with these early behavioral categories, the earliest categories of persons may be simply those who are liked and those who are disliked (or, at a more egocentric point in development, those who behave in ways that have a direct positive versus negative impact on the child). This suggests, then, that among younger children predictions about behavior may be based on the degree to which an actor is liked, rather than on conventional abilities or traits. The "liking" rule has not been investigated within the prediction paradigm, but evidence obtained by Feldman and Ruble (1988; see below) tentatively suggests its relevance.

Similar in some ways to valence matching, a third way in which expectations may be formed is by matching observed behavior and to-be-predicted behavior in terms of semantic–dispositional category membership. To use the simplest version of this rule, cross-situational consistency is predicted when both the observed and predicted behaviors can be accurately labeled with the same dispositional term. For example, if any two behaviors can both be characterized as altruistic, then the occurrence of either one increases the subjective probability of the occurrence of the other. (In more complex versions of this rule, the probability of a new behavior occurring varies as a function of the relationships of the observed and new behavior to the criteria that define membership in the category in question.) With this rule, the conceptual similarity between the behaviors dominates the expectancy formation process, independently of any consideration of the psychological constitution of the actor. It is not clear whether a prediction derived from this type of process should be regarded as a true dispositional prediction, since it occurs without a clear focus on the actor's psychological makeup. Presumably the answer depends on the way in which the dispositional concept is defined. If it is defined—as it is by Buss and Craik (1983), for instance—as simply a trend or regularity in behavior, then predictions that ignore the internal qualities of the actor are indeed dispositional. On the other hand, if dispositions are defined—as they are by Alston (1975) and, in our opinion, by lay adult perceivers—as closely associated with internal causes of behavior, then such predictions are not fully dispositional in nature.

Finally, predictions may be made on the basis of the internal causal structures, such as values and beliefs, that appear to underlie and motivate an actor's behavior. A principal difference between this process and the previous categorization-based one is the focus on the actor's personal qualities (although this approach is also dependent upon the predictor's having an understanding of conceptual relationships among different behaviors). This process differs from the third one above, however, in more than focus. The developmental processes involved in the acquisition of the ability to carry out the third and fourth rules are quite different. With the third rule, the task is to construct categories of conceptually related behaviors. Just as young children must construct natural object categories (e.g., the category "bird") and come to understand the sometimes intricate relationships between specific instances of the category and the defining criteria, so must they construct dispositional categories and come to understand the relationship of specific instances (behaviors) of these categories to one another and the categories' defining criteria. With the fourth rule, in contrast, the major acquisition task appears to involve sorting out deep, abiding psychological causes from more transient, phenomenologically accessible ones, as we discuss below (Nicholls, 1978).

The third and fourth rules are interesting in part because they relate to different aspects of dispositions. In order for children to achieve a full understanding of dispositions, in our opinion, both of these elements of dispositions have to be understood. However, it is not clear, first, that they are understood at exactly the same point in development. At least some conceptual relationships, for instance, may be grasped well before the internal, causal component of dispositions is understood. Moreover, it is also unclear whether the consequences of understanding each of the parts of the overall concept are the same. It is possible that development in the conceptual category area may affect processes (e.g., constructive memory) that are not closely related to the internal-force component of the dispositional concept, and vice versa. In the sections that follow, we discuss a number of motivational phenomena in light of the dispositional concept; although direct evidence is not available, our working hypothesis is that it is the invariant-causal-force component of the concept that is most important for developmental differences in motivation. (In a later section on gender constancy, we further develop the idea that social concepts are multifaceted and that different components may have different effects on developmental changes in behavior.)

The prediction studies described above typically have not been concerned with discriminating among the rules we listed, and do not take a clear position on the way in which predictions are made. Most seem to assume implicitly that the prediction measure taps into children's perceptions about and understanding of the personal qualities of the actor that underlie behavior. On the whole, the findings discussed above, particularly the convergence between cross-situational predictions and the increasing concern with the psychological qualities revealed in free descriptions, seem most consistent with that view. However, it also seems clear that other rules may sometimes be operative, and that research needs to be more explicit about the processes that are being measured by predictions and sensitive to the possibility that multiple processes may be assessed by prediction measures. It would be a mistake to confuse the prediction measure with the underlying construct of dispositional invariance or to use it exclusively as an assessment method.

Causes of Change in the Dispositional Concept

Any conceptualization of the nature of changes in children's understanding of dispositions ultimately must be linked to an analysis of the processes underlying change. Although there has been little empirical work directed toward this effort to date, a number of plausible processes have been proposed. The dominant accounts described in reviews to date (Kassin, 1981; Ruble & Rholes, 1981; Shantz, 1983) generally consider the development of person perception to be one aspect of general cognitive development (e.g., Livesley & Bromley, 1973; Peevers & Secord, 1973). In keeping with the theme of the present volume, however, we not only review these traditional accounts, but consider social and motivational alternatives to them and illustrate how such alternatives may also interact with cognitive-developmental changes to influence children's perceptions of people in stable, dispositional terms.

Cognitive-Developmental Factors

Livesley and Bromley (1973), in one of the first and most extensive discussions of this topic, have written about changes in the dispositional concept from a Piagetian cognitive-developmental point of view. Their basic assertion (pp. 214–216) is that children's growing powers of abstraction and generalization, and the capacity to perceive without being dominated by the proximal, concrete situation, allow children to go beyond the immediate stimulus situation and to infer stable and constant features in a person's behavior. Similar hypotheses have been advanced by Flavell (1977) and Rotenberg (1982), and this general orientation receives at least a small measure of support from Rotenberg's finding that, independent of age, invariant conceptions of dispositions are associated with superior performance on Piagetian conservation tasks. Other theoretical perspectives also suggest that development of the dispositional concept is dependent upon broad changes in cognitive capacities. For instance, Higgins (1989), borrowing heavily from Case's (1985) theory of intellectual change, suggests that the ability to coordinate values along two distinct dimensions is a prerequisite to representing temporally stable and cross-situationally consistent person attributes. For example, only by being able to consider simultaneously differences in outcome and effort can one make attributions of relative ability. Like Livesley and Bromley (1973), Peevers and Secord (1973) discuss the difficulties involved in integrating information acquired at different points in time in the person perception process. Indeed, the results of one recent study suggest that integrating trait-related information separated in time poses considerable difficulties for children under 7 years of age, particularly when the most recent information received is consistent with a positivity bias (Rholes & Ruble, 1986). Thus, because of such information-processing biases or limitations, young children may rarely "see" the consistencies in behaviors necessary to develop a concept of stable traits.

These various accounts provide quite compelling reasons why younger children may have problems perceiving others in terms of invariant traits and making predictions for future behavior on the basis of previous trait-relevant behavior. There are, however, elements of the dispositional concept that they do not address directly—namely, the recognition of the motivational or force component of traits. Although previous theoretical accounts have recognized the importance of this motivational component (e.g., Secord & Peevers, 1974), there have been few attempts to analyze the processes that underlie its development. Research by Nicholls and his colleagues (Nicholls, 1978; Nicholls & Miller, 1984) on children's understanding of ability and effort is suggestive in this connection, however. Effort, as a construct, differs from ability in two potentially important ways. First, it is part of phenomenological experience in a way that ability is not, and for this reason it may be easier for young children to appreciate its role in producing task outcomes. Second, it is unstable and perceived to be under stimulus regulation and voluntary control (i.e., one chooses to try hard when one encounters a situation that makes one want to do well). Nicholls finds that, while young children make use of both effort and ability terms, they do not distinguish ability from effort or even from outcomes. Until about age 7–9, effort is regarded as the prime cause of outcomes, and equal effort is expected to lead to equal outcomes. Ability, as a capacity that moderates the effectiveness of effort, is not understood. Thus, when a younger child uses a label like "smart," the true referent of the term is either an outcome ("has done well") or a level of effort ("has tried hard"), and not an invariant internal capacity.

An extension of Nicholls's observations to dispositions in general suggests that younger children may be unable to distinguish other disposition-based causal structures (e.g., personality traits) from more salient, proximal causes. The immediacy of proximal factors such as wishes, intentions, and goals, and their clear, direct covariation with behavior, often may overshadow dispositional factors—which are more remote and abstract—in the same way that effort seems to overshadow ability.

In addition to the difficulties suggested by Nicholls's (1978) research, children also may find it difficult to think about some dispositional forces because these forces undergo long periods during which they are not detectable in behavior. For example, many psychological needs (e.g., a need to be dependent) may influence behavior only in rare, atypical situations; however, despite being unobservable most of the time, they must be conceptualized as having a continuous existence by persons who view dispositions as invariant structures (Alston, 1975).

Social and Motivational Factors

Although cognitive factors provide a persuasive account, there are a number of reasons to believe that they are not sufficient to fully explain observed developmental changes in person perception. First, it has been suggested that the developmental changes described are at least partially culture-specific—in other words, that the tendency to attribute causality to the person and his or her traits may be magnified by a Western ideology that emphasizes the power and responsibility of the individual (Ross, 1981). Indeed, Miller (1984) reports that the emphasis on traits in explanations of others' behavior is not found in a non-Western culture, which emphasizes contextual determinants of behavior and a view of the person as interdependent with the environment. Miller found that approximately 40% of the reasons for behavior offered by Hindu adults were contextual, whereas dispositional explanations were only slightly more frequent than those in an 8-year-old American sample. For example, although a man's acts of cheating were typically explained by older American subjects in terms of competitiveness and self-absorption, a typical Hindu subject explained such behavior in terms of a temporary, uncontrollable state—the man's unemployment. Thus, as Miller (1984, 1986) suggests, although cross-cultural commonalities observed in younger groups of American and Hindu subjects may reflect similarities in cognitive processing, divergent developmental patterns are probably attributable to learned cultural differences in conceptions of people and associated modes of explanation.

Second, there is evidence that young children's perceptions of others are influenced by motivational factors. In a study by Feldman and Ruble (1988), children aged 5–6 and 9–10 viewed videotapes of target children that were designed to illustrate various dispositional characteristics. Motivation to diagnose the traits of the target children was manipulated by way of subjects' expectations for interaction with these children; half expected interaction and half did not. Descriptions of the target children made by the younger subjects in the former group contained a dramatically higher proportion of central/psychological, as opposed to peripheral (Livesley & Bromley, 1973), statements. In fact, the free descriptions of 5- to 6-year-olds expecting interaction were no less psychological than those of 9- to 10-year-olds not expecting interaction. These findings do not constitute a motivational "explanation" of developmental changes in person perception, because the motivational conditions also increased the dispositional perceptions of older children (Feldman & Ruble, 1988) and adults (Berscheid, Graziano, Monson, & Dermer, 1976; Monson, Keel, Stephens, & Genung, 1982). The results do indicate, however, that cognitive factors are not sufficient to explain the low proportion of psychological descriptors given by young children in previous free-description studies.

Finally, age-related changes in the way dispositions are understood may result from changes in children's life experiences. In all cultures, children usually pass through a predictable and orderly series of changes in their social experiences (Caspi, 1987; Higgins & Parsons, 1983). According to the "social life phase" perspective (Higgins & Parsons, 1983), such qualitative changes in the social lives and roles of children play an important role in developmental changes in social cognition. One of the most important life changes is entry into school at about age 5–6. A number of new experiences associated with this change in life phase may be related to person perception and the dispositional concept. Among them are the following: (1) children are exposed to a variety of new people with differing personal styles and trait-related behaviors; (2) companionship and social acceptance by peers become increasingly important; (3) there is an increased emphasis on relative standing on intellectual, physical, and social–behavioral traits; and finally (4) since children are expected to cooperate and coordinate their behaviors with other persons more extensively and more independently, the need for prediction and control of interpersonal situations increases. Although there is little direct evidence linking changes such as these to the dispositional concept (but see Feldman & Ruble, 1988), it seems reasonable to hypothesize that traits become increasingly important concepts to children in part because they are needed to adapt to and function effectively within an increasingly complex social environment.

Moreover, age-graded social interactions may also cause some dispositional constructs to become important before others. Wright and Mischel (1988) report differences between children and adults in their sensitivity to aggressive behaviors versus those relating to social withdrawal. This was reflected in the content of their descriptions of target persons at a summer camp for emotionally disturbed children. No fewer than 42% of the 8-year-olds' statements referred to aggression, as opposed to only 6% for social withdrawal. For adults at the camp, the corresponding proportions were 26% and 20%. The authors suggest that both children and adults may have dispositional categories reflecting the important aspects of their interactions, and that some behavioral categories may be more important during earlier periods. Children, more than most adults, live in a world in which people get hit. In fact, we (Newman, Ruble, & Higgins, 1987) found that kindergarten and fourth-grade children in describing other children they "never want to be around" used a great many aggression-related concepts. (These observations, of course, are closely related to the suggestion above that some of the inconsistency among prediction studies may result from differences in the traits or abilities examined in the various studies.)

A final hypothesis stemming from the "social life phase" perspective is that perhaps the belief in invariant dispositions is influenced by a slowdown in growth in later childhood that leads to increased consistency in the behavior of self and peers. Higgins and Parsons (1983) note that because preschoolers are acquiring new skills and knowledge so rapidly, perhaps they are correct in assuming that their own past behavior is not a very good predictor of future behavior. Similar considerations seem to have led Buss and Finn (1987) to offer separate conceptual classifications of personality traits for adults and 5-year-olds. Some of the adult traits do not appear in the latter list, as they require a level of cognitive ability not yet attained by such young children. More relevant to the life phase hyopthesis, others are omitted because the 5-year-olds' display of the relevant behaviors is not sufficiently consistent to infer invariant traits.

Although previous descriptions of the process of developmental change in person perception have considered interactions among different causal influences (e.g., Higgins & Parsons, 1983), it is our position that such interactions are not only possible but probably central to these changes. The cognitive × cultural interaction described by Miller (1986), discussed earlier, is a case in point. Cognitive development affects the nature and development of social goals, which in turn accelerate and direct cognitive development. This interaction takes place in a specific social context, the structure and demands of which determine the accessibility of the various goals and social constructs involved. As a result of these processes, a new class of person constructs ultimately emerges in early childhood.

IMPLICATIONS FOR SOCIAL MOTIVATION AND BEHAVIOR

Among the major reasons to be interested in developmental change in perception of dispositional characteristics are the likely implications of such change for social motivation and behavior. Once children recognize that behavior or outcomes may have long-term implications, their reactions to and evaluations of their behavior and experiences are likely to be transformed. Indeed, such a change may be considered as fundamental to children's social development as the recognition of physical constancy (i.e., conservation) is to their cognitive development.

The logic of this analysis linking perceived trait invariance to behavior builds on the literature concerning a related form of invariance—gender constancy. According to Kohlberg's (1966) cognitive-developmental theory, structural cognitive changes that allow children to perceive constancy of gender serve as organizers of sex-role behaviors. Some research supports the idea that once children become aware of the inevitability of their gender (usually between 5 and 6 years of age), sex-role information becomes more personally relevant and their orientations toward such information change. For example, gender-constant boys have been shown to be differentially attentive to same-sex models in a movie (Citron, Serbin, & Conner, 1979; Slaby & Frey, 1975), and the behavior of gender-constant versus gender-nonconstant children was found to be differentially affected by the sex of a televised model (Ruble, Balaban, & Cooper, 1981). Other studies, however, suggest that gender constancy may not represent the gender-organizing stage of development that Kohlberg (1966) hypothesized. Even children at low levels of constancy display preferences for same-sex activities and imitation (e.g., Bussey & Bandura, 1984; Marcus & Overton, 1978). Thus, a slight modification of the theory has been proposed—namely, that gender constancy heightens interest in and responsiveness to gender-related information, rather than initiating the organization of such information (Stangor & Ruble, 1987).

Similar links between developing social knowledge and behavior may be predicted with respect to perceiving invariance in personal dispositions. In the realm of interpersonal relations, for example, the recognition of invariant dispositions suggests the emergence of considerations other than physical characteristics and possessions in the establishment of similarities in the development of friendships (Gottman, 1987). Thus, during the process of becoming acquainted, a child may become motivated to try to discover more invariant underlying characteristics and orientations of the other child; consequently, different types of friends may be selected before and after a change in the dispositional concept has occurred. Similarly, in the realm of achievement, one or two failure experiences, though not consistent with desires, are not likely to be perceived as having implications for future performance or for a sense of underlying abilities until children become generally aware of invariant dispositional characteristics. Thus, there would be fewer reasons to respond to such failure experiences with embarrassment, or to give up trying on subsequent attempts at the same or a related task.

As suggested by these examples, changing perceptions about the nature of persons may have far-reaching consequences. In this section, we examine the nature of the evidence linking perceptions of invariant dispositional characteristics to three types of social motives and behaviors: (1) the meaning of achievement outcomes for self-evaluation and motivation; (2) internalization of prosocial motivation; and (3) interpersonal interactions. It is important to point out that in many cases the evidence linking behavior to changes in cognition is indirect, and that many of the studies are correlational in nature, with all of the difficulties associated with such work. Nevertheless, when taken as a whole, the evidence that can be marshaled suggests that important, age-related changes in behavior stem from changes in the way dispositions are understood.

The Meaning of Achievement Outcomes for Self-Evaluation and Motivation

Evaluative Judgments and Achievement Behavior

Once children become aware of underlying stable characteristics such as ability, their reactions to success and failure experiences, as well as to the feedback that conveys ability information, are likely to change in a number of ways. Not only does information about task outcomes convey a new sense of one's competence and chances for future success, but some forms of feedback are likely to be perceived as more informative than others. Social comparison, for example, may be particularly relevant to assessing ability as an invariant characteristic, at least during the early elementary school years. Relative standing is the basis for most external evaluations of competence (such as grades), and the conclusions from it about most emerging abilities at this stage are much less likely to change than are those that would be drawn from comparison with one's own past performance (temporal comparison) or with absolute standards. Thus, once children become aware of the invariant properties of ability, social comparison should be relatively more influential, and evaluative feedback of any type should have a more profound influence on self-assessment and subsequent motivation. Of course, in threatening circumstances the changing meaning of ability may lead to an avoidance of evaluation (Ruble & Frey, 1987; see below).

Several types of findings support this idea of changing evaluative standards, though most of the evidence is indirect. First, children show a dramatic drop in positive self-evaluations across the same ages that perceptions of invariant dispositional characteristics are developing (Benenson & Dweck, 1986; Eccles, Midgley, & Adler, 1984; Stipek, 1984). Interestingly, such age differences even emerged in a study of spontaneous verbal exchanges in the classroom. Younger children were more likely to make positive (vs. critical) self-evaluative statements than were older children (Frey & Ruble, 1987). Second, several studies also show that the impact of social comparison on self-evaluation of general ability increases after 7 years of age (Ruble, 1987), suggesting perhaps that such information becomes more meaningful once ability begins to be conceptualized in invariant terms. Similarly, the results of one observational study (Frey & Ruble, 1985) showed that for children in second and fourth grades, but not for younger children, there was a relation between frequency of social comparison and self-esteem. Specifically, the older children, but not younger ones, who more frequently engaged in social comparison exhibited more negative self-esteem. Finally, several studies suggest that evaluative feedback has relatively little impact on young (under 6–7 years of age) children's predictions for future performance, as noted above (Parsons & Ruble, 1977; Stipek & Hoffman, 1980). Thus, younger children apparently do not view poor performance, even multiple failures, as having implications for subsequent performance. Taken together, these findings suggest that the use of evaluative standards (especially social comparison), at least after the age at which children begin to conceive of ability in invariant terms, may inject realism into what otherwise are quite optimistic self-perceptions (Higgins, 1989; Stipek, 1984).

Research on children's motivational reactions to successful and unsuccessful achievement efforts has also found marked age differences (e.g., Miller, 1985; Rholes, Blackwell, Jordan, & Walters, 1980). In these studies, younger and older children worked on school-like tasks and were given success or failure feedback to determine whether task outcomes would affect subsequent motivation in the same way among different age groups. Both studies found that they did not: Younger children's motivation was less strongly affected by prior task outcomes than was older children's. Rholes et al. (1980) found that only among children in the fifth grade did failure feedback, relative to success feedback, significantly undermine subsequent task motivation; Miller (1985), contrasting second- and sixth-graders, found that sixth-graders were more strongly affected. Moreover, Rholes et al. also found that failure feedback had an impact on affective state only among the fifth-graders. The age trends in these studies generally parallel trends in the development of the dispositional concept, and the results are at least consistent with the hypothesis that changes in achievement behavior over age are contingent upon the development of the dispositional concept.

Only a few studies have made more direct tests of the hypotheses discussed above by including measures of children's conceptions of stable traits; in general, however, the results support the tentative conclusions drawn from the more indirect tests. One recent study found that differences in preferred standards of performance assessment (i.e., comparisons over time vs. social comparisons with others) were related to measures of stable conceptions of ability both for self and for others (Ruble & Flett, 1988). Consistent with results from the previous literature, there was an increase with age between second and sixth grades in the perception that ability level in general (i.e., when evaluating other children) is stable over time and consistent across situations. It was expected that this social-cognitive change would increase the salience and importance of information about levels of competence, just as reaching an understanding of the constancy of gender appears to increase the salience and importance of information relevant to defining young children's own sex roles. Moreover, it was hypothesized that the information most useful to children at high levels of ability constancy would be social comparison. As expected, ability constancy was positively related to interest in social comparison information, though the correlation within age groups was significant only for the oldest children, sixth-graders.[2]

Other evidence linking change in the process of self-evaluation to the dispositional concept comes from a study involving observations of spontaneous verbal exchanges in the classroom. The results of this study suggest that relatively blatant statements about performance tend to diminish in later grades, and that this decrease is associated with the perception of ability as a global, dispositional characteristic (Frey & Ruble, 1985; Ruble & Frey, 1987). This pattern of data is compatible with the hypothesis that once children have developed a belief that ability is a general factor observable in all academic performance, a new self-consciousness regarding performance evaluation may result. Thus, although children's *interest* in self-evaluative information may increase at this time, they may inhibit public evaluation in order to avoid possible embarrassment to themselves or others (Brickman & Bulman, 1977).

Also relevant to self-evaluation is a recent study by Rholes and Wade (1989), which found that among 7- to 8-year-olds higher self-evaluative standards were evident among children who viewed dispositions in more invariant terms. In this study children made predictions, as in other studies, and filled out questionnaires about their ideal self and their real self. There was no relation between perceptions of the real self and the invariance concept, but there was for the ideal self. Specifically, although all children strongly wished to avoid negative behaviors and characteristics, children whose predictions suggested invariance were even more extreme in this desire.

Finally, some studies have shown a direct link between dispositional concepts and performance following positive and negative outcomes. Rholes et al. (1988) studied this issue in a group of 7- to 8-year-olds. In the study's first session, approximately half of the children made predictions for the behavior of hypothetical actors indicative of an invariant dispositional concept and half did not. In a second session, the children worked on a series of puzzle-like tasks, with half receiving initial success feedback and half receiving initial failure feedback. Consistent with the hypothesis outlined above, children whose predictions suggested an invariant dispositional concept were affected more strongly by the feedback than were the other children. Among the invariant group, failure, relative to success, substantially undermined subsequent motivation, but among the other children in the other group it had little effect. In other words, the invariant subjects responded like the older children in previous studies (e.g., Rholes et al., 1980), whereas the other subjects responded like the younger children. Because the two groups did not themselves differ in age, the results appear to indicate that changes in the dispositional concept partially mediate age changes in responses to success and failure feedback.

Additional comparisons in the Miller (1985) study also support this conclusion. Miller assessed children's conceptions of ability through an interview (Nicholls, 1978) that concerns the child's differentiation of the concept of ability from the concept of effort. Consistent with the results of previous research, second-graders showed less differentiation than sixth-graders; somewhat surprisingly, however, even some sixth-graders showed incomplete differentiation. An analysis comparing sixth-graders showing more versus less differentiation revealed that outcomes had a stronger motivational impact on those children who had more clearly distinguished ability from effort. This finding is conceptually consistent with that of Rholes et al. (1988) and suggests that in some cases at least, conceptual development may not be completed until relatively late in childhood (Stipek & MacIver, 1989). Alternatively, the relation observed in sixth grade may reflect individual differences in motivational orientations associated with perceiving ability as relatively more or less fixed in its level, rather than differences in developmental level (Dweck & Leggett, 1988; Nicholls, 1984). From the developmental perspective we have been proposing, however, an additional theoretical point should be added—namely, the possibility that such an individual difference may only occur once children are capable of perceiving ability in invariant terms.

To summarize, developmental studies have found age differences in the impact of achievement task outcomes on self-evaluations, expectations, and subsequent motivation. In each case, outcomes have a stronger impact among older children, and additional recent evidence suggests that these differences may be mediated by changes in the dispositional concept.

Self-Evaluative Emotions

Although self-evaluation itself is fundamentally a cognitive process, it is nevertheless closely linked with affective responses to self-relevant events and outcomes. Consequently, it seems reasonable to suggest that changes in self-evaluative processes that occur with the development of the dispositional concept are paralleled by changes in children's affective experience. Specifically, it seems likely that children will become more emotionally responsive to events that have implications for the self-concept. Some studies of children's responses to task success and failure feedback report findings that are consistent with this expectation. Just as younger children are less likely than older children to revise their self-evaluations in response to task failures (Ruble, Parsons, & Ross, 1976), they also appear not to experience negative emotional reactions to such events that are as strong as those of older children (Rholes et al., 1980). Consistent with these findings, Glasberg and Aboud (1982) reported that kindergartners were less likely than second-graders to indicate having felt sad in response to negative life events such as task failures, and were less likely to view sadness as part of their emotional disposition. Glasberg and Aboud also found that the events that children regarded as having the potential to cause sadness changed with age. Specifically, the second-graders seemed to have a clearer understanding that sadness may result from psychological events, such as interpersonal rejection, than the kindergartners did.

Unfortunately, there are no studies of emotional experience that link age-related changes directly to the development of the concept of invariant dispositions, but a recent study by Stipek and DeCotis (1988) is suggestive in this regard. They asked children to predict the emotions of an actor following achievement failures that resulted from lack of ability, from lack of effort, or from bad luck. In contrast to older children (12- to 13-year-olds), 6- and 7-year-olds did not expect the actor to feel more ashamed when failure resulted from lack of ability than when it was caused by bad luck or lack of effort. In other words, this self-evaluative emotion was not specifically related to outcomes linked to the self-concept. Moreover, additional findings indicated that the younger children did not view ability as any less controllable than effort (cf. Nicholls, 1978). These findings are consistent with the idea that younger children do not view ability as an invariant entity, and, according to Stipek and DeCotis (1988), may partially explain why younger children did not predict highly differentiated self-evaluative emotions.

Interestingly, clinical research with depressed children has yielded findings that are generally consistent with the ones just described. Several studies have found that depressive symptoms are less common in younger children (Rutter, 1983). Moreover, when depression is observed, its character seems different among children of different ages. Most relevant to the present concerns is some evidence suggesting that it is not until later in childhood (approximately 8 years of age or older) that one commonly begins to see negative self-evaluations and self-regard as part of the depressive reaction (Arieti & Bemporad, 1978; McConville, Boag, & Purohit, 1973). These findings seem generally to be in accord with the findings described above from studies of normal populations, and they tentatively suggest that changes in the frequency and symptomology of childhood depression may be related to the development of the dispositional concept.

The Internalization of Prosocial Behavior

There is probably no process more central to the study of socialization and social motives than that of internalization—the incorporation of the moral principles and values of society as one's own (Hoffman, 1983; Maccoby, 1983). Recent approaches to the study of this process have emphasized self-attributions of morality, in the belief that children's self-attributions concerning moral traits may serve as guides for behavior in the absence of external pressure (Grusec, 1983; Lepper, 1983). For instance, Grusec and her colleagues have suggested that altruistic behavior can be encouraged by leading children to categorize themselves as altruistic. The fundamental hypothesis guiding this work is that such a view of oneself, in conjunction with basic consistency motives (i.e., to behave in ways that are consistent with one's views; Festinger, 1957; Heider, 1958) will enhance motivation to behave in altruistic ways (Grusec, Kuczynski, Rushton, & Simutis, 1978; Grusec & Redler, 1980). Several studies provide supportive evidence for this position (Grusec et al., 1978; Grusec & Redler, 1980; Jensen & Moore, 1977; Lepper, 1973; Miller, Brickman, & Bolen, 1975). For example, in a study by Grusec and Redler (1980), children were subtly induced to donate prize winnings to needy children and were then either reinforced socially for doing so or labeled as generous by an adult. In subsequent tests of generosity, the children who had been labeled were substantially more likely to behave altruistically than were the children who had received social reinforcement that was unrelated to their sense of self. Presumably, the labeling affected the way children in the study understood their own characteristics, which in turn conditioned their responses to opportunities to behave altruistically.

Interestingly, the effects of labeling in the Grusec and Redler (1980) study were much stronger for 8- to 10-year-olds than for 5-year-olds. In fact, among the 5-year-olds, the labeling procedure was not superior at all to the social reinforcement one. This was explained by the authors in terms that are directly relevant to the present chapter. They speculated that younger children were not strongly affected by the labeling manipulation because they "have difficulty in thinking of themselves in terms of enduring dispositional traits that produce consistency in behavior" (p. 532).

Like Grusec and Redler (1980), we would suggest that the self-consistency motive does not operate upon children's sense of their own characteristics until they develop a conception of traits or abilities as invariant entities. This would seem to have a number of interesting implications. First and most obviously, one mode of socialization (i.e., through modification of the self-concept) would not be applicable to younger children, and consequently external agents and behavior control processes would have proportionately more influence. Second, consistent with analyses of gender development, processes of self-socialization may begin to operate in connection with personality and ability categorizations once these are conceptualized as invariant. As suggested by Kohlberg's (1966) analysis of gender, this implies that children may become increasingly interested in determining which trait or ability categorizations are relevant to themselves and (in increasing detail) what such categorizations imply for their behavior—for example, what it means to be a good student, an altruistic person, and so on (Ruble, 1987).

The most direct evidence currently available linking the consistency motive and the dispositional concept is contained in a recent study of consistency pressures as manifested in the "foot-in-the-door" effect (Eisenberg et al., 1987). In this study, groups of kindergartners, second-graders, and fifth-graders were first induced to comply with a request to behave altruistically. Later, they were given a second opportunity to perform an altruistic act, in order to test the potential effects of the initial altruistic behavior on subsequent behavior. Children's understanding of trait stability was assessed, as was their personal preference for consistent behavior. The hypothesis of the study was that the foot-in-the-door manipulation would not influence children's behavior until they could understand the relevance of trait labels for future behaviors. Once this condition had been met, children's personal preference for consistency would then moderate the strength of the manipulation. The results were consistent with these expectations. The kindergartners did not show a clear understanding of invariant traits and were unaffected by the foot-in-the-door procedure. The second- and fifth-graders, in contrast, showed a substantial appreciation of the stable traits concept; and especially for those with a strong preference for consistency, the foot-in-the-door manipulation had a significant impact on subsequent behavior. This was the case even though the kindergartners indicated personal preferences for consistency that were as high as those of the older children. Apparently then, it is the interaction of this preference and the understanding of trait stability that determines the impact of the foot-in-the-door procedure.

In summary, two studies (Eisenberg et al., 1987; Grusec & Redler, 1980) suggest that trait-related consistency pressures have greater impact on the prosocial behavior of older children. Moreover, Eisenberg et al. provide evidence linking age differences to the development of notions about invariant dispositions.

Finally, the general implications of these studies are consistent with Kohlberg's (1966) hypothesis regarding the impact of gender-based self-consistency processes.

Interpersonal Interactions

As reflected in our review, although much of the research documenting the development of the dispositional concept examines children's descriptions of and judgments about other people, most of the research touching on the consequences of this development focuses on children's understanding of their own characteristics. Some recent research, however, illustrates how the ability to make inferences about other persons based on their dispositions may also affect responses to these others.

In one recent study (Camhy & Ruble, 1989), 7- to 8-year-old children were given the opportunity to select questions that they might ask a child their age who was visiting their school. The questions were selected on the basis of preratings to represent central/psychological versus peripheral characteristics of others, as defined by Livesley and Bromley (1973). Some subjects thought they would get a chance to play games with the target child, whereas others did not expect future interaction. In addition, subjects completed a measure of a tendency to make predictions consistent with previous disposition-relevant information, modified from that used by Rholes et al. (1988). It was hypothesized that children who expected future interaction would select more central than peripheral questions as a way to understand the target better, and that this would be particularly true for children who scored high on the measure assessing conceptions of dispositional invariance. Consistent with these predictions, there was a significant interaction between the future interaction condition and the tendency to make trait-consistent predictions. Children high on the trait prediction measure who expected future interaction were least interested in asking questions about peripheral, as opposed to central, characteristics. That is, only children who perceived others in invariant trait terms were differentially interested in finding out about the target child's central-psychological versus peripheral characteristics when they anticipated meeting him or her. Thus, these findings suggest that the development of the dispositional concept may have a profound effect on children's approaches to becoming acquainted with peers.

Two other recent studies have examined age differences in the importance of peripheral and central characteristics. In a study by Boggiano, Klinger, and Main (1986), children aged 5, 7, and 9 were asked whether they wanted to play with another child who was described either as having a new game (peripheral) or as being nice (dispositional). The results indicated that the peripheral reason undermined the 9-year-olds' interest in the playmate and dispositional information enhanced it, relative to the interest of a control group. Younger children's interest, in contrast, was enhanced by the information about the game, but was unaffected by the dispositional information. We (Newman & Ruble, 1988) asked children to predict the likelihood that pairs of children would become friends when the reason for one of the children choosing to play with the other was either that he or she had been told that (1) the other child had good toys (peripheral) or (2) the other child was nice (dispositional). Older children (9- to 10-year-olds) predicted a greater likelihood of friendship when the first child selected the other on the basis of personal characteristics rather than toys, but younger children did not make this distinction. This suggests that older children have a greater appreciation of the role of dispositional characteristics in social relationships.[3]

The studies described above suggest that children who understand dispositions to be invariant structures value others for their central or dispositional characteristics rather than for their possessions or other peripheral qualities. This suggests, in turn, that they may be particularly interested in discovering their dispositional characteristics. It also suggests that such children may form relationships that are more stable and less strongly influenced by the transient positive or negative aspects of the other's behavior. Finally, it suggests that after the transition to a more invariant conception of dispositions, children may tend to end old friendships and form new ones because of a shift in the basis upon which friends are evaluated (less peripheral and more central/dispositional).

A final study relevant to interpersonal issues (Feldman & Ruble, 1988) examined a variety of interpersonal choices and behaviors in relation to dispositional inferences. In this study, children aged 5–6 and 9–10 observed a videotaped sequence of behavior that revealed another child to have good or poor motor coordination or to be generous or selfish. Half of the children expected to interact with the children they observed in activities that were related to coordination and generosity, and half did not expect future interactions. After the observations, children described the other children and selected partners for the coordination- and generosity-related activities. It was hypothesized that expecting interaction would activate a need for prediction and control that would enhance children's use of dispositional information in both descriptions and partner choices. The results showed the predicted impact on descriptions for both ages, as described earlier, and on the older children's partner choices. For the younger children, however, increased use of dispositions in descriptions was not paralleled by increased use of dispositional information to select partners who would maximize their chances of winning the game. Instead, younger children's selections were more strongly influenced by the other's likeability than by his or her dispositional qualities.

A second study replicated this finding and showed further that expecting interaction even increased younger children's likeability bias. However, this study also provided direct evidence that dispositional information does influence at least some of the behaviors of young children: The 5-year-olds who expected interaction shared toys with the other child more generously when he or she had previously been observed to share and help others. Thus, these data suggest that motivational factors affect person perception processes and related social interaction consequences (behavior and choices) of children at both age levels. The nature of the consequences may be age-dependent, however: Older children may make more strategic use of the dispositional information to select partners who will help them win, but younger children may be more oriented toward affective or liking consequences. This pattern of findings raises questions about the nature of the social interaction decisions that younger children make on dispositional grounds. In this study, reciprocal sharing seems to have had a dispositional base, but choices that required children to match the other's characteristics with task demands did not. Differences of this sort suggest that children's understanding of the relevance of dispositions to social behavior accumulates gradually and may begin with situations such as reciprocal sharing, which are common in children's daily experience and perhaps are also targeted by adults for discussion and instruction within the socialization process.

Interpretational Issues: Lessons from the Study of Gender Constancy

This last observation suggests that considerable care must be exercised in specifying expected cognition–behavior links. Partner choice may not have been an effective outcome variable, because the trait information provided by the manipulations were not relevant to young children's goals in selecting partners. Thus, in initial attempts to examine the social and motivational consequences of developing social concepts, it may be necessary to evaluate the meaning of null findings quite carefully.

Recent literature in the area of gender constancy provides some relevant lessons along these lines. The idea that gender constancy leads to heightened responsiveness to gender implies that gender-constant children should be more attentive to and prefer same-sex objects and activities. Several studies, however, have failed to find an association between constancy and such measures (e.g., Bryan & Luria, 1978; Marcus & Overton, 1978). Moreover, attempts to relate gender constancy to measures of gender-related information processing have been unsuccessful (Carter & Levy, 1988). Such observations have led to recent conclusions that gender constancy may not be an important aspect of early sex-role development, after all, and that sex-role acquisition may be better conceptualized in terms of the development of gender schemas (Carter & Levy, 1988).

Two points, involving both methodological and conceptual issues, need to be raised concerning such null findings. First, it is not clear that gender constancy (or gender schema) should necessarily be related to all aspects of gender-role development. Indeed, gender schema and gender constancy may be conceptualized as representing different underlying processes, such that they would be expected to affect different aspects of gender-role development. A schema functions as an organizing system that facilitates efficient storage and retrieval of information (Fiske & Taylor, 1984). Thus, gender schemata may be most clearly conceptualized in terms of effects on information processing, such that as the schema becomes more comprehensive, gender-role information is better organized and remembered. In contrast, gender constancy may be better conceptualized as a motivational variable. Kohlberg (1966) argued that once children develop a conception of a constant categorical gender identity, they become motivated to learn what behavior is appropriate for their gender and to act accordingly.

If, indeed, two different processes are involved, one might expect that they would affect different dependent variables. Specifically, the growth of the gender schema—conceptualized as breadth and depth of knowledge, not as salience (Bem, 1984)—should be more closely associated with standard schema-driven processes, such as organization and memory. In contrast, the growth of gender constancy might instead be expected to affect more motivationally relevant variables, such as activity choice and behavior. Consistent with these predictions, one recent study found that these two types of social cognitions differentially predicted different aspects of gender development. The development of gender schemata, but not gender constancy, was positively associated with better recall of gender-stereotypic versus counterstereotypic information. In contrast, gender constancy, but not gender schema, predicted more motivationally relevant variables, such as preference for same-sex toys (Stangor & Ruble, 1989).

The second point raised by the null findings mentioned above is that careful consideration must be given to the way in which this motivational shift may be reflected in behavior. The failures to relate constancy to attention or preference have typically provided no alternative behaviors. Bryan and Luria (1978), for example, did not find differential attention to same-sex pictures. Their stimuli were presented sequentially, however, and thus did not require selective attention, as in the Slaby and Frey (1975) study, where male and female models were presented simultaneously. Moreover, there were no alternaive targets for the children to attend to other than the models themselves, which may have resulted in ceiling effects. Similarly, studies failing to find an association between constancy and same-sex preference have not provided children with alternative dimensions along which to make their selections. Thus, virtually, all children show preferences for same-sex activities. When a competing dimension is presented, however, such as the activity level of the toy, then a clear association between constancy and same-sex preference is found (Eaton, Von Bargen, & Keats, 1981), even when age is controlled for (Stangor & Ruble, 1989). Moreover, the results of a recent related study suggest that the effects of constancy on preferences may be shown most clearly when the same-sex choice involves a conflict, such as involving a less attractive option (Frey & Ruble, 1989).

In summary, the present analysis suggests that the development of the recognition of a stable gender does have important motivational and behavioral consequences. The scope of the influence of this change in social-cognitive understanding is limited, however, and is easily missed if the underlying process is not carefully conceptualized and the relevant dependent variables are not carefully selected. Such admonitions may serve as useful guides in a continuing analysis of consequences of the understanding of dispositions.

Processes Linking the Dispositional Concept to Social Motivation and Behavior

We have suggested that there appear to be many diverse consequences of children's developing perceptions of people in invariant dispositional terms. Why do these changes occur? Although it is widely recognized that developmental changes in social cognition should influence social motivation and behavior in predictable ways, there has been little theoretical guidance as to how this process might occur. In this section, we attempt to provide a preliminary conceptualization of how developmental shifts in social cognition should relate to behavioral consequences, based on the examples described in the preceding review of the empirical literature. Three distinct processes may be identified in this way: (1) desire for consistency; (2) a change in the impact or meaning of events; and (3) a change in motivation for or interest in acquiring certain kinds of information. We describe each in turn and indicate which kinds of empirical relations seem best described by each process.

Desire for Consistency

The need for consistency has a long and important history in social-psychological theories of motivation (Festinger, 1957; Heider, 1958). Moreover, recent reviews of the literature have noted a renewed interest in consistency-based processes (Cooper & Croyle, 1984). The operation of the consistency motive has been studied in connection with a wide variety of behavioral systems, and it may be used to explain a number of the relations between social cognition and behavior reviewed earlier.

Kohlberg (1966) was one of the first to suggest the relevance of this type of motive to such social-developmental concerns. According to his theory of sex-role development, once children are able to categorize themselves in terms of gender and realize the long-term significance of that categorization, they become subject to internal (as opposed to exclusively environmental) pressures to behave in ways that are consistent with their gender. Thus, in this way one can explain previously described relations between gender constancy and certain measures of sex typing.

Consistency motives are also the favored explanation of relations observed in the area of prosocial behavior. Grusec and Redler (1980), for example, have argued that needs "to maintain some kind of cognitive consistency" (p. 532) probably account for findings that older children who are induced to label themselves as generous subsequently behave more generously. Theoretically, consistency processes should also be relevant to developmental changes in children's responses to others' behavior. To our knowledge, however, there is no such research in the area of prosocial behavior, but there is supportive evidence in the literature on sex-role development. Children who have reached gender constancy are more likely to erroneously "remember" a videotaped character as behaving consistently with his or her sex than children who have not reached gender constancy (Stangor & Ruble, 1989).

Although the operation of a consistency motive seems to be a reasonably straightforward account of many relations between social cognition and behavior, there is no direct evidence concerning its mediating role, and a number of unanswered questions concerning how it might operate remain. First, as Eisenberg et al. (1987) note, it does not necessarily follow that a self-perception of an invariant trait by itself should lead to subsequent consistent responding. A desire for consistency may also be necessary and is probably best conceptualized as an independent or at least a partially independent entity. Indeed, Eisenberg et al. (1987) demonstrated empirically that the relation of the invariance concept to behavior is moderated by an individual difference in preference for consistency.

Second, it is not clear whether perceptions of people in mature dispositional terms play a role in initiating motives for consistency or only change their form. On the one hand, one might argue that perceptions of attributes as invariant are necessary before a consistency motive can be relevant. On the other hand, preferences for consistency might be viewed as fundamental, with changes in social cognition resulting primarily in a more global expression of existing needs for consistency. The consistency motives of young children, for example, may be expressed in a very specific need "to share with my brother" or "not to cry at the doctor's office" rather than in the need to be "generous" or "brave." Indeed, findings by Eisenberg et al. (1987) that kindergartners reported preferences for consistency as high as those of older children may support this latter interpretation of the operation of the consistency motive.

Finally, the source of the consistency motive is not completely clear. Are children motivated to maintain consistency between their behavior and their perceptions of their own characteristics (trait consistency), or are they motivated to maintain consistency between their actions and valued standards of behavior (cf. Higgins, in press; Higgins, Tykocinski, & Vookles, in press)? In connection with the studies of Eisenberg et al. (1987) and Grusec and Redler (1980), the basic question is whether the critical changes that took place involved changes in children's values and standards or in perceptions concerning their traits and sense of self. To argue in terms of a need for trait consistency means that one should in theory make similar predictions for positive and negative traits—for example, that children who label themselves as "stingy" would be motivated to behave in ways consistent with the label, in spite of the negative quality of the label, the potential costs to self-esteem, and the conflict with internalized values and standards. Although support for this negative aspect of consistency motives has been found with adults (Swann & Read, 1981), it has not been examined with children. The case for connecting social-cognitive development and consistency motives would be considerably strengthened if such data were to be obtained, because this would more clearly specify the nature of the motive in question.

Results described earlier concerning gender development suggest that research on the tendency to behave consistently with negative self-attributes may be an extremely important point in connection with the role of consistency motives in social development. Children who were not gender-constant showed a preference for toys depicted as gender-appropriate only when the toys were attractive. In contrast, children who were at the stage of gender constancy showed a preference for gender-appropriate toys even when they were unattractive (Frey & Ruble, 1989). Thus, the point at which children are willing to behave consistently with negative attributes or cases in which consistent behavior is associated with significant "costs" may most clearly indicate a true internalization of a self-perception.

Changes in the Impact or Meaning of Events

A second way in which developmental shifts in social cognition may be linked to social motivations and behaviors concerns changes in the meaning of events associated with changes in the perceived invariance of personal attributes. In the preceding review, such a process has seemed most clearly relevant to findings in the area of achievement and self-evaluation. That is, a new interpretation of events in terms of constancies means that a school-related failure implies something more consequential for a child's sense of self and future expectations than previously; indeed the findings reviewed earlier are consistent with such predictions. An interpretation in terms of change in meaning leads to similar predictions in the area of interpersonal relations, though, to our knowledge, such issues have not been addressed. For instance, being rejected by a peer no longer means just the loss of a playmate or a set of attractive toys for the moment; it may also signal a more basic personal inadequacy that will carry over to other occasions. Similarly, with respect to perceptions of others, another's unfriendly actions may now be expected to continue and lead to avoidance behaviors that would not have been anticipated previously. Evidence supporting the importance of this process is available in studies linking changes in the meaning of traits to achievement-related behaviors and self-evaluations, as reviewed earlier.

Changes in the Motivation for or Interest in Acquiring Relevant Information

A third possible process underlying relations between social cognition and behavior concerns the way in which perceptions of invariance may affect *interest* in information relevant to the self or other. A new realization of the impact of underlying personal stabilities implies that there is a previously unrecognized set of material one must learn in order to master one's social environment. Thus, at this point in development, a child may show a heightened interest in dispositional characteristics or information relevant to them. This emphasis on an active, constructive orientation toward the social environment and self-concept is consistent with self-socialization perspectives applied to gender development by Kohlberg (1966) and more recently to other aspects of self-definition (Ruble, 1987).

A number of the findings reviewed earlier are consistent with this perspective. First, with respect to gender constancy, greater attention and responsiveness to same-sex others suggests an orientation toward active information seeking. Similarly, in achievement settings, shifts in preferred standards of evaluation, such as social comparison, may indicate changes in interest in information relevant to invariant characteristics in oneself or others. Finally, differences between children who perceive others in invariant terms and children who do not in the kinds of questions selected when becoming acquainted with a peer (Camhy & Ruble, 1989) may reflect a changed interest in the kinds of characteristics perceived as relevant to becoming friends. Of course, such findings do not provide direct evidence concerning the role of self-initiated, active information seeking. As with the other two proposed processes, therefore, future research should provide opportunities to contrast these motivational explanations with alternative possibilities.

In summary, we have identified three possible processes linking emerging conceptions of person invariance with changes in social motivation and behavior. Taken together, these three processes can explain the observed relations reviewed earlier, and they also suggest other relations to be examined in future research. Moreover, conceptual and empirical limitations in the interpretations of some of these observed relations have been described, particularly with respect to the motivation for consistency. At present, progress in research on all three processes is impeded somewhat by our dependence upon less than ideal measures of invariance. As discussed above, though the different measures used in past research correlate, none is by itself unambiguous. The number and proportion of traits included in open-ended person descriptions may be confounded with verbal fluency; in addition, interpretation of prediction measures is not without problems because, as noted above, cross-situational prediction may reflect use of various matching rules that rely on perceptions of valence or situations or on semantic category structure rather than on underlying causal forces. Consequently, a simple prediction measure may underestimate the extent to which development of invariance affects the perceived meaning of events. Using it may be analogous to trying to predict gender-related behavior on the basis of a measure reflecting the development of *both* gender schema and gender constancy. In short, as in the work on gender concepts, more precise specification of cognition–behavior links will require more precise measurement of cognitions.

In addition to measurement concerns, future attention to direct demonstrations of process also seems important—not only to clarify the nature of links between social cognition and behavior (an issue common to social and developmental literatures), but also to identify the possibility of processes that may be unique to *emerging* social cognitions, such as heightened information seeking at certain points during development. Longitudinal studies are thus necessary to complement studies examining the effects of direct manipulations of these three hypothesized processes.

Notes

1. Note that central characteristics are not simply those that are stable or internal. Emotional states (e.g., "happy") are internal, and physical appearance (e.g., "pretty") typically is stable. Neither of them are dispositional concepts in the sense discussed above, though in some studies references to such qualities are classified as trait descriptions/explanations.

2. Interestingly, in the same study children's perceptions of the invariance of their own ability showed quite a different pattern. These perceptions were positively related to interest in temporal comparison, but negatively related to interest in social comparison, though once again this pattern was significant only for the oldest children. Thus, in seeming contradiction to our general hypothesis, children who were *least* certain of the invariance of their own ability level preferred social comparison over temporal comparison information. Perhaps among children who are mature enough to have a "concept" of invariant ability, factors that influence their level of certainty or uncertainty about

themselves determine their level of interest in relative standing (Trope, 1986). The difference in patterns for perceptions of the stability of one's own versus others' ability is intriguing. It seems quite possible that a focus on self-perceptions involves processes other than a straightforward application of one's conceptions of ability. That is, as in other domains, self-judgments differ from other-judgments in arousing, for example, self-esteem concerns (Damon & Hart, 1982). Thus, in evaluating the motivational implications of the understanding of invariant characteristics as a developmental variable, it would seem prudent to utilize measures based on perceptions of others.

3. It is also possible, however, that the effect reflected differences in perceived goals of the target as a function of the target's age—that if given the chance, for example, younger subjects would predict different bases for friendship for younger versus older targets.

References

Abramson, L. Y., Seligman, M. E. P., & Teasdale, J. (1978). Learned helplessness in humans: Critique and reformulation. *Journal of Abnormal Psychology, 87*, 49–74.

Allen, B. P., & Smith, G. F. (1980). Traits, situations, and their interaction as alternative "causes" of behavior. *Journal of Social Psychology, 111*, 99–104.

Allen, J. L., Walker, L. D., Schroeder, D. A., & Johnson, D. E. (1987). Attributions and attribution-behavior relations: The effects of level of cognitive development. *Journal of Personality and Social Psychology, 52*, 1099–1109.

Allport, G. W., & Odbert, H. S. (1936). Trait names: A psycholexical study. *Psychological Monographs: General and Applied, 47* (1, Whole No. 211).

Alston, W. P. (1975). Traits, consistency, and conceptual alternatives for personality theory. *Journal for the Theory of Social Behavior, 5*, 17–47.

Arieti, S., & Bemporad, J. (1978). *Severe and mild depression.* New York: Basic Books.

Barenboim, C. (1977). Developmental changes in the interpersonal cognitive system from middle childhood to adolescence. *Child Development, 48*, 1467–1474.

Barenboim, C. (1981). The development of person perception in childhood and adolescence: From behavioral comparisons to psychological constructs to psychological comparisons. *Child Development, 52*, 129–144.

Bem, S. L. (1984). Androgeny and gender schema theory. In T. B. Sonderegger (Ed.), *Nebraska Symposium on Motivation* (Vol. 32, pp. 179–226). Lincoln: University of Nebraska Press.

Benenson, J., & Dweck, C. (1986). The development of trait explanations and self-evaluations in the academic and social domains. *Child Development, 57*, 1179–1187.

Berscheid, E., Graziano, W., Monson, T., & Dermer, M. (1976). Outcome dependency: Attention, attribution, and attraction. *Journal of Personality and Social Psychology, 34*, 378–389.

Bigner, J. J. (1974). A Wernerian developmental analysis of children's descriptions of siblings. *Child Development, 45*, 317–323.

Boggiano, A. K., Klinger, C. A., & Main, D. S. (1986). Enhancing interest in peer interaction: A developmental analysis. *Child Development, 57*, 852–861.

Brickman, P., & Bulman, R. J. (1977). Pleasure and pain in social comparison. In J. M. Suls & R. L. Miller (Eds.), *Social comparison processes: Theoretical and empirical perspectives* (pp. 149–186). Washington, DC: Hemisphere.

Bryan, J. W., & Luria, Z. (1978). Sex role learning: A test of the selective learning hypothesis. *Child Development, 49*, 13–23.

Buss, A. H., & Finn, S. E. (1987). Classification of personality traits. *Journal of Personality and Social Psychology, 52*, 432–444.

Buss, D. M., & Craik, K. H. (1983). The act frequency approach to personality. *Psychological Review, 90*, 105–126.

Bussey, K., & Bandura, A. (1984). Influence on gender constancy and social power on sex-linked modeling. *Journal of Personality and Social Psychology, 47*, 1292–1302.

Calveric, B. R. (1979). *Conceptualizing others: A developmental investigation.* Unpublished doctoral dissertation, Clark University.

Camhy, M., & Ruble, D. N. (1989). *Becoming acquainted with a peer: Social-cognitive and motivational influences.* Manuscript in preparation, New York University.

Carter, D. B., & Levy, G. D. (1988). Cognitive aspects of early sex-role development: The influence of gender schemas on preschoolers memories and preferences for sex-typed toys and activities. *Child Development, 59,* 782–792.

Case, R. (1985). *Intellectual development: Birth to adulthood.* New York: Academic Press.

Caspi, A. (1987). Personality in the life course. *Journal of Personality and Social Psychology, 53,* 1203–1213.

Chaplin, W. F., John, O. P., & Goldberg, L. R. (1988). Conceptions of states and traits: Dimensional attributes with ideals as prototypes. *Journal of Personality and Social Psychology, 54,* 541–557.

Citron, C. C., Serbin, L. A., & Conner, J. M. (1979, March). *Children's observational learning of same and opposite sex models' behaviors.* Paper presented at the conference of the Association for Women in Psychology.

Cooper, J., & Croyle, R. T. (1984). Attitudes and attitude change. *Annual Review of Psychology, 35,* 395–426.

Crocker, J., Hannah, D. B., & Weber, R. (1983). Person memory and causal attributions. *Journal of Personality and Social Psychology, 44,* 55–66.

Damon, W., & Hart, D. (1982). The development of self-understanding from infancy through adolescence. *Child Development, 53,* 841–864.

DiVitto, B., & McArthur, L. Z. (1978). Developmental differences in the use of distinctiveness, consensus, and consistency information for making causal attributions. *Developmental Psychology, 14,* 474–482.

Dix, T., & Grusec, J. E. (1983). Parental influence techniques: An attributional analysis. *Child Development, 54,* 645–652.

Dweck, C. S., & Leggett, E. L. (1988). A social-cognitive approach to motivation and personality. *Psychological Review, 95,* 256–273.

Eaton, W. O., Von Vargen, D., & Keats, J. G. (1981). Gender understanding and dimensions of preschooler toy choice: Sex stereotype versus activity level. *Canadian Journal of Behavioral Science, 13,* 203–209.

Eccles, J. E., Midgley, C., & Adler, T. (1984). Age-related changes in the school environment: Effects on achievement motivation. In J. Nicholls (Ed.), *The development of achievement motivation* (pp. 283–331). Greenwood, CT: JAI Press.

Eisenberg, N., Cialdini, R., McCreath, H., & Shell, R. (1987). Consistency-based compliance: When and why do children become vulnerable? *Journal of Personality and Social Psychology, 52,* 1174–1181.

Epstein, S., & Teraspulsky, L. (1986). Perception of cross-situational consistency. *Journal of Personality and Social Psychology, 50,* 1152–1160.

Feldman, N. S., & Ruble, D. N. (1988). The effect of personal relevance on psychological inference: A developmental analysis. *Child Development, 59,* 1339–1352.

Ferguson, T. J., Olthof, T., Luiten, A., & Rule, B. G. (1984). Children's use of observed behavioral frequency vs. behavioral covariation in ascribing dispositions to others. *Child Development, 55,* 2094–2105.

Ferguson, T. J., van Roozendaal, J., & Rule, B. G. (1986). Informational basis for children's impressions of others. *Developmental Psychology, 22,* 335–341.

Festinger, L. (1957). *A theory of cognitive dissonance.* Stanford, CA: Stanford University Press.

Fiske, S. T., & Cox, M. G. (1979). Person concepts: The affects of target familiarity and descriptive purpose on the process of describing others. *Journal of Personality, 47,* 136–161.

Fiske, S. T., & Taylor, S. E. (1984). *Social cognition.* Reading, MA: Addison-Wesley.

Flavell, J. H. (1977). *Cognitive development.* Englewood Cliffs, NJ: Prentice-Hall.

Fletcher, G. J. O. (1984). Psychology and common sense. *American Psychologist, 39,* 203–213.

Frey, K. S., & Ruble, D. N. (1985). What children say when the teacher is not around: Conflicting goals in social comparison and performance assessment in the classroom. *Journal of Personality and Social Psychology, 48,* 550–562.

Frey, K. S., & Ruble, D. N. (1987). What children say about classroom performance: Sex and grade differences in perceived competence. *Child Development, 58*, 1066–1078.

Frey, K. S., & Ruble, D. N. (1989). *Gender constancy and the "cost" of sex-typed behavior: A test of the conflict hypothesis.* Manuscript submitted for publication.

Glasberg, R., & Aboud, F. (1982). Keeping one's distance from sadness: Children's self-reports of emotional experience. *Developmental Psychology, 18*, 287–293.

Gnepp, J., & Chilamkurti, C. (1988). Children's use of personality attributions to predict other people's emotional and behavioral reactions. *Child Development, 59*, 743–754.

Gollin, E. S. (1958). Organizational characteristics of social judgment: A developmental investigation. *Journal of Personality, 26*, 139–154.

Gordon, S. E., & Wyer, R. S. (1987). Person memory: Category-set-size effects on the recall of a person's behavior. *Journal of Personality and Social Psychology, 53*, 648–662.

Gottman, J. M. (1987). Same-sex and cross-sex friendships in children. In J. M. Gottman & J. Parker (Eds.), *Conversations of friends* (pp. 110–141). New York: Cambridge University Press.

Grusec, J. (1983). The internalization of altruistic dispositions: A cognitive analysis. In E. T. Higgins, D. N. Ruble, & W. W. Hartup (Eds.), *Social cognition and social development: A sociocultural perspective* (pp. 275–293). New York: Cambridge University Press.

Grusec, J. E., Kuczynski, L., Rushton, J. P., & Simutis, Z. (1978). Modeling, direct instruction, and attributions: Effects on altruism. *Developmental Psychology, 14*, 51–57.

Grusec, J. E., & Redler, E. (1980). Attribution, reinforcement, and altruism: A developmental analysis. *Developmental Psychology, 16*, 525–534.

Hayden, T., & Mischel, W. (1976). Maintaining trait consistency in the resolution of behavioral inconsistency: The wolf in sheep's clothing? *Journal of Personality, 13*, 141–154.

Heider, F. (1958). *The psychology of interpersonal relations.* New York: Wiley.

Heller, K. A., & Berndt, T. J. (1981). Developmental changes in the formation and organization of personality attributions. *Child Development, 52*, 683–691.

Higgins, E. T. (1989). Continuities and discontinuities in self-regulatory processes. *Journal of Personality, 57*, 407–444.

Higgins, E. T. (in press). Development of self-regulatory and self-evaluative processes: Costs, benefits, and trade-offs. In M. R. Gunnar & L. A. Sroufe (Eds.), *Self processes in development: Minnesota Symposium on Child Psychology* (Vol. 23). Minneapolis: University of Minnesota Press.

Higgins, E. T., & Parsons, J. E. (1983). Social cognition and the social life of the child: Stages as subcultures. In E. T. Higgins, D. N. Ruble, & W. W. Hartup (Eds.), *Social cognition and social development: A sociocultural perspective* (pp. 15–62). New York: Cambridge University Press.

Higgins, E. T., Tykocinski, O., & Vookles, J. (in press). Patterns of self-belief: The psychological significance of relations among the actual, ideal, ought, can, and future selves. In J. M. Olson & M. P. Zanna (Eds.), *Self-inference processes: The Ontario Symposium* (Vol. 6). Hillsdale, NJ: Erlbaum.

Hoffman, M. L. (1983). Affective and cognitive processes in moral internalization. In E. T. Higgins, D. N. Ruble, & W. W. Hartup (Eds.), *Social cognition and social development: A sociocultural perspective* (pp. 236–274). New York: Cambridge University Press.

Jackson, D. N. (1974). *Personality Research Form manual.* Port Huron, MI: Research Psychologists Press.

Jensen, A. M., & Moore, S. G. (1977). The effect of attribute statements on cooperativeness and competitiveness in school-age boys. *Child Development, 48*, 305–307.

Josephson, J. (1977). *The child's use of situational and personal information in predicting the behavior of another.* Unpublished doctoral dissertation, Stanford University.

Kassin, S. M. (1981). From laychild to "layman": Developmental causal attribution. In S. S. Brehm, S. M. Kassin, & F. X. Gibbons (Eds.), *Developmental social psychology* (pp. 169–190). New York: Oxford University Press.

Kelley, H. H. (1972). Causal schemata and the attribution process. In E. E. Jones, D. E. Kanouse, H. H. Kelley, R. E. Nisbett, S. Valins, & B. Weiner (Eds.), *Attribution: Perceiving the causes of behavior* (pp. 151–174). Morristown, NJ: General Learning Press.

Kohlberg, L. (1966). A cognitive-developmental analysis of children's sex-role concepts and attitudes. In E. E. Maccoby (Ed.), *The development of sex differences* (pp. 82-172). Stanford, CA: Stanford University Press.

Lepper, M. R. (1973). Dissonance, self-perception, and honesty in children. *Journal of Personality and Social Psychology, 25,* 65-74.

Lepper, M. R. (1983). Social-control processes and the internalization of social values: An attributional perspective. In E. T. Higgins, D. N. Rubles, & W. W. Hartup (Eds.), *Social cognition and social development: A sociocultural perspective* (pp. 294-330). New York: Cambridge University Press.

Livesley, W. J., & Bromley, D. B. (1973). *Person perception in childhood and adolescence.* Chichester, England: Wiley.

Maccoby, E. E. (1983). Let's not overattribute to the attribution process: Comments on social cognition and behavior. In E. T. Higgins, D. N. Ruble, & W. W. Hartup (Eds.), *Social cognition and social development: A sociocultural perspective* (pp. 356-370). New York: Cambridge University Press.

MacLennan, R. N., & Jackson, D. N. (1985). Accuracy and consistency in the development of social perception. *Developmental Psychology, 21,* 30-36.

Marcus, D. E., & Overton, W. F. (1978). The development of cognitive gender constancy and sex role preferences. *Child Development, 52,* 1119-1134.

McConville, B. J., Boag, L. C., & Purohit, A. P. (1973). Three types of childhood depression. *Canadian Psychiatric Association Journal, 18,* 133-138.

Miller, A. T. (1985). A developmental study of the cognitive basis of performance and improvement after failure. *Journal of Personality and Social Psychology, 49,* 529-538.

Miller, J. G. (1984). Culture and the development of everyday social explanation. *Journal of Personality and Social Psychology, 46,* 961-978.

Miller, J. G. (1986). Early cross-cultural commonalities in social explanation. *Developmental Psychology, 22,* 514-520.

Miller, R. L., Brickman, P., & Bolen, D. (1975). Attribution versus persuasion as a means for modifying behavior. *Journal of Personality and Social Psychology, 31,* 430-441.

Mischel, W. (1973). Toward a cognitive social-learning reconceptualization of personality. *Psychological Review, 80,* 252-283.

Mohr, D. M. (1978). Development of attributes of personal identity. *Developmental Psychology, 14,* 427-428.

Monson, T. C., Keel, R., Stephens, D., & Genung, V. (1982). Trait attributions: Relative validity, covariation with behavior, and prospect of interaction. *Journal of Personality and Social Psychology, 42,* 1014-1024.

Newman, L. S. (1990). *The stable disposition concept and spontaneous trait inference: Developmental and individual differences.* Unpublished doctoral dissertation, New York University.

Newman, L. S., & Ruble, D. N. (1988, April). *Children's friendships and the discounting principle: Age and motivational-experiential differences.* Paper presented at the annual meeting of the Eastern Psychological Association, Buffalo, NY.

Newman, L. S., Ruble, D. N., & Higgins, E. T. (1987). [Children's interaction goals]. Unpublished research data, New York University.

Nicholls, J. (1978). The development of the concepts of effort and ability, perceptions of academic attainment and the understanding that difficult tasks require more ability. *Child Development, 49,* 800-814.

Nicholls, J. G. (1984). Achievement motivation: Conceptions of ability, task choice, and performance. *Psychological Review, 91,* 328-346.

Nicholls, J. G., & Miller, A. T. (1984). Development and its discontents: The differentiation of the concept of ability. In J. G. Nicholls (Ed.), *The development of achievement motivation* (pp. 138-159). Greenwich, CT: JAI Press.

Nisbett, R. E. (1980). The trait construct in lay and professional psychology. In L. Festinger (Ed.), *Retrospections on social psychology.* New York: Oxford University Press.

Parsons, J. E., & Ruble, D. N. (1977). The development of achievement-related expectancies. *Child Development, 48*, 1075–1079.

Peevers, B. H., & Secord, P. F. (1973). Developmental changes in attribution of descriptive concepts to persons. *Journal of Personality and Social Psychology, 27*, 120–128.

Reeder, G. D., & Spores, J. M. (1983). The attribution of morality. *Journal of Personality and Social Psychology, 44*, 736–745.

Rholes, W. S., Blackwell, J., Jordan, C., & Walters, C. (1980). A developmental study of learned helplessness. *Developmental Psychology, 16*, 616–624.

Rholes, W. S., Jones, M., & Wade, C. (1988). Children's understanding of personal dispositions and its relationship to behavior. *Journal of Experimental Child Psychology, 45*, 1–17.

Rholes, W. S., & Ruble, D. N. (1983). *Information processing influence on the development of stable trait concepts.* Unpublished manuscript, Texas A&M University.

Rholes, W. S., & Ruble, D. N. (1984). Children's understanding of dispositional characteristics of others. *Child Development, 55*, 550–560.

Rholes, W. S., & Ruble, D. N. (1986). Children's impression of other persons: The effects of temporal separation of behavioral information. *Child Development, 57*, 872–878.

Rholes, W. S., & Wade, C. (1989). Unpublished data, Texas A&M University.

Rholes, W. S., & Walters, J. (1982). Schematic patterns of causal evidence. *Child Development, 53*, 1046–1057.

Ross, L. (1977). The intuitive psychologist and his shortcomings: Distortions in the attribution process. In L. Berkowitz (Ed.), *Advances in experimental social psychology* (Vol. 10, pp. 173–220). New York: Academic Press.

Ross, L. (1981). The "intuitive scientist" formulation and its developmental implications. In J. H. Flavell & L. Ross (Eds.), *Social-cognitive development: Frontiers and possible futures* (pp. 1–42). Cambridge: Cambridge University Press.

Rotenberg, K. J. (1980). Children's use of intentionality judgments of character and disposition. *Child Development, 51*, 282–284.

Rotenberg, K. J. (1982). Development of character constancy of self and other. *Child Development, 53*, 505–515.

Ruble, D. N. (1987). The acquisition of self-knowledge: A self-socialization perspective. In N. Eisenberg (Ed.), *Contemporary topics in developmental psychology* (pp. 243–270). New York: Wiley.

Ruble, D. N., Balaban, T., & Cooper, J. (1981). Gender constancy and the effects of sex-typed televised toy commercials. *Child Development, 52*, 667–673.

Ruble, D. N., Feldman, N. S., Higgins, E. T., & Karlovac, M. (1979). Locus of causality and the use of information in the development of causal attributions. *Journal of Personality, 47*, 595–614.

Ruble, D. N., & Flett, G. L. (1988). Conflicting goals in self-evaluative goal seeking: Developmental and ability level analysis. *Child Development, 59*, 97–106.

Ruble, D. N., & Frey, K. S. (1987). Social comparison and self-evaluation in the classroom: Developmental changes in knowledge and function. In J. C. Masters & W. P. Smith (Eds.), *Social comparison, social justice, and relative deprivation: Theoretical, empirical, and policy perspectives* (pp. 81–104). Hillsdale, NJ: Erlbaum.

Ruble, D. N., Newman, L. S., Rholes, W. S., & Altshuler, J. (1988). Children's naive psychology: The use of behavioral and situational information for the prediction of behavior. *Cognitive Development, 3*, 89–112.

Ruble, D. N., Parsons, J., & Ross, J. (1976). Self-evaluative responses of children in an achievement setting. *Child Development, 47*, 990–997.

Ruble, D. N., & Rholes, W. S. (1981). The development of children's perceptions and attributions about their social world. In J. H. Harvey, W. Ickes, & R. F. Kidd (Eds.), *New directions in attribution research* (Vol. 3, pp. 3–36). Hillsdale, NJ: Erlbaum.

Rutter, M. (1983). Developmental psychopathology. In E. M. Hetherington (Vol. Ed.), *Handbook of child psychology* (4th ed.): *Vol. 4. Socialization, personality, and social development* (pp. 689–779). New York: Wiley.

Scarlett, H. H., Press, A. N., & Crockett, W. H. (1971). Children's descriptions of peers: A Wernerian developmental analysis. *Child Development, 42,* 439–453.

Secord, P. F., & Peevers, B. H. (1974). The development and attribution of person concepts. In T. Mischel (Ed.), *Understanding other persons* (pp. 100–121). Totowa, NJ: Rowman & Littlefield.

Shantz, C. U. (1983). Social cognition. In J. H. Flavell & E. M. Markman (Vol. Eds.), *Handbook of child psychology* (4th ed.): *Vol. 3. Cognitive development* (pp. 495–555). New York: Wiley.

Slaby, R. G., & Frey, K. S. (1975). Development of gender constancy and selective attention to same sex models. *Child Development, 45,* 849–856.

Smetana, J. G. (1985). Children's impressions of moral and conventional transgressors. *Developmental Psychology, 21,* 715–724.

Stangor, C., & Ruble, D. N. (1987). Development of gender role knowledge and gender constancy. In L. S. Liben & M. L. Signorella (Eds.), *New directions for child development: Vol. 39. Children's gender schemata* (pp. 5–22). San Francisco: Jossey-Bass.

Stangor, C., & Ruble, D. N. (1989). Differential influence of gender schemata and gender constancy on children's information processing and behavior. *Social Cognition, 7,* 353–372.

Stipek, D. J. (1984). The development of achievement motivation. In R. E. Ames & C. Ames (Eds.), *Research on motivation in education: Vol. 1. Student motivation* (pp. 145–174). New York: Academic Press.

Stipek, D., & Daniels, D. (1987). *Children's use of dispositional attributions in predicting the behavior of classmates.* Paper presented at the convention of the Society for Research in Child Development, Baltimore.

Stipek, D. J., & DeCotis, K. M. (1988). Children's understanding of the implications of causal attributions for emotional experiences. *Child Development, 59,* 1601–1610.

Stipek, D., & Hoffman, J. (1980). Development of children's performance-related judgments. *Child Development, 51,* 912–914.

Stipek, D., & MacIver, D. (1989). Developmental change in children's assessment of intellectual competence. *Child Development, 60,* 521–538.

Swann, W. B., & Read, S. J. (1981). Self-verification processes: How we sustain our self-conceptions. *Journal of Experimental Social Psychology, 17,* 351–372.

Trope, Y. (1986). Self-enhancement and self-assessment in achievement behavior. In R. M. Sorrentino & E. T. Higgins (Eds.), *Handbook of motivation and cognition: Foundations of social behavior* (Vol. 1, pp. 350–378). New York: Guilford Press.

Uleman, J. S. (1987). Consciousness and control: The case of spontaneous trait inferences. *Personality and Social Psychology Bulletin, 13,* 337–354.

Wimer, S., & Kelley, H. H. (1982). An investigation of the dimensions of causal attribution. *Journal of Personality and Social Psychology, 43,* 1142–1162.

Weiner, B. (1985). An attributional theory of achievement motivation and emotion. *Psychological Review, 92,* 548–573.

Wood, M. E. (1978). Children's developing understanding of other people's motives for behavior. *Developmental Psychology, 14,* 561–562.

Wright, J. C., & Mischel, W. (1988). Conditional hedges and the intuitive psychology of traits. *Journal of Personality and Social Psychology, 55,* 454–469.

Yarrow, M. R., & Campbell, J. D. (1963). Person perception in children. *Merrill-Palmer Quarterly, 9,* 57–72.

Zuroff, D. C. (1982). Person, situation, and person-by-situation interaction components in person perception. *Journal of Personality, 50,* 1–14.

Zuroff, D. C. (1986). Was Gordon Allport a trait theorist? *Journal of Personality and Social Psychology, 51,* 993–1000.

CHAPTER 12

To Be Adored or to Be Known?
The Interplay of Self-Enhancement and Self-Verification

WILLIAM B. SWANN, JR.
University of Texas–Austin

Every man is inescapably a *Machtmensch*; his most coveted experience is the enhancement of his self-esteem, and his most ineradicable trait is vanity. —*Gordon Allport* (1937, p. 169)

Many people find it hard to believe that a person will defend and strive to maintain an idea [about himself] which is not to his advantage. But the evidence allows of no other conclusion.—*Prescott Lecky* (1945, p. 124)

What do people want to think of themselves? The founders of social and personality psychology generally assumed, as did Allport, that people want to think well of themselves. In fact, until the early 1950s, virtually every major theory of social behavior held that people are strongly motivated to enhance their self-images.

Yet during the 1950s and 1960s—what some regard as the "golden years" of social and personality psychology—a very different view of human organism prevailed, one that placed Lecky's lofty desire for cognitive consistency or balance at the center of the person's psychological universe (e.g., Aronson, 1968; Festinger, 1957; Heider, 1946; 1958; McGuire, 1960; Newcomb, 1956; Osgood & Tannenbaum, 1955; Rosenberg & Abelson, 1960; Secord & Backman, 1965). For nearly two decades, the concepts of "balance," "congruity," and especially "dissonance" so dominated the field of social psychology that some onlookers were moved to complain that "no behavioral phenomena were safe from the ravages of the imperialistic dissonance hordes" (Sears & Ables, 1969, p. 263).

The days of imperialism that inspired such ire are history now. In fact, even if the few remaining advocates of cognitive-consistency approaches *were* the ravaging type, any signs of pugnacity on their part would not go unchecked for long. This rather drastic shift in intellectual climate has stunned and perplexed many workers in the field (e.g., Aronson, 1989; Berkowitz & Devine, 1989), who have somewhat wistfully asked why the cognitive-consistency community, so prosperous only two decades ago, has deteriorated into an intellectual ghost town.

There are, of course, many factors responsible for this complex phenomenon. Students of the more circumscribed consistency and balance theories (e.g., Heider, 1958; McGuire, 1960; Newcomb, 1956; Osgood & Tannenbaum, 1955) quickly answered the important questions that the theories raised. The broader, bolder, and more provocative theories such as dissonance suffered a very different fate, with some critics complaining that empirical support was weak and contradictory (e.g., Sears & Ables, 1969), others proposing alternative explanations of key effects (e.g., Bem, 1967; Chapanis & Chapanis, 1964; Schlenker, 1980; Tedeschi, Schlenker, & Bonoma, 1971), and still others protesting the emphasis on experimental ingenuity at the expense of theoretical explicitness (e.g., Smith, 1968). Yet I believe that the most fundamental problem was that the Festingerians neglected an extraordinarily important component in the cognitive-consistency process: people's *enduring* self-concepts. This defect so weakened the theory that researchers, armed with dissonance alone, were unable to explain the provocative phenomena that were of interest to them. Rather than turn away from interesting phenomena, they discreetly spiced up the dissonance recipe with the very motive that it had eclipsed: self-enhancement. Eventually, outsiders spotted the self-enhancement wolf lurking beneath the cognitive-consistency fleece; this signaled the beginning of the end of social psychology's torrid love affair with dissonance theory.

My interpretation of the reasons underlying the demise of consistency theories is, of course, nothing more than that. To my mind, though, the real question is not so much why cognitive-consistency approaches have slipped into the backwaters of social psychology, but whether we should allow them to remain there. Here I can speak more confidently; although past consistency approaches may have been flawed in certain respects, I am convinced that it would be premature to let the cognitive-consistency *perspective* go the way of phlogiston, ether, and the four humors. At the same time, I am also convinced that the desire for self-enhancement is every bit as important as the desire for consistency, and must therefore be given its due in any serious treatment of human social behavior.

My purpose here, then, is not to banish or subsume *either* the self-enhancement or self-consistency approaches, but to suggest how these two motivational forces interactively guide behavior. First, however, I attempt to put my model in context by describing the intellectual traditions from which it sprang—namely, self-enhancement, self-consistency, and self-verification theories. In so doing, I ignore other alternatives to self-enhancement theory and devote a disproportionate share of attention to the self-consistency and self-verification formulations. Although I fear that this will be construed as a shameless display of favoritism, my real intent is to offer consistency approaches some recognition in an era so dominated by self-enhancement theories.

HISTORICAL INFLUENCES

The Desire for Self-Enhancement

Behavioral scientists have always clutched the self-enhancement assumption close to their hearts. Indeed, the notion that people strive to maintain high levels of self-esteem has been endorsed by philosophers (e.g., Hobbes, Nietzsche, Rousseau, Russell), anthropologists (e.g., Becker), sociologists (e.g., Goffman, Rosenberg), and psychiatrists and psychologists (e.g., Adler, Allport, Horney, James, Koffka, McDougall, Sullivan).

Over the last several decades two distinct versions of self-enhancement theory have emerged (e.g., Shrauger, 1975). What I will refer to as "simple" self-enhancement theory suggests that all people strive to systematically promote the perception that they are worthwhile persons. What I will refer to as "compensatory" or "defensive" self-enhancement theory (Baumeister & Jones, 1978) assumes that people with negative self-concepts rarely receive positive feedback and attempt to compensate for this deficit by intensifying their efforts to acquire positive feedback (Hull, 1943). The two versions differ, then, in that the simple version assumes that all people are motivated to self-enhance to an equal degree, and the compensatory version assumes that people with negative self-views are *especially* motivated to self-enhance.[1]

Researchers have attributed a wide range of empirical findings to self-enhancement strivings (e.g., Jones, 1973). For example, self-enhancement strivings have been used to explain self-presentational strategies (e.g., Baumeister, 1982; Jones, 1964; Jones & Pittman, 1982; Schlenker, 1980, 1985; Tedeschi & Lindskold, 1976), self-attributions (e.g., Bradley, 1978; Greenwald, 1980; Snyder & Higgins, 1988; Zuckerman, 1979), predictions of future success (e.g., Alloy & Abramson, 1988; Taylor & Brown, 1988; Weinstein, 1980), the targets to which people compare themselves (e.g., Taylor & Lobel, 1989; Tesser, 1986, 1988; Wills, 1981), and even belief change (e.g., Steele, 1988). In short, there can be little doubt that the self-enhancement motive is a potent determinant of human social behavior.

A close look at the self-enhancement literature raises three concerns, however. First, most of the evidence has supported the simple version of self-enhancement theory; the compensatory version of the theory has received relatively little support (e.g., Brown, 1986; Brown, Collins, & Schmidt, 1988; Campbell, 1986; Shrauger, 1975; Swann, 1987; Taylor & Brown, 1988). Second, researchers who have found evidence for self-enhancement theory have generally focused on "affective" reactions to social feedback, such as emotional responses to evaluations. Little evidence of self-enhancement is typically found when "cognitive" reactions to feedback are examined, such as memory for feedback or perceptions of its accuracy (e.g., Shrauger, 1975; Swann, Griffin, Predmore, & Gaines, 1987). Third, much of the research that has been taken as support for the existence of a self-enhancement motive may in reality reflect self-consistency strivings. Consider, for example, the tendency for most people to resist attempts to apply negative labels to them. Although such resistance *might* be fueled by a desire to feel good about themselves, it could also be a manifestation of the desire for self-consistency. That is, given that most people in our society have positive conceptions of themselves, the fact that most of an unselected sample of experimental participants resist negative labels may simply reflect a desire for others to see them as they see themselves (Swann, 1987). Therefore, evidence that people work to maintain positive self-views can be handled by self-consistency or self-enhancement theory; researchers can confidently identify self-enhancement strivings as such only if they can be sure that actor possesses a negative self-concept.

In summary, although there can be little doubt that people sometimes display a preference for favorable feedback over unfavorable feedback, the psychological mechanisms that underlie this preference are unclear, as is the generality of this preference. The model presented later in this chapter is designed, in part, to address both of these issues.

The Desire for Self-Consistency

Since Sumner (1907) discussed the "strain of consistency," there have been numerous proponents of the idea that people seek feedback that confirms their beliefs. Lecky (1945) offered what is probably the boldest and most radical self-consistency formulation. He not only argued for the existence of a unique self-consistency or "unity" motive, but granted superordinate status to this motive: "All pleasure appears to trace back to the primary motive for unification" (p. 66).

Lecky's theory can be seen as an extension of the gestalt theories of Wertheimer, Koffka, and Kohler (e.g., see Hall & Lindzey, 1970). That is, whereas the gestalt theorists argued that humans strive for order and symmetry in their *physical* worlds, Lecky suggested that people seek order and symmetry in their perceptions of *themselves* and of *social reality*. Lecky departed from gestalt theorists, however, in his holistic or organismic view of the person (e.g., Goldstein, 1939). He believed that people's idiosyncratic life histories and enduring conceptions of self channel the manner in which the gestalt principles of perceptual organization gain expression.

Of the many theorists who followed in Lecky's tradition, Festinger (1957), Heider (1958), Osgood and Tannenbaum (1955), Rosenberg (1968), and Secord and Backman (1965) were among the most visible. Like Lecky, these theorists sought to apply gestalt principles to social-psychological phenomena. With the exception of Secord and Backman, however, these theorists eschewed Lecky's emphasis on the importance of people's life histories and enduring self-conceptions. This characteristic of post-Leckyan consistency theories ultimately contributed to their demise, as is illustrated by the history of the most prominent of these theories, Festinger's (1957) theory of cognitive dissonance.

Festinger was interested in what happens when people realize that one of their cognitions is inconsistent with (i.e., does not logically follow form) one or more other cognitions. For instance, he supposed that dissonance would be aroused if a man believed that it was raining, despite the fact that he remained perfectly dry. He suggested further that dissonance is unpleasant and that people will work to reduce it by modifying relevant cognitions. The dry man who believed he was caught in a downpour, for example, might try to convince himself that it was not really raining or that he actually was getting wet (p. 14).

Students of dissonance theory generated a vast and rich literature that offered support for various aspects of the formulation (e.g., Aronson, 1968; Wicklund & Brehm, 1976). Unfortunately, as the research findings poured in, it became increasingly apparent that a pristine need for cognitive consistency would not of itself fuel the counterintuitive and compelling social behaviors that dissonance researchers were bent on studying: Something was needed to "warm up" the need for consistency. Although the precise nature of the "something" inspired years of debate—some investigators pointed to behavioral commitment, whereas others suggested ego investment or knowledge of consequences—the "something" that eventually emerged was none other than the desire for self-enhancement (e.g., Aronson, 1968; Brehm & Cohen, 1962; Cooper & Fazio, 1984; Greenwald & Ronnis, 1978; Wicklund & Brehm, 1976). This was bad news for the theory, for it introduced overlap between dissonance theory and the self-enhancement theories it had eclipsed: "The long and the short of it may be that the dissonance literature chiefly concerns the psychology of what people do to recover from experimentally engineered major embarrassments" (Abelson, 1983, p. 43; see also Greenwald & Ronnis, 1978).

To be sure, there were some valiant efforts to rescue dissonance phenomena from the clutches of the self-enhancement usurpers. In particular, Aronson (1968; Aronson & Carlsmith, 1962) articulated and tested a provocative version of dissonance theory that placed the motivational burden squarely on the shoulders of cognitive-consistency strivings. *Contrary* to self-enhancement theory, he suggested that people with negative self-views would prefer a consistent negative world to an inconsistent positive one. "If a person conceives of himself as a 'schnook,' he will expect to behave like a 'schnook.' One of the advantages of this kind of statement is that it allows us to separate the effects of dissonance from other hedonic effects" (1968, pp. 27–28).

But if Aronson knew precisely what was needed to save dissonance theory from an untimely death, he failed to get the word to subjects in the relevant experiments. A widely cited exception to this generalization was a clever experiment he conducted with Carlsmith (Aronson & Carlsmith, 1962). The experimenter asked subjects to determine whether a series of people pictured in photographs suffered from schizophrenia. After each of 100 trials, he delivered either positive or negative feedback to subjects. The crucial group of subjects received exclusively negative feedback throughout the study, followed by positive feedback on the last 20 trials. Shortly thereafter, the experimenter indicated that there had been an oversight, and asked subjects to take the final 20 trials of the test again. The major dependent variable was the extent to which subjects modified their responses to the last set of trials. The results were striking: Those who received unexpectedly positive feedback were particularly likely to undermine their outcomes by modifying their responses on the last set of trials! Apparently, the positive feedback aroused dissonance, causing subjects to modify their responses so they could obtain the negative feedback they expected.

If Aronson and Carlsmith's findings had proven to be robust, they may well have prevented researchers from concluding that dissonance theory was nothing more than a cleverly disguised version of self-enhancement theory. This was not to be: At last count (Dipboye, 1977), only 4 of 17 attempts to replicate Aronson and Carlsmith's findings had succeeded. This rather dismal track record was enough to convince most people that Aronson's (1968) version of dissonance theory was not tenable, and, more generally, that in a fair fight self-consistency striving were no match for self-enhancement strivings. Not surprisingly, then, many contemporary theorists tend either to subsume self-consistency strivings within a self-enhancement perspective (e.g., Backman, 1988; Schlenker, 1985; Steele, 1988) or to ignore them altogether.

Although the checkered history of the Aronson and Carlsmith study might give pause to even the staunchest advocate of cognitive-consistency strivings, I think this history says more about the frailities of the particular phenomenon they examined than it does about the limitations of consistency strivings. Influenced by the Festingerian–Lewinian emphasis on the importance of experimental control and associated disdain for personological or "class" variables (see Allport, 1937, p. 364, for a perspective on Lewin's views), Aronson and his followers tacitly assumed that the only inputs people consider in their quest for consistency are those given to them by the experimenter. They accordingly sought to *manipulate* self-views by presenting participants with unfavorable feedback regarding their ability to diagnose schizophrenics.

Although this tact of manipulating self-views is methodologically appealing, it is effective only insofar as people have no basis for evaluating themselves on the attribute being manipulated. Unfortunately, this is rarely the case. Participants in Aronson and Carlsmith's paradigm, for example, presumably had a lifetime of experience as person perceivers on which they could draw in interpreting the feedback that they received from the experimenter.[2] Given that people generally believe that they are quite capable person perceivers (e.g., Swann, 1987), most of the subjects were probably somewhat incredulous when they received negative feedback; at any rate, it is unlikely that they suddenly became invested in maintaining the belief that they were inept. From this perspective, the fact that Aronson and Carlsmith's manipulation was *ever* successful probably says more about the extraordinary skill of those investigators who made it work than it does about the relative ease of manipulating self-conceptions.

If Aronson erred, then, it was not in assuming that people would work to confirm negative self-views in the service of self-consistency; rather, it was in his implicit assumption that the typical experimenter could reliably bring people to become highly invested in negative self-views through a laboratory manipulation. If so, then, under what conditions *do* people become so invested in their negative conceptions of self that they work to confirm these conceptions? It was in an effort to answer this question that I developed the self-verification formulation.

THE SELF-VERIFICATION FORMULATION

Self-verification theory (Swann, 1983, 1987) is a consistency formulation, in that it assumes, like dissonance and balance theories, that people are embarked on a quest for cognitive symmetry. The self-verification formulation departs from these theories, however, in its analysis of the processes that fuel and organize this quest. In particular, self-verification theory assumes that people want to confirm their self-views *not* as an end in itself, but as a means of bolstering their perception that the world is predictable and controllable. From this perspective, self-verification processes are "warmed up" by a desire for prediction and control (rather than, e.g., a desire for self-enhancement). Moreover, self-verification theory assumes that, in their efforts to exert control over their current situation, people rely heavily on their chronic views of self. In this respect, self-verification theory is akin to Lecky's (1945) organismic theory, Secord and Backman's (1965) interpersonal congruency theory, and Epstein's (1985, in press) cognitive–experiential self-theory.

Self-verification theory also departs from previous consistency theories in its assumptions regarding the generality of self-consistency phenomena. With a few exceptions (e.g., Epstein, in press), theorists who embrace consistency principles have assumed that self-consistency is an "equal-opportunity" motive, a motive that does not discriminate among measures falling into different response classes. Because self-verification strivings presumably grow out of conceptual analyses designed to make the world seem predictable and controllable, it follows that responses associated with such conceptual analyses should be more heavily influenced by self-verification strivings than those that are not (see also Epstein, in press). In what follows, I therefore examine more closely the nature of the conceptual analyses that underlie self-verification.

Origins of Self-Verification

One of children's first tasks is to make sense of their worlds. To this end, they observe their own behavior (e.g., Bem, 1972), the reactions of others to them (e.g., Cooley, 1902; Shrauger & Schoeneman, 1979), and the relation of their own performances to those of others (e.g., Festinger, 1954; Goethals & Darley, 1977; Taylor & Lobel, 1989; Tesser, 1988). Eventually, they translate these observations into conceptions of themselves and their worlds (e.g., Epstein, 1973; Mead, 1934).

Soon after people form self-conceptions and become reasonably certain of them, they become invested in preserving these conceptions by eliciting self-verifying feedback. Like most robust psychological phenomena, the desire for self-verification is probably multiply determined or even overdetermined. At a general level, however, I believe that self-verification processes are driven by people's desire to maximize their perceptions of predictability and control. The desire for prediction and control presumably grows out of interpersonal (pragmatic) considerations as well as intrapsychic (epistemic) ones. From an epistemic perspective, stable self-conceptions act like the rudder of a ship, bolstering people's confidence in their ability to navigate through the sometimes murky seas of everyday life (cf. Epstein, 1973; Kelly, 1955; Lecky, 1945; Mead, 1934; Secord & Backman, 1965). For this reason, events that confirm people's self-conceptions fortify their feelings of security, and events that disconfirm their self-conceptions engender fear that they may not know themselves after all.[3]

The importance of bringing others to verify one's self-views can also be understood from a *pragmatic* perspective. Social interaction is in large measure predicated on an implicit agreement that people will honor identities to which they have laid claim (e.g., Athay & Darley, 1981; Carson, 1969; Goffman, 1959; Jones, 1964; Swann, 1984). Therefore, they should work to ensure that others do not form overly negative appraisals (which could cause others to patronize them, or to accuse them of false modesty) or overly positive appraisals (which could cause others to expect too much of them, or to place extravagant demands upon them).

In short, just as being perceived in a self-congruent manner may promote perceptions of control and grease the wheels of social interaction, being perceived in an incongruent manner may invite psychological and interpersonal anarchy. For these and other reasons, people should be motivated to ensure that others see them as they see themselves—even if it means bringing others to recognize their flaws and limitations (cf. Baumeister, Hamilton, & Tice, 1985; Baumgardner & Brownlee, 1987).

If the desire for prediction and control is truly fundamental, one would expect that it would manifest itself in many aspects of cognitive and emotional functioning. The research literature supports this proposition. Research on the effects of "mere exposure" (e.g., Zajonc, 1968; for a review, see Harrison, 1977), for example, suggests that there exists a relatively primitive, nonconscious preference for familiar and predictable phenomena. As a result, exposure to entities or people makes them more attractive, presumably because exposure makes them more familiar and predictable. This effect holds even when people cannot recognize the stimuli consciously (e.g., Kunst-Wilson & Zajonc, 1980).

People's desire for predictability also seems to skew their hypothesis-testing activities. When asked to test hypotheses about physical objects (e.g., Wason & Johnson-Laird, 1972) or other people (e.g., Snyder & Swann, 1978), people preferentially search for evidence that is likely to confirm rather than disconfirm their hypotheses. Presumably, such hypothesis-testing strategies reflect the fact that people regard positive or confirmatory instances of phenomena as particularly trustworthy, diagnostic, and easy to process (e.g., Bruner, Goodnow, & Austin, 1956; Klayman & Ha, 1987). In any event, this preference for positive instances of phenomena even seems to color their perceptions of self-relevant information. For example, people rate information that confirms their self-conceptions as more diagnostic than information that disconfirms their self-conceptions (Swann & Read, 1981a, Study 3).

A conscious preference for the familiar over the unfamiliar seems to influence various other decision-making strategies as well. For example, Kahneman and Tversky (1983) have shown that people prefer receiving $800 over taking an

85% chance of winning $1,000, despite the fact that the gamble has a higher mathematical likelihood of paying off (i.e., $850). Apparently, people are very unwilling to risk losing a sure or familiar thing—perhaps even a relationship partner who thinks poorly of them—even when taking such a risk would enhance the expected value of a payoff.

So basic are perceptions of predictability and control to living organisms that animals even seem to suffer when these perceptions are threatened. A study by Pavlov (1927) illustrates this principle. He began by feeding dogs while presenting an image of a circle, but not when presenting an image of an ellipse. After a few trials, the dogs could readily discriminate the two shapes, as shown by increased salivation when the circle was presented. Later, however, the experimenter presented a new series of ellipses that became increasingly circular. As the dogs began having difficulty discriminating the ellipse from the circle, they displayed a series of "neurotic" behaviors. Not only did they lose their ability to make the original circle–ellipse discriminations that they had mastered earlier; they began thrashing about, baring their teeth, and barking violently. Furthermore, their condition persisted even after they were taken to rest farms, leading Pavlov to conclude that they had suffered an "animal neurosis" (p. 291). Apparently, when the dogs recognized that their conceptual schemes were not up to the task at hand, their "faith" in these schemes collapsed, and psychological and emotional disorganization resulted (cf. Epstein, 1981; Lecky, 1945).

In short, there are sound reasons to believe that all organisms are strongly motivated to maintain their perception that the world is predictable and controllable. Given that self-conceptions are theoretically crucial to maintaining such perceptions (e.g., Epstein, 1973; Mead, 1934), people should think and behave in ways that promote the survival of their self-conceptions—even if their self-views happen to be negative. The research literature supports this proposition. For example, we (Swann & Read, 1981b) found that whether we examined looking time, overt interaction, or the extent to which participants paid attention to feedback, we encountered a clear preference for self-confirmatory feedback. Three additional investigations (Swann & Read, 1981a) showed that both males and females solicited self-confirmatory feedback preferentially. Furthermore, this was true whether the feedback pertained to valenced or neutral self-concepts. People were undaunted in their quest for self-confirmatory feedback even when they had reason to believe that it would make them depressed (Swann, Wenzlaff, Krull, & Pelham, 1990) and even when they had to spend their own money to get it (Swann & Read, 1981a).

This evidence that people are motivated to verify their self-views is immune to several rival hypotheses. For example, the notion that people seek self-confirmatory feedback simply as a means of self-improvement or reducing uncertainty (Trope, 1979, 1986) is undermined by evidence that they are more inclined to verify self-views of which they are certain (e.g., Maracek & Mettee, 1972; Pelham, 1989; Swann & Ely, 1984; Swann, Pelham, & Chidester, 1988). Similarly, the idea that people self-verify simply to avoid interaction partners who seem imperceptive is weakened by evidence that people seek self-verifying *feedback* as well as self-verifying interaction partners (Swann, Pelham, & Krull, 1989; Swann et al., 1990; Swann & Read, 1981a). The question remaining, then, is not *whether* people prefer self-confirmatory feedback, but *how* they translate this preference into thought and action.

Strategies of Self-Verification

The specific activities through which people manifest their desire for self-verifying feedback fall into two distinct classes (e.g., Swann, 1983, 1987). As can be seen in Figure 12.1, the first class of activities consists of the behavioral activities through which people strive to influence the reactions of others. Specifically,

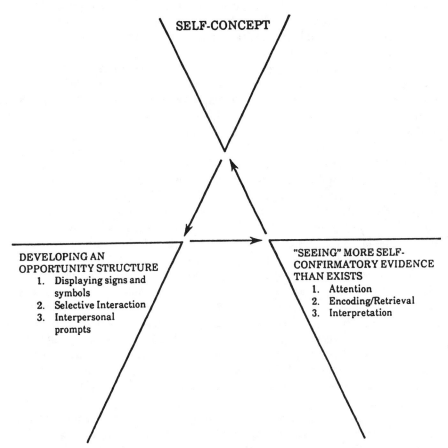

FIGURE 12.1 Self-verification processes. From "The Self as Architect of Social Reality" by W. B. Swann, Jr., 1985, in B. Schlenker (Ed.), *The Self and Social Life* (pp. 100–125), New York: McGraw-Hill. Copyright 1985 by McGraw-Hill Book Co. Reprinted by permission.

people work to create around themselves self-confirmatory social environments—that is, environments that provide them with support for their self-views (e.g., McCall & Simmons, 1966).

The second class of self-verification strategies contains the cognitive processes through which people's self-conceptions systematically distort their perceptions of social reality. In particular, people's thought processes produce the illusion of a social environment that is far more supportive of their self-views than is warranted by the objective evidence. I consider first the behavioral processes through which people alter the nature of the feedback available to them.

Developing a Self-Confirmatory Social Environment

Many biologists and ecologists have noticed that every living organism inhabits a "niche" that routinely satisfies its needs and desires (e.g., Clarke, 1954; Odum, 1963; Wilson, 1974). Human beings are no exception to this rule. Specifically, out of a concern for self-verification, people work to construct social environments that provide them with a steady diet of self-confirmatory feedback (McCall & Simmons, 1966).

In their efforts to construct self-verifying social environments, people may engage in three distinct sets of activities: They may strategically choose interaction partners and social settings; that may display identity cues; and they may adopt interaction strategies that evoke self-confirmatory responses (Swann, 1983, 1987). I consider each of these strategies in turn.

SELECTIVE INTERACTION   The notion that people seek social contexts that provide them with self-confirmatory feedback has been around for several decades (e.g., Secord & Backman, 1965; Wachtel, 1973, 1977). Until recently, however, much of the evidence for this hypothesis has been correlational in nature. Pervin and Rubin (1967), for example, found that students tended to drop out of school if they wound up in colleges that were incompatible with their self-views (see also Backman & Secord, 1962; Broxton, 1963; Newcomb, 1956).

Recent laboratory investigations have shown that people with negative self-views prefer interaction partners who unfavorably appraise them over those who favorably appraise them. For example, we (Swann et al., 1989) told some participants (targets) that two others (perceivers) had evaluated them on performance dimensions that targets had previously identified as their "worst" attribute (e.g., athletic ability, physical appearance, etc.). One perceiver offered an unfavorable evaluation and the other offered a favorable evaluation. Targets chose to interact with the unfavorable, self-verifying perceiver rather than with the favorable, non-self-verifying one.

In a somewhat similar vein, we (Swann et al., 1990) had depressed people choose between an interaction partner who thought poorly of them and one who thought well of them. We found that highly depressed people (but not mildly dysphoric ones) displayed a clear preference for negative evaluators over positive ones.

We (Swann & Pelham, 1988) showed that this tendency for people to prefer self-verifying interaction partners manifests itself in their choice of actual relationship partners. For example, targets were particularly inclined to remain in relationships with college roommates whose appraisals of them were congruent with their self-views and to drop roommates whose appraisals were incongruent with their self-views. The means plotted in Figure 12.2 show that this tendency was *symmetrical* with respect to self-concept. That is, just as targets with positive self-conceptions were poised to flee from highly unfavorable roommates, so too were targets with negative self-views inclined to flee from highly favorable roommates. Subsidiary analyses helped rule out several alternative explanations of this finding: The effects were *not* due to a tendency for targets in congruent relationships to be more similar to one another, to engage in more self-disclosure, or to spend more time with their roommates. Furthermore, the roommates for whom targets displayed a preference perceived them negatively not merely in a specific sense, but in a global sense as well. That is, these preferred roommates not only rated targets low on specific attributes; they also rated targets as relatively "worthless."

In two complementary investigations (Swann & Pelham, 1990), people

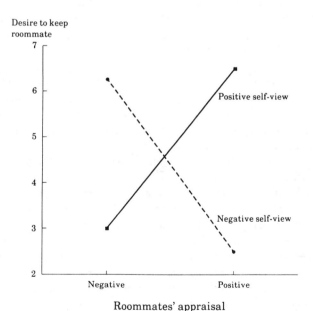

FIGURE 12.2 Selective interaction. From *The Social Construction of Identity: Self-Verification through Friend and Intimate Selection* by W. B. Swann, Jr., and B. W. Pelham, 1988, unpublished manuscript, University of Texas–Austin. Reprinted by permission of the authors.

involved in friendship relationships also showed a strong preference for congruent partners than people involved in roommate relationships. These investigations also revealed that only people who were highly certain of their negative self-views preferred unfavorable partners; those who were uncertain of their self-views displayed either a preference for favorable partners or no preference whatsoever. Apparently, as people become more certain of their self-conceptions, they are more inclined to rely on these conceptions to organize their experiences, predict future events, and guide behavior. For this reason, high certainty is associated with intensified efforts to self-verify through selective interaction.[4]

We (Swann & Pelham, 1990) also ruled out several additional alternative explanations of the self-verification effect. There was no evidence that people with negative self-views chose relationship partners who thought poorly of them as a means of improving themselves, or as a means of obtaining specific negative appraisals coupled with global acceptance; nor did they do so because they took expressions of favorability as signs of dull-wittedness or imperceptiveness.

Taken together, these data offer fairly clear evidence that people gravitate toward social relationships in which they think they will receive self-confirmatory feedback. An important characteristic of this selective interaction strategy is that once people enter a particular social relationship or institution, legal contracts and social pressures tend to keep them there. The power of such contractual arrangements is particularly salient in the case of marriage. Nevertheless, even dating couples are sometimes pressed by friends and family to maintain their relationships. From this vantage point, selective interaction strategies of self-verification often lock people into interpersonal feedback systems that are self-sustaining as well as self-verifying.

DISPLAYING IDENTITY CUES   Another way in which people can succeed in laying claim to a particular identity is by "looking the part." To be effective, identity cues must meet two criteria: They must be under the person's control, and they must characteristically evoke desired responses from others.

Physical appearance represents a particularly salient class of identity cues. The clothes one wears, for example, can be used to tell others whether one is liberal or conservative, wealthy or destitute, easygoing or meticulous, prudish or promiscuous. Similarly, through the skillful use of cosmetics and wigs, people can project dramatically different identities to onlookers. Even body posture and demeanor may be used to communicate various identities to others. Take, for example, the teenager who radiates anomie, the "punk" who projects danger, or the new father who exudes naiveté in the hope of avoiding responsibility.

If motivated enough, people may actually modify their body structure to convey various identities to others. Self-perceived athletes, for example, may diet and lift weights to keep their muscles bulging. Aging people may employ an array of contrivances designed to keep their youthful appearances alive: liposuction for the belly, implants for the breasts, and a plethora of potions for restoring the splendor of hair to balding pates. There is hope even for those who are squeamish about surgery or dubious about drugs, for material possessions may also serve to signal people's identities to others. The cars people drive, the homes they live in, and the trophies they display in their dens may all be used to tell others who they are and how they expect to be treated (see also Goffman, 1959; Schlenker, 1980).

If such physical contrivances do not suffice, people may ensure that they are understood by relying on social conventions such as titles and occupational labels. In this way, before they even open their mouths, people can tell others a great deal about the identities they wish to assume.

INTERPERSONAL PROMPTS   Even if people fail to gain self-confirmatory feedback through selective interaction, they may still acquire such feedback by adopting appropriate interaction strategies. We (Swann et al., 1990), for example, found that mildly depressed college students were more likely to solicit unfavorable feedback from their roommates than were nondepressed students. Moreover, students' efforts to acquire unfavorable feedback seem to have borne fruit: The more unfavorable feedback they solicited in the middle of the semester, the more their roommates were inclined to derogate them and to plan to terminate the relationship at the end of the semester (see also Coyne, 1976; Coyne et al., 1987).

If people are motivated to bring others to verify their self-conceptions, they should *intensify* their efforts to elicit self-confirmatory reactions when they suspect that they are misconstrued. We (Swann & Read, 1981b, Study 2) tested this proposition. The experimenter began by informing targets who perceived themselves as either likeable or dislikeable that they would be interacting with perceivers who had already formed impressions of them. Some targets learned that the perceiver had positive regard for them; some learned that the perceiver had negative regard for them; and still others learned nothing of the perceivers' evaluation of them.

There was an overall tendency for targets to elicit reactions that confirmed their self-views (see also Curtis & Miller, 1986). More important, the means in Figure 12.3 show that this tendency was especially pronounced when targets suspected that perceivers' appraisals might *disconfirm* their self-conceptions. Targets who thought of themselves as likeable elicited particularly favorable reactions when they thought perceivers disliked them, and targets who thought of themselves as dislikable elicited particularly unfavorable reactions when they suspected that perceivers liked them. In short, targets were especially inclined to elicit self-confirmatory feedback from perceivers when they suspected that perceivers' appraisals were incompatible with their self-views (see also Hilton & Darley, 1985).

We (Swann & Hill, 1982) obtained a similar pattern of results, using a different procedural paradigm and dimension of the self-concept (dominance). Targets began by playing a game with a confederate in which each player alternately assumed the dominant "leader" role or the submissive "assistant" role. During a break in the game, the experimenter asked the players to decide who should be the leader for the next set of games. This was the confederate's cue to

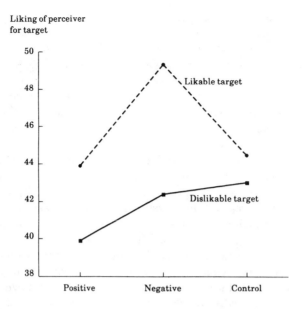

Liking of perceiver
for target

Likable target

Dislikable target

Positive   Negative   Control

Perceiver's alleged appraisal

FIGURE 12.3   Self-verification through interaction. Based on data from Swann and Read (1981b).

deliver feedback to the participant. In some conditions, the confederate said that the participant seemed dominant; in other conditions, the confederate asserted that the participant seemed submissive. If the feedback confirmed targets' self-conceptions, they seemed to passively accept the confederate's appraisal. If the feedback *dis*confirmed their self-conceptions, however, targets vehemently resisted the feedback and sought to demonstrate that they were not the persons the confederate made them out to be. Thus self-conceived dominants labeled as submissive became all the more dominant, and self-conceived submissives labeled as dominant became especially submissive.

An interesting feature of this study was that some people behaviorally resisted the discrepant feedback more than others. We (Swann & Ely, 1984) speculated that such differences in resistance might be due to differences in the extent to which people were certain of their self-conceptions. Specifically, we reasoned that increments in self-concept certainty would be associated with heightened investment in verifying such views, which would in turn lead to greater resistance in the face of disconfirmation.[5] To test this hypothesis, we (Swann & Ely, 1984) had perceivers interview targets who were either certain or uncertain of their self-conceived extraversion. They led perceivers to develop an expectancy about targets that was discrepant with the self-conceptions of targets.

This situation created the potential for a "battle of wills," with perceivers' experimentally manipulated beliefs vying against targets' chronic self-views.

Consistent with earlier research (Snyder & Swann, 1978; see also Swann & Giuliano, 1987; Swann et al., 1988), perceivers acted on their expectancies by soliciting responses that would confirm their own expectancies but *dis*confirm targets' self-conceptions. For example, perceivers who believed that the target was an extravert often asked questions such as "Do you like to go to lively parties?" Targets who were low in self-certainty generally answered in ways that confirmed perceivers' expectancies (but disconfirmed their own self-conceptions) when perceivers were highly certain of their expectancies. In contrast, targets who were high in self-certainty actively resisted the questions (regardless of the perceivers' level of certainty), thereby bringing perceivers' expectancies into harmony with their self-views. Thus, as long as targets were high in self-certainty, self-verification "won" over behavioral confirmation in the battle of wills. (For a further discussion of factors that influence the outcome of such battles, see Swann, 1987.)

Maracek and Mettee (1972) illustrated the importance of self-certainty in an achievement context. They recruited a group of people who possessed low self-esteem and were either low or high in self-certainty. The experimenter provided everyone with success feedback and then monitored their subsequent performance. There was no evidence of self-verification among persons who were low in certainty: They always sought to elicit highly positive evaluations by striving to perform well. In contrast, those who were high in self-certainty displayed substantial self-verification strivings. Apparently, those high in self-certainty regarded their success as a threat to their negative self-concepts and sought to bolster their conviction in their own incompetence by performing poorly. These data may help to explain why the Aronson and Carlsmith (1962) study has been so difficult to replicate: People work to maintain negative self-views *only* when these views are chronic self-conceptions of which they are certain.

Together, these findings suggest that targets work to bring perceivers to see them as they see themselves. As effective as such efforts may often be, however, people may sometimes fail to create a self-confirmatory opportunity structure through their *behavioral* self-verification strategies. When these self-verification strategies fail, the survival of people's self-views may hinge on the effectiveness of the three *cognitive* self-verification strategies described next.

Seeing More Self-Confirmatory Evidence than Actually Exists

Researchers have shown that expectancies in general and self-conceptions in particular can exert a powerful channeling influence on information processing (for reviews, see Higgins & Bargh, 1987; Kihlstrom & Cantor, 1984). This finding suggests that self-conceptions may guide the processing of social feedback so as to promote their own survival.

SELECTIVE ATTENTION   To the extent that people are motivated to acquire self-confirmatory feedback, they should be especially attentive to it. We (Swann &

Read, 1981b, Study 1) tested this hypothesis. Targets who perceived themselves as likeable or dislikeable learned that a perceiver had evaluated them. Some targets were led to suspect that the perceiver had formed a favorable impression of them; others were led to suspect that the perceiver had formed an unfavorable impression of them. All were then given an opportunity to examine some remarks that the perceiver had ostensibly made about them—remarks that were sufficiently vague and general as to apply to anyone.

The results showed that targets spent longer scrutinizing the remarks of the evaluator when they anticipated that the remarks would confirm rather than disconfirm their self-conceptions. That is, just as those self-perceived as likeable spent the most time looking when they expected the remarks would be favorable, those self-perceived as dislikeable spent the most time looking when they expected the remarks would be unfavorable. Hence, it appears that people are more attentive to social feedback when they suspect that it will confirm their chronic self-views (for related demonstrations, see Pyszczynski & Greenberg, 1987).

SELECTIVE ENCODING AND RETRIEVAL   Just as people may preferentially attend to self-confirmatory feedback, they may also encode and recall it selectively. Crary (1966) and Silverman (1964), for example, reported that people tended to recall more incidental information about experimental tasks in which they received self-confirmatory rather than self-discrepant feedback. Moreover, other research suggests that self-conceptions channel the *type* as well as the *amount* of feedback people recall. We (Swann & Read, 1981b, Study 3), for example, had targets who saw themselves as likeable or dislikeable listen to a perceiver make a series of positive and negative statements about them. Some targets expected that the statements would be generally positive; others expected that the statements would be generally negative. After a brief delay, targets attempted to recall as many of the statements as possible.

Overall, targets who perceived themselves as likeable remembered more positive than negative statements, and those who perceived themselves as dislikeable remembered more negative than positive statements. In addition, this tendency to recall more self-confirmatory statements than self-disconfirmatory statements was greatest when targets anticipated that the perceiver's statements would confirm their self-conceptions.[6]

SELECTIVE INTERPRETATION   When people receive feedback, they may ask themselves, "Is the feedback valid? Is the source of feedback reliable and trustworthy? What implications does the feedback have in light of what I know about myself? The research literature suggests that people typically supply answers to these questions that promote the survival of their self-views.

At least three independent investigations have demonstrated that people will endorse the validity of feedback only if it fits with their self-conceptions (Crary, 1966; Korman, 1968; Markus, 1977). Similarly, Shrauger and Lund (1975) reported that people expressed relatively more confidence in the perceptiveness of an evaluator when his impression confirmed their self-conceptions. We (Swann et al., 1987) replicated this effect and also found that people tended to attribute self-confirmatory feedback to characteristics of themselves and self-disconfirmatory feedback to the source of the feedback.

Together, the attentional, encoding, retrieval, and interpretational processes described in this section may prove formidable adversaries for self-discrepant feedback. This may be one reason why people's self-conceptions sometimes conflict with the actual appraisals of others (e.g., Felson, 1981a, 1981b) and, more specifically, why people overestimate the extent to which the appraisals of their friends and acquaintances confirm their self-conceptions (Miyamoto & Dornbusch, 1956; Orpen & Bush, 1974; Sherwood, 1967; Walhood & Klopfer, 1971). The fact that these cognitive self-verification strategies can lead to such misconceptions suggests that it is important that they do not work *too* well, since they may blind targets to perceivers' actual appraisals of them. In fact, if targets' misconceptions are serious enough, perceivers may avoid them (or, in extreme cases, recommend that they find their way to a therapist).

In closing this section, I would like to highlight some of the more important differences between the behavioral processes through which people create self-verifying social environments and those cognitive processes through which they "see" their social environments as offering more support than is warranted by the objective evidence. One difference is the sense in which the behavioral and cognitive activities are motivated by a desire to self-verify. For example, to some it might seem that behavioral resistance to self-discrepant feedback is evidence of a self-verification motive, but that selective recall of self-confirmatory feedback is produced by an "automatic" or "schematic" processing bias rather than by a self-verification motive.

Such concerns raise a host of heady issues, including the criteria that should be used to distinguish a motivated behavior from a nonmotivated one—issues that are obviously well beyond the scope of this chapter. Nevertheless, let me identify two reasons why at least some instances of selective attention, recall, and interpretation should be construed as manifestations of the desire to self-verify. First, some selective attention and recall processes are apparently produced by a tendency for the *anticipation* of self-confirming feedback to energize cognitive activity. In our (Swann & Read, 1981b) studies, for example, people looked at feedback longer (Study 1) and were more inclined to recall it (Study 3) when they suspected that it would confirm their self-views. Apparently, when people believe that self-confirmatory feedback is available, they intensify their efforts to acquire it through cognitive as well as behavioral activities.

In addition, even if a particular instance of information processing can be attributed to the structure of people's thought processes rather than to the vigor with which they engage those structures, self-verification processes may have been responsible for the formation of those structures in the first place. Thus, for example, a woman may preferentially recall feedback confirming her belief that she is an intellectual, because her success in eliciting such feedback in the past has led her to develop a finely honed concept of herself as an intellectual. In such instances, although memory structures may provide a *proximal* explanation for preferential recall, the *ultimate* explanation may be the self-verification activities that have led to the formation of those memory structures. This example brings us to the distinction between routine and crisis self-verification.

Routine versus Crisis Self-Verification

Most of us spend most of our time with people who have implicitly or explicitly agreed to honor the identities we have negotiated with them (e.g., Boissevain, 1974; Goffman, 1959; Swann & Predmore, 1985). Therefore, the bulk of the reactions people receive every day will be essentially preprogrammed, which means that people will rarely need to demonstrate that they want to be respected or coddled or dominated because their interaction partners will already know this. All they need to do is to remain in their self-verifying social environments, and their self-views will rarely be challenged.

Because of the automatic nature of such chronic self-verification activities, it is tempting to divorce them from the self and self-verification. This is a mistake, because *initially* people may have selected or "trained" their partners with an eye to acquiring self-confirmatory feedback. It is therefore perfectly appropriate to regard such routine self-verification activities as expressions of the self-concept and the desire to self-verify.

But if it is appropriate to regard such routine activities as members of a larger class of self-verification activities, it is also important to distinguish them from more active, "crisis" self-verification activities. Crisis self-verification activities differ from the relatively automatic, nonreflective activities that characterize routine self-verification, in that they involve self-focused attention and relatively specific and concerted efforts to elicit self-confirmatory reactions.

Probably the most common antecedent of crisis self-verification is the receipt of discrepant feedback. People may respond to such feedback in two ways. First, they may focus attention on the self-conception that has been threatened. Second, they may increase their efforts to learn about themselves by acquiring information that will be highly informative and diagnostic (e.g., Swann, Stephenson, & Pittman, 1981). Because people regard self-confirmatory feedback as particularly diagnostic (Swann & Read, 1981a), such intensified efforts to acquire *diagnostic* feedback will translate into attempts to acquire *self-confirmatory* feedback—that is, to self-verify.[7] In what follows, I present research that shows each of these processes at work.

Hill and I (Swann & Hill, 1986) illustrated that self-discrepant feedback causes people to focus attention onto relevant self-conceptions. Participants who perceived themselves as either emotional or unemotional were given "diagnoses," ostensibly written by student clinicians, that either confirmed or disconfirmed their self-views. A baseline control group received no feedback. Participants then moved to a different room for a "second experiment." Here the experimenter asked them to decide whether or not a series of adjectives described them. Some of the adjectives were emotionally-related; others were not. As participants made each judgment, the experimenter surreptitiously recorded their response latency.

As expected, the results revealed that those who received self-discrepant feedback were faster in making self-descriptive judgments than those who received either no feedback or self-confirmatory feedback. Furthermore, this pattern of results occurred only for the emotionally-related adjectives; the feedback manipulation had no impact on reaction times to the neutral adjectives. Apparently, self-discrepant feedback induced people to retrieve information relevant to the self-conception from memory, thereby making that information more cognitively accessible (e.g., Fazio, 1986; Higgins & King, 1981; Tversky & Kahneman, 1973).

To the extent that self-discrepant feedback makes people's self-conceptions more accessible, it should increase the probability that these self-conceptions guide subsequent behavior (e.g., Carver, 1975; Gibbons, 1978; Snyder & Swann, 1976; Wegner & Giuliano, 1982). This may explain why participants in the Swann and Hill (1982) and Swann and Read (1981b, Study 2) studies discussed earlier were most inclined to behave in a self-confirmatory manner when they were presented with self-discrepant feedback. From this perspective, the self-discrepant feedback apparently made their self-conceptions more cognitively accessible, in turn increasing the probability that they would act on these conceptions by behaving in a manner that elicited self-confirmatory reactions. (See also Fazio's [1986] analysis of the conditions under which attitudes guide behavior.)

Crisis self-verification may also emerge when people must make a decision with far-reaching implications (e.g., choosing a career, marriage partner, or home). Like discrepant feedback, such decisions focus attention on the self, but on a slightly different aspect of the self. That is, instead of causing people to ask, "Who am I?", highly consequential decisions often encourage people to ask, "Who am I and what does this suggest for the person I will become?" (see Markus & Nurius, 1986). In many ways, this question highlights one of the self-verifier's greatest struggles: reconciling the desire for stable self-conceptions with the fact that most of us must assume somewhat different identities over the course of our lives. I do not address this issue here, as I have dealt with it elsewhere (Swann, 1983, 1985, 1987). Rather, now that I have covered the essentials of self-verification theory, it is time to turn to the other great struggle with which self-verifiers must deal: that between the desire to self-enhance and the desire to self-verify.

BEYOND THE "MINE'S BIGGER" APPROACH TO THE SELF-ENHANCEMENT VERSUS SELF-VERIFICATION DEBATE

For people with positive self-views, favorable feedback is both self-enhancing and self-verifying, and thus the fact that such people prefer favorable over unfavorable feedback is consistent with both self-enhancement and self-verification theories. The two theories make competing predictions, however, regarding the behavior of people with negative self-views. Whereas the simple form of self-enhancement theory predicts that people with negative self-views should prefer favorable feedback, self-verification theory suggests that they should prefer unfavorable feedback.

Advocates of the two theories, enticed by the promise of a good fight, have taken up the challenge to eliminate the opposition. Some have attempted to subsume the opposing theory within their own framework. Lecky (1945), for example, argued that all self-enhancement strivings are *ultimately* in the service of self-consistency. Similarly, some (e.g., Backman, 1988; Schlenker, 1985; Steele, 1988) have suggested that self-consistency strivings are, in the final analysis, produced by a desire for self-enhancement. However parsimonious they may be, these efforts are rather like supposing that people sleep so that they can enjoy their next meal: Although there is surely some truth to them, they seem neither psychologically compelling nor empirically falsifiable.

Trope (1986) has also sought to embrace evidence of self-enhancement and self-verification within a single framework by suggesting that such behaviors are motivated by a desire to reduce uncertainty. His formulation has two limitations. First, as formulated, it deals with achievement behavior only. Second, it suggests that people who are uncertain of their self-views should be more inclined to seek self-verifying feedback than those who are certain of their self-views, when in fact the opposite is true.

Shrauger (1975) offered what is perhaps the most fruitful attempt to recon-cile evidence of self-enhancement and self-verification. He acknowledged that people are motivated to self-enhance as well as self-verify; he went on to suggest that "affective" responses (e.g., feelings about feedback) conform to self-enhance-ment theory and that "cognitive" responses (e.g., retention and appraisal of feedback) conform to self-consistency (or self-verification) theory. Subsequent re-search has generally supported Shrauger's thesis (e.g., McFarlin & Blascovitch, 1981; Moreland & Sweeney, 1984). For example, when my colleagues and I (Swann et al., 1987) presented participants with either favorable or unfavorable social feedback, participants with negative self-concepts indicated that unfavor-able feedback was more self-descriptive than favorable feedback (as suggested by self-verification theory), but that it also made them depressed (as suggested by self-enhancement theory).

However insightful it may be, the power of Shrauger's distinction between affective and cognitive measures is ultimately limited by ambiguity inherent in the terms themselves (e.g., Buck, 1985; Epstein, 1985; Lazarus, 1984; Zajonc, 1984). That is, because any two psychologists are apt to define the terms "affective" and "cognitive" differently, the task of classifying the many important behaviors that have both affective and cognitive components (e.g., feedback seeking, choice of relationship partners) is hazardous.

Ambiguity inherent in the affective–cognitive distinction has also clouded subsequent theoretical statements in which it plays a major role. Raynor and McFarlin (1986), for example, have suggested that when "affective value" is high, behavior will be influenced by self-enhancement strivings, and that when "infor-mational value" is high, behavior will be driven by self-verification strivings. One problem with this approach is that, like Shrauger, these authors fail to provide operational criteria for affective versus informational value. Perhaps related to this, Raynor and McFarlin have made predictions that have since been disconfirmed. They suggested, for example, that people will seek negative feedback only in experimental settings in which information value is high (1986, pp. 339–340). This prediction has been falsified by evidence that people seek negative feedback and relationship partners in field settings (e.g., Swann et al., 1990; Swann & Pelham, 1988, 1990). Finally, although Raynor and McFarlin can offer post hoc explanations of the tendency for people to seek favorable feedback in some situations but not others, their theory cannot explain why the very same people seek favorable feedback about their positive attributes and unfavorable feedback about their negative attributes (while the "information value" and "affective value" of the situation are held constant; Swann et al., 1989).

A related formulation developed by Sorrentino and Short (1986) assumes that some people concentrate on maximizing "affective value" and others concentrate on maximizing "cognitive value." Although it is certainly useful to identify individual differences in the extent to which people self-enhance versus self-verify, the difficulty of operationalizing affective and cognitive value plagues this formulation as it does the ones mentioned above.

The formulation advanced in this chapter represents an effort to tie the constructs employed by earlier investigators to a relatively specific set of operational definitions. That is, people strive to nourish their sense of self-worth (i.e., to maximize affective value) through self-enhancement processes, and they strive to maintain their self-conceptions (i.e., to maximize informational value) through self-verification processes. Furthermore, distinct psychological processes seem to underlie self-enhancement and self-verification processes. In what follows, I discuss these processes.

The Mental Processes Underlying Self-Enhancement, Self-Verification, and Strategic Self-Presentation

What is the minimal number of cognitive computations that can lead to a self-enhancing response as compared to a self-verifying one? Obviously, any given self-relevant stimulus (e.g., an evaluation by potential interaction partner) is psychologically meaningful only to the extent that one knows what that stimulus is. Therefore, both self-verifying and self-enhancing behaviors require that a person initially categorize self-relevant feedback as either favorable or unfavorable. And, in fact, self-enhancing behavior should require nothing more! That is, simply identifying feedback as favorable or unfavorable should be enough to enable people to self-enhance by embracing the former and avoiding the latter (e.g., Swann, Hixon, Stein-Seroussi, & Gilbert, in press).

Self-verifying behavior, on the other hand, should require additional mental work. That is, if people are to accept feedback only when it confirms or matches their self-view, then the feedback must be categorized, the relevant self-view must be retrieved, and the two must be compared. In short, self-verification should, like self-enhancement, require the initial categorization of self-relevant feedback;

however, only self-verification should require the additional comparison between the feedback and a self-conception.

The logic of this claim becomes apparent when one expresses these processes as implementation rules for a logical processor. In the case of self-enhancement, the implementation rule can be written as a simple conditional statement with two logical operators: "*If* the feedback is unfavorable, then avoid it." Two such rules (one for favorable feedback and one for unfavorable feedback) are all that are needed to build a self-enhancing device. A self-verifying device, however, requires implementation rules of the form: "*If* the feedback is unfavorable *and* the self-concept is favorable, *then* avoid it." Not only is this rule itself more complex (because it requires the additional logical operator "*and*"); in addition, four such rules are required to build a self-verifying device, rather than the two needed to build a self-enhancing device.

In short, self-enhancement merely requires the simple categorization of feedback, and self-verification requires that people categorize the feedback and then compare it with their self-concept. This distinction is presented schematically in the upper half of Table 12.1. Four predictions follow from this analysis of self-enhancement and self-verification:

1. *Insofar as self-verification is predicted on a more lengthy and complex set of mental operations than is self-enhancement, it should require more processing resources (cf. Baddeley & Hitch, 1974) than should self-enhancement. The experimental depletion of a person's processing resources should therefore interfere with self-verification, but should have relatively little impact on self-enhancement.*

There is evidence that experimentally depleting people of cognitive resources tends to truncate the normal information-processing sequence (Ben Zur & Breznitz, 1981), thereby forcing behavior to be based on the output of early

TABLE 12.1   Self-Enhancement, Self-Verification, and Strategic Self-Presentation

Stimulus			*Probable outcome*
I. Categorization phase (Is feedback positive or negative?)	⟶	Emotional reaction (happiness–sadness)	⟶ Self-enhancement
II. Comparison phase (How does feedback compare with relevant self-view?)	⟶	Emotional reaction (anxiety vs. comfort)	⟶ Self-verification
III. Strategic phase (Given the nature of the feedback, my self-view, and the situation, what will happen if _____, or _____, or _____, etc.?)	⟶	Emotional reaction	⟶ Strategic self-presentation

operations (see Norman & Bobrow's [1975] "principle of graceful degradation," Tversky & Kahneman's [1974] "anchor/adjust heuristic," or Gilbert's [1989] "principle of premature output"). Insofar as self-verification is just such a sequential operation, resource-deprived people should have difficulty comparing self-relevant feedback to their self-concepts to assess its accuracy. As a result, a person's behavior may be guided solely by the portion of the operation that he or she was in fact able to complete (i.e., the assessment of the positivity of the feedback). Depriving people of cognitive resources by, for example, encouraging them to rush their decisions should therefore leave them time to perform the operations involved in self-enhancement, but not those involved in self-verification.

To test this hypothesis, we (Swann et al., in press) examined the effect of depriving people of cognitive resources while they chose between interaction partners who evaluated them in a relatively favorable or unfavorable manner. The experimenter encouraged some participants to rush their choice of interaction partner and others to make their choice at leisure. Participants in the rushed condition tended to self-enhance—that is, to display a strong preference for the favorable evaluator over the unfavorable evaluator—presumably because they lacked the cognitive resources (i.e., time) to perform the computations underlying primary self-verification. In contrast, participants in the unrushed condition, who presumably possessed the cognitive resources required for self-verification, tended to self-verify.

A follow-up study provided further support for the hypothesis that depriving people of cognitive resources diminishes people's tendency to self-verify but not their tendency to self-enhance. In this study, people who were deprived of resources by being placed under cognitive load were particularly likely to self-enhance rather than self-verify. The results of this study also indicated that when participants were liberated from the load manipulation, they repudiated their self-enhancing responses in favor of self-verifying ones. This finding suggests that the cognitively loaded participants in Study 1 tended to self-enhance because they lacked the cognitive resources required by self-verification, not because the load manipulation somehow prevented them from picking up the information needed to perform the computations underlying primary self-verification.

The results of this study cast doubt upon the common assumption that self-enhancement processes are necessarily strategic (e.g., Baumeister, 1982; Jones, 1964; Jones & Pittman, 1982; Schlenker, 1980; Tedeschi & Lindskold, 1976). Indeed, in this research, it appeared that the more cognitive resources people had available to them (and, presumably, the more opportunity for strategic analysis), the *less* inclined they were to self-enhance.

This research may also lend insight into Shrauger's (1975) and Zajonc's distinction between affective and cognitive responses. Zajonc (1980), for example, has suggested that when people encounter a stimulus, they experience an immediate affective reaction before engaging in any higher-order cognitive analysis. He has argued that such affective reactions are propelled by a relatively primitive neurological system that enables organisms to perform rudimentary analyses of their worlds and to take rapid action to avoid threats to their well-being (see also Epstein, 1985, in press; Gazzaniga, 1985; Greenwald, 1989; Tomkins, 1981; Wilson, 1985; Zajonc, 1980, 1984). When organisms apprehend stimuli, for example, they theoretically make an initial favorable–unfavorable discrimination, and use output from this computation to guide action while more complex analyses continue (see also Lazarus's [1966] discussion of primary and secondary reactions to stressors.).

Our data seem to fit with the notion that a unique set of cognitive operations underlies self-enhancement and self-verification. That is, when we forced participants to act quickly or while under concurrent task demands, we gave them no recourse but to act on the basis of their immediate, self-enhancing reactions. In contrast, when we allotted subjects sufficient time and energy, they pondered their choices and subsequently attempted to self-verify.

2. *Depriving people of cognitive resources should prevent them from assessing the extent to which feedback is congruent with their self-conceptions.*

In theory, the manipulation of resource deprivation used in our research (Swann et al., in press) promoted self-enhancement because it prevented people from comparing feedback to their self-views and recognizing the extent to which it was self-congruent. Consistent with this interpretation, we (Hixon & Swann, 1989) found that people used the self-congruency of feedback to estimate its accuracy only when they had time for reflection. In a somewhat similar vein, Paulhus and Levitt (1987) found that increments in affective arousal increased subjects' propensity to endorse positive trait adjectives as self-descriptive. Presumably, affective arousal (which has many of the properties of cognitive load; e.g., Easterbrook, 1959; Kahnemann, 1973) blocked the comparison process that ordinarily allows people to reject overly positive adjectives.

3. *Self-enhancement should emerge earlier in development than self-verification.*

A tendency to gravitate toward people who are accepting rather than rejecting emerges much earlier in development than anything resembling self-verification processes. For example, within mere weeks of developing the ability to discriminate facial characteristics, 5-month-olds attend more to smiling faces than to nonsmiling ones (Shapiro, Eppler, Haith, & Reis, 1987). Similarly, as early as 4½ months of age, children tend to orient to voices that have the melodic contours of acceptance instead of nonacceptance (Fernald, 1989). Contrary to Rogers's (1951) notion that self-enhancement processes are learned, this research suggests that self-enhancement processes grow out of a very basic, "hard-wired" propensity to approach superficially accepting organisms and avoid threatening ones.

The cognitive prerequisites for self-verification do not emerge until much later in development. Most importantly, it is not before the 18th month of age that an integral component of the comparison process emerges: the sense of self as object (e.g., Lewis, 1987). Even after children develop rudimentary self-conceptions, self-verification will not occur reliably until they accumulate enough evidence that they become certain of them. Such well-articulated self-views probably do not emerge until several years later, particularly if the content of such views is abstract, negative, or both.

Although no one has actually tested the notion that active strategies of self-enhancement emerge before active strategies of self-verification, we do know that young children endorse positive descriptions of themselves well before they accept negative ones (e.g., Benenson & Dweck, 1986; Eshel & Klein, 1981; Nicholls, 1978, 1979; Stipek, 1981; Stipek & Daniels, 1988; Stipek & Tannatt, 1984). To the extent that feedback seeking is driven by the same processes that channel feedback acceptance, this evidence can be taken as indirect support for the idea that self-enhancement emerges earlier in development than does self-verification.

   4. Self-enhancement should not require conscious recognition of self.

Several investigators have suggested that self-enhancement strivings may influence the self-ratings of adults even in the absence of conscious self-recognition (Huntley, 1940; Wolff, 1933). Huntley, for example, surreptitiously photographed relatively innocuous aspects of his participants' bodies, such as the backs of their hands and their profiles. Six months later he had participants return to the laboratory and rate photos of their own hands and silhouettes as well as those of several other people. He found that participants tended to rate photos of themselves more favorably than the photos of others, and that this tendency was particularly strong when they failed to recognize the photos as their own. Thus it appeared that self-enhancement unfolded nonconsciously and that, if anything, self-recognition *diminished* self-enhancement processes. These findings offer further evidence that self-enhancement can occur without elaborate, self-relevant information processing.

Taken together, this research offers converging evidence that self-enhancement is a computationally simple tendency to approach and embrace friendly stimuli and avoid and reject unfriendly stimuli. Furthermore, it appears that this tendency is triggered by the mere categorization of feedback. Self-verification, in contrast, is a relatively complex process that grows out of the comparison of social feedback with representations of self stored in memory.

The categorization and comparison phases associated with self-enhancement and self-verification generate output (probably in the form of affect or emotional readout; see Buck, 1985; Pittman & Heller, 1987) that provides the person with two fundamentally distinct mandates; one emanating from the simple positivity of the feedback, the other from its subjective veridicality. These mandates then serve as inputs to a strategic or cost–benefit analysis. As can be seen in the lower portion of Table 12.1, this strategic analysis uses information about the self, the feedback, and social-contextual factors in the generation of hypothetical "if–then" scenarios. Such analyses may either bolster or undermine decisions emanating from the primary phase of the process (Hoffman, 1986). Some of the factors that enter into this cost–benefit analysis, as well as self-enhancement and self-verification reactions, are considered below. Although there are obviously many factors that influence these processes, four classes of factors are especially important: (1) the relationship of the evaluator and recipient of the feedback; (2) the recipient's conceptions of self; (3) the nature of the evaluation; and (4) the nature of the response.

Determinants of Self-Enhancement, Self-Verification, and Strategic Self-Presentation

Nature of the Relationship between Evaluator and Recipient of Feedback

Social norms tell us that some people should be more favorably disposed toward us than others. Just as intimates are supposed to spare the feelings of their partners, even if this requires obscuring the truth, teachers or superordinates are expected to be perfectly honest, even if this means communicating truths that hurt. The general principle here seems to be that increments in the intimacy of the relationship foster increments in self-enhancement. In support of this idea, we (Swann & Pelham, 1988) found that people preferred their intimates to view them most favorably, followed by their friends, followed by their casual acquaintances.

The existence of such social norms places people with negative self-views between a rock and a hard place. That is, although their knowledge of these norms encourages them to seek intimates who think well of them, their desire for self-verification urges them to seek intimates who think poorly of them. The situation is further complicated by the fact that if people with negative self-views locate relationship partners who think poorly of them, they risk being rejected; if they fail to find such partners, they will themselves want to leave. Not surprisingly, then, people with negative self-views tend to be in shorter-term friendships than those with positive self-views (Swann & Pelham, 1988).

Nature of Recipient's Conceptions of Self

POSITIVITY OF SPECIFIC SELF-CONCEPTIONS   The research reviewed above makes it clear that people will work to confirm their self-views, even if those self-views are negative. This means that people with negative self-views will be less likely to self-enhance (by, e.g., seeking positive feedback) than those with positive self-views.

POSITIVITY OF GLOBAL SELF-ESTEEM   Because people with low self-esteem typically have a wealth of negative self-views (Pelham & Swann, 1989), they will be less inclined than people with high self-esteem to self-enhance *overall*. This does not mean, however, that people with low self-esteem suffer from deficits in self-enhancement motivation (see, e.g., Taylor & Brown, 1988). We (Swann et al., 1989), for example, proposed that the self-concept is sufficiently differentiated that even people with low self-esteem possess positive attributes for which they can seek verification in the form of social feedback. We found that when people sought feedback pertaining to positive attributes, people with low self-esteem were just as inclined as people with high self-esteem to seek favorable feedback. Apparently, people with low self-esteem tend to seek unfavorable feedback because (1) they possess a wealth of negative self-conceptions and (2) they are faithful to self-verification principles; it is *not* that they have a poorly developed self-enhancement motive.

SALIENCE OF SELF-CONCEPTIONS   People are probably more inclined to verify self-views that are relatively accessible. One of the most direct ways to increase the accessibility of self-views is simply to ask people to think about themselves. We (Snyder & Swann, 1976), for example, found that asking people to think about their attitudes toward women increased their tendency to act on these beliefs (see also Fazio, 1986). Similarly, Sherman and Gorkin (1980) found that making the beliefs of feminists accessible by challenging their beliefs increased the likelihood that they would engage in profeminist behavior. Finally, Mori, Chaiken, and Pliner (1987) reported that women whose self-perceived femininity was threatened by false feedback behaved in a manner consistent with their image of femininity: They ate less than did controls.

We (Swann & Read, 1981b) showed that self-discrepant feedback intensified people's efforts to self-verify even when the relevant self-views were negative. That is, when their self-views were challenged, people who perceived themselves as likeable intensified their efforts to elicit *favorable* reactions, and those who perceived themselves as dislikeable intensified their efforts to elicit *unfavorable* reactions.

CERTAINTY OF SELF-CONCEPTIONS   People are more apt to verify self-views of which they are certain than ones they are uncertain about (e.g., Maracek & Mettee, 1972; Pelham, 1989; Swann & Ely, 1984; Swann & Pelham, 1990; Swann et al., 1988). Presumably, this effect reflects a tendency for relatively certain self-views to be particularly likely to promote people's perceptions of prediction and control. One mediator of this effect may be that certainty narrows people's latitude of acceptance (Pelham, 1989). Thus, for example, people who are relatively certain of their negative self-views may be particularly inclined to solicit unfavorable feedback because they are more likely to recognize and be repelled by the self-discrepant character of favorable feedback.

Sorrentino and Short (1986) have noted that some people (certainty-oriented) are more inclined to verify their self-views than others (uncertainty-oriented). Although it is tempting to hypothesize that people who are certain of their self-views are certainty-oriented and people who are uncertain of their self-views are uncertainty-oriented (see also Sorrentino & Hancock, 1987), an individual-difference approach cannot explain evidence that *within persons*, people are more inclined to verify those self-views of which they are certain as compared to uncertain (Swann & Pelham, 1990).

IMPORTANCE OF SELF-CONCEPTIONS   The more important a self-attribute is, the more people want feedback about it, even if that attribute is negative (Pelham, 1989). This finding probably reflects the fact that people regard as important those attributes that relate to their significant goals and plans. Academics, for example, tend to regard intelligence as important because they have, in a sense, "staked their beings" on being intelligent (e.g., James, 1890). At the same time, it seems reasonable to suppose that people are more motivated to seek verification for self-views that are highly important to them. Although this obviously poses problems for people who possess important self-views that are negative; it turns out that people rarely encounter such a dilemma because important self-views are almost always positive (Pelham, 1989).

DISCREPANCY BETWEEN REAL AND IDEAL SELF   In general, people will be motivated to self-enhance insofar as their self-views fall short of (1) the persons *they* wish they were or (2) the persons that *significant others* wish they were (e.g., James, 1890; Linville, 1987; for insightful discussions of these and other forms of self-discrepancy, see Higgins, 1987, in press).

Nature of the Evaluation

People should be particularly likely to self-verify insofar as they regard the evaluation or evaluator as credible. That is, from an epistemic perspective, relatively credible evaluations will be particularly comforting if they are self-verifying and particularly unsettling if they are not. For this reason, any variable that might increase the credibility of an evaluation—such as expertise, knowledgeability, or intelligence of the source—should increase the probability that people will seek self-confirming feedback. The converse is also true: Any variable that decreases the credibility of an evaluation or evaluator should increase self-enhancement strivings.

Nature of the Response

RELATION OF RESPONSE TO ANTECEDENTS OF SELF-ENHANCEMENT AND SELF-VERIFICATION   Responses that are closely allied with people's immediate, "affective" reactions should conform to self-enhancement theory. An elegant series of experiments by Tesser (1988) supports the former proposition: Affective responses (as measured by physiological reactions) conform to Tesser's "self-evaluation maintenance model" (a self-enhancement theory). Furthermore, my colleagues and I have shown that verbal measures of affective reactions to feedback also conform to self-enhancement theory (Swann et al., 1987).

By default, self-enhancement strivings should also influence any response that is logically unrelated to the considerations that underlie self-verification strivings. We (Swann et al., 1989), for example, asked people whether they would like to interact with someone who had formed an accurate appraisal of one of their strengths or one of their weaknesses. Even subjects with low global self-esteem chose to interact with the person who had evaluated one of their strengths, presumably because acquiring praise regarding one particular attribute does not necessarily threaten the notion that one is worthless in a general sense (especially if one devalues that attribute as people with low self-esteem generally do).

Social comparison processes are also logically unrelated to the considerations underlying self-verification strivings. That is, there is no logical (or, for that matter, social-psychological) reason why people with negative self-views should make themselves feel bad by comparing themselves to their superiors. For this reason, people who perceive themselves as unintelligent can self-enhance by comparing themselves to reptiles without suffering the epistemic and pragmatic consequences associated with failure to self-verify (e.g., Taylor & Lobel, 1989; Tesser, 1986, 1988; Tesser & Campbell, 1983; Wills, 1981).

Brown et al.'s (1988) research on "indirect" strategies of self-enhancement offers another example of a self-enhancing response that is logically unrelated to self-verification considerations. For instance, Brown et al. found that people with low self-esteem promoted their own group when they were *indirectly* but not *directly* responsible for the group's performance. In this way, people with low self-esteem could bask in the glory of their group without claiming to be better than they actually were and thereby leaving themselves open to the negative consequences associated with failure of self-verification (see also Cialdini & Richardson, 1980).

Still another example of a self-enhancing response that is not constrained by self-verification strivings has been offered by Baumgardner under the rubric of "affect regulation." She and her colleagues (Baumgardner, Kaufman, & Levy, 1989) reported that among people whose responses were relatively public, those who had low self-esteem were especially inclined to compliment persons who liked them and derogate persons who disliked them. Presumably, by publicly "putting others in their place," victims of chronic negative feedback can improve their affective states without claiming to be persons that they are not. As noted above, of course, other classes of responses *are* constrained by the epistemic and pragmatic considerations underlying self-verification strivings: (1) ratings of the diagnosticity and accuracy of feedback, attributions regarding feedback, and perceptions of the evaluator (Swann et al., 1987); (2) within-attribute feedback seeking (Swann et al., 1989, 1990; Swann & Read, 1981a, 1981b); (3) overt interaction strategies (Curtis & Miller, 1986; Swann & Ely, 1984; Swann & Hill, 1982; Swann, et al., 1988; Swann & Read, 1981b); and (4) choice of partners with whom to interact or pursue a relationship (e.g., Swann et al., 1989, 1990, in press; Swann & Pelham, 1988, 1990).

Yet another class of responses includes those that are only somewhat related to the epistemic and pragmatic considerations underlying self-verification strivings. Examples of such behaviors include ratings of the attractiveness of evaluators (e.g., Swann et al., 1987), preferences regarding future performances (e.g., McFarlin & Blascovitch, 1981), and preferences regarding the appraisals of relationship partners (e.g., Pelham & Swann, 1989).

COGNITIVE RESOURCES AVAILABLE IN FORMULATING THE RESPONSE   As noted earlier, depriving people of cognitive resources while they are making a behavioral choice should increase the likelihood of self-enhancement and diminish the likelihood of self-verification. Thus when people make a decision hurriedly or when their attentions are divided, they will be especially likely to self-enhance (e.g., Swann et al., in press). In contrast, when people have time to think before making a decision, they will tend to self-verify.

A caveat is in order here, however. Although self-verifying behavior is predicated on a relatively complex set of cognitive operations, this does not mean that *all* reasoned action will therefore be self-verifying. Indeed, after much reflection, a person may well decide that self-enhancing behavior has fewer costs and more benefits than does a self-verifying response. For example, an unathletic professor may encourage his students to believe he was once "jock" because, after considerable thought, he realizes that there will be few undesirable epistemic or pragmatic consequences associated with such a masquerade. Thus, although depriving people of cognitive resources will make them more likely to behave in a self-enhancing manner, allowing them to reflect will promote self-verification only if the epistemic and pragmatic considerations that theoretically underlie self-verification override competing considerations. If, upon reflection, people decide that they can acquire unrealistically favorable feedback without suffering the epistemic and pragmatic consequences that usually accompany failures to self-verify, they may well do so.

These observations suggest that the interplay between people's immediate "affective" preferences and reasoned decisions may be thought of in terms of a three-step process: an initial, minimally cognitive phase (self-enhancement); a second phase of somewhat more complex cognitive operations (self-verification); and finally a third, reflective stage during which the initial affective preference may or may not resurface (strategic self-presentation).

Research by Wilson and his colleagues offers some support for such a three-step process in a different context (e.g., Wilson & Dunn, 1986; Wilson, Dunn, Draft, & Lisle, 1989; Wilson & Lisle, 1990). These investigators have shown that although people initially form preferences for stimuli (e.g., pens) based on superficial qualities (e.g., color), if encouraged to reflect on their decision they will focus on objective attributes of the stimuli that seem plausible (e.g., durability) and thus revise their initial judgments. Later, however, they may experience a resurgence of the initial preference that causes them to regret the reasoned decision. The analogy in the interpersonal sphere would be the woman with a negative self-concept who, after some reflection, chooses a contemptuous but self-verifying relationship partner. After a bit more reflection, she may decide that life is too short to spend with someone who constantly makes her miserable. The lesson here is that although impulsive or "thoughtless" decisions may sometimes be the source of difficulty (e.g., Janis & Mann, 1977; Koriat, Lichtenstein, & Fischhoff, 1980; Langer, 1978, 1989), thought is by no means an antidote to unhappiness in social relations.

IMPORTANCE OF THE RESPONSE   When it comes to consequential decisions (choosing a spouse, close friend, or associate), people tend to take their time. Given that time promotes self-verification (at least up to a point), it is perhaps not surprising that when people with negative self-views select relationship partners, they self-verify by choosing persons who appraise them negatively (Swann & Pelham, 1988). This research also makes it easy to understand why laboratory investigators have typically found that people are more attracted to self-enhancing evaluators. That is, expressing attraction for a stranger who seems to have an inappropriately favorable appraisal of oneself is one thing. It is quite another to pursue a relationship with such a person (e.g., Huston & Levinger, 1978), since an incongruent relationship partner may frustrate the epistemic and pragmatic needs that drive self-verification processes. For example, the same flattering remarks that seem harmless and pleasant when delivered by a stranger may seem disturbing and unsettling when delivered by someone who should know one well. Thus, the fact that self-enhancement processes may be primary (in a temporal sense) does not necessarily mean that they influence important life decisions more strongly.

"COGNITIVE" VERSUS "AFFECTIVE" RESPONSES   The foregoing analysis may take some of the mystery out of evidence suggesting that affective responses are generally self-enhancing and cognitive responses are generally self-verifying (e.g., Shrauger, 1975; Swann et al., 1987). That is, just as "affective responses" are typically rapid and unrelated to the considerations that underlie self-verification, "cognitive responses" tend to be relatively slow and thus more apt to be influenced by the considerations that underlie self-verification.

CONCLUSION

Past attempts to reconcile self-enhancement and self-verification have resembled what members of the business community refer to as a "hostile takeover": Advocates of one theory have attempted to use their own theory's principles to explain the other theory's phenomena, and in so doing to eliminate the other theory. Some (e.g., Backman, 1988; Schlenker, 1985; Steele, 1988), for example, suggest that people strive for consistency in the service of a superordinate desire for self-enhancement. In a similar manner, Lecky (1945) asserted that, by definition, all behavior grows out of a desire for unity (consistency). Either approach makes one motive capable of predicting anything (e.g., a tendency to seek positive *or* negative feedback). Yet they both suffer from a major shortcoming: They are difficult, if not impossible, to disconfirm.

In my opinion, efforts to resolve the self-enhancement versus self-verification (self-consistency) debate have made it clear that we cannot do without *either* motive. Although each of these propensities ultimately promotes the survival of the organism, it makes no more sense to equate them than it does to equate the desires to eat, to sleep, and to drink. Clearly, people want to be praised and loved, but they also want their worlds to be predictable and controllable. The task of future researchers will be to develop a more complete understanding of how these two basic social motives control behavior.

Acknowledgments

The preparation of this chapter was supported by National Institute of Mental Health Grant Nos. MH 37598 and MH 00498 to William B. Swann, Jr. This chapter was prepared while I was a fellow at the Center for Advanced Study in the Behavioral Sciences. I am grateful to the John D. and Catherine T. MacArthur Foundation, which helped support my stay there. I am also grateful to Ann Baumgardner, Daniel Gilbert, Tory Higgins, Kathleen Much, Brett Pelham, Dave Sears, Dick Sorrentino, Deborah Stipek, and Shelley Taylor for their helpful comments on the chapter.

This chapter incorporates material that originally appeared in "Identity Negotiation: Where Two Roads Meet" by W. B. Swann, Jr., 1987, *Journal of Personality and Social Psychology*, 53, 1038–1051, and "From Self to Health: Self-Verification and Identity Disruption" by W. B. Swann, Jr., and J. D. Brown, 1990, in I. Sarason, B. Sarason, and G. Pierce (Eds.), *Social Support: An Interactional View*, New York: Wiley. Reprinted by permission of the American Psychological Association and John Wiley & Sons.

Notes

1. Applied to simple self-enhancement, the term "self-enhancement" is thus misleading, in that some theorists (e.g., Tesser, 1988) have argued that people work to *maintain* (rather than enhance) their (typically positive) self-views. The crucial distinction, however, is that no self-enhancement researchers suggest that a person would work to maintain a negative self-view, as does self-verification theory.

2. I am not denying that laboratory manipulations may influence people's momentary views of self (e.g., Jones, 1990). Rather, I am merely suggesting that chronic self-views color people's interpretation of social feedback and anchor momentary self-images.

3. At first blush, this emphasis on the importance of prediction and control may seem incompatible with the fact that people are fascinated by novel and unfamiliar stimuli and become bored with phenomena that are too predictable (e.g., Berlyne, 1971; White, 1959). Nevertheless, social stimuli are probably sufficiently labile that they are almost never construed as *too* predictable. In addition, when stimuli are self-relevant, people may eschew the luxury of novelty because prediction and control are so essential within this domain. Finally, there are individual differences in the extent to which people prefer novelty versus predictability (Sorrentino & Short, 1986).

4. Although previous investigations obtained self-verification effects without relying on self-certainty as a moderator variable (Swann & Pelham, 1988; Swann et al., 1989, 1990), these investigations found self-verification only among people whose self-views were relatively extreme, and such people tended to be more certain of extreme self-views.

5. In principle, a person who is *extremely* high in self-certainty may simply dismiss discrepant feedback out of hand. Thus far, however, my colleagues and I have not encountered participants who are sufficiently certain of their self-views that they are inclined to do this.

6. These data may seem incompatible with Hastie and Kumar's (1979) contention that people are especially likely to recall expectancy-*in*consistent evidence. Recent research, however, has indicated that Hastie and Kumar's findings were influenced by a confound between set size and expectancy. Reseachers who have avoided this confound (e.g., Bargh & Thein, 1985; Hemsley & Marmurek, 1982) have found that people preferentially recall information that confirms well-formed beliefs (for further details, see Higgins & Bargh, 1987).

7. Although self-verification is essentially epiphenomenal in such instances, at other times it is theoretically motivated by epistemic or pragmatic considerations.

References

Abelson, R. P. (1983). Whatever became of consistency theory? *Personality and Social Psychology Bulletin, 9*, 37-54.

Alloy, L. B., & Abramson, L. Y. (1988). Depressive realism: Four theoretical perspectives, In L. B. Alloy (Ed.), *Cognitive processes in depression* (pp. 223-265). New York: Guilford Press.

Allport, G. W. (1937). *Personality: A psychological interpretation.* New York: Holt.

Andrews, J. (1989). Psychotherapy of depression. A self-confirmation model. *Psychological Bulletin, 96*, 576-607.

Aronson, E. (1968). A theory of cognitive dissonance: A current perspective. In L. Berkowitz (Ed.), *Advances in experimental social psychology* (Vol. 4, pp. 1-34). New York: Academic Press.

Aronson, E. (1989). Analysis, synthesis, and the treasuring of the old. *Personality and Social Psychology Bulletin, 15*, 508-512.

Aronson, E., & Carlsmith, J. M. (1962). Performance expectancy as a determinant of actual performance. *Journal of Abnormal and Social Psychology, 65*, 178-182.

Athay, M., & Daley, J. M. (1981). Toward an interaction-centered theory of personality. In N. Cantor & J. F. Kihlstrom (Eds.), *Personality, cognition, and social interaction* (pp. 281-308). Hillsdale, NJ: Erlbaum.

Backman, C. W. (1988). The self: A dialectical approach. *Advances in Experimental Psychology, 21*, 229-260.

Backman, C. W., & Secord, P. F. (1962). Liking, selective interaction, and misperception in congruent interpersonal relations. *Sociometry, 25*, 321-335.

Baddeley, A. D., & Hitch, G. (1974). Working memory. In G. H. Bower (Ed.), *The psychology of learning and motivation: Advances in research and theory* (Vol. 7, pp. 47-89). New York: Academic Press.

Bargh, J. A., & Thein, R. D. (1985). Individual construct accessibility, person memory and the recall-judgment link: The case of information overload. *Journal of Personality and Social Psychology, 49*, 1129-1146.

Baumeister, R. F. (1982). A self-presentational view of social phenomena. *Psychological Bulletin, 91*, 3-26.

Baumeister, R. F. (1988). *The optimal margin of illusion.* Paper presented at the annual meeting of the American Psychological Association, Atlanta.

Baumeister, R. F., Hamilton, J. C., & Tice, D. M. (1985). Public versus private expectancy of success: Confidence booster or performance pressure? *Journal of Personality and Social Psychology, 48*, 1447-1457.

Baumeister, R. F., & Jones, E. E. (1978). When self-presentation is constrained by the target's knowledge: Consistency and compensation. *Journal of Personality and Social Psychology, 36*, 606-618.

Baumgardner, A. H., & Brownlee, E. A. (1987). Strategic failure in social interaction: Evidence for expectancy disconfirmation processes. *Journal of Personality and Social Psychology, 52*, 525-535.

Baumgardner, A. H., Kaufman, C. M., & Levy, P. E. (1989). Regulating affect interpersonally: When low self-esteem leads to greater enhancement. *Journal of Personality and Social Psychology, 56*, 907-921.

Bem, D. J. (1967). Self-perception: An alternative interpretation of cognitive dissonance phenomena. *Psychological Review, 74*, 183-200.

Bem, D. J. (1972). Self-perception theory. In L. Berkowitz (Ed.), *Advances in experimental social psychology* (Vol. 6, pp. 1-62). New York: Academic Press.

Benenson, J., & Dweck, C. (1986). The development of trait explanations and self-evaluations in the academic and social domains. *Child Development, 57*, 1179-1187.

Ben Zur, H., & Breznitz, S. J. (1981). The effects of time pressure on risky behavior. *Acta Psychologica, 47*, 89-104.

Berkowitz, L., & Devine, P. G. (1989). Research tradition, analysis, and synthesis in social psychological theories: The case of dissonance theory. *Personality and Social Psychology Bulletin, 15*, 493-507.

Berlyne, D. (1971). *Psychobiology and aesthetics.* New York: Appleton-Century-Crofts.

Boissevain, J. (1974). *Friends of friends: Networks, manipulators and coalitions.* Oxford: Blackwell.

Bradley, G. W. (1978). Self-serving biases in the attribution processes: A reexamination of the fact or fiction question. *Journal of Personality and Social Psychology, 36*, 56-71.

Brehm, J. W., & Cohen, A. R. (1962). *Explorations in cognitive dissonance.* New York: Wiley.

Brown, J. D. (1986). Evaluations of self and others: Self-enhancement biases in social judgments. *Social Cognition, 4*, 353-376.

Brown, J. D., Collins, R. L., & Schmidt, G. W. (1988). Self-esteem and direct versus indirect forms of self-enhancement. *Journal of Personality and Social Psychology, 55*, 445-453.

Broxton, J. A. (1963). A test of interpersonal attraction predictions derived from balance theory. *Journal of Abnormal and Social Psychology, 66*, 394-397.

Bruner, J. S., Goodnow, J. J., & Austin, G. A. (1956). *A study of thinking.* New York: Wiley.

Buck, R. (1985). Prime theory: An integrated view of motivation and emotion. *Psychological Review, 92*, 111-135.

Campbell, J. D. (1986). Similarity and uniqueness: The effects of attribute type, relevance, and individual differences in self-esteem and depression. *Journal of Personality and Social Psychology, 50*, 281-294.

Carson, R. C. (1969). *Interaction concepts of personality.* Chicago: Aldine.

Carver, C. S. (1975). Physical aggression and function of objective self-awareness and attitudes toward punishment. *Journal of Experimental Social Psychology, 11*, 510-519.

Chapanis, N. P., & Chapanis, A. (1964). Cognitive dissonance: Five years later. *Psychological Bulletin, 61*, 1-22.

Cialdini, R. B., & Richardson, K. D. (1980). Two indirect tactics of image management: Basking and blasting. *Journal of Personality and Social Psychology, 39*, 406-415.

Clarke, G. L. (1954). *Elements of ecology.* New York: Wiley.

Cooley, C. S. (1902). *Human nature and the social order.* New York: Scribner's.

Cooper, J., & Fazio, R. H. (1984). A new look at dissonance theory. In L. Berkowitz (Ed.), *Advances in experimental social psychology* (Vol. 17, pp. 229-266). Orlando, FL: Academic Press.

Coyne, J. C. (1976). Toward an interactional description of depression. *Psychiatry, 39*, 28-40.

Coyne, J. C., Kessler, R. C., Tal, M., Turnbull, J., Wortman, C. B., & Greden, J. F. (1987). Living with a depressed person. *Journal of Consulting and Clinical Psychology, 55*, 347-352.

Crary, W. G. (1966). Reactions to incongruent self-experiences. *Journal of Consulting Psychology, 30*, 246-252.

Curtis, R. C., & Miller, K. (1986). Believing another likes or dislikes you: Behavior making the beliefs come true. *Journal of Personality and Social Psychology, 51*, 284-290.

Dipboye, R. L. (1977). A critical review of Korman's self-consistency theory of work motivation and occupational choice. *Organizational Behavior and Human Performance, 18*, 108-126.

Easterbrook, J. A. (1959). The effect of emotion on cue utilization and the organization of behavior. *Psychological Review, 66*, 183-200.

Epstein, S. (1973). The self-concept revisited: Or a theory of a theory. *American Psychologist, 28*, 404-416.

Epstein, S. (1981). The unity principle versus the reality and pleasure principles, or the tale of the scorpion and the frog. In M. D. Lynch, A. A. Norme-Hebeisen, & K. J. Gergen (Eds.), *Self-concept: Advances in theory and research* (pp. 27-37). Cambridge, MA: Ballinger.

Epstein, S. (1985). The implications of cognitive-experiential self-theory for research in social psychology and personality. *Journal for the Theory of Social Behavior, 15*, 282-309.

Epstein, S. (in press). Cognitive-experiential self-theory: Implications for developmental psychology.

In M. R. Gunnar & L. A. Sroufe (Eds.), *Self-processes in development: Minnesota Symposium on Child Psychology* (Vol. 23). Hillsdale, NJ: Erlbaum.

Eshel, Y., & Klein, Z. (1981). Development of academic self-concept of lower-class and middle-class primary school children. *Journal of Educational Psychology, 73*, 287-293.

Fazio, R. H. (1986). How do attitudes guide behavior. In R. M. Sorrentino & E. Tory Higgins (Eds.), *Handbook of motivation and cognition: Foundations of social behavior* (Vol. 1, pp. 204-243). New York: Guilford Press.

Felson, R. B. (1981a). Self and reflected appraisal among football players. *Social Psychology Quarterly, 44*, 116-126.

Felson, R. B. (1981b). Social sources of information in the development of the self. *Sociological Quarterly, 22*, 69-79.

Fernald, A. (1989). *Emotion and meaning in mothers' speech to infants.* Paper presented at the annual meeting of the Society for Research in Child Development, Kansas City, KS.

Festinger, L. (1954). A theory of social comparison processes. *Human Relations, 7*, 117-140.

Festinger, L. (1957). *A theory of cognitive dissonance.* Evanston, IL: Row, Peterson.

Gazzaniga, M. S. (1985). *The social brain.* New York: Basic Books.

Gibbons, F. X. (1978). Sexual standards and reaction to pornography: Enhancing behavioral consistency through self-focused attention. *Journal of Personality and Social Psychology, 36*, 976-987.

Gilbert, D. T. (1989). *How mental systems believe.* Unpublished manuscript, University of Texas–Austin.

Goethals, G. R., & Darley, J. M. (1977). Social comparison theory: An attributional approach. In J. M. Suls & R. L. Miller (Eds.), *Social comparison processes: Theoretical and empirical perspectives* (pp. 259-278). Washington, DC: Hemisphere.

Goffman, E. (1959). *The presentation of self in everyday life.* Garden City, NY: Doubleday/Anchor.

Goldstein, K. (1939). *The organism.* New York: American.

Greenwald, A. G. (1980). The totalitarian ego: Fabrication and revision of personal history. *American Psychologist, 35*, 603-618.

Greenwald, A. G. (1989). Self-knowledge and self-deception. In J. S. Lockard & D. L. Paulhus (Eds.), *Self-deception: An adaptive mechanism?* (pp. 113-131). New York: Prentice-Hall.

Greenwald, A. G., & Ronnis, D. L. (1978). Twenty years of cognitive dissonance: Case study of the evolution of a theory. *Psychological Review, 85*, 53-57.

Hall, C. S., & Lindzey, G. (1970). *Theories of personality.* New York: Wiley.

Harrison, A. A. (1977). Mere exposure. In L. Berkowitz (Ed.), *Advances in experimental social psychology* (Vol. 10, pp. 39-83). New York: Academic Press.

Hastie, R., & Kumar, P. (1979). Person memory: Personality traits as organizing principles in memory for behaviors. *Journal of Personality and Social Psychology, 37*, 25-38.

Heider, F. (1946). Attitudes and cognitive organization. *Journal of Psychology, 21*, 107-112.

Heider, F. (1958). *The psychology of interpersonal relations.* New York: Wiley.

Hemsley, G. D., & Marmurek, H. C. (1982). Person memory: The processing of consistent and inconsistent person information. *Personality and Social Psychology Bulletin, 8*, 433-438.

Higgins, E. T. (1987). Self-discrepancy: A theory relating self and affect. *Psychological Review, 94*, 319-340.

Higgins, E. T. (in press). Development of self-regulatory and self-evaluative processes: Costs, benefits, and trade-offs. In M. R. Gunnar & L. A. Sroufe (Eds.), *Self-processes in development: Minnesota Symposium on Child Psychology* (Vol. 23). Hillsdale, NJ: Erlbaum.

Higgins, E. T., & Bargh, J. A. (1987). Social cognition and social perception. *Annual Review of Psychology, 38*, 369-425.

Higgins, E. T., & King, G. (1981). Accessibility of social constructs: Information-processing consequences of individual and contextual variability. In N. Cantor & J. F. Kihlstrom (Eds.), *Personality, cognition, and social interaction* (pp. 69-121). Hillsdale, NJ: Erlbaum.

Hilton, J. L., & Darley, J. M. (1985). Constructing other persons: A limit on the effect. *Journal of Experimental Social Psychology, 21*, 1-18.

Hixon, J. G., & Swann, W. B., Jr. (1989). *Timing and perceptions of accuracy.* Manuscript in preparation.

Hoffman, M. L. (1986). Affect, cognition, and motivation. In R. M. Sorrentino & E. T. Higgins (Eds.), *Handbook of motivation and cognition: Foundations of social behavior* (Vol. 1, pp. 244–280). New York: Guilford Press.

Hull, C. L. (1943). *Principles of behavior.* New York: Appleton-Century-Crofts.

Huntley, C. W. (1940). Judgments of self based upon records of expressive behavior. *Journal of Abnormal Social Psychology, 35,* 398–427.

Huston, T. L., & Levinger, G. (1978). Interpersonal attraction and relationships. *Annual Review of Psychology, 29,* 115–156.

James, W. (1890). *The principles of psychology* (2 vols.). New York: Henry Holt.

Janis, I. L., & Mann, L. (1977). *Decision making: A psychological analysis of conflict, choice and commitment.* New York: Free Press.

Jones, E. E. (1964). *Ingratiation.* New York: Appleton-Century-Crofts.

Jones, E. E. (1990). Constrained behavior and self-concept change. In J. Olson & M. P. Zanna (Eds.), *Self-inference processes: The Ontario Symposium* (Vol. 6). Hillsdale, NJ: Erlbaum.

Jones, E. E., & Pittman, T. S. (1982). Toward a general theory of strategic self-presentation. In J. Suls (Ed.), *Psychological perspectives on the self* (Vol. 1, pp. 231–262). Hillsdale, NJ: Erlbaum.

Jones, S. C. (1973). Self and interpersonal evaluations: Esteem theories versus consistency theories. *Psychological Bulletin, 79,* 185–199.

Kahneman, D. (1973). *Attention and effort.* Englewood Cliffs, NJ: Prentice-Hall.

Kahneman, D., & Tversky, A. (1983). Choices, values and frames. *American Psychologist, 39,* 341–350.

Kelly, G. A. (1955). *The psychology of personal constructs.* New York: Norton.

Kihlstrom, J. F., & Cantor, N. (1984). Mental representations of the self. In L. Berkowitz (Ed.), *Advances in experimental social psychology* (Vol. 12, pp. 1–47). New York: Academic Press.

Klayman, J., & Ha, Y.-W. (1987). Confirmation, disconfirmation, and information in hypothesis testing. *Psychological Review, 94,* 211–228.

Koriat, A., Lichtenstein, S., & Fischhoff, B. (1980). Reasons for confidence. *Journal of Experimental Psychology: Human Learning and Memory, 6,* 107–118.

Korman, A. K. (1968). Task success, task popularity, and self-esteem as influences on task liking. *Journal of Applied Psychology, 52,* 484–490.

Kunst-Wilson, W. R., & Zajonc, R. B. (1980). Affective discrimination of stimuli that cannot be recognized. *Science, 207,* 557–558.

Langer, E. J. (1978). Rethinking the role of thought in social interaction. In J. H. Harvey, W. Ickes, & R. F. Kidd (Eds.), *New directions in attribution research* (Vol. 2, pp. 35–58). Hillsdale, NJ: Erlbaum.

Langer, E. J. (1989). *Mindfulness.* Reading, MA: Addison-Wesley.

Lazarus, R. S. (1966). *Psychological stress and the coping process.* New York: McGraw-Hill.

Lazarus, R. S. (1984). On the primacy of cognition. *American Psychologist, 39,* 124–129.

Lecky, P. (1945). *Self-consistency: A theory of personality.* New York: Island Press.

Lewis, M. (1987). Social development in infancy and early childhood. In J. D. Osofsky (Ed.), *Handbook of infant development* (pp. 419–493).

Linville, P. W. (1987). Self-complexity as a cognitive buffer against stress-related illness and depression. *Journal of Personality and Social Psychology, 52,* 663–676.

Maracek, J., & Mettee, D. R. (1972). Avoidance of continued success as a function of self-esteem, level of esteem certainty, and responsibility for success. *Journal of Personality and Social Psychology, 22,* 90–107.

Markus, H. (1977). Self-schemas and processing information about the self. *Journal of Personality and Social Psychology, 35,* 63–78.

Markus, H., & Nurius, P. (1986). Possible selves. *American Psychologist, 41,* 954–969.

McCall, G. J., & Simmons, J. L. (1966). *Identities and interactions: An examination of human associations in everyday life.* New York: Free Press.

McFarlin, D. B., & Blascovitch, J. (1981). Effects of self-esteem and performance on future affective preferences and cognitive expectations. *Journal of Personality and Social Psychology, 40,* 521-531.

McGuire, W. J. (1960). Cognitive consistency and attitude change. *Journal of Abnormal and Social Psychology, 60,* 345-353.

Mead, G. H. (1934). *Mind, self and society.* Chicago: University of Chicago Press.

Miyamoto, S. F., & Dornbusch, S. A. (1956). Test of the symbolic interactionist hypothesis of self-conception. *American Journal of Sociology, 61,* 399-403.

Moreland, R. L., & Sweeney, P. D. (1984). Self-expectancies and reaction to evaluations of personal performance. *Journal of Personality, 52,* 156-176.

Mori, D., Chaiken, S., & Pliner, P. (1987). "Eating lightly" and the self-presentation of femininity. *Journal of Personality and Social Psychology, 53,* 693-702.

Newcomb, T. M. (1956). The prediction of interpersonal attraction. *American Psychologist, 11,* 575-586.

Nicholls, J. (1978). The development of the concepts of effort and ability, perceptions of academic attainment and the understanding that difficult tasks require more ability. *Child Development, 49,* 800-814.

Nicholls, J. (1979). The development of the perception of own attainment and causal attributions for success and failure in reading. *Journal of Educational Psychology, 71,* 94-99.

Norman, D. A., & Bobrow, D. G. (1975). On data-limited and resource-limited processes. *Cognitive Psychology, 7,* 44-64.

Odum, E. P. (1963). *Ecology.* New York: Holt, Rinehart & Winston.

Orpen, C., & Bush, R. (1974). The lack of congruence between self-concept and public image. *Journal of Social Psychology, 93,* 145-146.

Osgood, E. E., & Tannenbaum, P. H. (1955). The principle of congruity in the prediction of attitude change. *Psychological Review, 62,* 42-55.

Paulhus, D. L., & Levitt, K. (1987). Desirable responding triggered by affect: Automatic egotism? *Journal of Personality and Social Psychology, 52,* 245-259.

Pavlov, L. P. (1927). *Conditioned reflexes* (G. V. Antrep, Ed. and Trans.). Oxford: Oxford University Press.

Pelham, B. W. (1989). *Of confidence and consequence: On the certainty and importance of social knowledge.* Manuscript submitted for publication.

Pelham, B. W., & Swann, W. B., Jr. (1989). From self-conceptions to self-worth: The sources and structure of self-esteem. *Journal of Personality and Social Psychology, 57,* 672-680.

Pervin, L. A., & Rubin, D. B. (1967). Student dissatisfaction with college and the college dropout: A transactional approach. *Journal of Social Psychology, 72,* 285-295.

Pittman, T. S. & Heller, J. F. (1987). Social motivation. *Annual Review of Psychology, 38,* 461-489.

Pyszczynski, T. A., & Greenberg, J. (1987). Self-regulatory perseveration and the depressive self-focusing style: A self-awareness theory of reactive depression. *Psychological Bulletin, 102,* 122-138.

Raynor, J. O., & McFarlin, D. B. (1986). Motivation and the self-system. In R. M. Sorrentino & E. T. Higgins (Ed.), *Handbook of motivation and cognition; Foundations of social behavior* (Vol. 1, pp. 315-349). New York: Guilford Press.

Rogers, C. R. (1951). *Client-centered therapy: Its current practice, implication, and theory.* Boston: Houghton Mifflin.

Rosch, E. (1975). Cognitive reference points. *Cognitive Psychology, 7,* 532-547.

Rosenberg, M. (1965). *Society and the adolescent self-image.* Princeton, NJ: Princeton University Press.

Rosenberg, M. J. (1968). Hedonism, inauthenticity, and other goads toward expansion of a consistency theory. In R. Abelson, E. Aronson, W. McGuire, T. Newcomb, M. Rosenberg, & P. Tannenbaum (Eds.), *Theories of cognitive consistency: A sourcebook* (pp. 73-111). Chicago: Rand McNally.

Rosenberg, M. J., & Abelson, R. P. (1960). An analysis of cognitive balancing. In M. J. Rosenberg & C. I. Hovland (Eds.), *Attitude organization and change* (pp. 112-163). New Haven, CT: Yale University Press.

Schlenker, B. R. (1980). *Impression management.* Belmont, CA: Wadsworth.

Schlenker, B. R. (1985). Identity and self-identification. In B. R. Schlenker (Ed.), *The self and social life.* (pp. 65-99). New York: McGraw-Hill.

Sears, D. O., & Ables, R. P. (1969). Attitudes and opinions. *Annual Review of Psychology, 20,* 253-289.

Secord, P. F. & Backman, C. W. (1965). An interpersonal approach to personality. In B. Maher (Ed.), *Progress in experimental personality research* (Vol. 2, pp. 91-125). New York: Academic Press.

Shapiro, B., Eppler, M., Haith, M., & Reis, H. (1987). *An event analysis of facial attractiveness and expressiveness.* Paper presented at the meeting of the Society for Research in Child Development, Baltimore.

Sherman, S. J., & Gorkin, L. (1980). Attitude bolstering when behavior is inconsistent with central attitudes. *Journal of Experimental Social Psychology, 16,* 388-403.

Sherwood, J. J. (1967). Self-identity and referent others. *Sociometry, 30,* 404-409.

Shrauger, J. S. (1975). Responses to evaluation as a function of initial self-perceptions. *Psychological Bulletin, 82,* 581-596.

Shrauger, J. S., & Lund, A. (1975). Self-evaluation and reactions to evaluations from others. *Journal of Personality, 43,* 94-108.

Shrauger, J. S., & Schoeneman, T. J. (1979). Symbolic interactionist view of self-concept: Through the looking glass darkly. *Psychological Bulletin, 86,* 549-573.

Silverman, I. (1964). Self-esteem and differential responsiveness to success and failure. *Journal of Social Psychology, 69,* 115-119.

Smith, M. B. (1968). The self and cognitive consistency. In R. P. Abelson, E. Aronson, W. J. McGuire, T. M. Newcomb, M. J. Rosenberg, & P. H. Tannenbaum (Eds.), *Theories of cognitive consistency: A sourcebook* (pp. 366-372). Chicago: Rand McNally.

Snyder, C. R., & Higgins, R. L. (1988). Excuses: Their effective role in the negotiation of social reality. *Psychological Bulletin, 104,* 25-35.

Snyder, M., & Swann, W. B., Jr. (1976). When actions reflect attitudes: The politics of impression management. *Journal of Personality and Social Psychology, 34,* 1034-1042.

Snyder, M., & Swann, W. B., Jr. (1978). Hypothesis testing processes in social interaction. *Journal of Personality and Social Psychology, 36,* 1202-1212.

Sorrentino, R. M., & Hancock, R. D. (1987). The role of information and affective value for social influence: A case for the study of individual differences. In M. P. Zanna, J. Olson, & P. Herman (Eds.), *Social influence: The Ontario Symposium* (Vol. 5, pp. 244-268). Hillsdale, NJ: Erlbaum.

Sorrentino, R. M., & Short, J. C. (1986). Uncertainty, motivation, and cognition. In R. M. Sorrentino & E. T. Higgins (Eds.), *Handbook of motivation and cognition: Foundations of social behavior* (Vol. 1, pp. 379-403). New York: Guilford Press.

Steele, C. M. (1988). The psychology of self-affirmation: Sustaining the integrity of the self. In L. Berkowitz (Ed.), *Advances in experimental social psychology* (Vol. 21, pp. 261-302). New York: Academic Press.

Stipek, D. (1981). Children's perceptions of their own and their classmates' ability. *Journal of Educational Psychology, 73,* 404-410.

Stipek, D. J., & Daniels, D. H. (1988). Declining perceptions of competence: A consequence of changes in the child or in the educational environment? *Journal of Educational Psychology, 80,* 352-356.

Stipek, D., & Tannatt, L. (1984). Children's judgments of their own and their peers' academic competence. *Journal of Educational Psychology, 76,* 75-84.

Sumner, W. G. (1907). *Folkways.* Boston: Ginn.

Swann, W. B., Jr. (1983). Self-verification: Bringing social reality into harmony with the self. In J. Suls & A. G. Greenwald (Eds.), *Psychological perspectives on the self* (Vol. 2, pp. 33-66). Hillsdale, NJ: Erlbaum.

Swann, W. B., Jr. (1984). Quest for accuracy in person perception. A matter of pragmatics. *Psychological Review, 91,* 457-477.

Swann, W. B., Jr. (1985). The self as architect of social reality. In B. Schlenker (Ed.), *The self and social life* (pp. 100-125). New York: McGraw-Hill.

Swann, W. B., Jr. (1987). Identity negotiation: Where two roads meet. *Journal of Personality and Social Psychology, 53,* 1038-1051.

Swann, W. B., Jr., & Ely, R. J. (1984). A battle of wills: Self-verification versus behavioral confirmation. *Journal of Personality and Social Psychology, 46,* 1287-1302.

Swann, W. B., Jr., & Giuliano, T. (1987). Confirmatory search strategies in social interaction: When, how, why and with what consequences. *Journal of Clinical and Social Psychology, 5,* 511-524.

Swann, W. B., Jr., Griffin, J. J., Predmore, S., & Gaines, B. (1987). The cognitive–affective crossfire: When self-consistency confronts self-enhancement. *Journal of Personality and Social Psychology, 52,* 881-889.

Swann, W. B., Jr., & Hill, C. A. (1982). When our identities are mistaken: Reaffirming self-conceptions through social interaction. *Journal of Personality and Social Psychology, 43,* 59-66.

Swann, W. B., Jr., & Hill, C. A. (1986). *Some cognitive consequences of threats to the self.* Unpublished data, University of Texas–Austin.

Swann, W. B., Jr., Hixon, J. G., Stein-Seroussi, A., & Gilbert, D. T. (in press). The fleeting gleam of praise: Cognitive processes underlying behavioral reactions to self-relevant feedback. *Journal of Personality and Social Psychology.*

Swann, W. B., Jr., Wenzlaff, R. M., Krull, D. S., & Pelham, B. W. (1990). *Seeking truth, reaping despair: Depression, self-verification, and the quest for negative feedback.* Manuscript submitted for publication.

Swann, W. B., Jr., & Pelham, B. W. (1988). *The social construction of identity: Self-verification through friend and intimate selection.* Unpublished manuscript, University of Texas–Austin.

Swann, W. B., Jr., & Pelham, B. W. (1990). *Embracing the bitter truth: Positivity and authenticity in social relationships.* Manuscript submitted for publication.

Swann, W. B., Jr., Pelham, B. W., & Chidester, T. (1988). Change through paradox: Using self-verification to alter beliefs. *Journal of Personality and Social Psychology, 54,* 268-273.

Swann, W. B., Jr., Pelham, B. W., & Krull, D. S. (1989). Agreeable fancy or disagreeable truth? Reconciling self-enhancement and self-verification. *Journal of Personality and Social Psychology, 57,* 782-791.

Swann, W. B., Jr., & Predmore, S. C. (1985). Intimates as agents of social support: Sources of consolation or despair? *Journal of Personality and Social Psychology, 49,* 1609-1617.

Swann, W. B., Jr., & Read, S. J. (1981a). Acquiring self-knowledge: The search for feedback that fits. *Journal of Personality and Social Psychology, 41,* 1119-1128.

Swann, W. B., Jr., & Read, S. J. (1981b). Self-verification processes: How we sustain our self-conceptions. *Journal of Experimental Social Psychology, 17,* 351-372.

Swann, W. B., Jr., Stephenson, B., & Pittman, T. S. (1981). Curiosity and control: On the determinants of the search for social knowledge. *Journal of Personality and Social Psychology, 40,* 635-642.

Taylor, S. E, & Brown, J. D. (1988). Illusion and well being: Some social psychological contributions to a theory of mental health. *Psychological Bulletin, 103,* 193-210.

Taylor, S. E., & Lobel, M. (1989). Social comparison activity under threat: Downward evaluation and upward contacts. *Psychological Review, 94,* 564-575.

Tedeschi, J. T., & Lindskold, S. (1976). *Social psychology: Interdependence, interaction, and influence.* New York: Wiley.

Tedeschi, J. T., Schlenker, B. R., & Bonoma, T. V. (1971). Cognitive dissonance: Private rationalization or public spectacle. *American Psychologist, 26,* 685-695.

Tesser, A. (1986). Some effects of self-evaluation maintenance on cognition and action. In R. M. Sorrentino & E. T. Higgins (Eds.), *Handbook of motivation and cognition: Foundations of social behavior* (Vol. 1, pp. 435-464). New York: Guilford Press.

Tesser, A. (1988). Toward a self-evaluation maintenance model of social behavior. In L. Berkowitz (Ed.), *Advances in experimental social psychology* (Vol. 21, pp. 181-227). New York: Academic Press.

Tesser, A., & Campbell, J. (1983). Self-definition and self-evaluation maintenance. In J. Suls & A. G. Greenwald (Eds.), *Psychological perspectives on the self* (Vol. 2, pp. 1-31). Hillsdale, NJ: Erlbaum.

Tomkins, S. S. (1981). The quest for primary motives: Biography and autobiography of an idea. *Journal of Personality and Social Psychology, 41,* 306-329.

Trope, Y. (1979). Uncertainty-reducing properties of achievement tasks. *Journal of Personality and Social Psychology, 37*, 1505-1518.

Trope, Y. (1986). Self-enhancement and self-assessment in achievement behavior. In R. M. Sorrentino & E. T. Higgins (Eds.), *Handbook of motivation and cognition: Foundations of social behavior* (Vol. 1, pp. 350-378. New York: Guilford Press.

Tversky, A., & Kahneman, D. (1973). Availability: A heuristic for judging frequency and probability. *Cognitive Psychology, 5*, 207-232.

Tversky, A., & Kahneman, D. (1974). Judgment under uncertainty: Heuristics and biases. *Science, 185*, 1124-1131.

Wachtel, P. (1973). Psychodynamics, behavior therapy, and the implacable experimenter: An inquiry into the consistency of personality. *Journal of Abnormal Psychology, 82*, 324-334.

Wachtel, P. L. (1977). *Psychoanalysis and behavior therapy.* New York: Basic Books.

Walhood, D. S., & Klopfer, W. G. (1971). Congruence between self-concept and public image. *Journal of Consulting and Clinical Psychology, 37*, 148-150.

Wason, P. C., & Johnson-Laird, P. N. (1972). *Psychology of reasoning: Structure and content.* London: D. T. Batsford.

Wegner, D. M., & Giuliano, T. (1982). The forms of social awareness. In W. J. Ickes & E. S. Knowles (Eds.), *Personality, roles, and social behavior.* New York: Springer.

Weinstein, N. D. (1980). Unrealistic optimism about future life events. *Journal of Personality and Social Psychology, 39*, 806-820.

White, W. (1959). Motivation reconsidered: The concept of competence. *Psychological Review, 66*, 297-333.

Wicklund, R. A., & Brehm, J. W. (1976). *Perspectives on cognitive dissonance.* Hillsdale, NJ: Erlbaum.

Wilis, T. A. (1981). Downward comparison principles in social psychology. *Psychological Bulletin, 90*, 245-271.

Wilson, E. O. (1974). *Sociobiology: The new synthesis.* Cambridge, MA: Harvard University Press.

Wilson, T. D. (1985). Strangers to ourselves: The origins and accuracy of beliefs about one's own mental states. In J. H. Harvey & G. Weary (Eds.), *Attribution in contemporary psychology* (pp. 9-36). New York: Academic Press.

Wilson, T. D., & Dunn, D. S. (1986). Effects of introspection on attitude-behavior consistency: Analyzing reasons versus focusing on feelings. *Journal of Experimental and Social Psychology, 47*, 249-263.

Wilson, T. D., Dunn, D. S., Draft, D., & Lisle, D. J. (1989). Introspection, attitude change, and attitude-behavior consistency: The disruptive effects of explaining why we feel the way we do. In L. Berkowitz (Ed.), *Advances in experimental social psychology* (Vol. 22, pp. 287-343). Orlando, FL: Academic Press.

Wilson, T. D., & Lisle, D. J. (1990). *Some undesirable effects of self-reflection.* Unpublished manuscript, University of Virginia.

Wolff, W. (1933). The experimental study of forms of expression. *Character and Personality, 2*, 168-176.

Zajonc, R. B. (1968). The attitudinal effects of mere exposure. *Journal of Personality and Social Psychology Monograph Supplement, 9*, (Pt. 2), 1-27.

Zajonc, R. B. (1980). Feeling and thinking: Preferences need no inferences. *American Psychologist, 35*, 151-175.

Zajonc, R. (1984). On the primacy of affect. *Journal of Social Psychology, American Psychologist, 39*, 117-123.

Zuckerman, M. (1979). Attribution of success and failure revisited, or: The motivational bias is alive and well in attribution theory. *Journal of Personality, 47*, 245-287.

PART IV

Theories Relating Motivation and Cognition

CHAPTER 13

An Episodic View of Motivation
Unconscious Influences of Memory

LARRY L. JACOBY
McMaster University
COLLEEN M. KELLEY
Williams College

OVERVIEW

The central theme of this chapter is that behavior is often guided by unconscious influences of memory for prior episodes. The presence of such unconscious influences places limits on conscious, intentional control of behavior. The term "unconscious" may evoke a comparison to the psychodynamic approach to motivation. Unlike psychodynamic theorists, however, we have not been concerned with unconscious influences that represent widespread effects of traumatic experiences or unresolved conflicts. Rather, we are interested in unconscious influences that originate from a myriad of mundane experiences. By "unconscious influences of memory," we refer to effects of prior experience on the performance of some task that arise even though a person does not consciously remember the relevant prior experience.

Other cognitive approaches to motivated behavior have been based on an underlying conception of cognition that stresses abstraction. Dynamic approaches to motivation also focus on factors that have wide-ranging effects, such as the arousal of needs that are expressed in a variety of situations. In contrast, our episodic view of motivation predicts that behavior is locally controlled by the specific configuration of a situation that elicits the retrieval of similar prior events. Unconscious influences of memory are much more context-bound than would be predicted by the psychoanalytic tradition or by many other current theories of social cognition.

The most dramatic examples of unconscious influences of memory are shown by amnesics. Amnesics show effects of prior experience on their performance of a variety of tasks, although, by definition, they are severely impaired in their ability to recognize or recall earlier experiences. Unconscious influences of memory in the domain of perceptual–motor skills occur in amnesics (e.g., Cohen & Squire, 1980; Corkin, 1968; Warrington & Weiskrantz, 1974). Amnesics also reveal effects of recent prior experience in their performance of verbal tasks. We

(Jacoby & Witherspoon, 1982) found that Korsakoff patients' interpretation of the meaning of a homophone (e.g., "read–reed") was influenced by memory for its recent prior presentation. Homophones were presented auditorily in the context of questions that biased interpretation toward the less frequent meaning of the homophone (e.g., "Name a musical instrument that employs a reed"). Subjects were later asked to spell several words; no mention was made that some of the words were homophones that had been presented in the earlier phase of the experiment. Amnesics showed evidence of memory for the prior presentation of homophones by spelling those homophones in line with the meaning biased by their prior presentation (e.g., "reed"). Effects on spelling were as large for amnesics as for normal subjects, although the amnesics were generally unaware that the homophones had earlier appeared in the questions. Indeed, many of the amnesics did not remember the question at all. Amnesics also acquire affective reactions, although they are less able than normal subjects to consciously recollect the prior experience that gave rise to those reactions (Johnson, Kim, & Risse, 1985).

Unconscious influences of memory can be found in the behavior of normal subjects as well as that of amnesics. Evidence of memory is often shown by performance on an indirect test, although a direct test reveals no evidence of memory (see Johnson & Hasher, 1987, and Richardson-Klavehn & Bjork, 1988, for reviews). Spelling, as used in our experiment with amnesics, is an indirect test of memory because the instructions refer only to the task at hand and do not refer back to a particular prior event, although the subject's performance on the task may be influenced by memory for that prior event. Recognition and recall are direct tests of memory because the instructions refer to a target event in the personal history of the subject and ask the subject to consciously recollect that earlier event.

We consider it likely that the unconscious influences of prior episodes that we find so prevalent in perception, problem solving, and judgment also play an important role in motivated behavior. What an episodic view means for predicting the effects of motivational variables and other social factors is that effects are more controlled by local circumstances than would be expected if an abstract representation of knowledge, such as a schema, were responsible for directing behavior. An advantage of using the term "episodic" to name the view is that it makes obvious the relevance of factors that influence episodic memory. As is true for episodic memory, factors that affect encoding and those that affect retrieval should be important for motivation. In particular, factors influencing retrieval can be responsible for inconsistency in performance across situations, because retrieval factors determine the particular prior episodes that are retrieved from memory to guide later behavior.

Use of the term "episodic" carries the disadvantage that "episodic memory" usually refers to aware uses of the past, such as performance on a test of recognition memory or recall. Although we refer to influences of memory for a prior episode, we do not mean to imply that people are aware of memory for that prior episode or its effects on later performance. Later, we argue that the subjective experience of remembering relies on inference or attribution processes, and so a particular prior event can affect performance of an ongoing task independently of conscious recollection or the subjective experience of remembering.

To illustrate what we mean by an episodic view of motivation, we briefly describe the different functions with which motivation is credited, and the theories that have emphasized those functions. For each function of motivation, we argue that the interpretation of that function changes when one considers the role of unconscious influences of prior episodes.

FUNCTIONS OF MOTIVATION

Motivation as Plans

One approach to motivation holds that behavior is intentional, directed toward the attainment of consciously held goals. According to this account, the major function of motivation is to guide the selection and performance of actions. Miller, Galanter, and Pribram (1960) presented the paradigmatic theory of goal-directed behavior in their notion of "TOTE" sequences. A person first tests (T) the difference between the environment and a goal; operates (O) on the environment to reduce the discrepancy; tests (T) again to determine whether there is still a discrepancy between the environment and the goal; and then exits (E) if the goal has been met. A number of cognitive theories of motivation (e.g., Cantor, Markus, Niedenthal, & Nurius, 1986; Schank & Abelson, 1977; Srull & Wyer, 1986) also focus on the goal-directed control of behavior.

Although Miller et al. (1960) put in a disclaimer that goals need not be held consciously, their examples clearly refer to conscious goals and plans. Certainly cybernetic models illustrate how biological and computational systems can be goal-directed without reference to consciousness. However, psychological models of intentional control implicate consciousness, often by linking consciousness and attention (Posner & Snyder, 1975; Shiffrin & Schneider, 1977) or consciousness and an executive function (Johnson-Laird, 1983; Shallice, 1972).

Kuhl (1986) outlines a theory of how intentions control action. People formulate particular intentions when a situation matches the contextual aspects of the propositional representation of that action. If the difficulty of carrying out an action is high, and yet an actor perceives himself or herself as capable of the action, then the actor will use self-regulatory strategies to help maintain the intention against competing action tendencies. These self-regulatory strategies include selective attention to goal-relevant information and active avoidance of distraction (Mischel, Ebbesen, & Zeiss, 1972). One can also attempt to self-regulate by actively restructuring the environment, as when one makes a social commitment to stop smoking so as to create social pressure in support of the intention (Thoresen & Mahoney, 1974).

However, not all behavior is consciously directed toward goals. We do not always plan and then act. We sometimes act and then, if necessary, make our excuses. The theme of a great deal of recent research is that people are unable to report the factors that were important for controlling their behavior (e.g., Nisbett & Wilson, 1977). Behavior is often subject to unconscious influences that people either fail to notice or fail to comprehend (Bowers, 1984). One powerful source of unconscious influences is memory for prior episodes. When the current situation is very similar to a past situation, it effectively functions as a retrieval cue for the past situation. However, retrieval of the past situation need not be experienced as conscious remembering. Instead, the prior experience can unconsciously guide responses to the current situation.

Our suggestion that behavior is controlled by unconscious influences of the past may remind the reader of standard theories of automaticity, whereby unconscious behavior develops only after extended practice (e.g., Schneider & Shiffrin, 1977). The difference between that view of automaticity and our episodic view is in the specificity of the effects one would expect. An episodic view holds that performance is mediated by unconscious retrieval of memory for *particular* prior episodes. Thus, behavior will be sensitive to situational control because changing details of a situation create different cues for retrieval. The situation-as-retrieval-cue determines the particular prior episodes that are brought forward to influence interpretation and behavior in a current situation. If memory for a relevant prior episode is easily accessible, then the choice and enactment of a response may appear automatic. People's experience is that a particular response comes immediately to mind when they encounter a situation. Thus, automaticity reflects the match between the current situation and memory for a prior episode, rather than an abstract representation that is used in an invariant way across situations. Logan (1988) presents a theory that automaticity is the use of memory for particular prior responses rather than the formation of an abstract procedure.

Actions controlled unconsciously by memory for prior episodes produce far more situationally specific behaviors than would be predicted by abstract conceptions of automaticity. Furthermore, the episodic control of behavior implicates memory variables such as encoding specificity, distinctiveness, and delay. We think that these sorts of factors may be responsible for the inconsistencies in social research on automaticity reviewed by Bargh (1989). To know what prior episode will be unconsciously retrieved in a particular situation, one needs to know how past experiences were coded, and thus what aspects must be reinstated in the current situation before a past experience will be retrieved.

Behavior is subject to multiple levels of control (see, e.g., Shallice, 1988; Wegner & Vallacher, 1986). When behavior is affected by the unconscious retrieval of prior episodes, control can be considered local. The situation structures behavior by determining which past experiences will be retrieved. In contrast, when behavior is controlled by conscious intentions, control is more global or external to the situation. How might these two sources of control interact?

We propose that an important function of conscious control is the inhibition of responses that would otherwise occur as the result of unconscious influences of the past. The unconscious use of past episodes may determine one's first reaction to a situation. Consciousness serves to "edit" those first reactions by anticipating consequences and generating alternatives. Another important function of consciousness is to produce greater consistency across situations. If left to unconscious influences, behavior would vary with the details of situations. Consciousness counteracts that variation by introducing a more abstract standard against which behavior can be judged. For example, one may consciously reject some action because it is inconsistent with a higher-level goal. In line with this argument, manipulations that increase self-awareness can increase the degree to which behavior is consistent with a person's self-image (e.g., Buss, 1980). It should be noted here that unconscious memory for prior episodes works in a way opposite to that usually credited to automatic, unconscious influences. We hold memory for prior episodes responsible for variation in behavior across situations, whereas an automatic response that relies on some abstract representation would produce consistency across situations. In theories such as Shiffrin and Schneider's (1977), conscious intervention is responsible for variations in performance. In an episodic view, consciousness serves the equally important function of imposing consistency on behavior across situations.

An observer often cannot tell whether behavior is guided intentionally or unintentionally by unconscious use of prior experiences. Both levels of control could produce behavior that appears orderly and well structured. Furthermore, one cannot use an actor's retrospective report that a particular action was intentional, because intention can be an attribution that follows rather than causes behavior (Gazzaniga, 1988; Nisbett & Wilson, 1977). When a conscious intention produces effects in the same direction as those produced by the unconscious retrieval of prior episodes, it is impossible to know which is controlling behavior. This problem of separating unconscious from conscious influences is a general one (Holender, 1986; Richardson-Klavehn & Bjork, 1988). In a later section, we describe a method that we have found useful for separating conscious and unconscious influences of memory and perception.

Motivation as Category Accessibility

The central tenet of the "New Look" movement in perception (e.g., Bruner, 1957) was that perception is strongly influenced by psychological processes related to expectancies, values, attitudes, and needs. According to Bruner, perception involves an act of categorization. The accessibility of categories, and thereby perception, are influenced by a person's needs and other motivational factors. When a person is confronted with a social situation that requires some action, categorization of the situation may be seen as a prerequisite for responding. The approach taken by Bruner and most other cognitive psychologists is to propose that categorization involves centralized, abstracted models of everyday knowledge. It is common to claim that a situation is first analyzed for cues that can be used to classify it as a member of a more general class, and is then responded to in terms of that more general category of situations. For example, a situation may be classified and responded to in terms of some schema that has been abstracted across experiences in situations that are similar to a present one (e.g., Hastie, 1981). However, being confronted with a situation can also be seen as providing retrieval cues for memory of particular prior episodes involving situations that are *very* similar to a current one. The difference between the schema and the episodic view is in the level of abstraction of the memory representation that is said to guide behavior.

The notion of differences in category accessibility advanced by Bruner has been very popular in social psychology. Individual differences have been explained in terms of chronic differences in category accessibility. For example, researchers have suggested that particular trait and attitude categories are more readily accessible for people who are chronically disposed toward processing information with reference to those categories (e.g., Bargh & Pietromonaco, 1982; Fazio, 1986). Recent prior experience using a category is said to "prime" that category temporarily, making it temporarily more accessible for future use. In a well-known investigation of priming effects in the social domain, Higgins, Rholes, and Jones (1977) showed that presenting subjects with positive- or negative-trait terms influenced the evaluative impression that subjects formed of an ambiguously described person. Similar effects have been reported by others (e.g., Bargh & Pietromonaco, 1982; Srull & Wyer, 1980). The priming of different styles of thinking is also said to be possible. LaRue and Olejnik (1980) primed either concrete or formal operational thinking and showed effects on a test of subjects' level of moral development.

The term "priming" is taken from theories of word perception, and so it is important to consider the assumptions carried by the term. Morton (1969) proposed a "logogen" model of word recognition to account for effects of frequency in the language and effects of recently seeing a word on later identification of that word. A "logogen" is an abstract representation that has been formed across repeated exposures to a word and that does not preserve any information about particular encounters. Words that occur frequently in the language (e.g., "cat") are identified more readily than are words that occur infrequently (e.g., "cot") and tend to be mistakenly reported when a low-frequency word is actually presented. These effects of frequency in the language are explained by the proposal that high-frequency words have a lower threshold, and so require less information for their identification than do low-frequency words. The form of the argument is the same as that made for chronic differences in category accessibility. Reading a word in the experimental setting makes that word easier to identify when it is later repeated. This effect is called "priming" and is explained by claiming that reading a word temporarily lowers the threshold of its corresponding logogen. It is important that the effects of priming be considered temporary. If priming were long-term, all logogens eventually would be primed, so the basis for explaining the difference in the identification of high- and low-frequency words would be lost. Similarly, if priming of social categories is considered to be long-term, chronic differences in category accessibility cannot be explained in terms of differences in thresholds. The use of the term "priming" in theories of social cognition is generally consistent with its use in theories of word perception (see Broadbent, 1977). Differences in category accessibility are explained in a way equivalent to claiming that logogens vary in their thresholds.

According to an episodic view, it is (often unconscious) retrieval of memory for prior episodes, rather than differences produced by priming or chronic differences in the thresholds of abstract representations, that is responsible for the effects of prior experience on later perception and behavior. A priming view predicts that effects of prior experience will be relatively context-free because it is an abstract representation that is said to be primed. Later, we briefly review experiments that we have done to show effects of prior experience on perception that are too context-bound to be produced by the priming of an abstract representation.

Smith (1990) provides a review of effects on social judgments that are too specific to result from the use of schemas or other abstract representations. The framework that Smith proposes to interpret those effects is, in some ways, similar to our episodic view. Elsewhere, we (Jacoby, Marriott, & Collins, 1990) comment on similarities and differences between the two views. One difference is that Smith draws a distinction between content specificity and procedural or processing specificity. In contrast, we see memory as being for material as processed, so a distinction between content and processing of the sort implied by a procedural-declarative distinction is not useful (cf. Kolers & Smythe, 1979). Unlike Smith, we rely heavily on theorizing about episodic memory and use manipulations taken from experiments on episodic memory to explore effects on perception and judgment. We explain the variability in performance across situations in terms of differences in the encoding and the retrieval of memory for prior episodes.

The episodic view emphasizes the importance of the details of particular prior situations and experiences. In an episodic view, knowledge and motivation are decentralized, being spread across memory for prior episodes rather than being carried by a set of rules or general categories. The use of memory for episodes to direct the interpretation of later events and behavior is similar to that of the use of legal precedent in court cases. A current decision is made or a conflict is resolved by invoking the precedent of some earlier very similar situation. In this vein, our argument for the importance of memory for prior episodes is similar to arguments that case-based reasoning is often necessary because of the insufficiency of rules or other more abstract knowledge (e.g., Kolodner, 1984; Schank, 1982). Our emphasis on the importance of memory for prior episodes is also generally consistent with the discussions of exemplar or instances accounts of concept learning advanced by Brooks (1978), Medin (Medin & Schaffer, 1978; reviewed in Medin & Smith, 1984) and Hintzman (1986). McClelland and Rumelhart's (1981) discussion of the word superiority effect and Kahneman and Miller's (1986) discussion of judgment tasks also emphasize the importance of generalizing around prior instances.

The argument for the importance of memory for prior episodes is *not* an argument that only "surface" or literal characteristics of events are important. Rather, it is memory for the prior episode or event *as interpreted* that guides the interpretation of later events and behavior. Memory for prior processing episodes can preserve some overall interpretation of the earlier situation, as well as the organization of the perceptual stimulus and "semantic" aspects of the situation.

The motivation that was present during an earlier episode is likely to be important for memory of the episode. Again, the example of legal precedent is useful. Legal precedent rests on the overall similarity between a current case and some earlier case. Inferences about traits of the defendant and other sources of motives, as well as evidence used as a basis for those inferences, are likely to be preserved and enter into decisions about precedent. Unlike legal precedent, the use of memory for prior episodes does not necessarily involve conscious comparison of a present situation with some record of past situations. Memory for a prior event can produce unconscious influences on the perception and the interpretation of later events. That is, although a person does not recall or recognize an event as previously experienced, memory for that event can influence later judgments.

For a priming view to work, a category must retain its meaning and be used in an invariant fashion across situations. It might be tempting to solve the problem of specificity of effects by proposing subcategories or subtypes (e.g., Brewer, Dull, & Lui, 1981) that can be primed. However, at the extreme, subcategories would correspond to memory for particular episodes. Also, if subcategories are proposed, factors determining the level of categories that subjects use must be specified. According to our episodic view, use of particular prior episodes to interpret and guide behavior in a current situation depends on encoding–retrieval interactions of the sort that have been revealed by investigations of memory.

Consistency across situations must also be explained. For example, individual differences in achievement motivation have been used successfully to predict behavior in a wide variety of situations (e.g., Sorrentino & Short, 1986). Also, as described earlier, there do seem to be chronic differences in category accessibility. Abstractionist views are very well suited to explain stability in performance across situations, along with very general effects of a prior experience. How does an episodic view account for consistency in behavior across situations? Consistency can arise from generalization around memory for prior episodes (cf. Brooks, 1987; Hintzman, 1986; Medin & Schaffer, 1978). A person who is classified as being success-oriented, as compared to failure-threatened, has probably behaved frequently in a success-oriented manner in a wide variety of situations. This means that for the success-oriented person, a new situation is more likely to be similar to an old situation in which the person's behavior was success-oriented. Memory for that similar prior episode can be used to produce success-oriented behavior in the new situation; that is, behavior is directed by memory for prior episodes, rather than by some general trait that is then translated into behavior. How did the success-oriented person originally come to behave in a success-oriented way in a variety of situations? As described earlier with reference to the executive function of consciousness, behavior may have originally been consciously controlled by the person or even directed by others. Once success-oriented behavior has been started by whatever means, an episodic view holds that memory for prior episodes of such behavior breeds more of such behavior. Akin to Logan's (1988) account of automaticity, effects of prior experience can be carried by memory for prior episodes, rather than by an influence on the status of some abstract representation or trait.

The notion of priming seems particularly poorly suited to describe differences in styles of thinking (cf. LaRue & Olejnik, 1980). Abstractions such as concrete versus formal operations seem more likely to be drawn upon by the theoretician to describe behavior than to be unitary memory representations in the head of the subject that guide behavior and that can be primed. That is, it seems unlikely that there is a "logogen-like" representation of formal operational thinking that can be primed and that is invariably applied across situations. In this vein, concrete versus formal operations in thought seem to be context-bound (Gelman, 1978). One's strategy or plans for dealing with a problem may often rely on prior experience with similar problems in similar situations—memory for prior episodes.

Effects on category accessibility can be explained by other theories as well as by an episodic view. We have earlier mentioned Smith's (1990) approach and noted its similarity to an episodic view. Also, Higgins (1989) has proposed a model that includes episodic, procedural, and general declarative knowledge to explain category accessibility effects. The commentaries accompanying Smith's (1990) book chapter describe other models and provide very useful discussions of concerns for choosing among models. The various models may be formally indistinguishable (Barsalou, 1990), so that the choice must be made on the grounds of parsimony and heuristic value. We believe that the major advantage offered by an episodic view is its heuristic value. The use of research and theories about episodic memory to guide research leads one to ask questions and to seek contrasts that would probably be ignored if one held an abstractionist view of cognition. Later, we briefly describe a few lines of research that have grown out of our episodic view of cognition.

The Energizing Function of Motivation

Motivation has been credited with providing the energy or the "push" for behavior and is often treated as separate from other factors that control behavior. For example, drive has been said to combine with habit to determine performance. We argue that the source of energy for a behavior is often not separate from the control of behavior by prior experience. Once again, the question concerns the level of abstraction of the memory representation that controls behavior. Habit is an abstractionist notion, in that habit is said to cumulate across experiences. Claims that experiences are pooled to determine the "strength" of an association rest on many of the same assumptions as do claims for the existence of an abstract representation of a category. In contrast, an episodic view holds that memory for the particular experiences are retained and serve as a source of control for future behavior. An episodic view emphasizes the possibility of motivational variables configuring with other details of a situation. We first illustrate the importance of this possibility for the separability of habit and drive, and then argue that the same concerns apply to expectancy–value theories of motivation.

For drive to be treated as separate from habit, the one has to remain constant across variations in the other. A given number of hours of food deprivation, for example, must give rise to the same amount of hunger across a wide range of situations. Also, for any given situation, the stimuli to which a response is attached must remain constant across different levels of hunger. The simplest theory of this sort would hold that drive plays no role in defining either the stimulus to which a response is attached or the strength of the association formed between the stimulus and response. Drive would be said to influence only performance, not learning. The proposal (Spence, 1956) of a multiplicative relation between drive and habit as determinants of responding conveys this learning-performance distinction. A multiplicative relation between habit and drive means that when drive is at zero a response will not be observed, regardless of the strength of the association between a present stimulus and that response.

However, eating depends not only on number of hours of food deprivation, but also on factors such as the particular foods available, the time of day, and the social facilitation produced by others' eating. The effect of number of hours of food deprivation is likely to configure with those other factors. For example, the stimulus characteristics of a pizza might differ if one has not eaten for several hours and is surrounded by others who are rapidly devouring the pizza, as compared with a situation in which one has recently eaten another pizza and is not required to compete for the present one. There is good evidence to show the presence of interactions in palatability (e.g., Grill & Berridge, 1985). If configurations involving the effects of food deprivation dominate, it is no longer useful to talk about hunger separately from the other details of the situation. Indeed, the experience of hunger probably results from an interpretation of the whole situation, rather than from number of hours of food deprivation alone (e.g., Schachter, 1971). If so, only predictions that are very specific to the details of the situation can be made, because of the variability in performance produced by changes in configurations across situations. However, varying food deprivation surely produces some consistency across situations. One way of describing that consistency is in terms of similarity among configurations or situations. The claim would then be that an animal learns what to do in particular situations, and that hours of food deprivation configure with other stimulus properties to define those situations.

An episodic view of motivation is well equipped to describe configural relations between drive and other stimulus aspects of a situation, because an episodic view describes effects on behavior as depending on the similarity of the present situation to memory for prior episodes. We have illustrated arguments about drive by using the example of food deprivation. However, the same arguments apply to theorizing about dynamic processes and other sources of motivation that are typically investigated by social psychologists, and to descriptions of energizing functions of motivation that sound different from the classic notion of drive. For example, Bruner (1957) suggested that needs, task goals, and so on influence category accessibility by producing certain kinds of search sets. Rather than changing search sets, manipulations of motivation can be seen as influencing the cues that are available for unconscious retrieval of memory for prior episodes. We say "unconscious retrieval" because, as we discuss later, the retrieved memories influence subjective experience of the present instead of being experienced as memories. Manipulations of motivation may often have effects that configure with other factors to influence perception of a situation as a whole, rather than effects that are invariant across situations.

The possibility of configurations also creates problems for expectancy–value theories of motivation. According to those theories, choice is determined by the probability of obtaining a given outcome multiplied by the value of that outcome. The difficulties come when one describes how the probability of an outcome is estimated. Those probabilities are typically given to subjects in experiments, but would often have to be estimated outside the laboratory. People could estimate probabilities based on abstract representations that record the frequency of different classes of events—a notion similar to that of habit strength. Models of this form were called into question by Tversky and Kahneman's (1973) demonstrations that people use an "availability heuristic" to estimate probabilities. This means that people estimate the probability of an outcome as high if they can easily think of a prior occurrence of that outcome. Memory for particular experiences, rather than an abstract representation, serves as a basis for estimating probabilities. Expectancy and value are then no longer separate. The value of an outcome would configure with other details of a situation to determine which prior episodes would be retrieved, and consequently would influence the estimated probability of the outcome. Even when the probabilities of an outcome are given along with the outcome, the one is likely to influence interpretation of the other. Kuhl (1986) criticizes expectancy–value theories of motivation by noting that choice behavior is highly context-specific. Context specificity is to be expected if behavior relies on memory for prior episodes.

Motivation as Orientation

Another approach to motivation focuses on people's general orientation or mode of operation, as in Wicklund's (1986) distinction between "dynamic" and "static" orientations and Kuhl's (1986) conception of "action" versus "state" orientation. In particular, Wicklund proposes that one has a dynamic orientation to the environment when there is a press from the environment toward certain behaviors and one can enter into a "good fit" with those environmental demands. For example, a highly skilled engineer may have a "flow" experience when given the task of designing a bridge, because he or she has the skill to accomplish the task and can proceed immediately to solving the problem. In contrast, much less skilled engineers given the same task may have a poor fit with the environment and their performance may quickly derail, leading them to shift to a static mode in which they reflectively consider what sort of person could succeed in the task. Kuhl (1986) uses the difference between action and state orientation as an individual-difference dimension.

Orientation can lead to qualitative differences in the processing of information. We have found Polanyi's (1958) distinction between "tool" and "object" useful for thinking about the consequences of orientation or set for memory.

Polanyi has illustrated his distinction in an anecdote about reading his morning correspondence. He is multilingual and reports that it is necessary for him to look back at the language in which a letter is written before passing it to his son, who reads only English. When he is reading the letter, the language serves as a tool to convey meaning. When used as a tool, the language is transparent, used without awareness of the particular words being read. To specify the language, he has to make language the object of attention. Polanyi has also applied his distinction between tool and object to describe skilled performance. When one is driving a car, one's focus is on the road, rather than on the specifics of driving such as shifting gears. When accomplished drivers attempt to describe the particulars of driving to a beginner, they often are unable to do so. Also, treating the skill as an object for description can destroy skilled performance.

Polanyi's distinction between tool and object can be applied to two functions of memory (Jacoby & Kelley, 1987; Jacoby, Kelley, & Dywan, 1989). In conscious recollection, memory is treated as an object that can be inspected and described to others. Direct tests of memory, such as recognition and recall, request that people treat memory as an object by focusing on the past. Memory can also be used as a tool in a present task. When memory is used as a tool, people's attention is focused on the present rather than on the past, and memory for prior episodes is unconsciously incorporated into the ongoing task, altering perception, interpretation, and performance. The description of memory used as a tool is similar to Bransford, McCarrel, Franks, and Nitsch's (1977) notion that memory sets the stage for perception and interpretation of later events. The notion of memory as an object is similar to Johnson's (1983) description of "reflection."

One implication of the tool versus object metaphor is that treating memory as an object for recall or recognition, as compared with using memory as a tool, requires a different focus of attention and different types of processing. The two uses of memory can be antagonistic because of this difference in focus of attention. Later, we report data showing that the use of memory as a tool produces unconscious influences of the past. People can use memory for a specific prior episode as a tool in the perception and interpretation of events, although they are unable to recall or recognize the relevant prior episode. The use of memory as a tool can unconsciously affect subjective experience. As we discuss later, unconscious influences of this sort are important because people often use their subjective experience as a basis for judgment.

Unconscious influences of memory can arise simply because one is oriented toward the present rather than the past. Although people may shift orientations and focus on consciously remembering, they also may simply unconsciously use past experiences as a tool in their interpretation of the present. As an example, consider the effect of seeing an automobile accident while driving. Tversky and Kahneman (1973) note that people typically drive very carefully immediately after viewing an accident. They propose that the accident is readily available in memory for some time, and so increases people's estimates of the probability of an automobile accident by means of an availability heuristic. Tversky and Kahneman's (1973) use of the driving example implies that the careful driving results from people's conscious reflections upon their memory of the accident in order to arrive at an estimate of the probability of an accident. However, the effect seems better described as treating memory as a tool rather than as an object. Memory for a recently viewed accident seems to make people see danger in a current situation that would otherwise not seem dangerous. The focus is on the present, not the past. Indeed, focusing on the past—reflecting on one's memory for the automobile accident—may even be antagonistic to its effects on interpretation of the present. The use of memory as a tool may produce unconscious influences that are somewhat analogous to those described as "projection" in the psychoanalytic tradition.

One can also consider motives in light of the tool versus object metaphor. Experiments designed to manipulate attitudes and to induce cognitive dissonance often produce changes in performance that supposedly are mediated by attitudes or dissonance without corresponding changes in self-reports (e.g., Nisbett & Wilson, 1977; but see Quattrone, 1985). Similarly, individual differences in motives such as need for achievement or uncertainty orientation produce differences in behavior without accompanying differences in subjects' reports of their motives (R. M. Sorrentino, personal communication, May 1989). Self-report requires one to treat one's motives or attitudes as objects for reflection and observation, whereas performance measures allow one to use motives as tools in the production of behavior.

From an episodic perspective, people with a high need for achievement have repeatedly acted in ways that have furthered their power over people or things. Memory for those prior episodes may be used unconsciously as a tool in the perception and interpretation of Thematic Apperception Test (TAT) cards, as well as in the production of responses to situations that are similar to the prior episodes. However, people may later be unable to report their motives for an action, because a motive was not part of their conscious experience or a prerequisite for their behavior in the situation. To the extent that behavior is controlled unconsciously by memory for prior episodes, motives, intentions, trait terms, or higher-level descriptions of behavior play no role in controlling behavior and do not enter into one's subjective experience of a current episode. Wicklund (1986) makes a similar point that the dynamic (motivation-as-tool) and static (motivation-as-object) orientations are incompatible. Only people who cannot enter into a dynamic relation with their environment will attempt to formulate behavior in that environment in general trait terms, whereas people who are competent allow the environment to dynamically guide their actions (Wicklund & Braun, 1987). Those who can, do; those who can't, talk about abstractions.

Elsewhere, we discuss the difficulty of separating behavior that is controlled by consciously held intentions from behavior that is controlled by unconsciously used memory for prior episodes (Kelley & Jacoby, in press). Self-report cannot be relied upon as an indicator of conscious control, because intentions (and, we suspect, conscious motives) are attributions that can follow rather than cause behavior. Methods such as placing conscious intentions in opposition to unconscious influences allow one to separate the two.

EMPIRICAL ISSUES

There is a danger associated with being very speculative and providing interesting examples, as we have attempted to do up to this point in the chapter. The danger is that the reader may come to expect one's experiments to be as interesting as one's examples. Unfortunately, some of the experiments that we describe here are related only indirectly to questions about motivation, and none of the experiments used materials that are particularly relevant to social settings. However, many of the issues for the effects of motivation on social cognition are the same as issues in other areas of cognitive psychology. For example, some of the experiments we describe investigated the effects of recent prior experience on word perception. Those experiments show that effects on perception can rely on memory for a prior episode, rather than on the priming of an abstract representation such as a logogen. The results relate to the notion of priming as used by investigators of social cognition. Effects of memory for a prior episode should be more difficult to obtain in word perception than in person perception. The large amount of experience that undergraduates have in reading should favor the development of abstract representations that are used for word identification. Consequently, the finding of effects of memory for prior episodes on word identification is impressive and encourages looking for similar effects on social cognition.

In the first part of this section, we describe experiments that revealed unconscious influences of memory on perception. Next, we present experiments to show that awareness often serves the function of opposing unconscious influences that, if left unopposed, would arise from using memory for a prior episode as a tool. We then describe effects on subjective experience that are produced by using memory as a tool. We argue that subjective experience serves as one basis for judgments. The problem of explaining effects on subjective experience is similar to that of explaining causal attributions in social settings. Noting this similarity leads to a discussion of memory attributions.

The description of our research is brief, because much of it has recently been reviewed elsewhere (e.g., Jacoby, 1988; Jacoby & Kelley, 1987; Jacoby, Kelley, & Dywan, 1989, Kelley & Jacoby, in press). The main thing that we hope a social psychologist can take away from reading about our research is a set of questions and procedures that can be translated into research on social cognition. We have attempted to develop procedures that can be used to isolate effects of different sorts. For example, we argue that both aware and unaware effects of motivational variables and other factors can be observed. The trick is to separate those effects.

Many of the effects on perceptual identification performance that we describe have also been obtained using other indirect tests of memory, such as tests requiring completion of picture or word fragments and lexical-decision tests. Research done by Roediger and his colleagues (e.g., Blaxton, 1989; Roediger & Blaxton, 1987) is particularly relevant to some of the issues discussed here and leads to conclusions that are consistent with the ones we draw. Richardson-Klavehn and Bjork (1988) provide a more complete review of the literature comparing performance on indirect and direct tests of memory.

Unconscious Influences on Perception Produced by Memory for Prior Episodes

We have used effects of prior experience on perceptual identification of words as an indirect test of memory. Like the amnesic subjects, who heard words in the study reported earlier (Jacoby & Witherspoon, 1982), normal subjects show effects of earlier reading a word on its later perceptual identification, although they are unable to consciously recollect having earlier read the word. We briefly describe a few experiments to illustrate those effects and to show that they arise from unconscious influences of memory for prior episodes, rather than from the priming of some abstract representation.

Typically, in our experiments (e.g., Jacoby & Dallas, 1981), subjects were given a long list of words to read and were then given two types of tests. One test was a test of list recognition, for which previously read words were mixed with new words. In this direct test of memory, subjects were to indicate whether or not they recognized each word as read in the earlier list. The second type of test was a perceptual identification test that served as an indirect test of memory. Old and new words were mixed, and each word was flashed for a very brief duration (e.g., 35 milliseconds), followed by a visual mask. Subjects were to identify the flashed words by saying them aloud, and the dependent variable was the probability of identification. An advantage for old words in perceptual identification provides evidence of an influence of memory for a prior presentation of a word on its later perception. However, it is not logically necessary for old words to be recognized as previously presented for those words to hold an advantage in perceptual identification performance. For the perceptual identification task, our subjects were only asked to report the word that was presented, without reference to whether it was an old or a new word.

In these experiments, previously reading a word had a large effect on its later identification, sometimes doubling the probability that the word would be identified when flashed. This effect on identification performance was observed even when people were unable to recognize words as ones that were read in the earlier-presented list of words. Also, some manipulations that were important for list recognition performance were unimportant for effects on perceptual identification performance. Dealing with the meaning of a word rather than with more superficial characteristics, such as the appearance or the sound of a word, enhanced later list recognition performance (cf. Craik & Lockhart, 1972) but provided no advantage for perceptual identification performance (Jacoby & Dallas, 1981). Effects on perceptual identification performance were also specific to the modality of presentation of a word. Reading a word had a large effect, but hearing a word or producing a word as a name of a picture had little, if any, effect on later visual–perceptual identification of the word (e.g., Jacoby & Dallas, 1981; Morton, 1979). Effects on perceptual identification were long-lasting, persisting for at least 5 days (Jacoby, 1983a).

Effects of reading a word on its later identification are, in some ways, similar to the effects of priming on person perception (e.g., Higgins et al., 1977).

However, the effects on word perception are too long-lasting to be produced by the priming of some abstract representation. The same might be said for effects on person perception. Srull and Wyer (1979) observed that unscrambling sentences that had hostile content led subjects later to judge ambiguous descriptions of people as more hostile; the authors attributed that effect on person perception to the priming of the abstract trait of hostility. However, this effect on impression formation remained even when the test was delayed for 24 hours. In a later paper, Wyer and Srull (1986) have suggested that the priming effect is restricted to occasions when the trait is applicable and the subject has the goal of forming an impression. We would restrict the effects even further: In our view, effects on person perception as well as effects on word identification reflect memory for prior episodes, and consequently depend on factors influencing encoding and retrieval.

Again, arguments for effects of past experience on word identification also ought to apply to effects observed in social settings. Effects on identification of words presented without context reflect primarily memory for the earlier visual processing of an item. However, the claim that effects on person perception rely on memory for prior episodes does not imply that those effects rely on the literal or surface characteristics of earlier-presented items. Unconscious influences having to do with the earlier processing of the meaning of an event have also been observed (Jacoby, Kelley, & Dywan, 1989). The spelling task used in the earlier-described experiment employing amnesics as subjects (Jacoby & Witherspoon, 1982) serves as one example of an indirect test of memory that shows effects of the earlier processing of meaning. The finding that effects of prior experience are long-lasting is one piece of evidence against an account in terms of priming; along with other evidence, it can be used to support an episodic view of cognition (e.g., Jacoby & Brooks, 1984).

Effects of prior experience on perception are also too context-specific to be produced by the priming of an abstract representation. If effects on perceptual identification are produced by priming, those effects should be general, not restricted by memory for details of a prior presentation. However, manipulations of study processing influence later perceptual identification performance. We have found that prior presentation of an item does most to enhance its later perceptual identification when the processing of the item during its prior presentation matches that required by the test of perceptual identification (e.g., Jacoby, 1983b). Manipulations of retrieval factors also influence the effect of previously presenting an item on its later perceptual identification (Allen & Jacoby, in press; Jacoby, 1983a). Smith and Branscombe (1987, 1988) report investigations of person perception that, like our investigations of word perception, show effects of recent experience that are too specific to be interpreted as due to priming.

The results of our perceptual identification experiments can be summarized as showing that the effects of recent experience cannot be produced by priming an abstract representation, but must involve a memory that can be accessed when the details of the experimental setting are reinstated. Depending on the relation between study and test processing, memory for a prior episode can be unconsciously retrieved and used as a tool to aid perception of a later event. Effects of priming on person perception may also depend on reinstating the experimental context. If retrieval factors are important for social judgments, judgments will vary across situations as changes in cues for retrieval produce changes in the particular prior episodes that are retrieved and used as guides for interpretation of later events. Also, the overall similarity between earlier and later events should be important. Effects on word identification show that memory for a prior episode can be used as a tool even when people are unable to treat memory as an object for a test of recall or recognition memory. That is, the dissociations between effects on recognition and perceptual identification performance provide evidence that effects on perceptual identification arise from unconscious influences of memory. A person need not be able to recall or recognize an earlier event for memory of that earlier event to influence later performance. These unconscious influences of memory place an important limitation on claims that behavior is consciously goal-directed.

The Advantages of Opposition for Revealing Unconscious Influences

The possibility of unconscious influences has held fascination for laypeople as well as for experimental psychologists, but the two groups have very different interests. For the layperson, the possibility of unconscious influences is fascinating because of its implication that one is open to influences that are not detected and consequently cannot be opposed. The possibility of unconscious influences seems sinister, leaving one vulnerable to control via subliminal advertising or brainwashing. Experimental psychologists have been preoccupied with countering such sensationalistic claims about the dangers of unconscious influences. The history of research on unconscious influences has been marked by supposed demonstrations of unconscious influences, followed by further research to uncover methodological flaws in those supposed demonstrations. Experimental psychology has commonly framed the question of unconscious influences in terms of differences in the sensitivity of tests. Are there measures of perception or memory that are more sensitive than verbal report (e.g., Eriksen, 1960)? If the differential sensitivity cannot be demonstrated, then claims of unconscious processes are dismissed.

In what follows, we side with the layperson to a greater extent than with the experimental psychologists. We are not ready to accept sensationalistic claims about subliminal perception or unconscious influences of the past. However, we agree with the layperson that it is the detection of, along with the possibility of opposing, a potential source of influence that is important. We argue that an important function of consciousness is to oppose influences that would otherwise prevail. This opposition of conscious and of unconscious influences also provides a useful tool for their investigation.

Recently, there have been controversial demonstrations both of unconscious perception and of unconscious forms of memory. For example, Marcel (1983) studied unconscious perception by flashing words for a brief duration, followed by a pattern mask. He claimed that priming words speeded lexical decisions regarding target words even when subjects were unaware of the primes. In the domain of memory, subjects can exhibit unconscious influences of the past when their performance is altered by experience, in the absence of conscious recollection of that experience. As described above, reading a list of words enhances later perceptual identification (e.g., Jacoby & Dallas, 1981) and fragment completion (e.g., Tulving, Schacter, & Stark, 1982) of those words, even when subjects do not consciously recognize the words as being from the earlier list.

These and other experimental demonstrations of unconscious perception and memory have been criticized on the grounds that the experimenter has mistakenly measured conscious rather than unconscious performance. Marcel's (1983) method of determining a threshold for unconscious perception was criticized as producing a stimulus duration so high that subjects were aware of the words. When the situation is such that aware and unaware perception produce effects that are in the same direction, results taken as evidence of unconscious perception may actually reflect aware perception that is undetected by the experimenter. Indeed, Holender (1986) argues that there is so far no convincing evidence for unconscious perception from either visual-masking paradigms or divided-attention paradigms. Similarly, in studies of memory, Richardson-Klavehn and Bjork (1988) note that many effects commonly ascribed to unconscious forms of memory may be contaminated by conscious recollection. For example, the enhanced fragment completion for old words relative to new ones may be accomplished by quite deliberate and conscious retrieval of studied words.

We (e.g., Jacoby, Woloshyn, & Kelley, 1989) have taken an alternative approach to the notion of differing thresholds or sensitivity of conscious and unconscious processes. We start by assuming that awareness serves an important function of opposing unconscious influences. A commonplace example of such a function is the problem of avoiding repeating oneself. One effect of telling a story is to later make that story come more readily to mind and be told repeatedly to the same audience. However, conscious recollection can be used to oppose this effect of the past. If we recognize that we have already told a story to someone, we can inhibit the tendency toward repetition. Similarly, conscious experience of an event can oppose unconscious influences of perception. In the apocryphal example of subliminal advertising in movies, the notion was that people could resist messages when they were aware of their source as advertisements. However, the effect of a subliminal message to "Drink Coke" was considered likely to be mistakenly attributed to one's own desire for a drink. More generally, behavior may often *not* originate from an intent or be goal-directed. Rather than serving as a prerequisite for effects of memory, awareness of the past may often serve to oppose effects that would otherwise arise.

We have adopted the strategy of placing conscious and unconscious processes in opposition so as to reveal unconscious influences. When the situation is such that aware and unaware perception or memory would produce effects that are in the same direction, effects that are taken as evidence of unconscious perception or memory may actually reflect aware processes (e.g., Holender, 1986). This possibility is ruled out when awareness produces effects that are in the opposite direction from those produced by unaware processes. Opposition allows a clear separation of consicous from unconscious influences. The strategy of looking for opposite effects is a variant of the strategy of searching for qualitative differences in performance produced by conscious versus unconscious perception (e.g., Cheesman & Merikle, 1986; Dixon, 1981; Marcel, 1983) or by conscious versus unconscious influences of memory (e.g., Jacoby & Dallas, 1981). The approach of looking for opposite effects has considerable heuristic value, particularly if one accepts our starting assumption that awareness often does oppose unconscious influences.

Becoming Famous without Being Recognized

We have used the strategy of looking for opposite effects to show that unconscious influences of memory can make nonfamous names seem famous. In those experiments, people first read a list of names that they were correctly told included only nonfamous names. Next, these old nonfamous names were mixed with new nonfamous and new famous names and were presented for fame judgments. People were asked to judge whether or not each name was a famous one. Aware and unaware uses of memory were expected to have opposite effects on fame judgments, much as conscious and unconscious influences do in the example of repeatedly telling a story. Memory for earlier reading a nonfamous name should have the unconscious influence of making the name seem familiar, and thereby should increase the probability of the name's mistakenly being called famous. Aware use of memory to recognize a name as read in the earlier list of nonfamous names should oppose this unconscious influence of memory. If a name was recognized as read in the earlier-presented list of nonfamous names, people could call the name nonfamous with certainty. A finding that old nonfamous names were more likely to be called famous than were new nonfamous names would provide evidence of an unconscious influence of memory, because awareness of having read a name in the earlier-presented list would produce the opposite effect.

Using the fame judgment task, we (Jacoby, Kelley, Brown, & Jasechko, 1989) found an effect similar to the "sleeper effect" that has been investigated by social psychologists (Cook, Gruder, Hennigan, & Flay, 1979; Hovland, Lumsdaine, & Sheffield, 1949; Pratkanis, Greenwald, Leippe, & Baumgardner, 1988). The sleeper effect is the finding that a message from a low-reliability source has a larger impact on a delayed than on an immediate test of attitude change. The effect has been explained as resulting from faster forgetting of the source than of the message gained from that source. We found that old nonfamous names were less likely to be called famous than were new nonfamous names on a test of fame judgments that came immediately after reading a list of nonfamous names. On that immediate test, people could easily recognize old nonfamous names as ones read earlier, and consequently could be certain that those names were nonfamous. However, old nonfamous names were more likely to be called famous than were new nonfamous names when the fame judgment test was delayed; this was similar to the sleeper effect found for attitude change. On the delayed test, old names remained familiar but the source of that familiarity was not consciously recollected, so the names were mistakenly called famous. Findings of a sleeper effect in attitude change have been controversial (e.g., Greenwald, Pratkanis, Leippe, & Baumgardner, 1986). The fame judgment task is potentially useful for specifying the combination of conditions that are necessary to produce a sleeper effect.

It has been claimed that the attention to an event that is necessary to produce later awareness of memory for the event differs from the attention that is necessary to produce unconscious influences. For example, memory for unattended events is said to be revealed in the form of dreams, although one is unable to recollect the event consciously (see Dixon, 1981, for a review). We (Jacoby, Woloshyn, & Kelley, 1989) have used the fame judgment task to show effects of this sort. Dividing attention by engaging in a listening task while reading a list of nonfamous names resulted in old nonfamous names' later being more likely to be mistakenly called famous than were new nonfamous names. The opposite was found when full attention was given to reading the list of nonfamous names. The results of further analyses showed that dividing attention reduced a person's ability to recognize a name as having been read earlier, but had no effect on gains in familiarity produced by that earlier reading of the name. Names can be called famous without being recognized either if attention is divided during the reading of names that one has been told are nonfamous, or if the delay between reading nonfamous names and the test of fame judgments is increased.

R. M. Sorrentino (personal communication, May 1989) has raised the possibility that unconscious influences can also lead to corrective action. To use his example, "I might think of a great dirty joke to tell, but my unconscious need for social approval brings to mind that I should not tell a dirty joke to a group of nuns." According to our view, one may first make the mistake of telling a dirty joke to a group of nuns or some other unappreciative audience. Later, in a similar situation with one's aged aunt, memory for that earlier episode may lead one to view the present audience as potentially unappreciative. Awareness of that possibility should oppose unconscious influences of other memories that push toward telling the joke. If one's attention is divided in the later situation, one may fail to consciously monitor performance, and consequently may tell the dirty joke to one's aunt. However, episodes in which one successfully opposes unconscious influences are represented as memory for prior episodes that also unconsciously influence later behavior. If one has inhibited the telling of dirty jokes on several occasions, memory for those prior episodes can have the unconscious influence of making one so virtuous that a dirty joke does not even come to mind in front of a group of nuns, saving one from telling the joke even if attention is divided. Memory for prior episodes can unconsciously influence what comes to mind, can unconsciously influence the interpretation of situations, and (if left unopposed) can control behavior. Consciousness can serve to oppose unconscious influences of memory. Our episodic view predicts that behavior should be less stable across situations than would be predicted by a general unconscious need for social approval.

Spontaneous versus Directed Recollection

According to our tool–object distinction, the treatment of memory as an object requires a different focus of attention and different types of processing than does the use of memory as a tool. This means that conscious recollection of an earlier event requires an act that is separate from using memory for the prior event as a tool in some ongoing task. If conscious recollection does require an attention-demanding, separate act, it should be possible to limit the opportunity for conscious recollection by dividing attention at the time of testing. In line with that possibility, we (Jacoby, Woloshyn, & Kelley, 1989) have shown that requiring people to divide attention by engaging in a listening task while making fame judgments results in old nonfamous names' being more likely to be called famous than are new nonfamous names. Dividing attention limits the opportunity for conscious recollection of the source of familiarity of old nonfamous names, and consequently leaves unopposed the effects on familiarity produced by reading those names earlier.

If the unconscious use of a message and recollection of its source are separate acts, it is important to determine the conditions that encourage people to attempt recollection of source. The problem is the same as that of determining the conditions that lead to spontaneous causal attributions (e.g., Hastie, 1984; Weiner, 1985). The procedure in our fame judgment experiments differs in an important way from that of most other experiments done to investigate memory for source. Most other investigations of memory for source direct people to recall the source of a message (e.g., Johnson & Raye, 1981). This requirement to recall source may overestimate the probability of its being recollected if people had not been instructed to do so. In contrast, fame judgments provide a measure of spontaneous monitoring of source. When people are only asked to make fame judgments, they must take the initiative to recollect the source. A failure to check whether a name was among those read earlier is shown in old nonfamous names' being called famous. That is, effects on fame judgments can be used to infer whether or not spontaneous recollection of source has occurred.

Dividing attention at the time of testing makes spontaneous monitoring of source more difficult and thus less likely, as do factors such as divided attention during study and increases in delay. Spontaneous recollection of source is also less likely when there is a low probability that a message came from a misleading source. In our fame judgment task, people were more likely to mistakenly call old nonfamous names famous when very few, rather than many, of the names presented for fame judgments were old nonfamous names (Jacoby, Kelley, Brown, & Jasechko, 1989). Attempts to recollect source consciously may not be worth the expense when retrieval is difficult and the probability of a message's coming from a misleading source is low. People can sometimes recollect source when directed to do so, although they may not spontaneously recollect source. The probability of calling an old nonfamous name famous is reduced when source recollection is directed by requiring people to judge whether or not each name is old (presented earlier in the list of nonfamous names), as well as to make fame judgments (Jacoby, Kelley, Brown, & Jasechko, 1989). It is likely that there are also large individual differences in the probability of spontaneous monitoring of source. Folklore has it that the aged are less likely than are younger people to spontaneously montior their performance. For example, a common complaint about the aged is that they repeatedly tell the same stories and more likely than are younger people to deal inappropriately with a message from a misleading source. We (Dywan & Jacoby, in press) have used the fame judgment task to show that the aged are less likely than younger people to monitor source spontaneously. In that experiment, the aged were more likely to mistakenly call old than new nonfamous names famous, whereas the opposite was true for younger people.

The factors that are important for spontaneous monitoring of source are also likely to be important for monitoring of other dimensions. Some theories of motivation emphasize the goal-directed nature of behavior and the control of behavior by comparison with some standard such as a self-concept (e.g., Cantor et al., 1986). However, the probability of spontaneous monitoring with reference to a self-concept may depend heavily on the details of the situation, as did spontaneous monitoring of source in our fame experiments. Awareness may often serve to oppose unconscious influences on behavior that would hinder attaining some goal. Placing aware and unaware effects in opposition is a strategy that should be generally useful for investigating effects on monitoring.

Memory Attributions

Historically, writings about the unconscious have emphasized that different laws govern unconscious and conscious processes. It was thought that unnoticed or unattended events can nonetheless be detected in free associations, fantasies, or dreams (e.g., Dixon, 1981; Ellenberger, 1970). It was further believed that conscious processes are more active, whereas unconscious influences are more likely to emerge when one is relaxed or distracted by some other task. Our distinction between memory-as-tool and memory-as-object partially captures these distinctions. When one is engaging in a particular task, memory can be used as a tool without any analysis or activity beyond performing the task itself. In contrast, treating memory as an object of conscious reflection generally requires more active, analytic processing. Using memory as a tool is a nonanalytic process that does not allow one control over what aspects of a memory are used. It is also nonanalytic in that one cannot identify the prior experiences that may be acting as a tool to accomplish the present task, or even which aspects are responsible for changes in performance. Therefore, using memory as a tool leaves one open to errors of interpretation regarding the source of influences on a task.

Awareness of the past is not an attribute of a memory representation. Instead, gaining awareness is an attention-demanding act. Conscious remembering as a separate act is analogous to the difference between looking at someone in a crowd and noticing that person. In both cases, one obviously is using the "representation" of the person. But it makes more sense to talk about the change in attention or analysis involved in noticing than to make noticing a characteristic of the thing noticed. Similarly, conscious remembering is better understood as a process rather than a product in the form of an attribute of a representation. We now briefly outline our approach to memory attributions (see also Jacoby & Kelley, 1987; Jacoby, Kelley, & Dywan, 1989; Kelley & Jacoby, in press).

Familiarity as an Attribution

We have noted that the use of memory as a tool is a nonanalytic process that does not specify the source of effects. For example, reading a word once allows it to be read later more fluently. Fluent processing can be correctly attributed to the past, and so can be experienced as a feeling of familiarity. More generally, we have argued that familiarity is the attribution of variations in perceptual and conceptual processing to a particular source (e.g., Jacoby, 1988; Jacoby & Dallas, 1981; Jacoby, Kelley, & Dywan, 1989). The fluency heuristic that we believe underlies the feeling of familiarity is in some ways similar to the availability heuristic that Tversky and Kahneman (1973) proposed as underlying judgments of probability. According to the availability heuristic, the probability of an event will be judged as high if one can easily bring to mind a prior occurrence of that class of events. Similarly, according to the fluency heuristic, an item seems familiar if it can be easily brought to mind or fluently processed. Familiarity is seen as the result of an inferential or attributional analysis; it is not present in the memory representation itself.

One implication of a fluency interpretation of familiarity is that it should be possible to create memory illusions. That is, fluency is the basis for familiarity, it should be possible to induce the feeling of familiarity by enhancing the processing of new items on a recognition memory test. We (Jacoby & Whitehouse, 1989) have done experiments on memory illusions that provide direct evidence for a fluency heuristic. Unconscious perception of a word flashed immediately prior to its presentation as a new word on a test of recognition memory produced an increase in the probability of false recognition. The flashed word produced more fluent perceptual processing of the new word, which was interpreted as familiarity. We could be certain that this effect resulted from unconscious perception of the flashed word: When conditions were changed so that people could "see" the flashed word, effects were opposite to those produced by unconscious perception. That is, we used the strategy of placing aware and unaware effects in opposition so as to reveal effects of unconscious perception on memory judgments.

Subjective Experience as a Basis for Judgments

Our distinction between analytic and nonanalytic processing is similar to distinctions found in theories that propose multiple bases for decisions (e.g., Atkinson & Juola, 1974). In a two-process theory of category membership decisions (e.g., Smith, Shoben, & Rips, 1974), there is a nonanalytic process of assessing overall similarity of an instance to a category on the basis of characteristic features. In addition, people can use a more analytic process of checking for defining features. Mandler (1980) proposed that recognition memory decisions can be based either on familiarity or on retrieval of study context. Familiarity serves as a nonanalytic basis for recognition memory judgments, in addition to the more analytic retrieval of study context. Elsewhere, we have discussed the differences between analytic and nonanalytic processes (Jacoby & Brooks, 1984; Jacoby & Kelley, 1987). The important distinction here is that nonanalytic processing is more global or wholistic, whereas analytic processing segments and selects.

The use of memory as a tool can influence subjective experience. These effects are important because subjective experience serves as a nonanalytic basis for judgments. The unconscious influence of past experience used as a tool can influence fluency of processing in a task. Subjects can misattribute this fluent processing to changes in physical parameters of the later presentation, such as longer visual duration (Witherspoon & Allan, 1985) or lower background noise (Jacoby, Allan, Collins, & Larwill, 1988). Fluent processing may also be misattributed to a statement's being true, an argument's seeming to flow, or a problem's being easy (Jacoby & Kelley, 1987). The effect of "mere exposure" in studies of aesthetic judgments may also be a case of the misattribution of fluent processing that is actually due to prior experience (Jacoby, 1984; Mandler, Nakamura, & Van Zandt, 1987; Seamon, Brody, & Kauff, 1983). Subjects prefer random polygons or melodies encountered in an earlier phase of the experiment to new items. Prior exposure produces more fluent processing of old items that may be misattributed to qualities of the items (e.g., that they have good form or are pleasing). People attribute effects on performance to whatever source is most obvious or plausible, which often depends on the question they are asked.

Multiple bases for judgments are probably also used in social situations (e.g., Zanna & Rempel, 1988). Tasks such as judging the level of background noise might be useful as a means for revealing nonanalytic judgments in those situations. To illustrate this possibility, let us further consider the effects of prior experience on the judgments of background noise. In one experiment, we (Jacoby et al., 1988) presented previously heard sentences and new sentences against a background of white noise of varying loudness. Subjects judged the background noise as less loud when the sentences were old rather than new. The difference in ease of perception of old and new sentences was misattributed to a lower level of background noise. That is, people were unable to separate out the contribution of memory to perception when judging noise level, and so experienced a change in their subjective experience of the noise. Later experiments by a student in our laboratory, Jane Collins, have shown that people are unable to avoid this effect of prior experience on judgments. Even when subjects were informed about the effect and told to avoid it, they continued to judge the background noise accompanying old sentences as less loud than that accompanying new sentences. Unlike the fame judgment experiments, in which people could use a simple rule to avoid the effects of prior experience ("If you recognize the name, it is nonfamous"), people in the noise experiment had no analytic basis for correcting their judgments. To correct noise judgments for the effect of prior experience, subjects would have had to regain the subjective experience of a naive listener. Doing so is apparently impossible.

The noise judgment task may show effects of motivational variables as well as effects of prior experience. For example, the background noise accompanying a statement of a belief may be judged as less loud if one agrees with the stated belief. Also, emotional reactions produced by a statement may be reflected by a difference in judged loudness of background noise accompanying that statement. Experiments of this sort are now underway.

Our use of effects on background noise as an indirect test of memory and of the effect of motivational variables is akin to the approach taken by advocates of the "New Look" movement in perception (e.g., Eriksen, 1966). We are using judgments of a physical dimension, such as the loudness of a background noise, in much the same way as one would use a projective test to reveal unconscious influences on judgments. The advantage of our procedure over the use of standard projective tests (e.g., a Rorschach test) is that judgments of a physical dimension can be scored easily and objectively. Also, our procedure does not ask for a report that can readily be taken as self-revealing, so people are less likely to be defensive than when taking standard projective tests. Even if people are defensive, our results show that they are unable to avoid showing effects of memory on noise judgments. Perhaps the same will be found for motivational variables. Our goal is to show dissociations between effects on direct and indirect tests of motivation that are similar to those shown on direct and indirect tests of memory. For example, noise judgments (an indirect test) may show that a presented statement gives rise to some emotional reaction, although, when directly asked, a person may deny that the statement provoked emotion. More rational, analytic bases for judgment may often produce judgments that differ from nonanalytic judgments evidenced by performance on an indirect test.

CONCLUDING COMMENTS

The possibility of unconscious influences of memory has, until recently, generally been ignored. Measures such as performance on tests of recognition memory or free recall were the standards for assessing memory for prior episodes. That this is true can be shown by considering Hastie and Park's (1986) distinction between memory-based and on-line judgments. Hastie and Park required that a judgment be correlated with memory as assessed by a test of free recall to qualify as a memory-based judgment. For example, they computed the correlation between subjects' judgment of the suitability of a described person for a job and indices computed from free recall of items of information favoring or opposing the person. If the correlation was high, Hastie and Park concluded that the judgments were based on memory, whereas if the correlation was low, they concluded that the judgments were made on-line. The difficulty is that a low correlation between judgments and a measure of memory may result from an experimenter's using the wrong measure of memory. Memory for a prior experience can have effects on performance even when a person is unable to recall or recognize the prior experience. Given that this is the case, assessing the correlation of judgments with free recall is inadequate as a means of determining whether or not judgments are based on memory.

The finding of unconscious influences of memory means that one cannot rely on a person's verbal report to determine whether or not the person has been influenced by memory for a prior event. A failure to recall or recognize an earlier event might be taken as evidence that any effect of that event on performance of a later task was produced by the priming of some abstract representation; however, effects of prior experience can be too long-lasting and too context-specific to be produced by priming. Factors that influence encoding and retrieval are important for unconscious influences of memory. An episodic view leads to the prediction that effects on perception and judgment will be specific to very local context. Unconscious influences of memory can be clearly separated from aware uses of memory by arranging a situation such that effects of the two types are placed in opposition. There are multiple bases for judgments. Nonanalytic judgments are more open to unconscious influences of memory than are analytic judgments.

At a very general level, we believe that a fundamental issue for theories of motivation is the relation between habit and reason. The limited success of learning theories can be taken as showing that habit alone is insufficient as an account for all of human behavior. Behavior is also too often unreasonable to be fully guided by reason. It is the conflict between reason and habit that we find most interesting. People often do behave, presumably because of habit, in ways that are obviously counter to any reasonable assessment of their own self-interests. Notions such as habit are identified with unconscious influences. The motivation for a behavior is most likely to be brought into question when the behavior appears to be irrational. The strategy that we are using is that of producing conflicts between reason and habit so as to separate the two as different sources of control for behavior. One reason for ending this chapter by using the very global terms "reason" and "habit" is that terms of this sort are often used to describe the different levels of control. What is needed is a better understanding of habit as well as a better understanding of reason. For us, habit is memory for prior episodes.

Acknowledgments

This research was supported by a National Science and Engineering Research Council Grant to Larry L. Jacoby. We thank R. M. Sorrentino and E. T. Higgins for their comments on an earlier draft of this chapter.

References

Allen, S. W., & Jacoby, L. L. (in press). Reinstating study context produces unconscious influences of memory. *Memory and Cognition.*
Atkinson, R. C., & Juola, J. F. (1974). Search and decision processes in recognition memory. In D. H.

Krantz, R. C. Atkinson, R. D. Luce, & P. Suppes (Eds.), *Contemporary developments in mathematical psychology: Vol. 1. Learning, memory and thinking* (pp. 243-293). San Francisco: W. H. Freeman.

Bargh, J. A. (1989). Conditional automaticity: Varieties of automatic influences in social perception and cognition. In J. S. Uleman & J. A. Bargh (Eds.), *Unintended thought* (pp. 3-51). New York: Guilford Press.

Bargh, J. A., & Pietromonaco, P. (1982). Automatic information processing and social perception: The influence of trait information presented outside of conscious awareness on impression formation. *Journal of Personality and Social Psychology, 43,* 437-449.

Barsalou, L. W. (1990). On the indistinguishability of exemplar memory and abstraction in category representation. In T. K. Srull & R. S. Wyer (Eds.), *Advances in social cognition* (Vol. 3). Hillsdale, NJ: Erlbaum.

Blaxton, T. A. (1989). Investigating dissociations among memory measures: Support for a transfer-appropriate processing framework. *Journal of Experimental Psychology: Learning, Memory, and Cognition, 15,* 657-668.

Bowers, K. S. (1984). On being unconsciously influenced and informed. In K. S. Bowers & D. Meichenbaum (Eds.), *The unconscious reconsidered* (pp. 227-273). New York: Wiley.

Bransford, D. E., McCarrel, N. S., Franks, J. J., & Nitsch, K. E. (1977). Toward unexplaining memory. In R. Shaw & J. Bransford (Eds.), *Perceiving, acting, and knowing* (pp. 431-466). Hillsdale, NJ: Erlbaum.

Brewer, M. B., Dull, V., & Lui, L. (1981). Perceptions of the elderly: Stereotypes as prototypes. *Journal of Personality and Social Psychology, 41,* 656-670.

Broadbent, D. E. (1977). The hidden preattentive processes. *American Psychologist, 32,* 109-118.

Brooks, L. R. (1978). Non-analytic concept formation and memory for instances. In E. Rosch & B. Lloyd (Eds.), *Cognition and categorization* (pp. 169-211). Hillsdale, NJ: Erlbaum.

Brooks, L. R. (1987). Decentralized control of categorization: The role of prior processing episodes. In U. Neisser (Ed.), *Categories reconsidered: The ecological and intellectual bases of categories* (pp. 141-174). Cambridge, England: Cambridge University Press.

Bruner, J. S. (1957). On perceptual readiness. *Psychological Review, 64,* 123-152.

Buss, A. H. (1980). *Self-consciousness and social anxiety.* San Francisco: W. H. Freeman.

Cantor, N., Markus, H., Niedenthal, P., & Nurius, P. (1986). On motivation and the self-concept. In R. M. Sorrentino & E. T. Higgins (Eds.), *Handbook of motivation and cognition: Foundations of social behavior* (Vol. 1, pp. 96-121). New York: Guilford Press.

Cheesman, J., & Merikle, P. M. (1986). Distinguishing conscious from unconscious perceptual processes. *Canadian Journal of Psychology, 40,* 343-367.

Cohen, N. J., & Squire, L. R. (1980). Preserved learning and retention of pattern-analyzing skill in amnesia: Dissociation of knowing how and knowing that. *Science, 210,* 207-210.

Cook, T. D., Gruder, C. L., Hennigan, K. M., & Flay, B. R. (1979). History of the sleeper effect: Some logical pitfalls in accepting the null hypothesis. *Psychological Bulletin, 86,* 662-679.

Corkin, S. (1968). Acquisition of motor skill after bilateral medial temporal lobe excision. *Neuropsychologia, 6,* 255-265.

Craik, F. I. M., & Lockhart, R. S. (1972). Levels of processing: A framework for memory research. *Journal of Verbal Learning and Verbal Behavior, 11,* 671-684.

Dixon, N. F. (1981). *Preconscious processing.* Chichester, England: Wiley.

Dywan, J., & Jacoby, L. L. (in press). Effects of aging on source monitoring: Differences in susceptibility to false fame. *Psychology and Aging.*

Ellenberger, M. F. (1970). *The discovery of the unconscious: The history and evolution of dynamic psychiatry.* New York: Basic Books.

Eriksen, C. W. (1960). Discrimination and learning without awareness: A methodological survey and evaluation. *Psychological Review, 67,* 279-300.

Eriksen, C. W. (1966). Cognitive responses to internally cued anxiety. In C. D. Spielberger (Ed.), *Anxiety and behavior.* New York: Academic Press.

Fazio, R. H. (1986). How do attitudes guide behavior? In R. M. Sorrentino & E. T. Higgins (Eds.),

Handbook of motivation and cognition: Foundations of social behavior (Vol. 1, pp. 204-243). New York: Guilford Press.

Gazzaniga, M. S. (1988). Brain modularity: Towards a philosophy of conscious experience. In A. J. Marcel & E. Bisiach (Eds.), *Consciousness in contemporary science* (pp. 218-238). Oxford: Clarendon Press.

Gelman, R. (1978). Cognitive development. *Annual Review of Psychology, 29*, 297-332.

Greenwald, A. G., Pratkanis, A. R., Leippe, M. R., & Baumgardner, M. H. (1986). Under what conditions does theory obstruct research progress? *Psychological Review, 93*, 216-229.

Grill, H. J., & Berridge, K. C. (1985). Taste reactivity as a measure of the neural control of palatability. In A. N. Epstein & J. Sprague (Eds.), *Progress in psychobiology and physiological psychology* (Vol. 2, pp. 1-61). New York: Academic Press.

Hastie, R. (1981). Schematic principles in human memory. In E. T. Higgins, C. P. Herman, & M. P. Zanna (Eds.), *Social cognition: The Ontario Symposium* (Vol. 1, pp. 39-88). Hillsdale, NJ: Erlbaum.

Hastie, R. (1984). Causes and effects of causal attribution. *Journal of Pesonality and Social Psychology, 46*, 44-56.

Hastie, R., & Park, B. (1986). The relationship between memory and judgment depends on whether the judgment task is memory-based or on-line. *Psychological Review, 3*, 258-268.

Higgins, E. T. (1989). Knowledge accessibility and activation: Subjectivity and suffering from unconscious sources. In J. S. Uleman & J. A. Bargh (Eds.), *Unintended thought* (pp. 75-123). New York: Guilford Press.

Higgins, E. T., Rholes, W. S., & Jones, C. R. (1977). Category accessibility and impression formation. *Journal of Experimental Social Psychology, 13*, 141-154.

Hintzman, D. L. (1986). "Schema abstraction" in a multiple-trace memory model. *Psychological Review, 93*, 411-428.

Holender, D. (1986). Semantic activation without conscious identification in dichotic listening, parafoveal vision, and visual masking: A survey and appraisal. *Behavioral and Brain Sciences, 9*, 1-23.

Hovland, C. I., Lumsdaine, A. A., & Sheffield, F. D. (1949). *Experiments on mass communications.* Princeton, NJ: Princeton University Press.

Jacoby, L. L. (1983a). Perceptual enhancement: Persistent effects of an experience. *Journal of Experimental Psychology: Learning, Memory, and Cognition, 9*, 21-38.

Jacoby, L. L. (1983b). Remembering the data: Analyzing interactive processes in reading. *Journal of Verbal Learning and Verbal Behavior, 22*, 485-508.

Jacoby, L. L. (1984). Incidental versus intentional retrieval: Remembering and awareness as separate issues. In L. R. Squire & N. Butters (Eds.), *Neuropsychology of memory* (pp. 145-156). New York: Guilford Press.

Jacoby, L. L. (1988). Memory observed and memory unobserved. In U. Neisser & E. Winograd (Eds.), *Remembering reconsidered: Ecological and traditional approaches to the study of memory* (pp. 145-177). Cambridge, England: Cambridge University Press.

Jacoby, L. L., Allan, L. G., Collins, J. C., & Larwill, L. K. (1988). Memory influences subjective experience: Noise judgments. *Journal of Experimental Psychology: Learning, Memory, and Cognition 14*, 240-247.

Jacoby, L. L., & Brooks, L. R. (1984). Nonanalytic cognition: Memory, perception and concept learning. In G. H. Bower (Ed.), *The psychology of learning and motivation: Advances in research and theory* (Vol. 18, pp. 1-47). New York: Academic Press.

Jacoby, L. L., & Dallas, M. (1981). On the relationship between autobiographical memory and perceptual learning. *Journal of Experimental Psychology: General 3*, 306-340.

Jacoby, L. L., & Kelley, C. M. (1987). Unconscious influences of memory for a prior event. *Personality and Social Psychology Bulletin, 13*, 314-336.

Jacoby, L. L., & Kelley, C. M., Brown, J., & Jasechko, J. (1989). Becoming famous overnight: Limits on the ability to avoid unconscious influences of the past. *Journal of Personality and Social Psychology, 56*, 326-338.

Jacoby, L. L., & Kelley, C. M., & Dywan, J. (1989). Memory attributions. In H. L. Roediger & F. I. M. Craik (Eds.), *Varieties of memory and consciousness: Essays in honour of Endel Tulving* (pp. 391-422). Hillsdale, NJ: Erlbaum.

Jacoby, L. L., Marriott, M., & Collins, J. (1990). The specifics of memory and cognition. In T. K. Srull & R. S. Wyer (Eds.), *Advances in social cognition* (Vol. 3, pp. 111-121). Hillsdale, NJ: Erlbaum.

Jacoby, L. L., & Whitehouse, K. (1989). An illusion of memory: False recognition influenced by unconscious perception. *Journal of Experimental Psychology: General, 118,* 126-135.

Jacoby, L. L., & Witherspoon, D. (1982). Remembering without awareness. *Canadian Journal of Psychology, 36,* 300-324.

Jacoby, L. L., Woloshyn, V., & Kelley, C. M. (1989). Becoming famous without being recognized: Unconscious influences of memory produced by dividing attention. *Journal of Experimental Psychology: General, 118,* 115-125.

Johnson, M. K. (1983). A modular model of memory. In G. H. Bower (Ed.), *The psychology of learning and motivation: Advances in research and theory* (Vol. 17, pp. 81-123). New York: Academic Press.

Johnson, M. K., & Hasher, L. (1987). Human learning and memory. *Annual Review of Psychology, 38,* 631-668.

Johnson, M. K., Kim, J. K., & Risse, G. (1985). Do alcoholic Korsakoff's syndrome patients acquire affective reactions? *Journal of Experimental Psychology: Learning, Memory, and Cognition, 11,* 22-36.

Johnson, M. K., & Raye, C. L. (1981). Reality monitoring. *Psychological Review, 88,* 67-85.

Johnson-Laird, P. N. (1983). *Mental models.* Cambridge, MA: Harvard University Press.

Kahneman, D., & Miller, D. T. (1986). Norm theory: Comparing reality to its alternatives. *Psychological Review, 93,* 136-153.

Kelley, C. M., & Jacoby, L. L. (in press). The construction of subjective experience: Memory attributions. *Mind and Language.*

Kolers, P. A., & Smythe, W. E. (1979). Images, symbols, and skills. *Canadian Journal of Psychology, 33,* 158-184.

Kolodner, J. L. (1984). *Retrieval and organizational structures in conceptual memory: A computer model.* Hillsdale, NJ: Erlbaum.

Kuhl, J. (1986). Motivation and information processing: A new look at decision making, dynamic change, and action control. In R. M. Sorrentino & E. T. Higgins (Eds.), *Handbook of motivation and cognition: Foundations of social behavior* (Vol. 1, pp. 404-434). New York: Guilford Press.

LaRue, A., & Olejnik, A. B. (1980). Cognitive "priming" of principled moral thought. *Personality and Social Psychology Bulletin, 6,* 413-416.

Logan, G. D. (1988). Toward an instance theory of automatization. *Psychological Review, 95,* 492-527.

Mandler, G. (1980). Recognizing: The judgment of previous occurrence. *Psychological Review, 87,* 252-271.

Mandler, G., Nakamura, Y., & Van Zandt, B. J. S. (1987). Nonspecific effects of exposure on stimuli that cannot be recognized. *Journal of Experimental Psychology: Learning, Memory, and Cognition 13,* 646-648.

Marcel, A. J. (1983). Conscious and unconscious perception: An approach to the relations between phenomenal experience and perceptual processes. *Cognitive Psychology, 15,* 238-300.

McClelland, J. L., & Rumelhart, D. E. (1981). An interactive activation model of context effects in letter perception: Part I. An account of basic findings. *Psychological Review, 88,* 375-407.

Medin, D. L., & Schaffer, M. M. (1978). Context theory of classification learning. *Psychological Review, 85,* 207-238.

Medin, D. L., & Smith, E. E. (1984). Concepts and concept formation. *Annual Review of Psychology, 35,* 113-138.

Miller, G. A., Galanter, E., & Pribram, K. (1960). *Plans and the structure of behavior.* New York: Holt, Rinehart & Winston.

Mischel, W., Ebbesen, E., & Zeiss, A. R. (1972). Cognitive and attentional mechanisms in delay of gratification. *Journal of Personality and Social Psychology, 21,* 204-218.

Morton, J. (1969). Interaction of information in word recognition. *Psychological Review, 76*, 165-178.

Morton, J. (1979). Facilitation in word recognition: Experiments causing change in the logogen model. In P. A. Kolers, M. E. Wrolstal, & H. Bonma (Eds.), *Processing of visible language* (Vol. 1, pp. 259-268). New York: Plenum.

Nisbett, R. E., & Wilson, T. D. (1977). Telling more than we can know: Verbal reports on mental processes. *Psychological Review, 84*, 231-259.

Polanyi, M. (1958). *Personal knowledge: Towards a post-critical philosophy.* Chicago: University of Chicago Press.

Posner, M. I., & Snyder, C. R. R. (1975). Attention and cognitive control. In R. L. Solso (Ed.), *Information processing in cognition: The Loyola Symposium* (pp. 55-85). Hillsdale, NJ: Erlbaum.

Pratkanis, A. R., Greenwald, A. G., Leippe, M. R., & Baumgardner, M. H. (1988). In search of reliable persuasion effects: III. The sleeper effect is dead. Long live the sleeper effect. *Journal of Personality and Social Psychology, 54*, 203-218.

Quattrone, G. A. (1985). On the congruity between internal states and action. *Psychological Bulletin, 98*, 3-40.

Richardson-Klavehn, A., & Bjork, R. A. (1988). Measures of memory. *Annual Review of Psychology, 39*, 475-543.

Roediger, H. L., & Blaxton, T. A. (1987). Retrieval modes produce dissociations in memory for surface information. In D. S. Gorfein & R. R. Hoffman (Eds.), *Memory and cognitive processes: The Ebbinghaus Centennial Conference* (pp. 349-379). Hillsdale: NJ: Erlbaum.

Schachter, S. (1971). Some extraordinary facts about obese humans and rats. *American Psychologist, 26*, 129-144.

Schank, R. C. (1982). *Dynamic memory.* Cambridge, England. Cambridge University Press.

Schank, R. C., & Abelson, R. P. (1977). *Scripts, plans, goals, and understanding.* Hillsdale, NJ: Erlbaum.

Schneider, W., & Shiffrin, R. M. (1977). Controlled and automatic human information processing: I. Detection, search and attention. *Psychological Review, 84*, 1-66.

Seamon, J. G., Brody, N., & Kauff, D. M. (1983). Affective discrimination of stimuli that are not recognized: Effects of shadowing, masking, and cerebral laterality. *Journal of Experimental Psychology: Learning, Memory, and Cognition, 9*, 544-555.

Shallice, T. (1972). Dual functions of consciousness. *Psychological Review, 79*, 383-393.

Shallice, T. (1988). Information-processing models of consciousness: Possibilities and problems. In A. J. Marcel & E. Bisiach (Eds.), *Consciousness in contemporary science* (pp. 305-333). Oxford: Clarendon Press.

Shiffrin, R. M., & Schneider, W. (1977). Controlled and automatic human information processing: II. Perceptual learning, automatic attending, and a general theory. *Psychological Review, 84*, 127-190.

Smith, E. E., Shoben, E. J., & Rips, L. J. (1974). Structure and process in semantic memory: A featural model for semantic decisions. *Psychological Review, 81*, 214-241.

Smith, E. R. (1990). Content and process specificity in the effects of prior experiences. In T. K. Srull & R. S. Wyer (Eds.), *Advances in social cognition* (Vol. 3). Hillsdale, NJ: Erlbaum.

Smith, E. R., & Branscombe, N. R. (1987). Procedurally mediated social inferences: The case of category accessibility effects. *Journal of Experimental Social Psychology, 23*, 361-382.

Smith, E. R., & Branscombe, N. R. (1988). Category accessibility as implicit memory. *Journal of Experimental Social Psychology, 24*, 490-504.

Sorrentino, R. M., & Short, J. C. (1986). Uncertainty orientation, motivation, and cognition. In R. M. Sorrentino & E. T. Higgins (Eds.), *Handbook of motivation and cognition: Foundations of social behavior* (Vol. 1, pp. 379-403). New York: Guilford Press.

Spence, K. W. (1956). *Behavior theory and conditioning.* New Haven, CT: Yale University Press.

Srull, T. K., & Wyer, R. S. (1979). The role of category accessibility in the interpretation of information about persons: Some determinants and implications. *Journal of Personality and Social Psychology, 37*, 1660-1672.

Srull, T. K., & Wyer, R. S. (1980). Category accessibility and social perception: Some implications for the study of person memory and interpersonal judgments. *Journal of Personality and Social Psychology, 38,* 841-856.

Srull, T. K., & Wyer, R. S. (1986). The role of chronic and temporary goals in social information processing. In R. M. Sorrentino & E. T. Higgins (Eds.), *Handbook of motivation and cognition: Foundations of social behavior* (Vol. 1, pp. 503-549). New York: Guilford Press.

Thoresen, C. E., & Mahoney, H. J. (1974). *Behavioral self-control.* New York: Holt, Rinehart & Winston.

Tulving, E., Schacter, D. L., & Stark, H. A. (1982). Priming effects in word-fragment completion are independent of recognition memory. *Journal of Experimental Psychology: Learning, Memory, and Cognition, 8,* 336-342.

Tversky, A., & Kahneman, D. (1973). Availability: A heuristic for judging frequency and probability. *Cognitive Psychology, 5,* 207-232.

Warrington, E. K., & Weiskrantz, L. (1974). The effect of prior learning on subsequent retention in amnesic patients. *Neuropsychologia, 12,* 419-428.

Wegner, D. M., & Vallacher, R. R. (1986). Action identification. In R. M. Sorrentino & E. T. Higgins (Eds.), *Handbook of motivation and cognition: Foundations of social behavior* (Vol. 1, pp. 550-582). New York: Guilford Press.

Weiner, B. (1985). "Spontaneous" causal thinking. *Psychological Bulletin, 97,* 74-84.

Wicklund, R. A. (1986). Orientation to the environment versus preoccupation with human potential. In R. M. Sorrentino & E. T. Higgins (Eds.), *Handbook of motivation and cognition: Foundations of social behavior* (Vol. 1, pp. 64-95). New York: Guilford Press.

Wicklund, R. A., & Braun, O. L. (1987). Incompetence and the concern with human categories. *Journal of Personality and Social Psychology, 53,* 373-382.

Witherspoon, D., & Allan, L. G. (1985). The effects of a prior presentation on temporal judgments in a perceptual identification task. *Memory and Cognition, 13,* 101-111.

Wyer, R. S., & Srull, T. K. (1986). Human cognition and its social context. *Psychological Review, 93,* 322-359.

Zanna, M. P., & Rempel, J. K. (1988). Attitudes: A new look at an old concept. In D. Bar-Tal & A. Kruglanski (Eds.), *The social psychology of knowledge.* New York: Cambridge University Press.

CHAPTER 14

Constructing and Reconstructing the Past and the Future in the Present

MARCIA K. JOHNSON
Princeton University

STEVEN J. SHERMAN
Indiana University

OVERVIEW: TIME AS ORIGAMI

We have been thinking about time and truth—about the relations among past, present, and future, and about the extent to which our memories of the past and anticipations of the future are veridical. It seems natural to think of time in terms of three major divisions—past, present, future—arrayed in a linear fashion in some infinite abstract space, through which we move in a single, forward direction. In this view, we may remember or forget the past and imagine or ignore the future, but both past and future are essentially beyond reach. Such a characterization, however, misses something fundamental about our relation as psychological (cognizing, feeling) beings to time. Past, present, and future are not discrete divisions among an orderly succession of life's events. Rather, past, present, and future fold backward and forward like Japanese origami. They collapse onto each other, emerge from each other, and constantly determine each other, as we construct and reconstruct both past and future in the present, and the past and future construct the present.[1]

This origami quality of time derives from many psychological factors. Among the most important are the preconceptions we hold, confusion among sources of information, our mood, what we focus on when we think about events, our thoughts about the future and about what we might be like, considerations of what might have been, and our strategies for seeking and evaluating information. In discussing these factors, we do not make a strong distinction between cognitive and motivational effects because, in origami time, cognition and motivation often have a mutually metamorphic relation. Yesterday's motivational effects become today's cognitive constraints, and today's cognitive constraints determine tomorrow's active motives. Given the inseparability of cognition and motivation, and their many potentially distorting effects, what prevents us from drifting into a world of fantasy pasts and futures? How do we remain anchored in reality, and what sort of autobiographical truth is possible? These are some of the factors and issues we explore.

Construction and Reconstruction

In this chapter, "construction" refers to creating a past and future in the present, and "reconstruction" refers to altering (distorting) our memory for or anticipation of what has been created. The past is constructed because each person's past is continually changing as "now" is amalgamated into the past. As the past expands, we can change it. We cannot change a particular event, but we can change the entire context or background we refer to as "the past" and in which a particular event is interpreted. Thus we may change the meaning or impact of a particular past event by constructing a new past now.

Similarly, we construct the future. What we may do in the future is determined in large part by what we have done (or imagined doing) in the past. The past, in turn, is an amalgamation of "nows." Because we are projected into the future by a past that consists of an amalgamation of nows, we are constantly constructing the future (putting constraints on it) by what we do now. Thus the past and future are constructions of the present.

We may or may not, however, remember or anticipate these initial constructions veridically (as they really were or actually will be). Errors or distortions may be introduced in our recollections of the past and anticipations of the future by reconstructive processes. Such distortions may have positive as well as negative consequences (e.g., Taylor & Brown, 1988).

Cognition and Motivation

Remembering and anticipating are typically organized around purposes, goals, or agendas. Some agendas (e.g., to protect self-esteem, to see the future as bright) seem motivated or "hot," and other agendas (e.g., to understand a story) seem more purely cognitive or "cold" (Markus & Zajonc, 1985). The role in our lives of motives—hopes, fears, needs, desires, and so forth—is particularly intriguing; however, the mechanisms by which goals affect cognition are probably similar, whether the goals are hot or cold. Whether hot or cold, cognition is affected by schemas, expectancies, and inferential processes that, by their very nature, create "vested interests." Both emotional and less emotional goals influence which cognitions take place, and vice versa. Cognitions may be biased to meet needs and desires, as well as less affectively toned goals of individuals, and cognitions can in turn instigate affect, motivation, and goals. One way in which goals determine cognitions is by activating relevant information (e.g., memories of recent successes to repair self-esteem). A motive may also operate more indirectly by providing the conditions for continuing a particular line of thought. That is, we are likely to keep cognitions going that satisfy an activated goal and to cut short others that do not. Cognitive, motivational, and affective processes are constantly interacting (e.g., see Pyszczynski & Greenberg, 1987).

Just as important as the interaction of cognition and motivation at any given moment in time is their interaction across time. For example, suppose that a desire to control events prompts problem-solving activities. These activities not only may result in solutions to particular problems, but may contribute to the development of a repertoire of problem-solving strategies for future problems that may be elicited later, whether or not a desire for control is an active motive. In turn, these ready cognitive schemas for characterizing situations in terms of the strategies they call for may later be more likely to activate some motives (e.g., exploration) than others (e.g., avoidance of failure). In short, activities driven by current motives affect future cognitions, which affect future motives, which affect future cognitions, and so forth. Given this tangle of forces over time, it is somewhat arbitrary to attribute some effects to motivation and some to cognition, although it is often analytically useful.

In the next section, we consider various mechanisms by which the past is constructed and reconstructed. Following this, we discuss constructive and reconstructive processes as they affect our anticipations of the future and our actual futures. Throughout the chapter, we consider the factors that produce veridical and distorted recollections of the past and anticipations of the future.[2]

THE PAST AS A CONSTRUCTION AND RECONSTRUCTION IN THE PRESENT

The primary way in which the past is constructed in the present is, of course, that our current actions and thoughts become the past. That is, what we do and experience now sets up the "reality constraints" for our future remembering. Although this is obvious, we often do not sufficiently appreciate the profound way in which our current actions and thoughts constrain the possibilities for future remembering. Similarly, we may fail to take into account the extent to which our current actions and thoughts constrain our current remembering.

As events occur, we frame them in terms of schemas, expectancies, attitudes, goals, motives, and emotions. During the retention interval, we experience other events (again as framed by the cognitive and emotional context we bring to them) that may affect our interpretation of earlier events or their accessibility, or that may become confused with earlier events. At retrieval, we are once again influenced by our schemas, motives, and so forth, as well as by the criteria we use in evaluating the accuracy of what we remember. Encoding, retention, and retrieval stages cannot be separated completely for analysis, because what will be an effective set of retrieval circumstances is not independent of what the initial encoding circumstances were (Tulving, 1983), and how we frame events during a retention interval is not independent of how we framed them before or how we will frame them later. In spite of the difficulty of clearly identifying a single point in time for certain memory effects, available evidence gives us some insight into the complex set of factors that may influence our sense of the past.

Preconceptions

Among this set of factors, perhaps the most important are the preconceptions we have that operate during encoding and retrieval. Preconceptions, whether described as schemas (Bartlett, 1932; Neisser, 1976), coding systems (Bruner, 1957a), cognitive contexts (Bransford & Johnson, 1972), frames (Minsky, 1975), or scripts (Abelson, 1976), serve to structure information, direct attention, and guide inferences. Without schematic processing, little of our experience would seem coherent, or would be understood or available for voluntary recall (e.g., Bransford & Johnson, 1972). That is, schematic knowledge underlies accurate recall of the past. But for this clear benefit there are potential costs—omissions and distortions introduced by schematic processing, or, at the least, a kind of shearing of experience to fit the outlines of our schemas.

There are now many demonstrations of the effects of preconceptions in processing and remembering information (e.g., Arkes & Freedman, 1984; Bower, Black, & Turner, 1979; Bransford & Johnson, 1973; Chase & Simon, 1973; Chiesi, Spilich, & Voss, 1979; Johnson, Bransford, & Solomon, 1973; Markus, 1977; Pichert & Anderson, 1977; Snyder & Uranowitz, 1978; Spiro, 1977; Sulin & Dooling, 1974). The overall empirical picture, however, is complex, and a summary of schema effects is beyond the scope of this chapter (see Alba & Hasher, 1983; Higgins & Bargh, 1987; Markus & Zajonc, 1985; Taylor & Crocker, 1981, for reviews).[3] For our purposes, what is important is that sometimes the schemas that are activated either at input or retrieval produce a selective bias in what is remembered or introduce distortions. For example, Spiro (1977) found that subjects recalling a story about a couple made intrusions consistent with whether they had been told that the couple split up or lived happily ever after. In addition to intrusions in recall, people may make different interpretations of events, depending on which schema is active (e.g., Bransford & Johnson, 1973; Pichert & Anderson, 1977); may falsely recognize information consistent with a schema (e.g., Sulin & Dooling, 1974); and may reorder events in line with a schema (e.g., Bower et al., 1979).

Preconceptions in the form of expectancies may produce effects on recall that promote and sustain group stereotypes. For example, Rothbart, Evans, and Fulero (1979) presented subjects with behavioral descriptions of men (e.g., "George was his class valedictorian"). Descriptions fell into several categories, including "intellectual" and "friendly." Although there were equal numbers of intellectual and friendly descriptions, subjects who had been led in advance of hearing the descriptions to expect that the group of men was friendly later gave higher frequency estimates for and recalled more descriptions having to do with friendliness. Similarly, subjects who had been led to expect that the group was intelligent gave higher frequency estimates for and recalled more descriptions having to do with intelligence. Thus, preconceptions about group stereotypes or about individuals (including the self) may be reinforced by selective noticing and remembering of information consistent with these expectancies.

Other preconceptions—for example, our current attitudes—affect how we recall our personal histories (Bem & McConnell, 1970; Goethals & Reckman, 1973; Ross, McFarland, & Fletcher, 1981; Ross & Shulman, 1973), and how we recall our past actions may affect our current attitudes (Chaiken & Baldwin, 1981; Salancik, 1974). For example, Ross et al. (1981) exposed subjects to tape recordings of "health officials" explaining either the reasons why one should or shouldn't brush one's teeth. Later, in a seemingly unrelated context, subjects who had heard the positive messages were more favorable toward toothbrushing than were subjects who heard the negative messages. Most important, subjects who heard the message against toothbrushing reported brushing their teeth fewer times during the previous 2 weeks than did subjects hearing the positive message. In a similar experiment (Ross, McFarland, Conway, & Zanna, 1983), subjects heard a message discouraging physical exercise from either a credible source (a world authority on effects of exercise) or a noncredible source (a spokesman for the local chapter of the "Fat is Beautiful" organization). The credible group later expressed a more negative opinion about vigorous exercise. More important, although subjects actually reported the same types of activities in the two conditions, subjects in the credible condition rated the exercises they engaged in as less vigorous than did subjects in the noncredible condition. These results suggest that people selectively recall and interpret past actions to make them consistent with current attitudes (Ross et al., 1983).

Ross (1989) argues that how current attitudes affect memory depends on the operation of implicit theories of stability and change. When people change but do not assume that they have changed, they tend to recall in ways that support their sense of consistency; when people do not change but assume that they have, they tend to recall in ways that support their idea of change. As an example of what happens when subjects expect consistency in themselves, McFarland and Ross (1987) used personality characteristics that people generally think of as stable and has subjects report their impressions of themselves on two occasions, 2 months apart. Subjects whose views of themselves had become more favorable recalled their earlier evaluations as more favorable than they had been, and subjects with more negative views recalled more negative evaluations than they had given.

Biased recall also occurs when people expect change but little or none occurs. McFarland, Ross, and DeCourville (in press; cited in Ross, 1989) asked women who were not menstruating to recall ratings of physical and affective symptoms they had given previously when they were menstruating. Their beliefs about the effects of menstruation were also assessed. The more strongly a woman believed that menstruation has negative effects, the more exaggerated her remembered distress was. Conway and Ross (1984) had subjects evaluate their study skills and then assigned them to either a study skills program or a waiting-list group. When subjects were later asked to recall their initial evaluations, program participants, compared to waiting-list subjects, retrospectively belittled their initial study skills. In addition, although grades were not affected by the program, participants recalled having received better grades than they had actually obtained for the term during which the program was conducted. Thus, in this case, subjects appeared to support an expectation or theory of change by exaggerating in recall how poorly off they were before the program and by misremembering evidence relevant to the effectiveness of the program. Ross and McFarland (1988) speculate that a similar phenomenon may produce overly favorable evaluations of certain diets and popular therapies (e.g., est). Of course, biased recollections may also contribute to subjective evaluations of self-improvement programs and treatments that clearly work by more objective measures.

Some biases arise from relatively cohesive and stable structures (e.g., stereotypes), and others may be determined by more transient factors. For example, how a question is asked may set up a biased search in memory about either oneself or others (Kunda, in press; Salancik, 1974). Sanitioso (1989) asked subjects to recall information about themselves; subjects asked whether they were extraverted recalled more extraverted material about themselves and judged themselves as more extraverted than did subjects asked whether they were introverted. Snyder and Cantor (1979) had subjects read an account of a person's behavior, and then later judge the person's suitability for a job. If they thought that the job required an extraverted personality, they were more likely to recall facts consistent with the idea that the person was extraverted; if they thought that the job required an introvert, they were more likely to recall facts consistent with the idea that the person was introverted.

Confusion among Sources of Information

In addition to errors and biases introduced by preconceptions operating at encoding and retrieval, our recollections may be distorted by failures in "source monitoring" (Johnson, 1988a; Lindsay & Johnson, 1987a). For example, people may attribute information from one external source to another, as in misremembering that something said by Fran was said by Chris (e.g., Foley, Johnson, & Raye, 1983; Lindsay, 1987; Raye & Johnson, 1980). People also confuse different types of self-generated memories; for example, they may fail to discriminate between what they imagined themselves doing or saying and what they actually did or said (Anderson, 1984; Foley & Johnson, 1985; Foley et al., 1983).

Reality monitoring (Johnson, in press; Johnson & Raye, 1981) is an especially critical type of source monitoring that involves discriminating between what has been generated and what has been perceived. People's current actions and thoughts create conditions that may later lead to errors and distortions in memory. For example, individuals may confuse what they said with what someone else said (e.g., Brown & Murphy, 1989; Voss, Vesonder, Post, & Ney, 1987), although subjects sometimes are remarkably good at this discrimination (see Foley et al., 1983; Hashtroudi, Johnson, & Chrosniak, 1989; Raye & Johnson, 1980; Ross & Sicoly, 1979). People confuse what they imagined with what they saw (e.g., Durso & Johnson, 1980), and the more often they think about something, the more often they think they saw it (Johnson, Raye, Wang, & Taylor, 1979; Johnson, Taylor, & Raye, 1977). People confuse what they imagined someone said with what the person actually said (Johnson, Foley, & Leach, 1988). And people may confuse their description of an event with the actual event (Carmichael, Hogan, & Walter, 1932; Higgins & Rholes, 1978; Schooler, 1987). Reality-monitoring failures are potentially insidious, because people are most likely to confuse what they generated themselves with what they perceived when the generation is relatively natural or effortless (Durso & Johnson, 1980; Finke, Johnson, & Shyi, 1988; Johnson, Raye, Foley, & Foley, 1981).

Reality-monitoring failures not only contribute to a reconstructed memory of events of the past, but also influence knowledge and beliefs (Johnson, 1988b; Wicklund, 1989). For example, given that people come to believe in the validity of statements they have heard repeatedly (Arkes, Blumer, & Boehm, 1987; Hasher, Goldstein, & Toppino, 1977), it seems likely that they would also come to believe the statements that they repeat to others (e.g., Higgins & Rholes, 1978) or to themselves. Reality-monitoring failures may also operate in the formation and maintenance of stereotypes (Slusher & Anderson, 1987). Strong expectations and beliefs, including stereotypes, determine representations of imaginary events. Thus, in imagining an upcoming basketball game for the state championship between two teams with which we are unfamiliar, we may see a lot of black players in our mind's eye. In imagining a social event involving women, we may see it as entailing emotional exchanges, compliments, and gossiping. On the other hand, imagination of an all-male social event may include assertive and aggressive behaviors, joking, and bragging. Our expectations constrain our mental simulation of events and the traits and behaviors exhibited by imagined group members. Subsequently, we may fail to distinguish things that we have imagined from things that we have actually observed. Instances that we have only imagined may be taken as actual instances and lead to inflated frequency estimates for stereotype-consistent behaviors; thus, they may verify our initial stereotypic beliefs. Such imagined scenarios may contribute to our beliefs about the characteristics of specific individuals (including ourselves), as well as about groups.

The critical importance of reality-monitoring processes is made especially apparent when they break down dramatically, as in the case of delusional syndromes (Johnson, 1988a) or in the striking instances of confabulation found in certain types of organic brain damage (Johnson, in press). Although such extreme disruption of normal reality-monitoring processes is rare, to some degree we all have a sense of the past contaminated by what we have previously imagined, hoped for, anticipated, and feared. In spite of the dangers of reality-monitoring failures (e.g., heated arguments between intimates about whether and how events occurred, controversies between colleagues over ownership of ideas, and severe disruption of everyday function in extreme cases), some inaccuracy in reality monitoring may be good for us. For example, the tendency to confuse our wishes with reality and thus perhaps to have an inflated idea of the number of good things that have happened to us may help protect us from depression or help us deal with stress (Alloy & Abramson, 1979; Taylor & Brown, 1988).

Potential confusions between memories for thoughts and memories for perceptions are not the only consequences of thoughts, of course. For example, mentally reviewing autobiographical events increases their accessibility. If we think of several different past autobiographical events from a given category (e.g., times we loaned people money), we are likely later to think that events of that type have been more frequent in our lives than if we think in detail about only one such event (Lindsay & Johnson, 1987b). That is, in estimating the frequency of various kinds of events in our personal history, we do not completely discount or correct for the heightened availability (Tversky & Kahneman, 1973) that we may create by reminiscing and ruminating. Again, this potential source of distortion from past thoughts may have benefits as well as costs. If we rehearse past successes when faced with a failure, we may keep our successes accessible for the future, add to their apparent frequency, and in so doing provide ourselves with resources to repair self-esteem when it is challenged (Liu & Steele, 1986).

Another consequence of thinking is that thresholds of particular concepts or schemas may be lowered, and thus they may be more likely to be used again (e.g., Bruner, 1957b; Higgins, 1989a; Higgins & Bargh, 1987). Especially important, we think, are the consequences of entertaining some hypotheses but not others, in attempting to understand or explain what has happened. Highly accessible hypotheses, or ones for which there is already evidence, may be the ones people continue to selectively examine. In collecting information for evaluating potential causes of events, people tend to engage in what Shaklee and Fischhoff (1982) call a "truncated search." That is, subjects look for evidence consistent with a particular sufficient cause (sometimes an already known cause), rather than looking for evidence about additional sufficient or contributing causes. It seems likely that people also engage in truncated searches of autobiographical memory when attempting to determine the causes of events in their own lives. Such truncated searches may make them satisfied with explanations that occur readily and fit their current expectations. Although initial explanations may often be relevant, truncated searches may prevent people from discovering other equally important causes as they remember their personal histories.

In some instances, accessibility effects involve source confusions—for example, when we falsely believe that our expectations or hypotheses veridically arise from what we have perceived, when in fact they arise from what we have thought. Source-monitoring failures, including reality-monitoring failures, may underlie a number of other memory phenomena, such as errors induced in eyewitness testimony by misleading questions (Loftus, 1979), "sleeper effects" (Greenwald, Pratkanis, Leippe, & Baumgardner, 1986), and schema-related intrusions and false recognitions (Alba & Hasher, 1983; Johnson & Raye, 1981; Lindsay & Johnson, 1989). Confusion among sources of information occurs when we generate a selective description of a person or event and later treat our generated description as if it were an unbiased representation of what we perceived. For example, we may slant our description of a person to fit the attitudes of listeners, and then later forget this contextual influence and distort our recall and evaluation of the person in the direction of our description (Higgins & Stangor, 1988).

Failure in source monitoring may give rise to the feeling that a name or a fact that is familiar from a recent exposure was known previously (e.g., Jacoby, Kelley, Brown, & Jasechko, 1989; Schacter, Harbluk, & McLachlan, 1984) and may contribute to the uncanniness of "hindsight" (Fischhoff, 1975, 1977; Fischhoff & Beyth, 1975). For example, Fischhoff and Beyth (1975) asked subjects to estimate the likelihood of various possible outcomes of Nixon's then-upcoming Peking and Moscow trips. After the trips, subjects were asked to remember their predictions and to state whether or not an event had actually happened (e.g., whether Nixon visited Lenin's tomb). Subjects remembered having given higher probabilities than they actually had given to events they believed had happened and lower probabilities to events they believed had not happened. Similarly, if subjects are given outcome information at the time they make initial judgments about histori- cal events, they cannot respond as if they did not know the outcome (Fischhoff, 1975). In effect, subjects think of themselves (i.e., their prior experience) as the source of knowledge that they in fact derived from other sources. Under many circumstances, this tendency to "know it all along" may be a form of relatively harmless self-flattery. But in some circumstances, such source confusion may make people particularly harsh judges of themselves and others. People who feel that certain predictions were obvious at the time (even if they were not) may then be left with regret or guilt about not having taken actions that they should have. Similarly, they may unfairly accuse others of failing to take obviously needed action. Furthermore, if people underestimate the extent to which they could not anticipate events in the past, they are unlikely to look for better ways of doing so in the future. Thus, hindsight bias reduces the chances that people will learn from the past (Fischhoff, 1975).

Moods

Moods are another potential source of selection and bias in remembering. Two types of mood effects have been investigated (Eich, 1989). "Mood dependence" refers to the phenomenon whereby events encoded in a particular mood are most retrievable in that mood, regardless of the events' affective valence or content. "Mood congruence" refers to the enhanced encoding or retrieval of events whose affective content is congruent with one's current mood (see Blaney, 1986, Eich, 1989, and Isen, 1984, for reviews).

With respect to the issue of mood-dependent effects, Eich (1989) makes the intriguing suggestion that previous findings showing state-dependent effects of drugs or physical context may have been mediated by mood effects. Drugs or physical context may affect mood, and the decrements in memory that result from changes in drug state or physical context between the initial event and attempted memory may be attributable to failures in the match between moods at encoding and retrieval. Another new idea regarding changes in mood state comes from work by Eich and Metcalfe (1989). They report evidence that internally generated events are less likely than externally derived events to be recalled following a shift in mood state. This finding suggests that memory for what has been previously thought may be more subject to mood effects than memory for what has been previously perceived. If so, people are likely to be particularly unreliable reporters of their own past feelings and beliefs.

With respect to mood congruence, Williams and Dritschel (1988) suggest that, although mood-congruent effects found with laboratory-learned materials have not been reliable (Bower & Mayer, 1986; Hasher, Rose, Zacks, Sanft, & Doren, 1985), the effects of mood congruency are more robust for autobiographical recall (Teasdale & Fogarty, 1979; Teasdale, Taylor, & Fogarty, 1980). The potential role of mood in autobiographical recall is far-reaching. Reus, Weingartner, and Post (1979) suggested that depressed patients may find it difficult to recall or elaborate on earlier periods of time when they felt better, because the positive feelings from the earlier time do not match the negative feelings of the current mood. Williams and Broadbent (1986) found that patients who had taken drug overdoses in attempting suicide took longer than controls to retrieve a memory when given a positive cue word, but were comparable to controls when given a negative cue—findings suggesting a mood-congruent bias.

Not only does current mood affect what people are likely to recall, but what they recall may affect their current mood and sense of well-being. Strack, Schwarz, and Gschneidinger (1985) asked subjects to think about three events that were either particularly positive and pleasant or particularly negative and unpleasant. Some subjects were asked to describe events from their present life (in effect, from their recent past), and others were asked to describe events from their past life. Subsequently, subjects answered some questions from which an index of subjective well-being was derived. Subjects who described recent events were happier and more satisfied if the events they recalled were positive than if they were negative. In contrast, subjects who described events from the more distant past rated themselves as less happy when the events were positive than when the events were negative. Strack et al. have suggested that, whereas the recent past is taken as representative, the more distant past may become a standard of comparison against which the present situation is evaluated. They also reported subsequent experiments suggesting that when subjects were induced to think about *how* past events came about, their subjective well-being was influenced in the direction (positive or negative) of the events they recalled, whereas if they thought about *why* events came about, their ratings of subjective well-being showed a contrast effect. Strack et al. have suggested that thinking about *how* induces people to think in a vivid, detailed way about events, whereas thinking about *why* induces people to think about the abstract causes of events. Vivid memories presumably produce affect, which directly contributes to ratings of current well-being; more pallid memories function as standards of comparison.

Focus

Consistent with the Strack et al. (1985) study, other findings illustrate that how people focus on events affects the impact of these events. For example, in thinking about current or past events, people can focus on perceptual or "factual" aspects or on apperceptive (thoughts and feelings) aspects. Suengas and Johnson (1988) report evidence suggesting that the type of focus people adopt in thinking about events has consequences for how the events are later remembered. Subjects either imagined or engaged in a number of "minievents," such as wrapping a package, having coffee and cookies, and writing a letter. Subsequently, some subjects were instructed to think about various perceptual aspects of the events (e.g., colors and sounds), and others were instructed to think about apperceptive aspects of the events (what they were thinking or feeling at the time). On a later test in which subjects rated various qualitative characteristics of their memories for these events, there was some evidence that thinking about apperceptive aspects of events decreased access to perceptual qualities of memories and reduced intial differences between perceived and imagined events in their apperceptive qualities. Ordinarily, perceptual qualities provide highly salient information for discriminating perceived from imagined events in memory (i.e., for reality monitoring; Johnson, Foley, Suengas, & Raye, 1988; Johnson & Raye, 1981). The results of the Suengas and Johnson study suggest that focusing on apperceptive aspects of experience might decrease one's ability to later discriminate real from imagined events (see Hashtroudi, Johnson, & Crosniak, 1990, for evidence consistent with this idea).

Other evidence that type of focus may have important implications for memory comes from work by Williams and his colleagues (Williams & Broadbent, 1986; Williams & Dritschel, 1988; Williams & Scott, 1988). People who had recently attempted suicide by drug overdose were presented with words (e.g., "humor," "devotion," "boredom," "sickness") and were asked to recall a specific autobiographical memory for each. Compared to controls, attempted-suicide patients tended to retrieve quite general memories (e.g., "when I was at school," "that hotel in Germany") rather than more specific episodes (Williams & Broadbent, 1986; Williams & Dritschel, 1988). Patients with diagnoses of major depressive disorder also tended to be inappropriately general in remembering (Williams & Scott, 1988). One possibility is that overgeneral recall is caused by transient factors related to immediate crisis. That this may not be the entire story is suggested by the results of a follow-up experiment with ex-suicide patients who had taken an overdose between 3 and 14 months previously. Even quite long after the crisis of attempted suicide, patients showed a tendency for overgeneral recall.

One provocative possibility suggested by Williams and Dritschel (1988) is that people who are vulnerable to depression and thoughts of suicide tend to encode events in a general rather than a specific way initially (cf. Abramson & Martin, 1981, and Beck, 1967). Furthermore, Williams and Dritschel suggest that affective significance is more likely to be attached to more general encodings, perhaps because it is at the more general level that particular events relate to long-term criteria. People with a tendency toward general encoding may later have difficulty recalling specific episodes, but the episodes may still have made a contribution to the accessibility of the general category to which the event was assigned (e.g., failures).

Williams and Dritschel (1988) discuss some clinical implications of overgeneral encoding. One is that

> the type of affect which is associated with generic memory is unhelpful for
> therapeutic process. . . . Greater benefit is obtained in cognitive therapy if
> depressed patients are able to go beyond the general statement "I've always been
> a failure" to describe the details of particular instances when they feel they have
> failed. (p. 33)

A similar point is made by the results of a study by Wahler and Afton (1980),
which Williams and Dritschel discuss. Mothers who were under multiple stresses
and who had problems with their children tended to give general descriptions of
their children's behavior rather than detailed accounts. Wahler and Afton (1980)
suggested that at the time the behaviors occurred, these mothers tended to ignore
aspects of the behavior that were specific to the situation and instead quickly
classified the behavior as naughty or malicious. As treatment progressed, the
mothers became more specific in their descriptions. Williams and Dritschel
(1988) raise the possibility that a cognitive style that results in overgeneral
memories may be linked to real world problems in living.

Frank and Gilovich (1989) discuss another type of focus phenomenon that
may contribute to a reconstruction of the past in the present. With the passage of
time, people tend increasingly to attribute their behavior to dispositional factors
rather than situational factors (Moore, Sherrod, Liu, & Underwood, 1979; Peterson, 1980; but see Miller & Porter, 1980). Based on observations that actors tend
to see their actions as determined by aspects of the situation, whereas observers
tend to see actors' behaviors as determined by traits or dispositions (Jones &
Nisbett, 1971), Moore et al. (1979) proposed that, with time, people may shift
from an actor's to an observer's visual perspective with respect to their own
behavior. Consistent with this idea that people's visual images of events become
more observer-like with the passage of time, Nigro and Neisser (1983) reported
that in remembering, people are more likely to adopt an observer perspective for
older memories.

Frank and Gilovich (1989) reported direct evidence for a relation between
perspective while remembering and type of attribution. Subjects were in a get-
acquainted conversation, then rated themselves on several characteristics (e.g.,
friendliness, nervousness) and indicated to what extent personality traits caused
them to behave as they did during the conversation and to what extent characteristics of the situation caused them to behave as they did. Three weeks later, they
filled out the same questionnaire and indicated whether their memory perspective
was as an observer or similar to what it was when the event occurred (a "field"
perspective). Attributions of people remembering from an observer's perspective
tended to become more dispositional and less situational with the passage of time,
compared to those subjects who recalled the conversation from a field perspective.
In a second study, subjects participated in the get-acquainted conversation and
then were randomly assigned to remember from either a field or an observer
perspective. Subjects in the observer-perspective condition tended to make more
dispositional attributions for their behavior than they had made initially; subjects

in the field-perspective condition tended to attribute their behavior less dispositionally.

Frank and Gilovich speculate that people develop an observer perspective because, as time passes, which visual perspective a person adopts in remembering becomes the most powerful determinant of a person's attributions. The implication of this suggestion is that, with the passage of time, other information that would support a field or participant perspective (e.g., initial thoughts and feelings) fades from memory at a faster rate than do visual qualities. Interestingly, Suengas and Johnson (1988) report evidence consistent with this line of thought; in that study, memory for thoughts and feelings seemed to decrease at a faster rate than memory for visual aspects of events.

The Frank and Gilovich (1989) findings raise the possibility that we tend to see our former selves as more guided by traits (e.g., shyness, lack of self-confidence, honesty) and less affected by situational factors than we actually were. If we see the past as a consequence of our dispositions rather than the situations we found ourselves in (or created for ourselves), and if we are not happy about the past, we may be tempted to try to change ourselves (try to be more extraverted) rather than to change the situations we seek out (find some people we want to talk to). If so, therapies directed at changing traits (promising dramatic changes in outlook or personality) may seem attractive, although therapies directed at changing situations may in fact be more effective.

Frank and Gilovich also raise the interesting question of whether there are people who chronically recall events from either a field or an observer perspective, and speculate that those who tend to recall events from an observer's perspective tend to see themselves as the primary cause or origin of their actions. If so, such people may also see themselves as having stable traits and may be more inclined to minimize differences between current and past attitudes by adopting a theory of no change (Ross, 1989).

The Issue of Veridicality

In a world open to multiple interpretations, confronted by a memory system that selects, edits, and otherwise reconstructs events, what is veridical memory? Perhaps the concept of truth is simply irrelevant to the issue of personal memory. Although much of the research in memory and cognition in the last 20–25 years has focused on errors and distortions in memory and has highlighted the reconstructive nature of memory, more recently researchers have emphasized that reconstructive processes are, after all, constrained by reality (e.g., Alba & Hasher, 1983; Brewer, 1988; Johnson & Raye, 1981; Kunda, in press; Ross & McFarland, 1988).

For example, in studies of both laboratory-learned materials and autobiographical recall, there are surprisingly few distortions and intrusions in recall of even fairly complex events (e.g., Alba & Hasher, 1983; Brewer, 1988; Johnson, Kahan, & Raye, 1984; Zangwill, 1972). Although misleading information reliably produces errors in memory, subjects are not as likely to be misled about central facts as they are to be misled about peripheral details (Loftus, 1979). Some distortion arises from the criteria subjects use when remembering: They may too readily accept a memory as truth. If people are induced to use more stringent criteria, they may avoid errors they would have made otherwise (e.g., Hasher & Griffin, 1978; Lindsay & Johnson, 1989; Raye, Johnson, & Taylor, 1980). Not surprisingly, whether one finds accuracy (e.g., Brewer, 1988) or distortion (e.g., Barclay & DeCooke, 1988) may have something to do with one's theoretical expectations (McCauley, 1988). It may also have to do with whether perceptual or reflective records of events are accessed in a given situation (e.g., Johnson, 1983).

The limits of reconstructive processes have also been noted in the social-cognitive literature (Ebbesen, 1981; Kunda, in press; Markus & Zajonc, 1985; Ross & McFarland, 1988). Ross and McFarland (1988) suggest that researchers may have exaggerated the degree of fabrication subjects engage in by focusing on bias rather than accuracy, and they point out that there may be limits to how much current attitudes reshape people's recollections of their prior histories. Recall of especially vivid or readily recalled events may be immune to changes induced by changes in attitudes (Ross et al., 1981). On the other hand, reconstruction may take place in quite subtle ways for even vivid memories. People

> need not reshape or falsify the more "objective" features of their past actions to produce consistency with current attitudes. They may more readily change their perceptions of how or why they did something, rather than whether or how often they did it. (Ross et al., 1983, p. 260)

Kunda (in press) makes a similar point. She argues that motivated reasoning is mediated by biased memory search and belief construction. She points out, however, that "people are not at liberty to believe anything they like—they are constrained by their prior beliefs." That is, desiring a particular conclusion is not sufficient to completely overwhelm the effect of prior knowledge. (Of course, that prior knowledge will vary, depending on the cognitive and motivational factors that operated when it was derived.)

Motives, schemas (including self-schemas), moods, temporary cognitive contexts, and type of focus or perspective contribute to selective access and produce biased or distorted memories. In addition, failures in reality monitoring and source monitoring contribute to error and distortion. But when we reconstruct the past in the present, either in remembering events, remembering prior attitudes, or for the purposes of reasoning about something, we are not free to construct any prior past. We are constrained by reality-monitoring processes (Johnson & Raye, 1981) that sort fact from fantasy and that, though subject to error, ordinarily serve us reasonably well (the Christs in mental hospitals and the confabulators suffering from organic brain damage are exceptions). That is, memory pursues past actualities, not the pure possibilities of imagination (Casey, 1987). Reality monitoring grounds us in these past actualities.

Reality-monitoring processes capitalize on aspects of the memory records of what we initially experienced, using, for example, characteristic differences in memories for perceived and imagined events to set heuristic criteria for distinguishing between them. In addition to the residual memory records of what happened, other reality-monitoring constraints on reconstruction derive from our knowledge of how the world works and of what plausibly could have happened (Johnson, in press; Johnson & Raye, 1981).[4] That is, prior knowledge may be a force for veridical memory as well as a cause of distorted memory. Still other constraints on reconstruction may derive from our understanding of ourselves as cognizing, feeling beings, and by extension from our understanding of others. Together, these various constraints allow us to monitor the origin of memories, knowledge, and beliefs; to consider a range of possibilities for what might have happened; and to estimate corresponding probabilities for these possibilities. In short, truthful remembering is constrained by what happened, and events are interpreted within a context of possibilities appropriately weighted by their corresponding probabilities.

It is especially important in remembering social information to consider the ways in which people's cognitive and motivational processes create possibilities for what happened. Suppose you claim that I make most of the decisions and I claim that you do. Is it reasonable to think that one person's memory may be more erroneous or distorted than the other's? Yes, if we could agree on what constitutes a decision and who made each one, then someone has the more accurate view of the true frequency with which each person made decisions. Thus the issue of veridicality about some social facts may be equivalent to issues of veridicality about physical facts (Were there two boxes or three? Were they all red or was one blue?). Alas, the issue of truth for much social information is complicated by many potential factors: We may not agree on what constitutes a decision; we may not agree about who made each decision; because of cognitive or motivational factors, we may fail to remember a representative sample of decisions and who made them; we may not agree about how each decision is to be weighted (even if you make three decisions to every one of mine, it may still seem to you as if I am making all the decisions if you regard those I make as more important).

We are plagued in interpersonal contexts by the problem of interpretation or appearance, and this is especially true with respect to reading other people's motives or emotions. Suppose I say you were angry with me last week and you claim you were not. Who has the veridical memory of the exchange? You may have been angry at the time and may now be misremembering your affective state. Or you may not have been angry, but I may have misperceived your affective state. Or you may not have been angry, and I may have perceived your affective state correctly at the time but now I am misremembering it. Assuming that we both know what anger is and when someone is experiencing it, then this (like the questions about the boxes) has an answer in principle. But chances are that neither of us recorded anywhere what your true state was at the time of the event. To remember veridically is to remember informed by the realization that disagreements that can only be resolved "in principle" (without benefit from further, converging evidence) cannot be resolved at all.

The fact that people do not always agree on what the same evidence means or even on the unit of analysis may further complicate the picture. "Being angry" in a social context is not simply a matter of one person's experience. People ordinarily think of emotions as being defined by the experience of the "emoter," but they are defined as much in a social context by the experience of the "emotee"—that is, by what is communicated.

Given that two people may not agree at the time about what each is feeling, either because they "misperceive" information or because they experience it differently, or that people may misremember later what they originally felt (or misremember what they thought at the time another person originally felt), how can we speak of veridical or nonveridical memory in such cases? To remember social information veridically is to see the full range of possibilities for remembering—to see the possibility that a person might not have been angry, but might have appeared angry while experiencing something else; or to see the possibility that a person might have been angry and have forgotten (or forgiven). In other words, social memory, like memory for more "factual" events, is veridical insofar as the remembering is constrained not only by "what happened," but by our understanding of the cognitive and motivational factors that may affect our remembering and that should keep us from too readily accepting any particular memory as truth, especially memories for social information.

To what extent, then, are we "revisionist historians" with respect to our personal pasts (Greenwald, 1980; Ross et al., 1981)? As we have seen, we do interpret initial experience selectively; we also revise in remembering according to the cues we confront, and according to our current mood, attitudes, motives, schemas, and so forth. But our revisions are constrained by memory records of what happened in combination with reality-monitoring processes that evaluate what we remember. This evaluation includes constraints imposed by whatever knowledge of memory, motivational, and social processes we can bring to bear on interpreting our past.

THE FUTURE AS A CONSTRUCTION AND RECONSTRUCTION IN THE PRESENT

Thus far, we have seen how people both construct and reconstruct the past in the present. With regard to thinking about the future, we might suppose that there should be important differences from thinking about the past with respect to construction, reconstruction, and constraints. In the first place, it would appear that the future can only be constructed and shaped rather than reconstructed. After all, the future has not yet occurred. How can it be reconstructed or be distorted or nonveridically perceived? But just as the past can be either constructed and shaped in the present without distortion or can be distorted or reconstructed, so too can judgments of the future be reasonable and "accurate" in terms of the perceived probabilities of the occurrence of possible events, or nonveridical when these judgments do not conform to the actual probabilities of occurrence of possible events. And, as we shall see, these veridical or nonveridical judgments of the future can shape that future, thus either constructing a future as it "should have been" or "reconstructing" and bringing about a future that "should not have occurred" in the absence of the judgments and their effects.

With regard to constraints in thinking about the future, we might suppose that there would be far fewer constraints than occur in thinking about the past. The past has already taken place; it is what it is. The future has yet to take place; anything is possible. Yet, as we shall see, there are indeed constraints in thinking about the future, of both a cognitive and a motivational nature, that have certain similarities with the constraints involved in thinking about the past.

Thoughts about the Future

For more than a decade, researchers have been interested in the effects of imagining and/or generating explanations for hypothetical future events and outcomes. In this work, a particular future is specified, and subjects are asked to think about and explain how and why such a future might have come about. In the first study of this sort, Ross, Lepper, Strack, and Steinmetz (1977) had subjects read detailed clinical case histories. Subjects were asked to find evidence in the case that would help them explain various possible (but not yet actually occurring) future events in the life of the clinical patient. In more recent studies, subjects have been asked to imagine and explain a variety of future occurrences: the outcome of an upcoming election (Carroll, 1978); the outcome of upcoming football games (Hirt & Sherman, 1985; Sherman, Zehner, Johnson, & Hirt, 1983); and the impact on people of watching televised aggression (Anderson & Sechler, 1986). In all cases, the hypothetical outcome that was imagined or explained was subsequently perceived as more likely to occur. For example, subjects who imagined a Ford victory in the then-upcoming 1976 Carter–Ford presidential election judged a Ford victory as far more likely than those who had imagined a Carter win (Carroll, 1978).

Thus, specifying a particular future for people to think about affects judgments of the likelihood of occurrence of such a future. These effects are generally interpreted in terms of the types of cognitive mechanisms we have discussed previously. It is assumed that when people are asked to imagine or explain a hypothetical future event, they access from memory facts and scenarios that are consistent with the outcome to be explained. It is further assumed that people are capable of easily accessing material consistent with any number of possible future outcomes. For example, people may hold in memory facts that would be consistent with a victory by either team in an upcoming basketball game or by either candidate in an upcoming election. Even when one team is a decided underdog, explanations of a victory by the underdog in terms of the gambler's fallacy (losing streaks have to end sometime) or in terms of overconfidence by the favorite team or heightened motivation by the underdog will suffice as reasonable explanations. When subsequently asked what is really likely to happen in the future, subjects will make judgments primarily on the basis of facts and impressions that are most accessible in memory. The facts and ideas generated during the recent explanation task ought to come to mind quickly and easily, and thus ought to serve as the basis of judgment.

Such a process is consistent with Tversky and Kahneman's (1973) ideas about availability and about the simulation heuristic (Kahneman & Tversky, 1982). Subjects will use the availability of information and the ease of constructing any scenario or outcome as an indication of likelihood. They may fail to recognize that the availability of certain facts in memory and the ease of construction of future scenarios may be based only on the fact that they were recently induced to access and use these facts and scenarios. As an indication of the validity of such an explanation, Sherman, Cialdini, Schwartzman, and Reynolds (1985) asked subjects to imagine contracting a (hypothetical) disease that had either easy-to-imagine or difficult-to-imagine symptoms. When the symptoms were easy to imagine, imagination led to an increase in the subjective likelihood of contracting the disease. However, when the symptoms were difficult to imagine, subjects evidently used this difficulty as a way of judging the likelihood of the disease, and the imagination task led to a decrease in the subjective likelihood of the disease. Similarly, as indicated previously, accessibility and ease of imagination or "simulation" affect our recall of the past (e.g., Finke et al., 1988; Lindsay & Johnson, 1987b).

Interestingly, specifying a particular future for people to think about not only increases judgments of the likelihood of such a future, but affects actual subsequent behavior as well. Sherman, Skov, Hervitz, and Stock (1981) asked subjects to imagine and explain either their own success or their own failure on an upcoming anagram task. Such explanations clearly affected subjects' judgments of how they were likely to do on the task. Accessibility of certain facts in memory (facts consistent with either success or failure at the task) was assumed to be the process underlying these effects. In addition, among subjects who explicitly stated their (biased) expectations, their actual performance on a subsequent anagram task was influenced. Those who had explained hypothetical success actually outperformed those who had explained hypothetical failure. Self-fulfilling prophecy effects (Darley & Fazio, 1980) were no doubt important in bringing about these results.

An additional finding from the Sherman et al. (1981) study indicated the possibility of important motivational effects of explaining undesirable future events. Subjects who had explained failure but who had not fully committed themselves to this possible future by explicitly stating expectancies actually performed best of all. It is as though the accessible possibility of future failure motivated them to avoid such a future outcome by putting more effort into the anagram task. Small doses of potential future failure may act to inoculate people against such a future by preparing them to behave in ways so as to avoid the outcome.

Thinking about specific possible futures has been shown to influence a number of other kinds of behaviors as well. Gregory, Cialdini, and Carpenter (1982) demonstrated that having people imagine enjoying the benefits of cable TV increased their likelihood of subscribing to a cable TV service. Meichenbaum and Goodman (1971) employed cognitive rehearsal and mental planning to alter the behavior of impulsive schoolchildren, and Marlatt (1978) reduced the relapse rate among alcoholics by using similar imagination and explanation techniques. More recently, R. T. Sherman and Anderson (1987) reduced premature termination of therapy among clients by having them initially imagine and explain staying in psychotherapy for at least four therapy sessions. Finally, imagination of the future has been used to enhance the performance of athletes (Feltz & Landers, 1983; Hall & Erffmeyer, 1983; Suinn, 1976).

Another way in which people think about the future is to try to predict the future: "Who will win the upcoming election, and what will the country be like in that case?" "Who will win the next Super Bowl?" "What will the stock market do in the next year?" "What is my life likely to be like 5 years from now?" People often engage in such self-generated predictions about the future. Sherman (1980) asked subjects to predict what they would do if they found themselves in several kinds of situations. For example, subjects were asked (in the context of a psychology experiment) to predict whether or not they would agree to volunteer 3 hours of time to collect money for the American Cancer Society if they were called and asked to do so. In one sense, subjects' predictions of their future behavior were very inaccurate. Whereas only 4% of a similar population agreed to volunteer their time when called directly by the American Cancer Society, 48% of experimental subjects predicted that they would agree to such a request if called. In another sense, however, these predictions were accurate. Having made the (mis)-predictions (mispredictions compared to the control group),[5] virtually all subjects who had predicted compliance actually did agree to a similar request to help for charity that was made 3 days later in a situation that was totally unconnected to the original prediction situation. Having made a prediction and having come to hold a certain view of what they would act like in a possible future situation, subjects indeed behaved in a way that was consistent with what they had imagined and what they had predicted.

Greenwald, Klinger, Van de Kamp, and Kerr (1988) asked registered voters in Seattle to predict whether they would vote in an upcoming election. The percentage of subjects who predicted that they would in fact vote was much higher than the actual rate of voter turnout. Greenwald et al. then collected actual voter turnout data. Those subjects who had predicted that they would vote did in fact vote at a high rate, thus rendering their predictions true.

But why were the predictions of subjects in the Sherman (1980) and Greenwald et al. (1988) studies inaccurate relative to the control subjects' behavior? What factors constrained their predictions and prevented subjects from "correctly" judging what they would likely do in a potential future situation? One possibility is that subjects may have failed to conceive of or construe the imagined situation appropriately, as it would actually seem "in real life." For example, in predicting their willingness to donate time to charity, Sherman's subjects may not have imagined the likely possibility of time pressures and alternative plans that they would have that would prevent such a commitment—pressures that they would feel strongly in the actual behavioral request situation. Moreover, subjects may have imagined the pressures for complying with a request to be stronger than they would actually be in the real request situation. These cognitive misconstruals would lead to a misprediction in the direction of a high compliance rate. Another possibility is that, in a purely hypothetical situation, when no actual effort or commitment is involved, subjects may be more motivated to appear socially desirable (to themselves or to others) than to be accurate in their predictions. They thus tend to make the low-cost, socially desirable prediction. (Social desirability, however, is not a necessary component of situations in which [mis]predictions come to guide future behavior; see Kahneman & Snell, 1988.)

In any case, regardless of why the initial misprediction is made, once subjects think about themselves in a certain way in a possible future scenario, they tend to act in that way when such a potential future actually becomes the present. In other words, certain cognitive and motivational factors constrain the way in which people make predictions about the future. These predictions, in turn, constrain the ways in which people act when the possible future comes to pass. A prediction thus acts as a type of commitment, rendering the subsequent behavior different from what it would have been if people had not thought about and predicted the future. In this way, (mis)predictions can turn into commitments and can alter the course of individuals' own history. The act of predicting the future can, interestingly, free people from the past and leave them *more* unconstrained by the past as they behave in new ways that are different from what they would have done without the act of prediction. On the one hand, then, predictions of the future are constrained by the past through the effects of expectancies, hopes, and wishes. Such constraints can lead to an inability to perceive the world correctly and thus to mispredictions. On the other hand, predictions once made serve a directive function and can free people from the past and lead them in new directions. This is yet another indication of the ways in which the past, the present, and the future collapse into and emerge from each other.

In recent years, there has been much discussion of the predictability of behavior from measures of behavioral intentions. Behavioral intentions are, of course, like behavioral predictions, in that a person is projecting into a future situation and making statements about what he or she will do in that situation. (One difference is that the person may predict behavior without intending for it to happen, as in a prediction of losing a tennis match or not doing well in an exam. In this sense, predictions are like expectations and intentions are more like wishes.)

Fishbein and Ajzen (1980) report that there is, under most circumstances, a strong relation between intention and behavior. In fact, a central methodological assumption in assessing the relation between intentions and behavior is that subjects who do not state their intentions have the same intentions as subjects that do. And yet, in studies on behavioral prediction, the behaviors of prediction subjects were markedly different from the behaviors of subjects who did not state their intentions. Fishbein and Ajzen were correct, however, about the correspondence of "intentions" and behavior for those subjects who did make predictions: Those subjects showed a strong association between what they said they would do and what they later did. High correspondence between intentions and behavior occurred when the stated intentions and the behaviors were obtained from the same subjects (see Fishbein & Ajzen, 1980, for a review). The prediction studies suggest that such correspondence may exist only when the behavior follows initial statements of intention, and may exist because of these statements. Thus there is a more dynamic interplay among past, present, and future than that reflected in Ajzen and Fishbein's (1970) original model.

As previously mentioned, inability to predict the future may sometimes result from a misconstrual of the future situation or scenario. L. Ross and his colleagues have recently investigated the role of social construals in the accuracy of the confidence that people place in their predictions about the future (Dunning, Milojkovic, & Ross, 1988; Griffin, Dunning, & Ross, 1988; Vallone, Griffin, Lin, & Ross, 1988). In their studies, subjects predicted the actions of their peers, their roommates, and themselves in a variety of hypothetical situations. For example, subjects made yes or no predictions about dropping courses, voting, breaking up with a boyfriend or girlfriend, and calling their parents a certain number of times during the semester. Subjects also indicated probability estimates reflecting their confidence in the accuracy of their predictions. Overconfidence was prevalent; that is, achieved levels of accuracy were far below the levels of confidence expressed. Like other investigators (Lichtenstein, Fischhoff, & Phillips, 1982), Ross and his colleagues demonstrated a lack of accurate calibration between subjective confidence and objective accuracy in predictions. Clearly, because people tend to act on things that they are confident about, overconfidence can be quite costly.

The fact that confidence exceeded accuracy, especially in cases where subjects were highly confident about their predictions, informs us about some of the constraints that may act on people's views of the future. Subjects seem constrained by their expectancies. Alternatives to events and acts that are likely are difficult to generate, and subjects predict that the future will be like the past. They appear to predict a future that is too normal, a future that is less surprising than it actually will be. That is, they predict a future where highly probable events occur too often and improbable events occur too infrequently. Even in attempting to generate random sequences, people fail to stray far enough from what is normal and expected (Kahneman & Tversky, 1972). Inertia prevails. Such a constraint may be related to the role of the anchoring and adjustment heuristic in overestimating the likelihood of high-probability conjunctive events and underestimating the likelihood of low-probability disjunctive events (Bar-Hillel, 1973). Even when the current situation is extreme, people make nonregressive predictions and believe that the world will continue to be as it is (Kahneman & Tversky, 1979).

We have seen how the act of (mis)prediction in itself can direct and determine the future. Similarly, overconfidence in predictions of the future can direct and constrain the future and can keep the future in line with the predictions. However, both in the case of predictions and in the case of overconfidence about the future, this directive and constraining function can occur only in the case of futures over which one has control. For example, predictions about one's own future charitable acts or one's voting behavior, or overconfidence in not breaking up with a boyfriend, can have an impact on these behaviors. However, predictions about the weather or about the outcome of an upcoming boxing match, or predictions about the behavior of others whom one cannot influence, cannot constrain the future. Some kinds of predictions can affect the future indirectly through the process of self-fulfilling prophecy, as when people predict a stock market crash and act in ways that increase the likelihood of a crash. (Over)confidence for controllable versus uncontrollable future events may have different functional consequences. For controllable events, the confidence may be well placed because one can change the future, and overconfidence may simply represent a misperception of how much one really wants to work to bring about a particular future. Overconfidence for uncontrollable events is less justified; rather than having the consequence of altering one's behavior, such overconfidence may simply make one a poor decision maker (as when a person backs out of a parking space without looking because he or she is overconfident that no other cars are coming).

Even though people are overconfident in their judgments of the future, such overconfidence may still lead to futures that are different and that occur more often than would have been the case without the expressions of confidence. Thus, overconfidence can increase the likelihood of circumstances and actions, even though the likelihood of such actions is still below the level of confidence. In addition, the act of expressing one's level of confidence in a prediction may operate above and beyond the act of predicting the future in its effects on determining that future.

Ross and his colleagues interpret their findings of overconfidence as indicating a tendency toward dispositionalism—inferring the dispositions of the actor and overestimating the impact of dispositions relative to situational pressures. In this sense, overconfidence is a result of the fundamental attribution error (Heider, 1958; Jones & Davis, 1965; Ross, 1977), because judges believe that knowing what people are like is reason enough to be very confident in their predictions. In addition, and related to the previously discussed explanation for mispredictions, the studies reporting overconfidence in judgments of the future suggest that subjects made predictions on the basis of construals of what the future would be like and that they failed to make adequate inferential allowance for the great uncertainty that ought to be associated with such construals. This uncertainty about how actors will actually attach meaning to a real situation should be reflected in more conservative confidence estimates, and a failure to do this is the reason for overconfidence (Griffin et al., 1988). Overconfidence related to dispositionalism may also help account for why people are particularly shaken by "uncharacteristic" behavior of someone they know well.

This failure to take into account the many possible construals of the future is related to our previous discussion of veridicality in memory and judgments about the past. In the first place, people rarely consider that their memories of the past may be inaccurate and that there is some likelihood that alternative pasts were actually true. That is, they do not generate several possible pasts, each with an associated likelihood. Rather, people take their memory of the past as what must have happened. In addition, both the past and the future are open to multiple interpretations, and judgments in both cases are subject to the problems of interpretation and appearance. Failure to recognize the possibilities of alternative construals of the past and of the future may lead to overconfidence about them, which can create both intrapersonal and interpersonal problems.

Perhaps people tend to think of the truth in too rigid a way. Believing that there was and is one truth may lead them to view the past as inevitable in hindsight and to have overconfidence in the one truth that will emerge in the future. In actuality, many possibilities are the truth before anything happens. In addition, assigning a high likelihood to an event that actually is highly probable is the truth prior to the occurrence—even if the likely event fails to occur. Similarly, the truth about the past (at least subjectively) should consist of many possibilities, because people should be aware of the likelihood of reconstructions and faded memories. Yet they are all too confident that they know the truth both about the past and about the future.

Moreover, a realization that there are many possibilities in the future means that the truth before an event is quite different from the truth after an event. The judgment of the quality of a decision should not be guided by the outcome that occurs. Good decisions (based on the truth at the time) can end in bad (but a priori unlikely) outcomes. And yet people have a strong tendency to rate the thinking as better, to rate the decision maker as more competent, and to be more willing to yield to future decisions by this person when the outcome is favorable—regardless of the "truth" of the decision prior to outcome knowledge (Baron & Hershey, 1988).

Overconfidence effects may be produced by dispositionalism and a failure to allow for uncertainty associated with situational construal, even when people have little at stake in a prediction. However, it is likely that motivational factors often play a role in overconfidence. For self-prediction items, subjects show overconfidence in the direction of desirable outcomes. For example, subjects are too certain that a current romantic relationship will not end in the near future. Overconfidence in items such as this may result from faulty construals in the service of strong desires. We suspect that most people would be overconfident about not contracting a fatal disease, about not getting divorced, about not having children with birth defects, and about not dying in the near future. In support of this, Weinstein (1980) reported that estimates of the likelihood of contracting diseases such as diabetes or cancer were far too optimistic. Perloff (1983) found similar overoptimism about not developing illnesses such as venereal disease and alcoholism. Subjects were most optimistic about their own lack of vulnerability and were more optimistic about friends than about strangers. Perloff and Fetzer (1986) refer to this effect as the illusion of "unique invulnerability."

These motivations for having a healthy and happy life in the future may lead people to be biased toward imagining and daydreaming about good things in the future (with the exception of depressed people; Alloy & Ahrens, 1987; Crocker, Alloy, & Kayne, 1988; Kuiper & Olinger, 1986). Such biased imaginings may in turn lead to an increase in the accessibility and ease of construction of good futures, and this increased accessibility may then lead to further confidence in good future outcomes. Thus, motivational and cognitive factors may combine to determine the overconfidence that people exhibit in certain predictions of the future. As noted before, such illusions of well-being, although capable of creating problems and disappointments, may be extremely important in keeping people happy and mentally healthy (Taylor & Brown, 1988).

Interestingly, the imaginings of depressed people may also be biased, but in a pessimistic rather than an optimistic way. These biased views of the future may indeed play a role in the etiology and maintenance of depression. In addition, realistic views of the future may prevent depressed individuals from developing the healthy (but unrealistic) optimism of their nondepressed counterparts (Alloy & Abramson, 1979). In support of this, Alloy and Ahrens (1987) reported that depressed individuals made more pessimistic predictions of the likelihood of future outcomes than did nondepressed individuals. In addition, whereas nonde-pressives showed a self-enhancing bias in overestimating probabilities of future success and in underestimating probabilities of future failure, depressives did not show either positive or negative biases in prediction. Differences in social comparison processes and attributional style are implicated in the differences in judgments of the future by depressive and nondepressives. Just as depressed and nondepressed people make different judgments about the future and bias their imaginings of the future in different ways, we have seen parallels in how these populations remember and reconstruct the past. The kinds of autobiographical memories retrieved by depressed people differ from those retrieved by nonde-pressives (Williams & Dritschel, 1988). These biases concerning both the past and the future may be in part responsible for dejection among depressives and healthy optimism among nondepressives.

Faulty perceptions of the future are thus apparent in the effects of imagining and explaining hypothetical future outcomes and in the effects of predicting the future. In addition, these erroneous views of the future, once they emerge, have effects on subsequent behavior and tend to persist. It is difficult to alter such judgments once they are made (Ross, Lepper, & Hubbard, 1975). Interestingly, the one manipulation that seems to be effective in eliminating these errors in judgment concerning the future is the same for cases of overconfidence and for the effects of explaining hypothetical future events. With regard to the former, Griffin et al. (1988) had a group of subjects consider alternative construals of potential future situations. These subjects were far less likely to exhibit overconfidence in their judgments of the future. Similarly, Anderson (1982; Anderson & Sechler, 1986) has demonstrated that the biasing effect of explaining a hypothetical event or a relation between variables can be dramatically reduced by having subjects engage in a counterexplanation task, in which the opposite outcomes or relations are explained. These findings indicate that, in thinking about the future, people generally do not consider the entire spectrum of possible outcomes. It is these failures to entertain the entire space of possibilities that are in large part responsible for subjects' misperceptions of and mispredictions about the future. In the preceding section of the chapter, we have noted that similar failures to recognize the range of possibilities in the past may occur, as when people engage in truncated searches for the causes of past events (Shaklee & Fischhoff, 1982) or fail to consider alternative interpretations of past events. Whether such failures are due to cognitive or motivational factors, some apparently can be remedied by forcing people to think about many possible futures rather than dwelling on the one that is most accessible or most desirable. People may similarly develop a more veridical view of the past from considering alternative versions of past events.

Thoughts about the Self

Although a good deal of our thinking about the future involves the external world around us (e.g., "What will transportation be like in 20 years?" or "What team will be the next football dynasty?") and involves other specific individuals (e.g., "How will the new president change over the next 4 years?"), clearly the bulk of our thinking about the future and our most important thoughts about the future involve the self. We are especially likely to think about our goals and about ourselves approaching and realizing these goals or failing to attain them. According to Markus and Nurius (1986), these goals occasion the construction of "possible selves" that may be different from the present self. Goals will serve as effective guides to present behaviors only if we can create and sustain effective possible selves.

Possible selves are thus our self-generated imaginings of what we could be like in the future. They are, according to Markus and Ruvolo (1989), the future-oriented components of the self-system—"what I might become," "what I would like to become," and, importantly, "what I am afraid of becoming." Possible selves impart structure and meaning to our personal futures in areas that are important to us. As with our other kinds of predictions and imaginings of the future, Markus sees important constraints on our generation of future possible selves. Because possible selves derive from our current involvements, expertise, limitations, and expectations, we are somewhat limited in our ability to imagine certain future possibilities. In addition, recent experiences, moods, or concerns can render different possible selves (e.g., a positive possible self or a feared self) dominant at any moment in time. The ease of imagination of any possible self is also a factor in the strength of representation of that self, in judgments of the likelihood of future possibilities, and in the impact on behavior. Increased subjective probabilities of becoming a possible self in the future should then be associated with increased effort toward realizing that possibility (Feather, 1963; Zajonc & Brickman, 1969).

Possible selves, as imaginings of the self in a future state, are important because of their role in goal-directed action. Thoughts, images, and senses of the self in the future are important cognitive–affective elements that incite and direct goal-relevant action. They are at the heart of motivation and action in the present. In this sense, just as our present self constrains our thoughts about the future, these thoughts about the future, in turn, have important effects on our present thoughts and actions.

Markus and her colleagues have shown some empirical consequences of possible selves. Ruvolo and Markus (in press) used guided imagery to activate either positive or negative possible selves. Subjects were asked to imagine themselves in the future as they succeeded or failed at a task as a result of either luck or hard work. The accessibility of one or the other type of possible self very much affected persistence at a task, as well as time taken to respond to things that would be possible for the self in the future. The similarity of these findings to those of Sherman et al. (1981), discussed earlier, should be noted.

Health researchers have proposed that thoughts and feelings about the future self and the representation of possible selves may play an important role in recovery from mental and physical illness. For example, Simonton, Matthews-Simonton, and Creighton (1978) found positive health effects of imagery in the treatment of cancer (but see Angell, 1985, for an opposing view). Simulating situations in the future can result in feelings of control and optimism. Taylor and Brown (1988) argue that optimism about the future (even unrealistic optimism) is characteristic of normal thought and that these illusions about the future are important for mental and physical health, happiness, and productivity. The existence of possible selves is also extremely important in our ability to cope. Unexpected events (events for which possible selves have not been considered) are the most difficult to cope with. Possible selves serve as a resource when stressful times arrive. They do this in two ways: by preparing us in advance to deal with the stressful situation while maintaining our current identity, and by allowing the easy construction of alternative life possibilities in a time of change, as when a job is lost (Markus, Cross, & Wurf, in press).

In cross-sectional and longitudinal studies of the role of possible selves in delinquency, Oyserman and Markus (in press) reported important differences between delinquent and nondelinquent adolescents. The best predictor of delinquency was the degree of balance in possible selves between hoped-for and expected selves on the one hand and feared selves on the other hand. "Balance" was defined as the extent to which expected positive selves were offset by countervailing feared selves in the same domain (e.g., expecting a well-paying job in the future but fearing unemployment). Delinquent youths had asymmetries in their configuration of possible selves; there was little balance between their expectations and hopes and their fears. This aspect of possible selves was a better predictor of delinquency than were current levels of self-esteem. Again, thoughts and images about the future may exert important effects in motivating current behavior.

With regard to hopes and wishes about the future, Higgins (1989b) has introduced some novel considerations. In his earlier work, Higgins (1987) developed a self-discrepancy model. This model predicts that certain negative affective states result from discrepancies between a person's cognitive representation of his or her actual self and certain self-guides. The self-guides consist of the "ideal" self (hopes, aspirations, and wishes) and the "ought" self (duties, obligations, and responsibilities). In particular, discrepancies between the ideal self and the actual self lead to depression, whereas discrepancies between the ought self and the actual self bring about anxiety.

In his more recent work, Higgins (1989b) considers not only the present state of the self, but a person's thoughts about his or her future selves. The "can" self refers to a person's perception of his or her potential and capability. The "future" self is the person's perception of what he or she will actually become in the future. Higgins considers the implications of relations between the ideal self and the can and future selves. When the ideal is better than the can self, that ideal is a dream, not a potential. When the ideal self equals the can self, the ideal is realistic. Chronic discrepancies between the actual and ideal selves are worse and produce more negative emotions when the ideal self equals the can self than when the ideal self is better than the can self. An unfulfilled potential hurts more than an unfulfilled dream. With respect to the future self, when the ideal self is greater than the future self, the ideal exists as a wish, a desirable end state that one does not expect to attain. When the ideal self is equal to the future self, the ideal exists as a hope, a desirable end state that one expects to achieve. Chronic discrepancies between the actual and ideal selves are worse for hopes than for wishes.

In short, unfulfilled potential and unmet hopes are more closely related to depression than are unfulfilled dreams and unmet wishes. In this way, Higgins has shown that emotional vulnerability is not simply a function of the discrepancy between one's present actual self and ideal self. One's conceptions of and predictions of the future self play a moderating role in causing negative emotional states. These can and future selves are, of course, subject to the same kinds of cognitive and motivational constraints that we have discussed previously.

Thoughts about What Might Have Been

Up to now, we have considered instances in which people think about the future itself. Either because they think about a particular future (as in the work concerning explaining and imagining hypothetical furture events) or because they self-generate potential futures as they plan, set goals, and simply daydream, people have thoughts about what the world will be like in the days and years to come. However, thoughts and feelings about the future and preparations for the future are not always achieved in such a direct way. Often people think about the present or the past, especially about alternatives to how things are or were, and such thoughts affect how they feel and how they think about and prepare for the future. Thinking about the past and present can open up possibilities for the future as well as close such possibilities.

For example, "counterfactuals" are mental simulations of alternatives to preceding and current events (e.g., thoughts about how an automobile accident might have been avoided "if only. . ."). According to Kahneman and Miller (1986), the experienced facts of reality evoke counterfactual possibilities, and the facts of reality are compared to these possibilities. These counterfactuals are postcomputed representations that are not held prior to an event but are generated post hoc. Whereas precomputed representations focus on what was expected or what should have been, postcomputed counterfactuals focus on what might have been (Miller, Turnbull, & McFarland, in press). The accessibility of counterfactuals (or of facts that would ease the generation of certain counterfactuals) is the major determinant of the alternatives to reality that are constructed (Kahneman & Miller, 1986). As such, counterfactuals, like memories of the past and predictions of the future, are determined by the characteristics of the evoking stimulus event and by the momentary mental and physical context in which the event occurs. There are thus clear constraints on the generation of counterfactuals.

In a sense, the past and the future are both alternatives to present reality. Counterfactuals are also alternatives to reality, but they do not necessarily reside in the past, the present, or the future. They are simply other possibilities to events that have happened or are happening. It may even be useful to think about counterfactuals to the future if a particular future seems so likely that it is virtually accepted as truth. Alternatives to expected, hoped-for, and dreaded futures also may be evoked in certain circumstances.

From the point of view of the present chapter, counterfactuals are important because they have implications for feelings, judgments, and future behaviors. Counterfactual generation can prepare us for maintaining our beliefs in the future; for coping with an uncertain, unexpected, or stressful future; and for paving the way for changing in the future.

Some of the work on counterfactual generation suggests that there are constraints on what will be generated. Certain aspects of reality are more easily changed than others in order to arrive at a counterfactual representation. Recent work suggests that exceptional features are more mutable than routine features (Hofstadter, 1985; Kahneman & Tversky, 1982; Wells, Taylor, & Turtle, 1987; but see Wells & Gavanski, 1989, for an alternative view); that changes toward an ideal are more likely than deteriorations (Read, 1985); that alternatives to effects are more easily generated than alternatives to causes (Kahneman & Miller, 1986); that focal items are more mutable than nonfocal items (Read, 1985); and that prior events and primary causes are more mutable than more recent events (Wells et al., 1987).

Aside from the question of which counterfactuals are likely to be generated, other work has addressed the question of the effects of counterfactual generation. In general, emotional responses to an event are more extreme to the extent that counterfactuals that have a very different evaluative impact from that produced by the event itself are easy to generate. Thus, one feels worse about negative events that easily generate positive counterfactuals, and one feels better about positive events that easily generate negative counterfactuals (Gleicher et al., in press; Landman, 1987). Similarly, because it is easier to imagine abstaining from an action than carrying out an action that was not performed, consequences of actions, as opposed to inactions, evoke stronger emotional reactions (Kahneman & Tversky, 1982).

It follows from this work that the abnormality of a victim's fate affects the sympathy and amount of compensation given to the victim, because it is easier to generate alternatives for an abnormal event (Miller & McFarland, 1986). Thus, victims who suffer in abnormal circumstances (e.g., victims who are injured in a store that they rarely frequent, as opposed to one that they often shop in) are extended more sympathy and are compensated more for their victimization. In a related way, people who narrowly miss out on good fortune are derogated—a stronger reaction when actions are exceptional and alternatives come to mind easily (J. T. Johnson, 1986). Finally, factual events are judged as causes to the extent that alternatives to those events that would have led to other outcomes are easily generated (Wells & Gavanski, 1989).

Counterfactuals are thus important in determining affective reactions to actual events and to judgments of responsibility and causality. (Perhaps one reason why we are more angered by betrayals by people we trust than by people we do not trust is that we can so easily imagine trusted people as behaving otherwise.) More than this, counterfactual generation is important because it affects the ways in which we think about the past and about the future. Without considering alternatives to reality, we must accept the past as having been inevitable and must believe that the future will be no different from the past. The generation of counterfactuals gives us flexibility in thinking about possible futures and prepares us better for those futures. Along these lines, Taylor and Schneider (1989) have proposed a theory of coping that focuses on the mental simulation of past, future, and hypothetical events. Such event simulation serves problem-solving and emotion-regulating functions for stressors by increasing the perceived validity of the imagined experiences, providing a framework for organizing experience, and providing a mechanism for mustering helpful emotions. In this way, counterfactual generation and the mental simulation of events can help in coping with ongoing, anticipated, or past stressful events.

It is thus clear that after-the-fact counterfactual reasoning affects feelings and judgments about the past, the present, and the future. Before-the-fact reasoning, in the form of expectancies, hopes, and wishes, likewise affects these feelings and judgments, as we have seen.

Strategies for Seeking and Evaluating Information

Information-gathering strategies in the service of hypothesis testing represent another set of processes in which consideration of the present has important effects on how one thinks about and prepares for the future, and can very much constrain that future. A number of researchers (e.g., Baron, Beattie, & Hershey, 1988; Klayman & Ha, 1987; Snyder & Swann, 1978) have suggested that when people test a hypothesis, they tend to seek out hypothesis-confirming information—information about characteristics that are more likely to be present if the hypothesis is true than if it is false. This preference for information that has a high probability of a positive result given the assumed hypothesis is referred to as "hypothesis confirmation bias" by Snyder and Swann (1978), as "congruence bias" by Baron et al. (1988), and as "positive test strategy" by Klayman and Ha (1987). In addition, subjects seem to seek information about aspects of the hypothesis that are extreme (either extremely likely or extremely unlikely; Skov & Sherman, 1986).

Skov and Sherman (1986) further note that this pattern of information seeking, combined with an insensitivity to the differential information value of various answers to the questions, often leads to overconfidence in the original hypothesis (Slowiaczek, Klayman, Sherman, & Skov, 1989). People thus end up perceiving (at a future time) that the world they originally believed in is actually true—that their hypotheses were well justified. It is interesting to note that our previous discussion of hindsight bias has indicated that people believe, in retrospect, that their views of the world were correct all along. Biases in information seeking and information use further ensure that people will continue to believe in the goodness of their hypotheses in the future. This makes it difficult for people to change their minds or alter their beliefs in the light of subsequent evidence.

These biases in information seeking and use may have both cognitive and motivational components (Higgins & Bargh, 1987; Slowiaczek & Sherman, 1987). People may prefer to seek particular information by asking only certain questions, because the answers to these questions are cognitively easier to process. For example, questions about the hypothesis rather than about the alternative (especially where a "yes" answer confirms the hypothesis) may be easier to process, because fewer transformations of the feedback are necessary for making inferences. It is also possible that certain questions are asked in a motivated attempt to make certain undesirable errors in judgment less likely to occur. That is, one may prefer to ask questions where the false rejection of a desirable a priori hypothesis is far less likely that the false acceptance of this desirable hypothesis.

People not only seek information in a biased fashion, but they may actually try, consciously or unconsciously, to control the "facts." For example, people want to believe that they are healthy now and will remain healthy in the future. They are likely to avoid, defend against, and misinterpret any evidence to the contrary. Thus, even when current objective indicators are unfavorable, people may distort their perceptions in order to maintain their beliefs and wishes about their health. Moreover, they may even try to manipulate the facts of the present in order to allow a belief in a healthy future. For example, a person who is concerned with high blood pressure during a visit to the doctor may try to relax prior to having blood pressure measured and may take several deep breaths. This may temporarily reduce (high) blood pressure, allowing the person to continue to believe in his or her health.

Quattrone and Tversky (1984), in fact, tested such a possibility empirically. In one of their experiments, they had subjects immerse their arms in ice water before and after exercise. Some subjects were led to believe that a long life expectancy was associated with increases in tolerance to ice water after exercise, and some subjects were led to believe that a long life expectancy was associated with decreases in tolerance. As predicted, subjects changed their tolerance in the direction correlated with a long, healthy life. Of course, if subjects had recognized the strategic nature of their behavior, such an action would not have been effective in giving them optimism about the future. When a behavior is chosen simply because it is correlated with (diagnostic of) a favorable future outcome, it should logically yield no information that such a favorable outcome is likely to occur in the future. However, subjects failed to recognize that they had "cheated" on the medical examination, and they deceived themselves into believing that the results of the test were indicators of a better future.

Similarly, Kunda and Sanitioso (1989) have demonstrated that the content of people's self-conceptions at any time is affected by the perceived desirability of various attributes. Subjects who were led to believe that a given attribute (extraversion or introversion) was predictive of academic success saw themselves as having higher degrees of that attribute. The authors argue that motivation provokes such changes in temporary self-conceptions by guiding the memory search to select those aspects of the self that are in fact consistent with a view of self that is predictive of a brighter future.

Kunda (1987) also showed how optimistic health beliefs can be maintained through self-serving biases in the evaluation of evidence. High and low caffeine consumers were told about possible future health risks due to caffeine use. High users were more likely to disbelieve the evidence, especially when the health risks were relevant to their gender and were serious in nature. Thus, it appears that people are motivated to evaluate and believe scientific theories differentially, depending upon the theories' implications for their own future.

Gilovich (1983) has also suggested that people will bias their views of current evidence in order to maintain a desired self-conception in the future. Gamblers represent a population that is consistently confronted with failure, and yet these people persist in gambling and persist in believing that they are competent gamblers and good decision makers. Gilovich analyzed the reactions of winners and losers of a gamble concerning a basketball game. The game involved a salient and important fluke play toward the end of the game. Losers used this play as an explanation for their loss, whereas winners did not attach much importance to the fluke play. Thus, both winning and losing subjects were able to maintain their beliefs in their gambling ability, and this would allow them to gamble confidently in the future. Of course, reconstructions of past gambles and a focus on past wins and successes rather than losses are related ways in which gamblers are able to maintain beliefs in their gambling ability.

It is thus clear that people's explanations and understandings of the present and of the past can help them to prepare for the future, and that these explanations determine how good such preparation will be. These attempts at explanation and understanding have been seen as people engage in generation of counterfactuals (Kahneman & Miller, 1986), as they generate theories to make sense of the world (Kunda, 1987), and as they engage in causal reasoning (Gilovich, 1983; Wells & Gavanski, 1989).

Interestingly, some of these attempts at explanation make people feel worse about a current negative situation but are beneficial for better preparing them for the future, so that similar negative situations are less likely to recur. For example, generating a positive counterfactual to a negative event makes one feel worse about the event (Kahneman & Miller, 1986). However, the realization of positive alternatives should make these positive outcomes more likely in the future. Likewise, the losers in Gilovich's (1983) study who focused on the fluke play no doubt felt worse about their "undeserved" loss; however, such perceptions allowed the maintenance of a positive self-view in the future. Findings concerning the reactions of rape victims (Janoff-Bulman, 1979) and of paralyzed victims of freak accidents (Bulman & Wortman, 1977) make a similar point: Victims who engaged in characterological self-blame ended up coping better with their traumatic experience, although blaming themselves may have made them feel worse about the incident itself. Self-blame gives one a feeling of more responsibility for the current event, but also gives a possibility for personal control of the future— similar events can be avoided.

On the other hand, certain mental constructions and attempts at explanation seem to leave people feeling better about themselves in the present, but perhaps at the cost of leaving them ill prepared to deal with events in the future. Hindsight bias (Fischhoff, 1975) has this flavor. Falsely believing that one understood the present before it occurred makes one feel smart and in control. However, such hindsight bias makes it difficult to learn from mistakes and ensures that one will continue to think about the future in the same error-prone ways. Similarly, Kunda's (1987) subjects who generated theories in a self-serving manner no doubt felt optimistic about the future and enhanced their current good feelings. However, such faulty theory construction may have left them vulnerable to unhappy surprises in the future.

Aside from theory construction and causal reasoning, there are other general processes by which people maintain positive views of the self in the future. Tesser and his colleagues (Tesser, 1986; Tesser & Campbell, 1983) have shown how the motivation to maintain positive self-evaluation guides judgments and guides the interpretation of information. For example, people will reduce the perceived relevance of tasks on which they are outperformed by others. Self-handicapping represents a similar kind of motivational process: Positive but tenuous self-images are sustained in the future by adopting behaviors that can serve as excuses for possible upcoming failures (Arkin & Baumgardner, 1985; Berglas & Jones, 1978). Thus, partying the night before an important exam or taking a performance-inhibiting drug prior to a task allows the maintenance of a positive self-concept in the face of possible failure.

Constraints on Imagined Futures

Most people seem to be motivated to attain or maintain a future self that is healthy, competent, happy, and successful. Subjects have been shown to bias their interpretations of past and current events and even to manipulate the current situation (as in self-handicapping or biased information search) in ways that allow them to maintain beliefs in a happy future and even to make a better future more likely by setting up constraints that will operate on that future. However, we have also seen cognitive processes that are involved in these biases and in the setting of situational constraints. In the first place, even when motives to be happy and healthy in the future lead to certain judgments and biases, people must still be able to make their judgments on the basis of reasonable inferential principles and must be able to maintain an illusion of objectivity about the way in which the judgments are made. The usual cognitive and reasoning processes underlying proper inference and judgment must be maintained. Any effects of the motivations must thus be subtle and difficult for both the self and others to detect. This means that the ability of motivation to have an impact on judgment and inference is constrained by plausibility and reality. Just as people are constrained by plausibility in their constructions and reconstructions of the past, in a similar way they cannot simply envision any old future. There are what we might call "reality-checking" processes that evaluate the reasonableness of imagined futures, just as there are reality-testing processes that evaluate current perceptions and reality-monitoring processes that evaluate memories (Johnson, 1988a).

Reality constrains constructions of the future. In fact, the reality that serves to constrain our generation of possible and likely futures is the past. It is the past that supplies expectancies and determines what is plausible. Without the past and the reality-checking processes that evaluate imagined futures against the backdrop of the past, people could make up and visualize any future. However, without a past, there could be little sense of a future because the feeling of a continuous, coherent, and meaningful life would be gone. Interestingly, dense amnesia may be accompanied by little sense of the future (Tulving, Schacter, McLachlan, & Moscovitch, 1988).

We may thus think of the future as a gradual construction of the past. At any moment in time, we can think about how things will be, based on the constraints set by the past. However, as each new event occurs, it interferes with this evolution of the past into the future and requires that we reconsider and reconstruct the future so that it takes into account the new aspects of the past. The unfolding of events in the present thus alters both our past and our future.

If happy, healthy, and successful futures are thought about more than failures and sad futures (in planning for and preparing for the future), these happy futures are more likely to be accessible. This, in turn, would affect the judgment of the likelihood of such futures through the availability heuristic. Expectancies for happy futures would also be more likely because of the kinds of encouragements and predictions that are made by friends and relatives. Accessability and expectancies can, of course, determine how current situations are interpreted and how situations are selected. In this way, thoughts about the future can affect judgments and behavioral choices in the present. The present may certainly help to determine the future, but thoughts about the future can also help determine the present, which in turn affects the future.

CONCLUSIONS

At any given moment, cognition is driven by vested interests that affect how we seek out and sample information, how we interpret ambiguous evidence, and how we remember it or use it to predict the future. Some of this mental activity is prompted by motives—our hopes, fears, desires, and needs. That is, cognitive processing may be initiated or sustained in the service of particular motives. But in the absence of defined motives, cognition is not disinterested; schemas, expectancies, inferential mechanisms, goals, and so forth constantly nudge processing in some directions at the expense of others.

Although the schemas and expectancies built up from past experience constitute vested interests, it may nevertheless make sense to think of the resulting biases as unmotivated or "purely cognitive." However, according to the conception of past, present, and future discussed here, it may be arbitrary to distinguish between cognitively produced and motivationally produced bias. First, the mechanisms that are involved are the same, whether they are set off by emotionally toned or less emotionally toned agendas. And second, previous motives may have determined which information was sought out and processed in the past. If so, although a particular motive may not currently be operating, we may pay a price in the present for the operation of that motive in the past. Similarly, we may pay a price in the future for the motives operating now. For example, if fear of rejection causes us to encode or remember selectively now, even if the fear of rejection motive later is inactive, certain information will be selectively more accessible because this information was activated earlier. Thus, it is difficult to separate motivated bias from unmotivated bias in remembering the past and anticipating the future, because the effects of motives may project forward and backward in time.

What we can be sure of is that whether or not they are directly or immediately in the service of ongoing feelings or motives, schemas and expectancies profoundly affect our view of the world and our own place in it, because they determine what we will notice at the time of an experience and what will be easily recalled later. In addition, the difference between a largely apperceptive and a largely perceptual focus at the time of an event (or when subsequently thinking about it) may affect how the event is incorporated into memory (e.g., a child's misbehavior may be remembered as another instance of the child's being malicious or as an event providing information about what situations the child does not know how to handle). Thus, how we think about events may determine whether we later have memories that could support specific learning, efforts to repair self-esteem, or a hopeful view of the future, or whether we have a less functional set of memories such as those characteristic of depressed individuals or attempted-suicide patients.

Schemas, expectancies, and apperceptive-perceptual focus are only the beginning of a long list of potential sources of bias in remembering. We are subject to both mood dependence and mood congruity effects. Our recollection of our past is influenced by our current attitudes and our current theories about whether we are changing or stable with respect to a particular domain. Over time, we may drift toward an observer rather than a participant perspective for our recollections, and the perspective we take may have consequences for whether we see our past behavior as determined by traits or by situations. We may confuse information from various sources, falling prey to misleading information effects or hindsight bias. Some of our most far-reaching errors in identifying the source of information come from failures in reality monitoring. We may confuse what we imagined with what happened, or count imagined events in estimates of the frequency of actual events. As is true of other cognitive and motivational bias effects, if such reality-monitoring errors sustain nonfunctional schemas ("I always fail") or stereotypes ("Most men do not care about women"), they operate against us. If they strengthen schemas that promote self-esteem and optimism, they may sometimes actually work to our advantage.

With respect to the future, we are also subject to the consequences of our cognitive and motivational processes. Mispredictions about the future derive from mistakes in reality-checking processes, for example, not taking into account base rate data; overconfidence in the probability of high-probability events; a tendency to overestimate dispositional factors and to underestimate the power of situational factors; a failure to take into account that situations are being construed and that there is much uncertainty associated with such construals; hypothesis-confirming strategies; and failures to consider the possible role of imperfect reality monitoring as we use the past to predict the future (including failures to distinguish what we imagined might happen in the future from what actually happened).

Some evidence suggests that we could judge the past and estimate the future more accurately by thinking of alternatives, thus protecting ourselves from overconfidence or hindsight bias. But there is a potential cost to considering all the alternatives: We lose the comfort of not seeing all the possibilities too clearly. For example, our sense of well-being may partly depend on not fully realizing the true probability of such things as divorce or cancer. On the other hand, realizing true probabilities may get us to behave in ways (e.g., reduce tension, quit smoking) that will protect our mental and physical health. Similarly, thinking of how things might have been (counterfactuals) may increase negative affect for bad outcomes as well as increase positive affect for good outcomes. The risk of experiencing powerful negative feelings generated by counterfactual thinking ("If only I hadn't made that thoughtless remark . . .") may be worthwhile if thinking of how things might have been otherwise generates possible alternatives that can be drawn upon if similar situations should arise again.

Thinking about a possible future increases our subjective likelihood estimates for that future. More important, it may also affect subsequent behavior, such as how long we will stick with a task, whether we will be successful at it, whether we will volunteer time for a cause, how our preferences will change, or whether we will vote. These behavioral effects occur because some predictions seem to act like commitments. Whether an imagined possible future self can operate like a commitment may depend on whether it is a dream (and thus not seen as realistic) or a hope (and thus seen as a possible end state). Because acts (including simply imagining something) that we engage in now may change the future from what it might have been, misprediction may become prediction.

In summary, there is no single truth about what was and what will be. A veridical representation of the past or future is one that depicts the entire space of possibilities, appropriately weighted for corresponding probabilities. It is tempting to see the future as open and the past as fixed. But the already-happened past as remembered consists only of possibilities because of the uncertainty of our own construal of the past, and the yet-to-be past is open to possibilities because we are in the process of constructing it. Conversely, the future may be more fixed than we realize by our failure to see the whole range of possibilities, including the way in which what we do now might reconstruct the future. In this chapter we have suggested some of the ways in which both past and future are open and fixed, and how these qualities of possibility and constraint emerge from an origami-like folding and refolding of past, present, and future as a consequence of cognitive and motivational processes. In this psychological time labyrinth of past, present, and future, our only point of entry is now. What we do now determines what will be the past in the future, and thoughts and actions we take now can reconstruct futures that would otherwise, without our intervention, unfold from the past. As the words from Carly Simon's song "Anticipation" insightfully remind us, the present is the past in the future—"these are the good old days."[6]

Acknowledgments

Preparation of this chapter was supported in part by National Science Foundation Grant No. BNS-8510633 to Marcia K. Johnson and by National Institute of Mental Health Grant No. MH 40058 to Steven J. Sherman. We would like to thank Ed Casey, Shelly Chaiken, Tory Higgins, Ned Jones, Mike Ross, and Dick Sorrentino for helpful comments on an initial draft of this chapter.

Notes

1. Many philosophers have struggled with the problem of time (e.g., see the collection of essays edited by Gale, 1968) and have considered such questions as these: To what does time refer? Are there three categories of time (past, present, and future), or only two (before and after)? Is the present a durationless "knife edge" that connects the past with the future? If there is a present, how long is it? In this chapter, we focus on relations among mental activities (remembering, perceiving, anticipating) that are inextricably linked to the concepts of past, present, and future, and that presuppose the functional importance of temporal concepts for defining an autobiographical self. We also assume that, for individuals, the meanings of past, present, and future are context-dependent (much as what constitutes an "event" is context-dependent; e.g., Hanson & Hirst, 1989; Neisser, 1986). For example, the "present" may refer to "11 A.M.–12 noon" if one is eating lunch, to "today" if one is cleaning the garage, and to "this summer" if one is commenting on the state of Hollywood movies. Similarly, whether a recent event (e.g., an argument) is assimilated to the past or present may depend on whether one is now engaged in related activity (e.g., nagging). Nevertheless, in considering the issue of veridicality, we assume that there is some reality "outside" an individual's mental activities to which the activities may (but do not necessarily) refer. Thus, in one sense, past, present, and future arise from cognitive and motivational processes; in another sense, they stand outside these processes.

2. This chapter is not a comprehensive review of the ways in which cognition and motivation affect our sense of the past, present, and future; nor is it an in-depth critical review of any particular factor. Some of the findings mentioned here are controversial, or hold for some situations but not others. Most of the issues mentioned have already been shown to be complicated or will undoubtedly soon be shown to be complicated. Rather, we draw on ideas and evidence from a variety of sources to illustrate the fundamental inseparability of past, present, and future in determining our thoughts and actions.

3. Similarly, we do not discuss the implications of schema effects for theoretical characterizations of the representation of information in memory. For example, it may be that schemas sometimes

operate by filtering out inconsistent information and not allowing it to be stored in memory at all. Or it may be that there are at least two types of representations generated by experience, one closer to the perceptual facts and another that is the consequence of more reflective processing, including inferences based on schematic knowledge (e.g., Alba & Hasher, 1983; Johnson, 1983; Johnson & Raye, 1981; Johnson-Laird, 1983; van Dijk & Kintsch, 1983). According to the multiple-representation view, which representation will be accessed (and whether we confuse the two) may depend on a number of factors, including the cues available, the goals we have, and the criteria we adopt while remembering.

4. In effect, reality monitoring is a set of processes for evaluating the persuasiveness of memories. As in the case of evaluating the persuasiveness of external messages, reality monitoring involves both "heuristic" and "systematic" processing whose relative contributions depend, in part, on what people regard as a sufficient degree of confidence in their judgments (Chaiken, Liberman, & Eagly, 1989).

5. A "misprediction" is a prediction that turns out to be wrong. A "(mis)prediction" is a prediction that is wrong compared to the performance of control subjects who do not make predictions, but that turns out to be right for the subject making the prediction.

6. Copyright 1971 by Quackenbush Music, Ltd., ASCAP.

References

Abelson, R. P. (1976). Script processing in attitude formation and decision making. In J. S. Carroll & J. W. Payne (Eds.), *Cognition and social behavior* (pp. 33–45). Hillsdale, NJ: Erlbaum.

Abramson, L. Y., & Martin, D. J. (1981). Depression and the causal inference process. In J. H. Harvey, W. Ickes, & R. F. Kidd (Eds.), *New directions in attribution research* (Vol. 3, pp. 117–168). Hillsdale, NJ: Erlbaum.

Alba, J. W., & Hasher, L. (1983). Is memory schematic? *Psychological Bulletin, 93,* 203–231.

Alloy, L. B., & Abramson, L. Y. (1979). Judgments of contingency in depressed students: Sadder but wiser? *Journal of Experimental Psychology: General, 108,* 441–485.

Alloy, L. B., & Ahrens, A. H. (1987). Depression and pessimism for the future: Biased use of statistically relevant information in predictions for self and others. *Journal of Personality and Social Psychology, 52,* 366–378.

Anderson, C. A. (1982). Inoculation and counter-explanation: Debiasing techniques in the perseverance of social theories. *Social Cognition, 1,* 126–139.

Anderson, C. A., & Sechler, E. S. (1986). Effects of explanation and counterexplanation on the development and use of social theories. *Journal of Personality and Social Psychology, 50,* 24–34.

Anderson, R. E. (1984). Did I do it or did I only imagine doing it? *Journal of Experimental Psychology: General, 113,* 594–613.

Angell, M. (1985). Disease as a reflection of the psyche. *New England Journal of Medicine, 312,* 1570–1572.

Arkes, H. R., Blumer, C., & Boehm, L. (1987). *The generality of the relation between familiarity and judged validity.* Unpublished manuscript, Ohio University.

Arkes, H. R., & Freedman, M. R. (1984). A demonstration of the costs and benefits of expertise in recognition memory. *Memory and Cognition, 12,* 84–89.

Arkin, R. M., & Baumgardner, A. H. (1985). Self-handicapping. In J. H. Harvey & G. Weary (Eds.), *Attribution: Basic issues and applications* (pp. 169–202). London: Academic Press.

Ajzen, I., & Fishbein, M. (1970). The prediction of behavior from attitudinal and normative variables. *Journal of Experimental Social Psychology, 6,* 466–487.

Barclay, C. R., & deCooke, P. A. (1988). Ordinary everyday memories: Some of the things of which selves are made. In U. Neisser & E. Winograd (Eds.), *Remembering reconsidered: Ecological and traditional approaches to the study of memory* (pp. 91–125). New York: Cambridge University Press.

Bar-Hillel, M. (1973). On the subjective probability of compound events. *Organizational Behavior and Human Performance, 9,* 396–406.

Baron, J., Beattie, J., & Hershey, J. C. (1988). Heuristics and biases in diagnostic reasoning: II.

Congruence, information, and certainty. *Organizational Behavior and Human Decision Processes, 42*, 88-110.

Baron, J., & Hershey, J. C. (1988). Outcome bias in decision evaluation. *Journal of Personality and Social Psychology, 54*, 569-579.

Bartlett, F. C. (1932). *Remembering*. Cambridge, England:Cambridge University Press.

Beck, A. (1967). *Depression: Clinical, experimental, and theoretical aspects*. New York: Hoeber.

Bem, D. J., & McConnell, H. K. (1970). Testing the self-perception explanation of dissonance phenomena: On the salience of premanipulation attitudes. *Journal of Personality and Social Psychology, 14*, 23-31.

Berglas, S., & Jones, E. E. (1978). Drug choice as a self-handicapping strategy in response to noncontingent success. *Journal of Personality and Social Psychology, 36*, 405-417.

Blaney, P. H. (1986). Affect and memory: A review. *Psychological Bulletin, 99*, 229-246.

Bower, G. H., Black, J. B., & Turner, T. J. (1979). Scripts in memory for text. *Cognitive Psychology, 11*, 177-220.

Bower, G. H., & Mayer, J. D. (1986). Failure to replicate mood-dependent retrieval. *Bulletin of the Psychonomic Society, 23*, 39-42.

Bransford, J. D., & Johnson, M. K. (1972). Contextual prerequisites for understanding: Some investigations of comprehension and recall. *Journal of Verbal Learning and Verbal Behavior, 11*, 717-726.

Bransford, J. D., & Johnson, M. K. (1973). Considerations of some problems of comprehension. In W. Chase (Ed.), *Visual information processing* (pp. 383-438). New York: Academic Press.

Brewer, W. F. (1988). Memory for randomly sampled autobiographical events. In U. Neisser & E. Winograd (Eds.), *Remembering reconsidered: Ecological and traditional approaches to the study of memory* (pp. 21-90). New York: Cambridge University Press.

Brown, A. S., & Murphy, D. R. (1989). Cryptomnesia: Delineating inadvertent plagiarism. *Journal of Experimental Psychology: Learning, Memory, and Cognition, 15*, 432-442.

Bruner, J. S. (1957a). Going beyond the information given. In H. E. Gruber, K. R. Hammond, & R. Jessor (Eds.), *Contemporary approaches to cognition* (pp. 41-69). Cambridge, MA: Harvard University Press.

Bruner, J. S. (1957b). On perceptual readiness. *Psychological Review, 64*, 123-152.

Bulman, R. J., & Wortman, C. B. (1977). Attributions of blame and coping in the "real world": Severe accident victims react to their lot. *Journal of Personality and Social Psychology, 35*, 351-363.

Carmichael, L., Hogan, H. P., & Walter, A. A. (1932). An experimental study of the effect of language on the reproduction of visually perceived form. *Journal of Experimental Psychology, 15*, 72-86.

Carroll, J. S. (1978). The effect of imagining an event on expectations for the event: An interpretation in terms of the availability heuristic. *Journal of Experimental Social Psychology, 14*, 88-96.

Casey, E. S. (1987). *Remembering: A phenomenological study*. Bloomington: Indiana University Press.

Chaiken, S., & Baldwin, M. W. (1981). Affective-cognitive consistency and the effect of salient behavioral information on the self-perception of attitudes. *Journal of Personality and Social Psychology, 41*, 1-12.

Chaiken, S., Liberman, A., & Eagly, A. H. (1989). Heuristic and systematic information processing within and beyond the persuasion context. In J. S. Uleman & J. A. Bargh (Eds.), *Unintended thought* (pp. 212-252). New York: Guilford Press.

Chase, W. G., & Simon, H. A. (1973). Perception in chess. *Cognitive Psychology, 4*, 55-81.

Chiesi, H. L., Spilich, G. J., & Voss, J. F. (1979). Acquisition of domain-related information in relation to high and low domain knowledge. *Journal of Verbal Learning and Verbal Behavior, 18*, 257-274.

Conway, M., & Ross, M. (1984). Getting what you want by revising what you had. *Journal of Personality and Social Psychology, 47*, 738-748.

Crocker, J., Alloy, L. B., & Kayne, N. T. (1988). Attributional style, depression, and perceptions of consensus for events. *Journal of Personality and Social Psychology, 54*, 840-846.

Darley, J. M., & Fazio, R. H. (1980). Expectancy confirmation processes arising in the social interaction sequence. *American Psychologist, 35*, 867-881.

Dunning, D., Milojkovic, J. H., & Ross, L. (1988). *The overconfidence effect in social prediction.* Unpublished manuscript, Stanford University.

Durso, F. T., & Johnson, M. K. (1980). The effects of orienting tasks on recognition, recall, and modality confusion of pictures and words. *Journal of Verbal Learning and Verbal Behavior, 19,* 416–429.

Ebbesen, E. B. (1981). Cognitive processes in inferences about a person's personality. In E. T. Higgins, C. P. Herman, & M. P. Zanna (Eds.), *Social cognition: The Ontario Symposium* (Vol. 1, pp. 247–276). Hillsdale, NJ: Erlbaum.

Eich, E. (1989). Theoretical issues in state dependent memory. In H. L. Roediger III & F. I. M. Craik (Eds.), *Varieties of memory and consciousness: Essays in honor of Endel Tulving* (pp. 331–354). Hillsdale, NJ: Erlbaum.

Eich, E., & Metcalfe, J. (1989). Mood dependent memory for internal versus external events. *Journal of Experimental Psychology: Learning, Memory, and Cognition, 15,* 443–455.

Feather, N. T. (1963). Mowrer's revised two-factor theory and the motive-expectancy-value model. *Psychological Review, 70,* 500–515.

Feltz, D. L., & Landers, D. M. (1983). The effects of mental practice on motor skill learning and performance: A meta analysis. *Journal of Sports Psychology, 5,* 25–57.

Finke, R. A., Johnson, M. K., & Shyi, G. C.-W. (1988). Memory confusions for real and imagined completions of symmetrical visual patterns. *Memory and Cognition, 16,* 133–137.

Fischhoff, B. (1975). Hindsight does not equal foresight: The effect of outcome knowledge on judgment under uncertainty. *Journal of Experimental Psychology: Human Perception and Performance, 1,* 288–299.

Fischhoff, B. (1977). Perceived informativeness of facts. *Journal of Experimental Psychology: Human Perception and Performance, 3,* 349–358.

Fischhoff, B., & Beyth, R. (1975). "I knew it would happen": Remembered probabilities of once-future things. *Organizational Behavior and Human Performance, 13,* 1–16.

Fishbein, M., & Ajzen, I. (1980). *Belief, attitude, intention, and behavior.* Reading, MA: Addison-Wesley.

Foley, M. A., & Johnson, M. K. (1985). Confusion between memories for performed and imagined actions: A developmental comparison. *Child Development, 56,* 1145–1155.

Foley, M. A., Johnson, M. K., & Raye, C. L. (1983). Age-related changes in confusion between memories for thoughts and memories for speech. *Child Development, 54,* 51–60.

Frank, M. G., & Gilovich, T. (1989). Effect of memory perspective on retrospective causal attributions. *Journal of Personality and Social Psychology, 57,* 399–403.

Gale, R. M. (Ed.). (1968). *The philosophy of time.* London: Macmillan.

Gilovich, T. (1983). Biased evaluation and persistence in gambling. *Journal of Personality and Social Psychology, 44,* 1110–1126.

Gleicher, F. H., Kost, K. A., Baker, S. M., Strathman, A., Richman, S. A., & Sherman, S. J. (in press). The role of counterfactual thinking in judgments of affect. *Personality and Social Psychology Bulletin.*

Goethals, G. R., & Reckman, R. F. (1973). The perception of consistency in attitudes. *Journal of Experimental Social Psychology, 9,* 491–501.

Greenwald, A. G. (1980). The totalitarian ego: Fabrication and revision of personal history. *American Psychologist, 35,* 603–618.

Greenwald, A. G., Klinger, M. R., Van de Kamp, M. E., & Kerr, K. L. (1988). *The self-prophecy effect: Increasing voter turnout by vanity-assisted consciousness raising.* Unpublished manuscript, University of Washington.

Greenwald, A. G., Pratkanis, A. R., Leippe, M. R., & Baumgardner, M. H. (1986). Under what conditions does theory obstruct research progress? *Psychological Review, 93,* 216–229.

Gregory, W. L., Cialdini, R. B., & Carpenter, K. M. (1982). Self-relevant scenarios as mediators of likelihood estimates and compliance: Does imagining make it so? *Journal of Personality and Social Psychology, 43,* 89–99.

Griffin, D. W., Dunning, D., & Ross, L. (1988). *The role of construal processes in overconfident predictions about the self and others.* Unpublished manuscript, Stanford University.

Hall, E. G., & Erffmeyer, E. S. (1983). The effect of visuo-motor behavior rehearsal with videotaped modeling of free throw accuracy of intercollegiate female basketball players. *Journal of Sport Psychology, 5,* 343-346.

Hanson, C., & Hirst, W. (1989). On the representation of events: A study of orientation, recall, and recognition. *Journal of Experimental Psychology; General, 118,* 136-147.

Hasher, L., Goldstein, D., & Toppino, T. (1977). Frequency and the conference of referential validity. *Journal of Verbal Learning and Verbal Behavior, 16,* 107-112.

Hasher, L., & Griffin, M. (1978). Reconstructive and reproductive processes in memory. *Journal of Experimental Psychology: Human Learning and Memory, 4,* 318-330.

Hasher, L., Rose, K. C., Zacks, R. T., Sanft, H., & Doren, B. (1985). Mood, recall, and selectivity effects in normal college students. *Journal of Experimental Psychology: General, 14,* 104-118.

Hashtroudi, S., Johnson, M. K., & Chrosniak, L. D. (1989). Aging and source monitoring. *Psychology and Aging, 4,* 106-112.

Hastroudi, S., Johnson, M. K., & Chrosniak, L. D. (1990). Aging and qualitative characteristics of memories for perceived and imagined complex events. *Psychology and Aging, 5,* 119-126.

Heider, F. (1958). *The psychology of interpersonal relations.* New York: Wiley.

Higgins, E. T. (1987). Self-discrepancy: A theory relating self and affect. *Psychological Review, 94,* 319-340.

Higgins, E. T. (1989a). Knowledge accessibility and activation: Subjectivity and suffering from unconscious sources. In J. S. Uleman & J. A. Bargh (Eds.), *Unintended thought* (pp. 75-123). New York: Guilford Press.

Higgins, E. T. (1989b). *Patterns of self-beliefs and suffering.* Paper presented at the Social Psychology Winter Conference, Park City, UT.

Higgins, E. T., & Bargh, J. A. (1987). Social cognition and social perception. *Annual Review of Psychology, 38,* 369-425.

Higgins, E. T., & Rholes, W. S. (1978). "Saying is believing": Effects of message modification on memory and liking for the person described. *Journal of Experimental Social Psychology, 14,* 363-378.

Higgins, E. T., & Stangor, C. (1988). Context-driven social judgment and memory: When "behavior engulfs the field" in reconstructive memory. In D. Bar-Tal & A. W. Kruglanski (Eds.), *The social psychology of knowledge* (pp. 262-298). New York: Cambridge University Press.

Hirt, E. R., & Sherman, S. J. (1985). The role of prior knowledge in explaining hypothetical events. *Journal of Experimental Social Psychology, 21,* 519-543.

Hofstadter, D. R. (1985). *Metamagical themas: Questions for the essence of mind and pattern.* New York: Basic Books.

Isen, A. M. (1984). Toward understanding the role of affect in cognition. In R. S. Wyer & T. K. Srull (Eds.), *Handbook of social cognition* (Vol. 13, pp. 179-236). Hillsdale: NJ: Erlbaum.

Jacoby, L. L., Kelley, C. M., Brown, J., & Jasechko, J. (1989). Becoming famous overnight: Limits on the ability to avoid unconscious influences of the past. *Journal of Personality and Social Psychology, 56,* 326-338.

Janoff-Bulman, R. (1979). Characterological versus behavioral self-blame: Inquiries into depression and rape. *Journal of Personality and Social Psychology, 37,* 1798-1809.

Johnson, J. T. (1986). The knowledge of what might have been: Affective and attributional consequences of near outcomes. *Personality and Social Psychology Bulletin, 12,* 51-62.

Johnson, M. K. (1983). A multiple-entry, modular memory system. In G. H. Bower (Ed.), *The psychology of learning and motivation* (Vol. 17, pp. 81-123). New York: Academic Press.

Johnson, M. K. (1988a). Discriminating the origin of information. In T. F. Oltmanns & B. A. Maher (Eds.), *Delusional beliefs: Interdisciplinary perspectives* (pp. 34-65). New York: Wiley.

Johnson, M. K. (1988b). Reality monitoring: An experimental phenomenological approach. *Journal of Experimental Psychology: General, 117,* 390-394.

Johnson, M. K. (in press). Reality monitoring: Evidence from confabulation in organic brain disease patients. In G. Prigatano & D. L. Schacter (Eds.), *Awareness of deficit after brain injury.* New York: Oxford University Press.

Johnson, M. K., Bransford, J. D., & Solomon, S. K. (1973). Memory for tacit implications of sentences. *Journal of Experimental Psychology, 98,* 203-205.

Johnson, M. K., Foley, M. A., & Leach, K. (1988). The consequences for memory of imagining in another person's voice. *Memory and Cognition, 16,* 337-342.

Johnson, M. K., Foley, M. A., Suengas, A. G., & Raye, C. L. (1988). Phenomenal characteristics of memories for perceived and imagined autobiographical events. *Journal of Experimental Psychology: General, 117,* 371-376.

Johnson, M. K., Kahan, T. L., & Raye, C. L. (1984). Dreams and reality monitoring. *Journal of Experimental Psychology: General, 113,* 329-344.

Johnson, M. K., & Raye, C. L. (1981). Reality monitoring. *Psychological Review 88,* 67-85.

Johnson, M. K., Raye, C. L., Foley, H. J., & Foley, M. A. (1981). Cognitive operations and decision bias in reality monitoring. *American Journal of Psychology, 94,* 37-64.

Johnson, M. K., Raye, C. L., Wang, A. Y., & Taylor, T. H. (1979). Fact and fantasy: The roles of accuracy and variability in confusing imaginations with perceptual experiences. *Journal of Experimental Psychology: Human Learning and Memory, 5,* 229-240.

Johnson, M. K., Taylor, T. H., & Raye, C. L. (1977). Fact and fantasy: The effects of internally generating events on the apparent frequency of externally generated events. *Memory and Cognition, 5,* 116-122.

Johnson-Laird, P. N. (1983). *Mental models: Towards a cognitive science of language, inference, and consciousness.* Cambridge, MA: Harvard University Press.

Jones, E. E., & Davis, K. E. (1985). From acts to dispositions: The attribution process in person perception. In L. Berkowitz (Ed.), *Advances in experimental social psychology* (Vol. 2, pp. 219-266). New York: Academic Press.

Jones, E. E., & Nisbett, R. E. (1971). The actor and the observer: Divergent perceptions of the causes of behavior. In E. E. Jones, D. E. Kanouse, H. H. Kelley, R. E. Nisbett, S. Valins, & B. Weiner (Eds.), *Attribution: Perceiving the causes of behavior* (pp. 79-94). Morristown, NJ: General Learning Press.

Kahneman, D., & Miller, D. T. (1986). Norm theory: Comparing reality to its alternatives. *Psychological Review, 93,* 136-153.

Kahneman, D., & Snell, J. (1988). *Predicting utility.* Unpublished manuscript, University of California-Berkeley.

Kahneman, D., & Tversky, A. (1972). Subjective probability: A judgment of representativeness. *Cognitive Psychology, 3,* 430-454.

Kahneman, D., & Tversky, A. (1979). Intuitive prediction: Biases and corrective procedures. *TIMS Studies in Management Science, 12,* 313-327.

Kahneman, D., & Tversky, A. (1982). The simulation heuristic. In D. Kahneman, P. Slovic, & A. Tversky (Eds.), *Judgment under uncertainty: Heuristics and biases* (pp. 201-208). New York: Cambridge University Press.

Klayman, J., & Ha, Y.-W. (1987). Confirmation, disconfirmation, and information in hypothesis-testing. *Psychological Review, 94,* 211-228.

Kuiper, N. A., & Olinger, L. J. (1986). Dysfunctional attitudes and a self-worth contingency model of depression. In P. C. Kendall (Ed.), *Advances in cognitive-behavioral research and therapy* (Vol. 5, pp. 115-142). New York: Academic Press.

Kunda, Z. (1987). Motivated inference: Self-serving generation and evaluation of causal theories. *Journal of Personality and Social Psychology, 53,* 636-647.

Kunda, Z. (in press). The case for motivated reasoning. *Psychological Bulletin.*

Kunda, Z., & Sanitioso, B. (1989). Motivated changes in the self-concept. *Journal of Experimental Social Psychology, 25,* 272-285.

Landman, J. (1987). Regret and elation following action and inaction. *Personality and Social Psychology Bulletin, 13,* 524-536.

Lichtenstein, S., Fischhoff, B., & Phillips, L. D. (1982). Calibration of probabilities: The state of the art to 1980. In D. Kahneman, P. Slovic, & A. Tversky (Eds.), *Judgment under uncertainty: Heuristics and biases* (pp. 306-334). New York: Cambridge University Press.

Lindsay, D. S. (1987). *Whence comes this memory?* Unpublished doctoral dissertation, Princeton University, Princeton, NJ.

Lindsay, D. S., & Johnson, M. K. (1987a). Reality monitoring and suggestibility: Children's ability to discriminate among memories from different sources. In S. J. Ceci, M. P. Toglia, & D. F. Ross (Eds.), *Children's eyewitness memory* (pp. 92-121). New York: Springer.

Lindsay, D. S., & Johnson, M. K. (1987b). *Thinking about autobiographical events affects subjects' estimates of the number of times they have experienced those events.* Paper presented at the annual meeting of the Eastern Psychological Association, Arlington, VA.

Lindsay, D. S., & Johnson, M. K. (1989). The eyewitness suggestibility effect and memory for source. *Memory and Cognition, 17,* 349-358.

Liu, J., & Steele, C. M. (1986). Attributional analysis as self affirmation. *Journal of Personality and Social Psychology, 51,* 531-540.

Loftus, E. F. (1979). *Eyewitness testimony.* Cambridge, MA: Harvard University Press.

Markus, H. (1977). Self-schemata and processing information about the self. *Journal of Personality and Social Psychology, 35,* 63-78.

Markus, H., Cross, S., & Wurf, E. (in press). The role of the self-system in competence. In R. Sternberg & J. Kolligan (Eds.), *Perceptions of competence and incompetence across the lifespan.* New Haven, CT: Yale University Press.

Markus, H., & Nurius, P. (1986). Possible selves. *American Psychologist, 41,* 954-969.

Markus, H., & Ruvolo, A. (1989). Possible selves: Personalized representations of goals. In L. A. Pervin (Ed.), *Goal concepts in personality and social psychology* (pp. 211-241). Hillsdale, NJ: Erlbaum.

Markus, H., & Zajonc, R. B. (1985). The cognitive perspective in social psychology. In G. Lindzey & E. Aronson (Eds.), *Handbook of social psychology* (3rd ed., Vol. 1, pp. 137-230). New York: Random House.

Marlatt, G. A. (1978). Craving for alcohol, loss of control, and relapse: A cognitive-behavioral analysis. In P. E. Nathan, G. A. Marlatt, & T. Loberg (Eds.), *Alcoholism: New directions in behavioral research and treatment* (pp. 271-314). New York: Plenum.

McCauley, R. N. (1988). Walking in our own footsteps: Autobiographical memory and reconstruction. In U. Neisser & E. Winograd (Eds.), *Remembering reconsidered: Ecological and traditional approaches to the study of memory* (pp. 126-144). New York: Cambridge University Press.

McFarland, C., & Ross, M. (1987). The relation between current impressions and memories of self and dating partners. *Personality and Social Psychology Bulletin, 13,* 228-238.

McFarland, C., Ross, M., & DeCourville, N. (in press). Women's theories of menstruation and biases in recall of menstruation symptoms. *Journal of Personality and Social Psychology.*

Meichenbaum, D. H., & Goodman, J. (1971). Training impulsive children to talk to themselves: A means of developing self-control. *Journal of Abnormal Psychology, 77,* 115-126.

Miller, D. T., & McFarland, C. (1986). Counterfactual thinking and victim compensation: A test of norm theory. *Personality and Social Psychology Bulletin, 12,* 513-519.

Miller, D. T., & Porter, C. A. (1980). Effects of temporal perspective on the attribution process. *Journal of Personality and Social Psychology, 39,* 532-541.

Miller, D. T., Turnbull, W., & McFarland, C. (in press). Counterfactual thinking and social perception: Thinking about what might have been. In M. P. Zanna (Ed.), *Advances in experimental social psychology* (Vol. 23). Orlando, FL: Academic Press.

Minsky, M. (1975). A framework for representing knowledge. In P. H. Winston (Ed.), *The psychology of computer vision* (pp. 211-277). New York: McGraw-Hill.

Moore, B. S., Sherrod, D. R., Liu, T. J., & Underwood, B. (1979). The dispositional shift in attribution over time. *Journal of Experimental Social Psychology, 15,* 553-569.

Neisser, U. (1976). *Cognition and reality: Principles and implications of cognitive psychology.* San Francisco: W. H. Freeman.

Neisser, U. (1986). Nested structure in autobiographical memory. In D. C. Rubin (Ed.), *Autobiographical memory* (pp. 71-81). Cambridge, England. Cambridge University Press.

Nigro, G., & Neisser, U. (1983). Point of view in personal memories. *Cognitive Psychology, 15,* 467-482.

Oyserman, D., & Markus, H. (in press). Possible selves and delinquency. *Journal of Personality and Social Psychology.*

Perloff, L. S. (1983). Perceptions of vulnerability to victimization. *Journal of Social Issues, 39,* 41-61.

Perloff, L. S., & Fetzer, B. K. (1986). Self-other judgments and perceived vulnerability to victimization. *Journal of Personality and Social Psychology, 50,* 502-510.

Peterson, C. (1980). Memory and the "dispositional shift." *Social Psychology Quarterly, 43,* 372-380.

Pichert, J. W., & Anderson, R. C. (1977). Taking different perspectives on a story. *Journal of Educational Psychology, 69,* 309-315.

Pyszczynski, T., & Greenberg, J. (1987). Toward an integration of cognitive and motivational perspectives on social inference: A biased hypothesis-testing model. In L. Berkowitz (Ed.), *Advances in experimental social psychology* (Vol. 20, pp. 297-340). New York: Academic Press.

Quattrone, G. A., & Tversky, A. (1984). Causal versus diagnostic contingencies: On self-deception and on the voter's illusion. *Journal of Personality and Social Psychology, 46,* 237-248.

Raye, C. L., & Johnson, M. K. (1980). Reality monitoring vs. discriminating between external sources of memories. *Bulletin of the Psychonomic Society, 15,* 405-408.

Raye, C. L., Johnson, M. K., & Taylor, T. H. (1980). Is there something special about memory for internally generated information? *Memory and Cognition, 8,* 141-148.

Read, D. (1985). *Determinants of relative mutability.* Unpublished research, University of British Columbia.

Reus, V. I., Weingartner, H., & Post, R. M. (1979). Clinical implications of state-dependent learning. *American Journal of Psychology, 136,* 927-931.

Ross, L. (1977). The intuitive psychologist and his shortcomings: Distortions in the attribution process. In L. Berkowitz (Ed.), *Advances in experimental social psychology* (Vol. 10, pp. 173-220). New York: Academic Press.

Ross, L., Lepper, M. R., & Hubbard, M. (1975). Perseverance in self-perception and social perception: Biased attribution processes in the debriefing paradigm. *Journal of Personality and Social Psychology, 32,* 880-892.

Ross, L., Lepper, M. R., Strack, F., & Steinmetz, J. L. (1977). Social explanation and social expectation: The effects of real and hypothetical explanation upon subjective likelihood. *Journal of Personality and Social Psychology, 35,* 817-829.

Ross, M. (1989). Relation of implicit theories to the construction of personal histories. *Psychological Review, 96,* 341-357.

Ross, M., & McFarland, C. (1988). Constructing the past: Biases in personal memories. In D. Bar-Tal & A. Kruglanski (Eds.), *Social psychology of knowledge* (pp. 299-314). New York: Cambridge University Press.

Ross, M., McFarland, C., Conway, M., & Zanna, M. P. (1983). Reciprocal relation between attitudes and behavior recall: Committing people to newly formed attitudes. *Journal of Personality and Social Psychology, 45,* 257-267.

Ross, M., McFarland, C., & Fletcher, G. J. O. (1981). The effect of attitude on the recall of personal histories. *Journal of Personality and Social Psychology, 40,* 627-634.

Ross, M., & Shulman, R. F. (1973). Increasing the salience of initial attitudes: Dissonance vs. self-perception theory. *Journal of Personality and Social Psychology, 28,* 138-144.

Ross, M., & Sicoly, F. (1979). Egocentric biases in availability and attribution. *Journal of Personality and Social Psychology, 37,* 322-336.

Rothbart, M., Evans, M., & Fulero, S. (1979). Recall for confirming events: Memory processes and the maintenance of social stereotypes. *Journal of Experimental Social Psychology, 15,* 343-355.

Ruvolo, A. P., & Markus, H. (in press). Possible selves and motivation. *Social Cognition.*

Salancik, G. R. (1974). Inference of one's attitude from behavior recalled under linguistically manipulated cognitive sets. *Journal of Experimental Social Psychology, 10,* 415-427.

Sanitioso, R. S. (1989). *Mechanisms of motivated changes in the self-concept.* Unpublished doctoral dissertation, Princeton University.

Schacter, D. L., Harbluk, J. L., & McLachlan, D. R. (1984). Retrieval without recollection: An experimental analysis of source amnesia. *Journal of Verbal Learning and Verbal Behavior, 23,* 593-611.

Schooler, J. W. (1987). *Verbalizing non-verbal memories: Some things are better left unsaid.* Unpublished doctoral dissertation, University of Washington.

Shaklee, H., & Fischhoff, B. (1982). Strategies of information search in causal analysis. *Memory and Cognition, 10,* 520-530.

Sherman, R. T., & Anderson, C. A. (1987). Decreasing premature termination from psychotherapy. *Journal of Social and Clinical Psychology, 5,* 298-312.

Sherman, S. J. (1980). On the self-erasing nature of errors of prediction. *Journal of Personality and Social Psychology, 39,* 211-221.

Sherman, S. J., Cialdini, R. B., Schwartzman, D. F., & Reynolds, K. D. (1985). Imagining can heighten or lower the perceived likelihood of contracting a disease: The mediating effects of ease of imagery. *Personality and Social Psychology Bulletin, 11,* 118-127.

Sherman, S. J., Skov, R. B., Hervitz, E. F., & Stock, C. B. (1981). The effects of explaining hypothetical future events: From possibility to probability to actuality and beyond. *Journal of Experimental Social Psychology, 17,* 142-158.

Sherman, S. J., Zehner, K. S., Johnson, J., & Hirt, E. R. (1983). Social explanation: The role of timing, set, and recall on subjective likelihood estimates. *Journal of Personality and Social Psychology, 44,* 1127-1143.

Simonton, O. C., Matthews-Simonton, S., & Creighton, J. (1978). *Getting well again.* New York: St. Martin's Press.

Skov, R. B., & Sherman, S. J. (1986). Information-gathering processes: Diagnosticity, hypothesis-confirmatory strategies, and perceived hypothesis confirmation. *Journal of Experimental Social Psychology, 22,* 93-121.

Slowiaczek, L. M., Klayman, J., Sherman, S. J., & Skov, R. B. (1989). *Information selection and use in hypothesis testing: What is a good question, and what is a good answer?* Unpublished manuscript, Loyola University of Chicago.

Slowiaczek, L. M., & Sherman, S. J. (1987). *Biases in information seeking and decision making.* Paper presented at the meeting of the Psychonomic Society, Seattle, WA.

Slusher, M. P., & Anderson, C. A. (1987). When reality monitoring fails: The role of imagination in stereotype maintenance. *Journal of Personality and Social Psychology, 52,* 653-662.

Snyder, M., & Cantor, N. (1979). Testing hypotheses about other people: The use of historical knowledge. *Journal of Experimental Social Psychology, 15,* 330-342.

Snyder, M., & Swann, W. B., Jr. (1978). Hypothesis-testing processes in social interaction. *Journal of Personality and Social Psychology, 36,* 1202-1212.

Snyder, M., & Uranowitz, S. W. (1978). Reconstructing the past: Some cognitive consequences of person perception. *Journal of Personality and Social Psychology, 36,* 941-950.

Spiro, R. J. (1977). Remembering information from text: The "state of schema" approach. In R. C. Anderson, R. J. Spiro, & W. E. Montague (Eds.), *Schooling and the acquisition of knowledge* (pp. 137-165). Hillsdale, NJ: Erlbaum.

Strack, F., Schwarz, N., & Gschneidinger, E. (1985). Happiness and reminiscing: The role of time perspective, affect, and mode of thinking. *Journal of Personality and Social Psychology, 49,* 1460-1469.

Suengas, A. G., & Johnson, M. K. (1988). Qualitative effects of rehearsal on memories for perceived and imagined complex events. *Journal of Experimental Psychology: General, 117,* 377-389.

Suinn, R. (1976, July). Body thinking: Psychology for Olympic champs. *Psychology Today,* pp. 38-43.

Sulin, R. A., & Dooling, D. J. (1974). Intrusion of a thematic idea in retention of prose. *Journal of Experimental Psychology, 103,* 255-262.

Taylor, S. E., & Brown, J. D. (1988). Illusion and well-being: A social psychological perspective on mental health. *Psychological Bulletin, 103,* 193-210.

Taylor, S. E., & Crocker, J. (1981). Schematic bases of social information processing. In E. T. Higgins, C. P. Herman, & M. P. Zanna (Eds.), *Social cognition: The Ontario Symposium* (Vol. 1, pp. 89-134). Hillsdale, NJ: Erlbaum.

Taylor, S. E., & Schneider, S. K. (1989). Coping and the simulation of events. *Social Cognition, 7,* 174-194.

Teasdale, J. D., & Fogarty, J. J. (1979). Differential effects of induced mood on retrieval of pleasant and unpleasant memories from episodic memory. *Journal of Abnormal Psychology, 88,* 248-257.

Teasdale, J. D., Taylor, R., & Fogarty, J. J. (1980). Effects of induced elation-depression on the accessibility of memories of happy and unhappy experiences. *Behaviour Research and Therapy, 18,* 339-340.

Tesser, A. (1986). Some effects of self-evaluation maintenance on cognition and action. In R. M. Sorrentino & E. T. Higgins (Eds.), *Handbook of motivation and cognition: Foundations of social behavior* (Vol. 1, pp. 435-464). New York: Guilford Press.

Tesser, A., & Campbell, J. (1983). Self-definition and self-evaluation maintenance. In J. Suls & A. G. Greenwald (Eds.), *Psychological perspectives on the self* (Vol. 2, pp. 1-31). Hillsdale, NJ: Erlbaum.

Tulving, E. (1983). *Elements of episodic memory.* New York: Oxford University Press.

Tulving, E., Schacter, D. L., McLachlan, D. R., & Moscovitch, M. (1988). Priming of semantic autobiographical knowledge: A case study of retrograde amnesia. *Brain and Cognition, 8,* 3-20.

Tversky, A., & Kahneman, D. (1973). Availability: A heuristic for judging frequency and probability. *Cognitive Psychology, 5,* 207-232.

Vallone, R. P., Griffin, D. W., Lin, S., & Ross, L. (1988). *The overconfident prediction of future actions and outcomes by self and others.* Unpublished manuscript, Stanford University.

van Dijk, T. A., & Kintsch, W. (1983). *Strategies of discourse comprehension.* New York: Academic Press.

Voss, J. F., Vesonder, G. T., Post, T. A., & Ney, L. G. (1987). Was the item recalled and if so by whom? *Journal of Memory and Language, 26,* 466-479.

Wahler, R. G., & Afton, A. D. (1980). Attentional processes in insular and non-insular mothers: Some differences in their summary reports about child problem behaviours. *Child Behaviour Therapy, 2,* 25-41.

Weinstein, N. D. (1980). Unrealistic optimism about future life events. *Journal of Personality and Social Psychology, 39,* 806-820.

Wells, G. L., & Gavanski, I. (1989). Mental simulation of causality. *Journal of Personality and Social Psychology, 56,* 161-169.

Wells, G. L., Taylor, B. R., & Turtle, J. W. (1987). The undoing of scenarios. *Journal of Personality and Social Psychology, 53,* 421-430.

Wicklund, R. A. (1989). The appropriation of ideas. In P. B. Paulus (Ed.), *Psychology of group influence* (2nd ed., pp. 393-423). Hillsdale, NJ: Erlbaum.

Williams, J. M. G., & Broadbent, K. (1986). Autobiographical memory in suicide attempters. *Journal of Abnormal Psychology, 95,* 144-149.

Williams, J. M. G., & Dritschel, B. H. (1988). Emotional disturbance and the specificity of autobiographical memory. *Cognition and Emotion, 2,* 221-234.

Williams, J. M. G., & Scott, J. (1988). Autobiographical memory in depression. *Psychological Medicine, 18,* 689-695.

Zajonc, R. B., & Brickman, P. (1969). Expectancy and feedback as independent factors in task performance. *Journal of Personality and Social Psychology, 11,* 148-156.

Zangwill, O. L. (1972). Remembering revisited. *Quarterly Journal of Experimental Psychology, 24,* 123-138.

CHAPTER 15

Feelings as Information
Informational and Motivational Functions of Affective States

NORBERT SCHWARZ

Zentrum für Umfragen, Methoden und Analysen, ZUMA
and University of Heidelberg

A key element in many theories of emotion is the often implicit assumption that "emotions exist for the sake of signaling states of the world that have to be responded to, or that no longer need response and action" (Frijda, 1988, p. 354). Surprisingly, this assumption has received little attention in psychological theorizing about the interplay of affect and cognition. Rather, recent research on emotional influences on cognitive processes has focused primarily on the impact of emotions on the valence of material that is recalled from memory (see Blaney, 1986, and Isen, 1984b, for reviews). Accordingly, studies on the impact of emotional states on reasoning and judgment have been characterized by attempts to trace the observed effects to selective recall.

In contrast to this research tradition, the present chapter focuses on the informative functions of affective states; it is based on the assumption that affective states inform us about the nature of the situation in which they are experienced. The first part of this chapter reviews research on the impact of affective states on evaluative judgments, presenting evidence that is difficult to reconcile with the assumption that emotional influences on social judgment are mediated by selective recall from memory. Rather, the presented research suggests that individuals frequently use their affective state at the time of judgment as a piece of information that may bear on the judgmental task, according to a "How do I feel about it?" heuristic (Schwarz & Clore, 1988). The second part of the chapter extends the informative-functions assumption to research on affective influences on decision making and problem solving, suggesting that affective states may influence the choice of processing strategies. Specifically, it is argued that negative affective states, which inform the organism that its current situation is problematic, foster the use of effortful, detail-oriented, analytical processing strategies, whereas positive affective states foster the use of less effortful heuristic strategies.

HOW DO I FEEL ABOUT IT?: AFFECTIVE STATES
AND EVALUATIVE JUDGMENTS

That our moods may strongly influence how we see the world is a familiar experience to most persons. Not surprisingly, it has been confirmed in a large number of experimental studies. Individuals' affective states have been shown to influence a wide range of evaluative judgments, ranging from satisfaction with consumer goods (Isen, Shalker, Clark, & Karp, 1978) and the evaluation of other persons (Clore, Schwarz, & Kirsch, 1983), selected activities (Carson & Adams, 1980), or past life events (Clark & Teasdale, 1982) to reports of happiness and satisfaction with one's life as a whole (Schwarz & Clore, 1983).

Findings of this type have usually been attributed to the impact of affective states on the recall of valenced material from memory. Specifically, memory research has demonstrated that positively valenced material is more accessible in memory when individuals are in positive rather than in negative moods, whereas negatively valenced material is more accessible when they are in negative rather than positive moods (e.g., Bower, 1981; Isen et al., 1978). Thus, a person who is asked to evaluate a specific target while in a good mood is likely to recall the positive aspects of the target before the negative ones. Because individuals rarely retrieve all the information that is potentially relevant, but rather truncate the search process as soon as enough information has come to mind for them to form a judgment (see Bodenhausen & Wyer, 1987, and Wyer, 1980, for reviews), mood-congruent recall results in a selective data base. Subsequent evaluations, based on the recalled information, are therefore bound to be more positive under more positive moods, because positive information about the target is overrepresented in recall. In addition, the ease with which that information came to mind may lend it additional weight (Tversky & Kahneman, 1974). These assumptions predict mood-congruent judgments to the extent that the judgment is based on material recalled from memory.

The same assumptions can be used to account for differences in the evaluation of people, events, and objects that are new in one's experience, because mood congruency of recall should also influence the accessibility of relevant interpretive concepts. New information, however, is encoded in terms of the most accessible applicable concepts, as has been found in a variety of studies (e.g., Higgins, Rholes, & Jones, 1977; see Higgins, 1989, for a review). Accordingly, the mood-induced differential accessibility of concepts should result in mood-congruent encodings of new information, at least if the newly acquired information is sufficiently ambiguous to allow for different interpretations. Therefore, the target stimulus will be considered more favorably under positive than under negative moods. Finally, the increased accessibility of mood-congruent material in memory may lead to mood-congruent associations that may further influence the evaluation of the target (e.g., Clark & Wadell, 1983).

Although the described logic of mood-congruent recall seems to provide a plausible account for mood-induced differences in evaluative judgments, the accumulating empirical evidence challenges some of the assumptions entailed in this position. On the one hand, mood-congruent recall has been found to be a rather fragile phenomenon that is sometimes difficult to obtain in empirical studies (cf. Blaney, 1986; Bower & Mayer, 1985). Most importantly, mood-congruent recall is most likely to be obtained for self-referenced material, and it is "impossible or difficult to demonstrate when stimulus exposure occurs under sets that are explicitly antithetical to self-referencing" (Blaney, 1986, p. 232). Moreover, mood congruency may be limited to relatively unstructured material and is difficult to find when material is presented in narrative form, such that positive and negative elements are interconnected (Hasher, Rose, Zacks, Sanft, & Doren, 1985; Mecklenbräuker & Hager, 1984) or otherwise well organized (Fiedler, Pampe, & Scherf, 1986). In addition, facilitated recall of *mood-incongruent* material has been observed in some studies (e.g., Laird, Wagener, Halal, & Szegda, 1982; Srull, 1983)—a finding that has been attributed to cue overload (Watkins, 1979): In the absence of additional recall cues, mood states may result in a diffused retrieval of mood-congruent information, rendering mood-incongruent material more distinct. Finally, numerous alternative explanations have been suggested to account for the effects of mood congruency, and a good many inconsistent findings have been reported (see Blaney, 1986, for a review). On the other hand, mood effects on evaluative judgments are rather robust and have frequently shown a pattern that is inconsistent with predictions generated by models of mood-congruent recall.

An alternative account of mood effects on evaluative judgments, one that provides a better fit with the available data, has been suggested by Schwarz and Clore (Schwarz, 1987, 1988; Schwarz & Clore, 1983, 1988). This account was stimulated by previous discussions by Wyer and Carlston (1979) and research on the misattribution of arousal (see Zanna & Cooper, 1976; Zillman, 1978). It focuses on the informative function of affective states in controlled inference processes, rather than on the automatic process of mood-congruent retrieval.

Specifically, it is suggested that individuals may use their perceived affective reactions as relevant information when making evaluative judgments. In fact, some evaluative judgments refer, by definition, to one's affective reaction to the stimulus. For example, when asked how "likeable" Mary is, individuals may interpret this question to refer to their feelings toward Mary. If so, they may not engage in detailed analyses of Mary's behaviors and traits, but may assess their own feelings toward Mary and use them as a basis for judgment. Other evaluative judgments may not refer directly to one's feelings about the target, but may pose a task that is very complex and demanding. Again, the judgmental task may be simplified by assessing one's own feelings about the target. Rather than computing a judgment on the basis of recalled features of the target, individuals may therefore ask themselves, "How do I feel about it?" (Schwarz & Clore, 1988). In doing so, they may mistake feelings due to a pre-existing state as a reaction to the target stimulus, and this may result in more positive evaluations under pleasant than under unpleasant moods.

This assumption generates a number of predictions that cannot be derived from the assumption that mood effects are mediated by selective recall of mood-congruent information. The first, and most important, prediction is that the impact of affective states on evaluative judgments is a function of their perceived informational value. If individuals attribute their current feelings to a source that is irrelevant to the evaluation of the target stimulus, the informational value of their affective state for evaluating the target should be discredited. If so, they should consider their feelings uninformative, and the feelings should not influence their judgments about the target. According to models of mood-congruent recall, on the other hand, the impact of affective states should depend only on the evaluative information retrieved from memory, rather than on information provided by the affective state itself. Therefore, models of mood-congruent retrieval predict that manipulations of the informational value of the affective state itself will not influence its impact on evaluative judgments.

A second prediction holds that the impact of affective states on evaluative judgments should be independent of the event that induced the affective state in the first place, unless this event discredits the informational value of one's feelings for the judgment at hand, as discussed above. In contrast, the mood-congruent recall hypothesis predicts that the more other conditions facilitate selective recall of relevant information, the more pronounced mood effects on evaluative judgments should be. Thus, mood effects should be more pronounced when potentially biasing material is activated *both* by the mood one is in and the event that elicited this mood in the first place. For example, a depressed mood that is induced through thoughts about a serious disease should affect judgments about diseases more strongly than a depressed mood that is induced by other thoughts, because negative information about diseases would be activated by both the content of one's thoughts and one's depressed mood. According to the informative-functions hypothesis, however, the nonemotional content of the mood-inducing stimulus should be irrelevant unless it influences the apparent informational value of the accompanying feelings. Mood effects on evaluative judgments should therefore generalize over a wide range of judgments, independently of whether the thought content associated with that mood does or does not bear on the judgment.

Finally, models of mood-congruent recall hold that mood effects on evaluative judgments should be more pronounced when the mood at the time of judgment matches the mood one was in when one originally acquired the relevant information. This prediction derives from the finding that recall is facilitated by matching mood states at the time of encoding and at the time of retrieval, according to the principles of state-dependent learning (Bower, 1981). By contrast, the hypothesis that affective states serve informative functions does not make this prediction. If individuals consult their feelings as a source of information, the effects of the mood should occur at the time of judgment, irrespective of the mood at the time of encoding.

The available empirical evidence favors the informative-functions hypothesis over the mood-congruent recall hypothesis with regard to all three predictions, as reviewed below.

The Informational Value of Moods and the Implications of Memories: (Mis)Attribution Studies

If individuals use their affective state at the time of judgment as information, the impact of feelings on judgments should depend on their perceived informational value. Feelings that are attributed to a source that is irrelevant to the judgment at hand should not be considered informative; they should therefore be disregarded and should have no effect.

The evidence bearing most clearly on this hypothesis comes from research on the impact of moods on judgments of subjective well-being—that is, judgments of happiness and satisfaction with one's life as a whole (see Schwarz, 1987, and Schwarz & Strack, in press, for detailed discussions). In general, respondents report being happier and more satisfied with their life as a whole when they are in an elated rather than in a depressed mood. For example, subjects who found a dime on a copy machine (Schwarz, 1983), or who were interviewed on sunny days (Schwarz & Clore, 1983, Experiment 2), reported higher well-being than subjects who did not find a dime or subjects who were interviewed on rainy days.

Different theoretical models may account for these findings. From the perspective of mood-congruent recall, subjects in good moods may have recalled more positive information about their lives, as has been reported by Bower and Gilligan (cited in Bower, 1981; see also Clark & Teasdale, 1982; Diener, Larson, & Emmons, 1984). If so, the more positive evaluations may have resulted from selective recall of more positive memories. Alternatively, subjects may have used their feelings at the time of judgment as heuristically relevant information. Facing the complex task of evaluating one's "life as a whole," for which too many facts are potentially relevant and for which judgmental criteria are ill defined, one may simply consider the target ("life as a whole") for a moment, using any affective reactions that result as a guide to an evaluation. When one is using feelings as information in this way, however, it is not generally possible to separate the feelings due to the object of judgment from those due to one's background mood state. Accordingly, feelings that were elicited by the experimental manipulations may be interpreted by subjects to reflect their reactions to the target, resulting in mood-congruent judgments that were *not* mediated by mood-congruent recall.

To test these alternative hypotheses, the perceived informational value of subjects' affective state was manipulated in various studies (Schwarz & Clore, 1983; Schwarz, Servay, & Kumpf, 1985). For example, in the weather study mentioned above (Schwarz & Clore, 1983, Experiment 2), some subjects were induced to attribute their current moods to a transient external source that was irrelevant to the evaluation of their lives. This was accomplished by directing their attention to the weather. In one condition, the interviewers—who collected the data on the telephone—pretended to call from out of town and asked at the beginning of the conversation, "By the way, how's the weather down there?" The idea was that in the process of answering the question (e.g., "It's terrible" or "It's very pleasant"), respondents would link their momentary feelings to the weather, with the result that they would not later see their feelings as a reaction to the process of considering the quality of their lives.

As predicted by the feelings-as-information hypothesis, subjects who were called on rainy days and were induced to attribute their bad mood to the weather reported being as happy and satisfied with their lives as subjects who were called on sunny days. When the weather was not mentioned, however, lower global well-being was reported on rainy than on sunny days. In other words, subjects who felt bad but attributed their momentary feelings to a transient, irrelevant source—namely, the weather—discounted their current affective state in evaluating the quality of their lives as a whole. Subjects who were called on sunny days and who were in a good mood, on the other hand, were not influenced by the situational explanation offered to them. This asymmetry is presumably due to the fact that positive affective states require less explanation than negative ones, as I elaborate in more detail in the second part of this chapter. If no explanation for one's positive feelings is sought to begin with, however, directing subjects' attention to a plausible source of their good mood is unlikely to show any effect.

With regard to the competing theoretical models, the discounting effect (Kelley, 1972) observed under bad-mood conditions clearly supports the hypothesis that affective states may serve informative functions: Facing the complex task of evaluating his or her life as a whole, a person may use whatever feelings are encountered at the time of judgment as an indication of his or her reaction to the question. This should not happen, however, when the informational value of the momentary feelings is called into question. Accordingly, a measure of subjects' current mood, administered at the end of the interview, was more strongly correlated with reported well-being when the weather was *not* mentioned than when it was mentioned. The valence and intensity of subjects' current mood itself, however, was not affected by directing subjects' attention to the weather; this suggests that the attributional manipulation did not influence respondents' current mood itself, but only their inferences based on it.

These findings are incompatible with predictions that can be derived from models of mood-congruent recall. According to these models, subjects who were interviewed on sunny days should have recalled more positive aspects of their lives than subjects who were interviewed on rainy days. Note, however, that attributing one's current feelings to the weather should not affect the evaluative implications of the recalled information. Rather, it should only limit the range of issues about which the feelings seem informative. Accordingly, models of mood-congruent recall would predict a main effect of subjects' affective state, rather than the observed interaction of subjects' mood and the source to which it was attributed. Therefore, the obtained findings render it unlikely that the impact of mood on reported well-being was mediated by selective recall of mood-congruent information, as retrieved models of affect and cognition would suggest.

This point is further supported by a study in which moods were induced by having each subject vividly recall and describe either a positive or a negative life event (Schwarz & Clore, 1983, Experiment 1). Generally, subjects who had to describe negative life events reported lower happiness and satisfaction with their lives as a whole than subjects who described positive events. Again, however, this difference was washed out when subjects who described negative events had a chance to misattribute the resulting negative mood to a transient external source—namely, features of the soundproof experimental room they were in. Under that condition, they reported being as satisfied as subjects who had not described negative events. This finding suggests that subjects did not base their evaluations of their lives on a review of life events, despite the fact that the mood manipulation had rendered a negative event highly salient. Rather, the effect seems to have depended on the informational implications of subjects' current affective states. In line with this assumption, a measure of subjects' current mood was again more strongly correlated with measures of general life satisfaction when their attention was not directed to the experimental room as a possible source of their current feelings than when it was.

In summary, these studies suggest that individuals evaluate their global well-being on the basis of their mood at the time of judgment, unless the informational value of their current feelings for that purpose has been called into question. That the impact of mood did depend on its perceived informational value, as is reflected in the observed discounting effects, is incompatible with models of mood-congruent recall, which hold that the judgment is a function of the evaluative implications of the recalled (mood-congruent) information. The implications of any memories that may have come to mind, however, should not have been affected by the source to which subjects attributed their current feelings. Obviously, this does not imply that mood-congruent recall may not have occurred. Given that recall data were not assessed, this issue cannot be addressed. The pattern of results renders it unlikely, however, that subjects used whatever they may have recalled as a basis of judgment; this parallels other research that suggests a relative independence of memory and judgment (cf. Fiske, Kenny, & Taylor, 1982; Hastie & Park, 1986). This issue is addressed in more detail in a subsequent section of this chapter.

Mood and Thought Content: Generalizing Affective Influences

According to models of mood-congruent recall, mood is just one of a multitude of variables that affects which information is retrieved, and the key variable in mood effects on judgment is the *content* of the retrieved information. Accordingly, mood effects on evaluative judgments should be most pronounced when the mood is induced by thoughts that are relevant to the judgment, because both the content of the mood induction and the mood itself should contribute to an increased accessibility of relevant material in memory. Several studies, however, have failed to confirm this prediction.

For example, in a study by Johnson and Tversky (1983), subjects read reports of negative events (e.g., descriptions of a case of cancer), which presumably induced a depressed and slightly anxious mood. Subsequently, they evaluated a large number of risks as more threatening than did subjects in a good mood. The impact of subjects' mood, however, was independent of the object of judgment or the content by which it was induced. Reading about cancer, for example, had equally strong effects on judgments of the risk of cancer and on judgments of the risk of accidents and divorce. This generalization of effects over dissimilar content domains is incompatible with existing models of mood-congruent recall, but does conform well with predictions derived from the feelings-as-information hypothesis.

According to this hypothesis, individuals who face the difficult task of evaluating unknown risks may cope with the judgmental task by consulting their current feelings. If they feel depressed and anxious, they may conclude that the risk they are asked to evaluate is indeed depressing and threatening, and may then evaluate it as being more severe than they would under a more elated mood. Note that this assumption predicts that the impact of the affective state should be the same for all judgments to which the state is relevant, regardless of the content by which the mood was induced. Mood effects should only be absent when subjects attribute their feelings to the story they read, which discredits the feelings' general informational value, as discussed in the context of the misattribution studies reported earlier.

Similar content-free generalizations of mood effects were observed in a study (Clore et al., 1983) that induced positive or negative moods through guided fantasies either about a pleasant or an unpleasant date (an interpersonal theme) or about a pleasant or an unpleasant vacation (a noninterpersonal theme). Subsequently, subjects read ambiguous passages either about another person (interpersonal theme) or about a vacation (noninterpersonal theme), modeled after materials used by Higgins et al. (1977). It was hypothesized that if mood states increase the accessibility of mood-congruent concepts, ambiguously described stimuli should be encoded in more positive terms in good moods than in bad moods. Moreover, it was thought that this effect should be more pronounced when the nonemotional cognitive content of the mood-inducing fantasy was relevant to the ambiguous description than when it was not. Accordingly, models of mood-congruent encoding and recall would predict additive effects of the quality of the mood and the thematic similarity of the fantasy and the ambiguous passage.

Such additive effects, however, were not obtained. Rather, subjects evaluated both the person and the vacation resort more positively when they were in a good rather than a bad mood, regardless of the content of the fantasy through which their mood was induced. Thus, their evaluations reflected only their mood at the time of judgment, as predicted by the hypothesis that feelings serve informative functions.

Mood at Encoding and Mood at Judgment: What's Crucial?

Following the rules of state-dependent learning, mood-congruent recall has been found to be most pronounced when the mood at encoding matches the mood at retrieval (Bower, 1981). If mood effects on evaluative judgments are mediated by mood-congruent recall, they should show the same pattern. If evaluative judgments are based on the implications of the mood state itself, however, rather than on the implications of any information that may be recalled from memory, mood effects on judgment should only be a function of the mood at the time of judgment, and the encoding mood should prove largely irrelevant.

In a study that addressed this issue (Clore, Parrott, & Wilkin, 1989; Schwarz & Clore, 1986), positive or negative moods were induced through vivid recall of a positive or a negative life event under hypnosis. Subsequently, subjects read an ambiguous person description and reported, in a forced-choice format, which traits of four pairs of traits best characterized the stimulus person. Not surprisingly, subjects in a negative mood chose more negative traits than subjects in a positive mood.

Following this first judgment, subjects were again hypnotized and put into a good or bad mood through the recall of another life event; this resulted in a design that crossed mood at the time of encoding (and first judgment) with mood at the time of retrieval (and second judgment). After completion of the second mood induction, subjects reported how well each of the traits presented earlier described the stimulus person.

According to models of mood-congruent recall, the information that subjects retrieve from memory should reflect their mood at the time of encoding. This should have been particularly likely in the present study, because subjects had already provided a first judgment at the time of encoding. Moreover, selective recall should be enhanced if the retrieval mood matches the encoding mood. In contrast to these predictions, however, the second judgment showed no impact of encoding mood whatsoever. Rather, it reflected only subjects' mood at the time of the second judgment, with subjects in a good mood evaluating the target person more positively than subjects in a bad mood. Thus, both judgments at Time 1 and judgments at Time 2 were solely a function of the mood the subjects were in at the time the respective judgments were made.

In combination with the previous findings, these results suggest that subjects did not engage in a detailed analysis of the evaluative implications of each piece of information presented about the target. Rather, they simplified the judgmental task by consulting their current feelings to determine whether the target person was likeable or not. Consistent with this conclusion, Fiedler et al. (1986) found pronounced effects of mood on judgments of liking, without any evidence for mood-congruent retrieval of information about the stimulus person, in their recall data.

Global Moods and Specific Emotions: Some Important Differences

Although the studies reviewed above demonstrate that global mood states serve informative functions, it is assumed that the same logic holds for specific emotions. However, some important qualifications may apply, as is suggested by a consideration of the characteristics of global moods and specific emotions.

The Informational Value of Moods and Emotions

A central characteristic of mood states is their diffuse and unfocused quality (cf. Clore, 1985; Ewert, 1983), which sets them apart from specific emotions. In contrast to moods, emotions are specific reactions to particular events. Most importantly, they have an identifiable cause, a sharp rise time, and a relatively short duration. Moods, on the other hand, may result from a series of mildly pleasant or unpleasant events, none of which needs to be sufficiently intense to produce an emotion by itself, but which collectively leave one in a generalized positive or negative feeling state. Moods, therefore, do not always have easily identifiable causes. They may come about gradually, and they tend to last longer than emotions. Moreover, a mood may develop as the residue of a specific emotion, once the emotion's intensity dissipates and its cause is no longer in the focus of attention (Bollnow, 1956). Thus, the cause of a mood tends to be more remote in time than the cause of an emotion and tends to be less clearly defined for the experiencer. These characteristics are reflected in our use of language that implies specific references for emotions, but not for global moods. Thus, we say that we are afraid "of" something and angry "about" something, but that we are "in" a happy or sad mood.

It is this undifferentiated and unfocused nature of mood states that renders them informative for a wide variety of different judgments. In fact, when subjects are induced to attribute their moods to specific causes—as in the weather experiment, described above (Schwarz & Clore, 1983)—the impact of mood on judgments that are unrelated to that source vanishes. These considerations suggest that the informational value of specific emotions is more restricted than the informational value of global moods (Clore, 1985). Given that the source of an emotion is more likely to be in the focus of attention, one's emotional feelings may be more likely to be attributed (correctly) to a specific event. This should reduce their potentially biasing role in judgments that are unrelated to this event.

This hypothesis is nicely supported by a study by Keltner and Audrain (1988, Experiment 2). Following our research (Schwarz & Clore, 1983), these authors induced a sad mood by having subjects vividly recall a negative life event. Subsequently, some subjects were asked to describe "what emotions" they currently felt, whereas others indicated where and when the negative event had taken place. Compared to the latter group, those subjects who had to label their current feelings with specific emotion terms were considerably less affected by the mood manipulation and reported significantly higher life satisfaction, despite being in a depressed mood. In a related study (Keltner & Audrain, 1988, Experiment 1), describing one's current emotions was at least as effective in reducing the impact of a sadness-inducing hypothetical event as was misattributing one's sad feelings to the experimental room. In combination, these studies suggest that labeling their current feelings with specific emotion terms induced subjects to identify specific causes for their current feelings, thus rendering the feelings uninformative for subsequent evaluative judgments that did not pertain to these specific causes.

A particularly interesting implication of this analysis is that specific emotions may be unlikely to affect unrelated judgments shortly after their onset, when the event that elicited them is still salient. Rather, their more general impact may be expected after the emotion dissipates, leaving the individual in a diffuse mood, as described by Bollnow (1956). This possibility awaits further research. Note, however, that these considerations do not imply that specific emotions would not serve informative functions; they only emphasize that their informational value is likely to be more restricted.

Misattributing Fear

That specific emotions do affect judgments to which they are relevant has, in fact, received empirical support. For example, in a study on the misattribution of fear (Schwarz et al., 1985), heavy smokers were exposed to a fear-arousing movie that vividly portrayed the negative side effects of smoking. Relative to a control group that was not exposed to the movie, subjects who saw the movie reported a stronger intention to cut down on the number of cigarettes they smoked. This intention was less pronounced, however, when subjects could misattribute their affective reactions to a placebo pill that was said to have arousing side effects. Subjects who were informed that the pill had tranquilizing side effects, on the other hand, reported a stronger intention to reduce smoking than subjects who did not expect side effects of the pill. In addition, daily self-reports of the number of cigarettes smoked over a 2-week period following the experiment still showed a significant impact of the misattribution manipulation.

These discounting and augmentation effects (see Kelley, 1972) suggest that subjects used their affective reactions to the movie as a basis for evaluating the described risk, resulting in the perception of the highest risk when they experienced arousal "despite" being tranquilized, and in the perception of the lowest risk when they could attribute their arousal to the pill.

Note, however, that the induced fear was relevant to the judgmental task—namely, evaluating the risks involved in heavy smoking. That is, fear is an affective reaction that carries with it information about the degree of perceived risk (Ortony, Clore, & Collins, 1988). Accordingly, judgments of risk should be influenced when made in the presence of fearful feelings, as the study of smokers indicated. For other judgments, however, feelings of fear may not be considered informative.

This assumption is supported by research on the differential impact of fear and anger (Gallagher & Clore, 1985). Whereas fear carries information about risk, anger involves in part disapproving of someone else's blameworthy action (Ortony et al., 1988). In line with this reasoning, Gallagher and Clore (1985) found that hypnotically induced feelings of fear affected judgments of risk but not of blame, whereas feelings of anger affected judgments of blame but not of risk. Thus, the induced emotions influenced evaluative judgments relevant to that specific emotion, but not evaluative judgments in domains relevant to a different emotion.

In combination, the findings reviewed in this section suggest that the impact of specific emotions is more limited than the impact of global moods. First, emotions usually have a clear referent, thus rendering them uninformative for judgments that do not pertain to this referent, as is suggested by the Keltner and Audrain (1988) findings. Second, specific emotions provide specific types of information (e.g., information bearing on risk or blameworthiness), thus rendering them uninformative for judgments that pertain to a different dimension. If a specific emotion is used as the basis for judgment, however, its impact follows the logic of discounting and augmentation, as has been shown for global moods.

When Are Judgments Based on One's Affective State Rather than on Other Information?

Now that considerable evidence has been reviewed for the informative functions of affective states, this question arises: Under which conditions are individuals likely to use the information that their feelings provide? That is, when do individuals follow a "How do I feel about it?" heuristic, and when are they likely to engage in more effortful, retrieval-based strategies?

That individuals base evaluative judgments on the information provided by their feelings seems particularly likely under the following four conditions: (1) when the judgment at hand is affective in nature (e.g., liking for another person); (2) when little other information is available; (3) when the judgment is overly complex, and cumbersome to make on the basis of a piecemeal information-processing strategy; and (4) when time constraints or competing task demands limit the cognitive capacity that may be devoted to forming a judgment. Whereas the first two variables pertain to the availability of competing information, the latter two pertain to processing load. Each of these aspects is discussed in turn before their implications for retrieval-based models of judgment are assessed.

Availability of Competing Information

A judgment that refers explicitly to how one feels about the object of judgment renders one's feelings highly relevant. Accordingly, it is not surprising that judgments of liking and preference have been found to be strongly influenced by respondents' feelings (cf. Clore & Byrne, 1974; Zajonc, 1980). Moreover, one's feelings are sometimes the only source of information that may be available to assist in forming a particular judgment. Suppose, for example, that subjects in an experiment are asked to evaluate whether an unknown Chinese ideograph means something good or something bad. Given the absence of any useful knowledge about the ideograph, subjects may be likely to turn to their affective response, asking themselves, "How do I feel about it?" If they encounter positive feelings, they may conclude that the ideograph may mean something positive, unless they have reason to doubt the informational value of their feelings.

In line with this reasoning, Zajonc (1989) found that subjects attributed a more positive meaning to Chinese ideographs when the ideographs were preceded by smiling rather than by frowning faces, which presumably elicited positive or negative affective reactions. However, this effect was only obtained when subjects' exposure to the smiling or frowning faces was subliminal, thus ensuring that subjects were unaware of the source of their affective reaction. Under supraliminal exposure conditions, subjects apparently attributed their affective reaction correctly to the facial stimuli, thus rendering it uninformative for evaluating the Chinese ideographs. This finding clearly coincides with other research reviewed in the present chapter, in illustrating that judgments may be based on individuals' affective states rather than on any specific features of the to-be-evaluated stimulus. This finding does *not* imply, however, that "preferences need no inferences," as the subtitle of Zajonc's (1980) paper suggested. As the preceding sections of this chapter have indicated, consulting one's affective state and determining its informational value for the judgment at hand are highly inferential strategies, which may result in augmentation and discounting effects as described by the most "reasoned" models in social-cognitive research, although these inferential steps may not necessarily be accessible to introspection (see Nisbett & Wilson, 1987).

In summary, one's apparent affective reaction to the object of judgment may be the most relevant information in making certain judgments, either because the judgment refers to one's feelings or because one's feelings are the only information available.

The latter argument also suggests that the impact of individuals' affective state decreases as the accessibility of competing information increases. The available evidence is in line with this assumption. For example, Srull (1983, 1984) reported that subjects' mood influenced their evaluations of unfamiliar, but not of familiar products. Moreover, the impact of the information provided by one's mood may be a function of the relative salience of one's mood and of competing information. Accordingly, we (Strack, Schwarz, & Gschneidinger, 1985, Experiments 2 and 3) observed that subjects who provided short, nonemotional reports of a past life event used this event as a standard of comparison, resulting in contrast effects on judgments of current life satisfaction. Subjects who had to report a past life event in an emotionally involving style, on the other hand, relied on the elicited mood state in evaluating their current life satisfaction, resulting in assimilation effects. This pattern of findings has been replicated in the area of relationship satisfaction (Collins & Clark, 1989). In combination, these findings suggest that other sources of information may be ignored in the presence of a salient mood state.

Processing Load

Although the discussion above suggests that individuals may consult their feelings because of a lack of other relevant information, they may also do so because too much information is available. In that case, asking oneself how one feels about the object of judgment may provide an efficient heuristic that greatly simplifies the judgmental task and limits the demands on cognitive capacity.

In line with this assumption, we (Schwarz, Strack, Kommer, & Wagner, 1987, Experiment 1) found pronounced mood effects (as a function of the outcome of games of the West German national soccer team) on judgments of general life satisfaction, but not on judgments of satisfaction with specific life domains, such as one's income. This is presumably due to the facts that evaluative criteria for specific life domains are well defined and that comparison information is easily available, whereas the evaluation of one's life as a whole requires a multitude of comparisons along many dimensions with ill-defined criteria (cf. Schwarz & Strack, in press). Thus, the more complex the judgmental task was, the more likely subjects were to rely on their feelings at the time of judgment.

In a related study, inducing a good or bad mood by testing subjects in a pleasant or an unpleasant room (Schwarz et al., 1987, Experiment 2) resulted in mood effects on judgments of general life satisfaction, but in contrast effects on judgments of housing satisfaction. This suggests that subjects evaluated their lives as a whole on the basis of their mood (resulting in *lower* life satisfaction in the unpleasant than in the pleasant room), but evaluated their housing satisfaction on the basis of salient comparison information provided by the room (resulting in *higher* housing satisfaction in the unpleasant than in the pleasant room). Again, this finding indicates that reliance on one's affective state may increase with increasing complexity of the task.

In addition, the notion that using one's feelings as information may simplify complex judgments according to a "How do I feel about it?" heuristic predicts that the less relevant a judgment is, the fewer consequences it has, and the higher the time pressure under which it is made, the more pronounced mood effects should be (cf. Kruglanski, 1980). Similarly, competing processing demands, which limit the available cognitive capacity, should increase reliance on this heuristic, as has been shown with regard to the use of other heuristics (see Sherman & Corty, 1984). These implications await further research.

On the Relationship of Recall and Judgment

As emphasized previously, the findings reviewed in the present chapter are incompatible with models that assume that mood effects on evaluative judgments are mediated by mood-congruent memory (e.g., Bower, 1981; Clark & Isen, 1982; Isen, 1984b). The results of the reported misattribution experiments cannot be accounted for by these models, and the impact of moods on evaluative judgments has been shown to be unaffected by variables that are likely to affect selective recall. As noted before, however, this does not necesssarily imply that models of mood-congruent recall are inadequate as models of *recall*. Rather, these findings simply suggest that evaluative judgments may frequently not be based on recalled information (see Schwarz, 1987, for a more detailed discussion).

As many authors have noted, the relationship between evaluative judgments and the recall of information upon which these judgments are presumably based is frequently weak (e.g., Anderson & Hubert, 1963; Bargh & Thein, 1985; Carlston & Skowronski, 1986; Dreben, Fiske, & Hastie, 1979; Lingle & Ostrom, 1979). This is usually interpreted to indicate that subjects are recalling a judgment that was made "on-line"—that is, at the time the relevant information was received, rather than at the time they are asked to report the judgment to the researcher (cf. Hastie & Park, 1986; Lichtenstein & Srull, 1985). Accordingly, the *currently* recalled behaviors may not be the ones that served as a basis of judgment in the first place, and this may result in weak relationships between both measures.

The present findings suggest, however, that the distinction between "on-line" and "retrieval-based" judgments is not exhaustive. Rather, there is a third type of judgment, which is based neither on on-line processing of features of the target nor on any retrieved features of the target. Specifically, evaluative judgments may be based on potentially unrelated information (such as one's own affective state) that is considered heuristically relevant. These "heuristic-based" judgments are likely to reduce the relationship between recall and evaluation even more than "on-line" judgments, given that their informational basis may potentially be *completely unrelated* to features of the object of judgment, as one might expect in the case of the weather (Schwarz & Clore, 1983), dime (Schwarz, 1983), or soccer (Schwarz et al., 1987) experiments discussed earlier.

Judgments as Recall Cues?

Finally, it is worth noting that a reversal of the generally assumed influence of affective states on the retrieval of valenced information is conceivable. As a considerable body of social cognition research indicates (see Martin & Clark, in press, for a review), individuals may use previously formed judgments as a basis for subsequent ones, independently of the information on which the judgment was originally based (e.g., Carlston, 1980; Lingle & Ostrom, 1979). More importantly, they may also use a judgment as a retrieval cue for reconstructing the information that presumably provided the basis of judgment in the first place, as was recently demonstrated by Higgins and colleagues (Higgins & Lurie, 1983; Higgins & Stangor, 1988).

Applied to the present reasoning, this raises the possibility that individuals' affective state may influence their evaluative judgments, which in turn may serve as mood-congruent retrieval cues, resulting in mood-congruent recall. To use one of Bower's (1981) examples, individuals who are asked to recall events from their kindergarten days may first ask themselves, "Well, kindergarten days. What were they like?" In doing so, they may form a global evaluation that is based on their current mood, as described above. Facing the task to report specific episodes, they may then use this global evaluation as a retrieval cue to guide the recall of specific information, resulting in an increased recall—or reconstruction—of mood-congruent information.

One important implication of this reasoning is that mood effects on recall should only be obtained under conditions that give rise to mood effects on evaluative judgments in the first place. Accordingly, misattribution manipulations of the type we used (Schwarz & Clore, 1983) should eliminate the impact of moods on the recall of mood-congruent information from memory. Although experimental tests of this possibility are not yet available, it is conceivable that variations in the perceived informational value of one's mood may underlie the inconsistent findings in the literature on mood-congruent memory.

Conclusions

In summary, the research reviewed in the first part of this chapter has demonstrated that affective states may serve informative functions, and that individuals may form evaluative judgments on the basis of their feelings. In doing so, however, they may misread feelings that were elicited by other causes as affective reactions to the object of judgment, resulting in more positive evaluations in the presence of positive rather than negative feelings. The assumption that feelings serve as information implies that the information that is provided by them is processed in the same way as any other piece of information is. In line with this assumption, the reviewed research indicates that the information provided by one's feelings is only used in making evaluative judgments if it is relevant to the judgment at hand, and if its informational value is not discredited. Accordingly, mood effects were not obtained when respondents were induced to attribute their current mood to a transient, external source, thus calling its diagnosticity into question (e.g., Schwarz & Clore, 1983; Schwarz et al., 1985). Moreover, moods have been found to influence a wide variety of evaluative judgments (e.g., Johnson & Tversky, 1983), whereas the information provided by specific emotions appears to be more specific, thus limiting the range of judgments likely to be influenced (e.g., Gallagher & Clore, 1985; Keltner & Audrain, 1988). In addition, the impact of affective states has been found to decrease as the salience (Collins & Clark, 1989; Strack et al., 1985) or amount (Schwarz et al., 1987; Srull, 1983, 1984) of other information relevant to the judgment at hand increases.

Although these findings have repeatedly been contrasted to predictions derived from mood-congruent recall models, it is also important to highlight their relationship to other, more closely related approaches. Most obviously, the present approach builds, both theoretically and experimentally, on previous misattribution research. Some of this research addressed the influence of perceived context on the interpretation of physical arousal (Schachter & Singer, 1962), whereas other research explored the impact of physical arousal on attitudinal judgments (e.g., Zanna & Cooper, 1974). In general, the latter research indicated that physical arousal will only influence judgments if the object of judgment is seen as the source of arousal. Although the original accounts for this finding were couched in somewhat different terms—they were related either to a dissonance framework (see Zanna & Cooper, 1976, for a review) or to an excitation transfer framework (see Zillman, 1978, for a review)—they indicate that perceived physical arousal will only influence evaluative judgments if its informational value for the respective judgment is not discredited.

The "feelings-as-information" approach presented in the present chapter is clearly compatible with these previous lines of research and extends this work in several ways. Most importantly, the work by Zanna, Cooper, and colleagues, as well as that by Zillman and colleagues, was primarily concerned with the subjective experience of arousal (often in the context of dissonance motivation), rather than the implications of the valence of the experienced state (but see Higgins, Rhodewalt, & Zanna, 1979, for an exception). Although the research procedures were tailored to discredit the implications of arousal states, the informational value of these states was not explicitly elaborated. Accordingly, this line of research did not invite differentiations between moods and emotions, explorations of the specific informational value of different affective states, or their linkage to information processing in general. This difference in focus reflects general differences in the theoretical orientation of social psychology in the early 1970s and the mid-1980s (see Markus & Zajonc, 1985). This becomes particularly apparent in the second part of this chapter, which addresses the impact of affective states on strategies of information processing.

AFFECTIVE STATES AND THE CHOICE OF PROCESSING STRATEGIES

So far, the discussion of the informative functions of affective states has focused on the impact of feelings on evaluative judgments. However, the informational value of one's affective state may be more fundamental than the preceding discussion of evaluative judgments may suggest. As many authors have pointed out (e.g., Arnold, 1960; Frijda, 1988; Higgins, 1987; Oatley & Johnson-Laird, 1987; Ortony et al., 1988), different affective states are closely linked to different psychological situations. In Nico Frijda's words (1988, p. 349), "emotions arise in response to the meaning structures of given situations, [and] different emotions arise in response to different meaning structures." In general, "events that satisfy the individual's goals, or promise to do so, yield positive emotions; events that harm or threaten the individual's concerns lead to negative emotions" (p. 349).

If we extend these arguments, it seems plausible to assume that the relationship between emotions and the "meaning structures" that constitute a "psychological situation" (Higgins, 1987) is bidirectional: Different psychological situations result in different emotions, but the presence of a certain emotion also informs the individual about the nature of his or her current psychological situation. At a general level, one may assume that a positive affective state informs the individual that the world is a safe place, one that does not threaten the person's current goals. That is, positive feelings tell the person that the current situation is characterized neither by a lack of positive outcomes nor by a threat of negative outcomes. Negative affective states, on the other hand, inform the individual that the current situation is problematic, and that it is characterized either by a lack of positive outcomes or by a threat of negative outcomes—a distinction that is elaborated on below. If this is so, one's affective state can serve as a simple but highly salient indicator of the nature of the situation one is in.

To the extent that individuals are motivated to obtain positive outcomes and to avoid negative ones, negative emotions do therefore inform the individual that some action needs to be taken. Positive emotions, on the other hand, may not signal a particular action requirement. Indeed, empirical evidence indicates that different emotions are associated with different states of action readiness; these are evident in physiological changes (e.g., Lacey & Lacey, 1970; Obrist, 1981) and overt behavior (e.g., Ekman, 1982; Izard, 1977), as well as in introspective reports (e.g., Davitz, 1969; Frijda, 1986, 1987). This evidence supports the assumption that "emotions exist for the sake of signaling states of the world that have to be responded to, or that no longer need response and action" (Frijda, 1988, p. 354).

The remainder of this chapter relates these considerations to a variety of differences in information processing that have been observed under the influence of positive and negative affective states. However, the reader should be fore-warned: Although the evidence bearing on the informational value of affective states for evaluative judgments is fairly persuasive, the following discussion of differences in processing strategy goes far beyond any data given.

Affect, Motivation, and Information Processing

The significance of the above-described considerations for information processing derives from the assumption that different psychological situations, reflected in different affect states, require different information-processing strategies.

If positive affective states inform the individual that his or her personal world is currently a safe and satisfactory place, the individual may see little need to engage in cognitive effort, *unless* this is required by other currently active goals. In pursuing these goals, the individual may also be willing to take some risk, given that the general situation is considered safe. Thus, simple heuristics may be preferred to more effortful, detail-oriented judgmental strategies; new procedures and possibilities may be explored; and unusual, creative associations may be elaborated. Accordingly, the thought processes of individuals in a positive affec-tive state may be characterized by what Fiedler (1988), borrowing a term from George Kelly (1955), has called "loosening."

By contrast, if negative affective states inform the individual about a lack of positive outcomes or a threat of negative outcomes, the individual may be moti-vated to change his or her current situation. Attempts to change the situation, however, initially require a careful assessment of the features of the current situation, an analysis of their causal links, detailed explorations of possible mechanisms of change, and anticipation of the potential outcomes of any action that might be initiated. Moreover, individuals may be unlikely to take risks in a situation that is already considered problematic, and may therefore avoid simple heuristics as well as novel solutions. Accordingly, their thought processes may be characterized by what Fiedler (1988) has termed "tightening"; again, the term is borrowed from Kelly (1955).

In summary, these considerations suggest that individuals' thought processes are tuned to meet the requirements of the psychological situation that is reflected in their feelings. Conceptually related to this argument, Heckhausen, Gollwitzer, and their collaborators (see Gollwitzer, Chapter 2, this volume, for a review) have shown that different motivational states, conceptualized in the context of a comprehensive action theory, elicit different "mind-sets" that are tuned to the requirements of the respective state. This tuning assumption has interesting implications for individuals' thoughts about the affect-eliciting situation, as well as for their performance on unrelated tasks. For the sake of simplicity, the following discussion of these implications focuses on the contributions of affective states; the impact of third variables, such as higher-order goals, is addressed in a later section.

Affective States and Event-Related Thoughts

Focus of Attention

As a first hypothesis, it follows that individuals in a negative affective state should be more likely to focus their attention on features of the situation that elicited their feelings. In fact, a large body of literature indicates a narrowing of attentional focus under negative affect (see Broadbent, 1971; Bruner, Matter, & Papanek, 1955; Easterbrook, 1959; Eysenck, 1976). As a recent example, Wegner and Vallacher (1986) observed that failures to obtain a desired outcome are more likely to elicit attention to details of one's action strategy than are successful actions.

In addition, one may expect individuals in a situation that elicits negative affect to be less likely to encode incidental information, and less likely to get distracted by other tasks. Consistent with this assumption, Fuhrman and Ostrom (1989) observed that subjects in a person memory experiment paid more attention to information that elicited a pronounced negative reaction, and presumably spent more time thinking about it, as had previously been observed by Fiske (1980) for negative person information in general. As a consequence, Fuhrman and Ostrom's subjects had excellent memory for the affect-eliciting information as well as related items, but missed subsequently presented information that was unrelated to the affect-eliciting items.

Finally, negative affect may also be accompanied by an increased readiness to engage in effortful strategies to obtain information that is relevant to the situation at hand. Although the available empirical evidence that bears on these hypotheses is scarce, the hypotheses are clearly testable.

Causal Reasoning

In addition, one may assume that individuals in a negative affective state are more likely to engage in causal reasoning about the affect-eliciting event than are individuals in a positive affective state. Such an asymmetry has repeatedly been observed in the attribution literature. Specifically, it has been found that negative events, which elicit negative feelings, are more likely to trigger causal explanations than are positive events (e.g., Abele, 1985; Schwarz, 1987; Weiner, 1985b; Wong & Weiner, 1980). In line with this assumption, the misattribution experiments reviewed above (Schwarz & Clore, 1983) revealed that subjects who were in a bad mood were more likely to search for a situational explanation of their mood than subjects in a good mood were; this resulted in the observed asymmetric impact of positive and negative moods on evaluative judgments.

In a related study (Schwarz, 1987, Experiment 9), college students who were asked to describe a positive or a negative life event were more likely to provide unelicited causal explanations for negative (38%) than for positive (18%) events. Moreover, if a causal explanation was offered, it was provided earlier in the description if the event was negative (specifically, after 10.2 words) than if the event was positive (after 41.0 words); this suggests that causal explanations are more accessible in the cognitive representation of negative rather than positive events.

However, findings of this type are difficult to interpret because of a natural confound of valence and expectancy: As many attribution theorists have noted, unpleasant events are seen as less likely than pleasant ones in everyday life. Accordingly, the subjective probability of the event and its hedonic quality are naturally confounded. The unexpectedness of an event, however, has been found to trigger causal explanations in its own right (see Hastie, 1984, for a review). To isolate the contribution of both variables, we (Bohner, Bless, Schwarz, & Strack, 1988) conducted a laboratory experiment that provided independent manipulations of the subjective probability of an event and its hedonic valence. Specifically, the subjects received either success or failure feedback about their performance on an ostensible "professional skills test." In addition, the subjective probability of success was varied by informing subjects that either 23% or 77% of a comparable student population had met the criterion. Following success or failure feedback, subjects were asked to write down everything that came to mind, and finally provided a direct rating of the intensity with which they tried to explain their test result.

These manipulations produced pronounced main effects of the valence of the outcome: As predicted by the current analysis, the number of possible reasons that subjects spontaneously reported for the outcome was greater after negative than after positive feedback, *regardless* of the outcome's a priori probability. In addition, subjects reported a higher intensity of causal reasoning after negative than after positive feedback. Additional correlational analyses indicated that the number of causal explanations reported, as well as the intensity ratings, increased with increasing negativity of subjects' current affective state.

In summary, these findings indicate that subjects were more likely to explain a negative event, which elicited negative feelings, than to explain a positive event, which elicited positive feelings. Given that the probability of the outcome was held constant, these findings demonstrate that the valence of the event, and its accompanying affective reaction, constitute a determinant of the degree of causal reasoning in their own right.

At a more general level, Holyoak and Nisbett (1988, p. 61) have observed that "people make inferences only when there is some triggering condition. An event or relationship must be problematic, unexpected, or at least interesting, before people begin to make inferences." The present argument holds that experiencing negative feelings may be one of the conditions informing individuals that an event or relationship is "problematic," and may thus serve as a triggering condition.

Generalization to Other Tasks

So far, the reviewed evidence has pertained to subjects' reasoning about the situation that elicited the affective state to begin with. Although this is interesting in its own right, it also raises the more intriguing possibility that the impact of affective states may generalize to other tasks that individuals work on while in that state. Why might such a generalization occur?

On the one hand, the discussion above suggests that different affective states may elicit different motivations (see Schaller & Cialdini, Chapter 8, this volume, for a related discussion). Most importantly, individuals in a negative state, for whom the situation is already defined as problematic, may be more motivated to avoid (additional) negative outcomes and less willing to engage in "risky" strategies than individuals in a positive affective state, for whom the current situation is defined as safe. In fact, individuals in an elated mood have been found to be more optimistic about future events than individuals in a depressed mood (e.g., Forgas & Moylan, 1987; Johnson & Tversky, 1983; Masters & Furman, 1976), to (erroneously) perceive more control over their current environment (e.g., Alloy & Abramson, 1979; Alloy, Abramson, & Viscusi, 1981), and to be more willing to take moderate risks (e.g., Isen, Means, Patrick, & Nowicky, 1982).

In addition to changes in individuals' motivational state, affective states may influence the cognitive accessibility of procedural knowledge in memory. If one assumes that analytic reasoning is helpful in handling negative situations, it should be highly adaptive if the negative affective states accompanying these situations increase the cognitive accessibility of relevant procedural knowledge. This should increase the speed with which adequate procedures can be applied to the negative situation. Moreover, it should decrease response competition between various applicable procedures, thus reducing the likelihood that other potentially applicable but less effective procedures will be selected.

However, any mechanism increasing the accessibility of analytic procedures to facilitate their application to the affect-eliciting situation may also increase the accessibility of the same procedures per se, resulting in a higher likelihood that they will be applied to *any* task to which they are applicable (see Higgins, 1989, for a review of research on accessibility effects). Accordingly, subjects in a bad mood should be more likely to apply analytic processing strategies to cognitive tasks that they work on while in that mood than subjects in an elated mood should be. Evidence from diverse areas of research is compatible with these assumptions.

Information Seeking

If being in a bad mood informs individuals that their current situation is problematic, it may increase their willingness to engage in effortful information seeking, and it may tune their attention to more diagnostic information. The current evidence bearing on this assumption is limited to depressed individuals, who are chronically in a bad mood. For example, in a study on social information gathering, Hildebrand-Saints and Weary (1989) observed that mildly depressed college students asked more highly diagnostic questions of their interaction partners than nondepressed college students did. Moreover, they did so independently of whether they expected having to answer subsequent questions about their interaction partner or not, whereas nondepressed subjects only asked highly diagnostic questions if that seemed useful for a later task. The authors assume that "this heightened information seeking and utilization are motivated by depressives' attempts to reduce the uncertainty and lack of control which accompanies their depression" (Marsh & Weary, 1989, p. 326). According to the present argument, simply being in a negative affective state may elicit the same motivation, regardless of individuals' chronic depressive state, although data bearing on this hypothesis are not yet available.

Focus of Attention and the Encoding and Organization of Information

With regard to the finding that negative events elicit a narrower focus of attention, the generalization hypothesis would predict that information that is encoded while the person is in a bad mood will be categorized more narrowly and stored in smaller chunks than information that is encoded while the person is in a good mood. Several studies bear on this prediction. For example, Leight and Ellis (1981) found that a depressed mood inhibited chunking, resulting in decreased recall of nonsense words. Conversely, Isen, Daubman, and Gorgoglione (1987) reported increased chunking and increased recall performance under positive mood.

As Isen (1984a, p. 535) observed, "positive affect results in an organization of cognitive material, such that either more or broader, more integrated, categories" are used. For example, items that are not generally considered good exemplars of a category (e.g., "cane" as a member of the category "clothing") were more likely to be assigned to that category by subjects in an elated mood than by subjects in a nonmanipulated mood (Isen & Daubman, 1984). Similarly, subjects in an elated mood were found to sort stimuli into fewer groupings, again suggesting the use of broader categories (Isen & Daubman, 1984). Related research by Sinclair (1988), conducted in a performance appraisal paradigm, confirmed that subjects in an elated mood used broader categories than subjects in a neutral mood, and indicated that subjects in a depressed mood categorized different performance behaviors most narrowly. Moreover, this narrow categorization elicited by a negative mood resulted in more accurate performance appraisals and less evidence for halo effects.

A particularly interesting example of encoding differences was reported by Fiedler et al. (1986), who crossed elated and depressed moods with memory and impression formation instructions in a person memory experiment. Although impression formation instructions usually result in increased recall, due to the organization format of the resulting representation (cf. Hamilton, Katz, & Leirer, 1980), Fiedler et al. observed an interaction of instructions and mood state: "Recall performance was superior when positive mood was combined with impression formation instructions, and when negative mood was combined with memory instructions" (Fiedler, 1988, p. 105). Presumably, the narrower focus of attention under negative mood, resulting in narrower categorizations, inhibited the organization of the material under impression formation instructions, but facilitated the effortful learning of the material under explicit memory instructions.

Analytic Reasoning

The propensity of negative affective states to elicit a higher degree of causal, analytic reasoning has repeatedly been observed to generalize to unrelated tasks that individuals work on while in a negative mood. For example, individuals in experimentally induced bad moods (e.g., Schwarz, Kommer, & Lessle, 1988), as well as subjects in naturally depressed moods (e.g., Alloy & Abramson, 1979) were found to provide more accurate contingency assessments than individuals in elated moods—a finding that has become known as "depressive realism" (see Ruehlman, West, & Pasahow, 1985, for a review). Although this finding is usually attributed to the impact of chronically or temporarily accessible depressive schemata, the finding that depressed moods facilitate covariation detection under conditions that are neither self-referential nor control-related suggests that it may be mediated by processing style rather than by the impact of depressive schemata.

For example, Sinclair (1987, Experiment 2) had subjects estimate correlation coefficients from scatterplots presented to them. He found that subjects in a depressed mood provided the most accurate estimates and subjects in an elated mood the least accurate ones, with subjects in a nonmanipulated mood falling in between. He concluded that "elated subjects are taking less care, processing more heuristically, [and] making more errors" (p. 16). Subjects in a depressed mood, on the other hand, "may process in a more algorithmic manner, leading to narrower categorization, weighing of more information, and less error in judgment" (p. 18). Consistent with this assumption, he found in a related study (Sinclair, 1988) that subjects in a depressed mood considered more information in making performance appraisals than did subjects in an elated mood, with subjects in a nonmanipulated mood again falling in between. Moreover, the performance appraisals provided by depressed subjects corresponded more closely to the number of positive or negative behaviors presented than did the performance appraisals provided by elated subjects; this suggested that elated subjects may "form sweeping global impressions," whereas depressed subjects may "assess more facts and make more discrete judgments" (p. 39).

In line with the assumption of more analytic and algorithmic processing under the influence of depressed moods, Fiedler and Fladung (1986; cited in Fiedler, 1988) observed that subjects in an induced bad mood produced fewer logical inconsistencies in a multiattribute decision task than subjects in a good mood. Specifically, the good-mood subjects, by producing inconsistent triads of the form "A > B and B > C, but A < C," were twice as likely to violate the transitivity of preference as the bad-mood subjects were.

Moreover, in the domain of persuasion research, individuals in depressed moods were shown to pay more attention to the quality of persuasive arguments. Specifically, they were influenced by strong but not by weak arguments. Individuals in a good mood, on the other hand, were equally persuaded by strong and by weak arguments, and cognitive response measures indicated that they were less likely to elaborate the quality of the arguments (Bless, Bohner, Schwarz, & Strack, in press; Worth & Mackie, 1987). In fact, subjects in a good mood only paid attention to the quality of the arguments when they were explicitly instructed to do so, whereas individuals in a bad mood did so spontaneously (Bless et al., in press, Experiment 1). Accordingly, introducing a distractor task inhibited message elaboration under bad-mood conditions, but not under good-mood conditions; this suggested that subjects in a good mood did not engage in extensive message elaboration to begin with (Bless et al., in press, Experiment 2).

Closely related to these findings, research on the impact of affective states on helping behavior (see Schaller & Cialdini, Chapter 8, this volume, for a review) suggests that individuals in a depressed mood base their helping decisions on a careful consideration of the involved costs and benefits. By contrast, subjects in an elated mood seem to take a less considered approach to helping, and have been shown to be relatively unaffected by perceived costs and benefits (e.g., Manucia, Bauman, & Cialdini, 1984; Weyent, 1978).

In combination, this diverse set of findings (see Fiedler, 1988, for additional examples) strongly suggests that being in a depressed mood increases, and being in an elated mood decreases, the likelihood of a more analytic, careful, and deliberate processing of the available information.

Creativity

So far, it seems that the hypothesis that negative affective states increase the cognitive accessibility of analytical reasoning procedures, as well as individuals' motivation to engage in these effortful procedures, can well account for increased analytic reasoning under negative affect. But how about the other side of the coin? It has also been observed that individuals in a good mood are more creative than individuals in a bad mood. For example, they were found to be better at solving Dunker's candle problem and to generate more unusual associations (see Isen, 1987, for a review).

If positive affective states inform individuals that no particular action is required by the current situation, they may be unlikely to activate any specific procedure. Accordingly, no response hierarchy that is tuned to the current situation may be elicited, and different procedures may be equally accessible. If so, individuals in a good mood may be more likely to access a diverse range of procedures, and to apply them in combination, than individuals in a bad mood may be. Moreover, if elated moods are associated with a wider focus of attention than negative moods, individuals in an elated mood may also draw upon a wider range of semantic and episodic knowledge. The combination and application of diverse strategies and heterogeneous knowledge bases, however, is exactly what is usually considered to be at the heart of creative problem solving (cf. Martindale, 1981; Mednick, 1962). In addition to these automatic influences of knowledge accessibility, persons in a good mood may be less likely to consciously constrain themselves, because their affective state informs them that their current environment is safe, and thus allows them to take the risk that is associated with novel solutions.

Individuals in a bad mood, on the other hand, may be more constrained in both respects. At the level of access to diverse procedural, semantic, and episodic knowledge, the problem-oriented set that is presumably activated by being in a bad mood may inhibit the accessibility of other bodies of knowledge (see Higgins & King, 1981, for a general discussion of temporary and chronic accessibility). At the motivational level, being in a bad mood may also reduce individuals' willingness to engage in risky novel solutions, in a situation that is already defined as problematic. Thus, mood-induced differences in creativity may also be plausibly accounted for in the current framework.

When Are Tuning Effects to Be Observed?

Do the arguments above imply that one should *always* find improved analytic performance when individuals are in a bad mood, and impaired analytic performance when they are in a good mood? Day-to-day experience suggests otherwise, rendering it necessary to consider conditions that seem incompatible with the predictions offered above. Regarding improved analytic performance in a bad mood, the two exceptions that seem most likely to come to mind pertain (1) to interference effects of negative affect and (2) to the apathy inherent in severe depression. In addition, exceptions to most hypotheses can be readily constructed by referring to the impact of other currently active goals that may interfere with the hypothesized processes. Each of these possibilities is considered in turn.

Processing Capacity

To the extent that handling the affect-eliciting situation binds a considerable degree of subjects' cognitive capacity, performance on unrelated tasks is likely to be inhibited. Given that negative situations need more attention than positive ones, this has been most clearly demonstrated for negative affect (see Easterbrook, 1959; Lazarus, 1966). Note, however, that this condition may be unlikely to be met in experimental studies, in which affective states are typically induced by vivid imagery of fictitious events, feedback on already completed tasks that may not be repeated, and similar procedures that foreclose real opportunities to change the negative situation eliciting one's feelings. Studies that vary the functionality of thoughts about the mood-inducing event are therefore obviously needed, but are not yet available. Most importantly, the impact of affective states on performance on unrelated tasks needs to be compared under conditions that do and do not allow subjects to change the affect-eliciting situation.

Similarly, some situations may require that individuals control their affective state itself, or at least their social display of their affective experiences. Again, this task may bind considerable cognitive capacity, resulting in impaired cognitive performance on *other* tasks. Unfortunately, experimental studies on the impact of affect control on performance on unrelated tasks are not available. However, regarding individuals' thoughts about the negative event itself, the available evidence suggests that an analytic reasoning style may not only serve to explain the event, but may also reduce its emotional impact. As different lines of research have demonstrated (see Schwarz, 1987, for a more detailed discussion), the emotional experience is less intense if individuals' processing style is characterized by a preponderance of analytic thoughts rather than vivid images (e.g., Leyens, Cisneros, & Hossey, 1976; Spiesman, Lazarus, Mordkoff, & Davidson, 1964; Strack et al., 1985). Accordingly, attempts to analyze one's feelings are likely to reduce their intensity, as James (1890/1950, p. 451) noted.

The Apathy Inherent in Severe Depression

Regarding cognitive performance under severe clinical depression, clinical experience as well as the literature on depressive realism (see Ruehlman et al., 1985) suggest that severe depression, in contrast to being in a "depressed mood," is *unlikely* to improve analytic performance. It is interesting to note, however, that phenomenological studies of the subjective experience of severe depression (see Tölle, 1982, p. 232 ff., for a review) indicate that the experience of "sadness" or of "being in a bad mood" is *not* part of the melancholic state that characterizes severe depression. As Lehmann (1985) noted, "persons who are deeply depressed cannot feel the sadness they used to be capable of feeling. . . . Although feeling an intolerable oppression, these persons tend to be incapable of normal grief or of feeling normal concern" (pp. 792–793). It is thus conceivable that the subjective experiences accompanying severe depression are different in nature from the "normal" negative affective states considered in the present chapter. Moreover, these experiences are likely to endure over very long periods of time with limited variation, and may therefore lose whatever informational value they may have had at their onset.

Finally, it is important to note that working on a task is a necessary prerequisite for any differences in performance to be manifested. If the individual does not engage in the task to begin with, as is likely to be the case under severe depression, any increased accessibility of adequate procedural knowledge, for example, will be of little value.

Currently Active Goals

However, aside from the specific issues raised above, it is obviously possible to construct plausible exceptions for most of the hypotheses offered. For example, an author who is trying to meet the deadline for a chapter revision may attempt to remain in an analytic processing mode, despite being in a good mood as a result of other events. It seems, however, that these counterexamples usually pertain to the potential impact of current goals that an individual may pursue. It is therefore important to acknowledge that other currently active goals or task requirements may override the impact of affective states. Of course, this possibility is highly compatible with the functionality assumption that underlies the present line of argument. Note, however, that one should expect an asymmetric impact of positive and negative states in this regard. If positive feelings inform the individual that no action is needed, overrriding this message because of other action requirements poses no problem. By contrast, if negative feelings inform the individual about current problems, ignoring this message would not be adaptive. Accordingly, one may expect that the impact of negative feelings on processing style will be more immune to the influence of other variables than the impact of positive feelings. Again, this implication remains to be tested.

Moreover, the short-term and long-term effects of positive and negative experiences need to be distinguished to avoid misleading conclusions. The arguments presented earlier suggest, for example, that a success that is accompanied by feeling good may decrease analytic processing while the person is in an elated mood, but this argument certainly does not imply that the person may not engage in analytic efforts to obtain additional successes. It seems likely, however, that these efforts will be invested after the most intense positive feelings dissipate, or that these feelings will be experienced as less intense once the individual engages in new efforts.

Specific Emotions and the Cognitive Asymmetry of Approach and Avoidance Situations

So far, the discussion has focused on the consequences of global "positive" or "negative" affective states. However, the present approach easily lends itself to the analysis of specific emotions; it suggests that a particular emotion's cognitive effects can be predicted on the basis of an analysis of the meaning structure that underlies the emotion (see Ortony et al., 1988; Stein & Levine, 1987), and the action requirements that are associated with it.

A particularly interesting possibility is suggested by Higgins's (1987) distinction between "agitated" and "dejected" negative emotions. According to his analysis, agitated negative states, such as fear, threat, anger, or edginess, result from a threat of negative outcomes. In contrast, dejected negative states, such as sadness or disappointment, result from a lack of positive outcomes. Accordingly, agitated states should be associated with a motivation to *avoid* negative outcomes, whereas dejected states should be associated with a motivation to *approach* positive outcomes.

Approach and avoidance situations, however, are characterized by a basic asymmetry in the amount of analytic reasoning that they require. When we want to obtain a certain positive outcome, it is usually sufficient to determine *one* of the many possible ways of obtaining the desired outcome. Knowing one way that is accessible to us guarantees that we will obtain the positive outcome, regardless of whether other ways do or do not exist. When we want to avoid a certain outcome, on the other hand, we need to determine *all* possible causal links that may produce this outcome in order to avoid it. Being aware of just one process that may bring about the negative outcome, and being able to block it, do not eliminate the threat as long as other processes may produce the same negative event. Thus, we need to determine *all* processes that may generate the negative outcome, and for all of them we need to find appropriate ways to block or to escape their impact. Accordingly, approach and avoidance situations show a natural asymmetry in the degree of analytic reasoning that they require (see Lewicka, 1986, for a related argument).

If so, it is conceivable that agitated negative affective states, which are usually associated with an avoidance motivation, are more likely to trigger an elaborate analytic processing style than are dejected negative affective states, which are usually associated with approach motivations; this may particularly be the case when avoidance in the form of leaving the field is impossible and an immediate response is not required. Moreover, one may assume that agitated negative states focus individuals' attention on information that is relevant to an avoidance motivation—namely, information that pertains to blocking or escaping a negative outcome—whereas dejected negative states focus their attention on information that is relevant to an approach motivation. Unfortunately, the experience of agitated and dejected states has been shown to be an interaction effect of situational and individual variables (cf. Higgins, 1987), and studies tailored to provide sensitive tests of the present hypotheses within this framework are not yet available.

Conclusions

In summary, the considerations offered in the second part of this chapter, and the limited evidence that bears on them, suggest that individuals' affective state may influence their style of information processing (for related claims, see Fiedler, 1988; Isen, 1987; Kuhl, 1983). These influences may be conceptualized by considering the informative functions of affective states and their implications for individuals' inferences about the nature of their psychological situation (Frijda, 1988; Higgins, 1987). If negative emotions inform the individual about a threat of negative or a lack of positive outcomes, they may activate the procedural knowledge that is relevant to handling these problematic situations. This procedural knowledge may therefore be more accessible in memory, increasing the likelihood that the respective procedures will be applied to other tasks to which they are applicable while the individual is in a negative affective state. Moreover, individuals in a negative state may appreciate opportunities to distract themselves from this state if the event that elicited it cannot be changed, as is typical of the experimental manipulations used in affect and cognition research, and they may be motivated to avoid risky novel solutions in a situation that is already characterized as problematic. As a result, one finds that individuals are more likely to use effortful, detail-oriented, analytical processing strategies spontaneously when they are put in a bad rather than in a good mood, but that their reasoning is characterized by a lower degree of originality, creativity, and playfulness.

Positive affective states, on the other hand, inform the individual that his or her current environment is a safe place. Accordingly, individuals in a good mood may be more likely to take risks and to use simple heuristics in information processing. Moreover, they may have better access to a variety of different procedural knowledge, given that no specific procedure is activated to cope with the current situation. In combination, this may facilitate that higher creativity that has been observed under elated-mood conditions, but may inhibit the spontaneous use of effortful, analytic processing strategies, unless those are required by other active goals.

Unfortunately, the currently available evidence that bears on these speculations is limited. Moreover, alternative accounts cannot be ruled out on the basis of the available data. But it is encouraging to note that the assumption that affective states may serve informative functions does provide a plausible and comprehensive framework for the conceptualization of affective influences on information processing.

Most importantly, the present review suggests that the informative-functions approach combines a number of advantages that may recommend it as a heuristically fruitful framework for future research. First, the basic assumption that affective states may serve informative functions is clearly in line with a long tradition of theorizing about the nature of emotions (see Frijda, 1986, 1987, for reviews). Second, the present approach invites an explicit consideration of what specific information may be provided by different moods and emotions. One may expect that current explorations of the conditions giving rise to different emotions (e.g., Higgins, 1987; Oatley & Johnson-Laird, 1987; Ortony et al., 1988; Scherer, 1984; Weiner, 1985a), as well as research on people's knowledge about their emotions (e.g., Stein & Levine, 1987), will result in a more precise understanding of emotions' respective informational value. Moreover, these links may foster a more fruitful exchange between basic emotion research and social-cognitive research than has been true for approaches that make less contact with mainstream theorizing in the emotions domain. Finally, the informative-functions approach potentially offers a parsimonious and unifying explanation not only for the impact of moods and emotions on various aspects of processing style, but also for their impact on evaluative judgments—two areas of research that have so far been treated as separate.

Accordingly, research into the interplay of affect and cognition may profit from a serious consideration of the informational implications of our feelings. Although the basic assumption is all but new, its potential has not yet been fully exploited.

Acknowledgments

Parts of the reported research were supported by Grant Nos. Schw. 278/1, Schw. 278/2, and Str. 264/3 from the Deutsche Forschungsgemeinschaft to myself and F. Strack, and by a Feodor Lynen Fellowship from the Alexander von Humboldt Foundation. I want to thank Herbert Bless, Gerd Bohner, Jerry Clore, Fred Kanfer, Bettina Scheuring, Dick Sorrentino, Fritz Strack, and especially Tory Higgins and Tom Ostrom, for their stimulating responses to a previous draft.

References

Abele, A. (1985). Thinking about thinking. Causal, evaluative and finalistic cognitions about social situations. *European Journal of Social Psychology*, 15, 315–332.

Alloy, L. B., & Abramson, L. Y. (1979). Judgment of contingency in depressed and non-depressed students: Sadder but wiser? *Journal of Experimental Psychology: General*, 108, 441–485.

Alloy, L. B., Abramson, L. Y., & Viscusi, D. (1981). Induced mood and the illusion of control. *Journal of Personality and Social Psychology, 41,* 1129–1140.

Anderson, N. H., & Hubert, S. (1963). Effects of concomitant verbal recall on order effects in personality impression formation. *Journal of Verbal Learning and Verbal Behavior, 2,* 379–391.

Arnold, M. B. (1960). *Emotion and personality* (2 vols.). New York: Columbia University Press.

Bargh, J. A., & Thein, R. D. (1985). Individual construct accessibility, person memory, and the recall–judgment link: The case of information overload. *Journal of Personality and Social Psychology, 49,* 1129–1146.

Blaney, P. H. (1986). Affect and memory: A review. *Psychological Bulletin, 99,* 229–246.

Bless, H., Bohner, G., Schwarz, N., & Strack, F. (in press). Mood and persuasion: A cognitive response analysis. *Personality and Social Psychology Bulletin.*

Bodenhausen, G. V., & Wyer, R. S. (1987). Social cognition and social reality: Information acquisition and use in the laboratory and the real world. In H. J. Hippler, N. Schwarz, & S. Sudman (Eds.), *Social information processing and survey methodology* (pp. 6–41). New York: Springer.

Bohner, G., Bless, H., Schwarz, N., & Strack, F. (1988). When do events trigger attributions? The impact of valence and subjective probability. *European Journal of Social Psychology, 18,* 335–345.

Bollnow, O. F. (1956). *Das Wesen der Stimmungen.* Frankfurt: Klostermann.

Bower, G. H. (1981). Mood and memory. *American Psychologist, 36,* 129–148.

Bower, G. H., & Mayer, J. D. (1985). Failure to replicate mood-dependent retrieval. *Bulletin of the Psychonomic Society, 23,* 39–42.

Broadbent, D. E. (1971). *Decision and stress.* London: Academic Press.

Bruner, J. S., Matter, J., & Papanek, M. L. (1955). Breadth of learning as a function of drive-level and maintenance. *Psychological Review, 62,* 1–10.

Carlston, D. E. (1980). The recall and use of traits and events in social inference processes. *Journal of Experimental Social Psychology, 16,* 303–328.

Carlston, D. E., & Skowronski, J. (1986). Trait memory and behavior memory: The effects of alternative pathways in impression judgment response times. *Journal of Personality and Social Psychology, 50,* 5–13.

Carson, T. P., & Adams, H. E. (1980). Activity valence as a function of mood change. *Journal of Abnormal Psychology, 89,* 368–377.

Clark, D. M., & Teasdale, J. D. (1982). Diurnal variation in clinical depression and accessibility of memories of positive and negative experiences. *Journal of Abnormal Psychology, 91,* 87–95.

Clark, M. S., & Isen, A. M. (1982). Toward understanding the relationship between feeling states and social behavior. In A. H. Hastorf & A. M. Isen (Eds.), *Cognitive social psychology* (pp. 73–108). New York: Elsevier.

Clark, M. S., & Wadell, B. (1983). Effects of mood on thoughts about helping, attraction, and information acquisition. *Social Psychology Quarterly, 46,* 31–35.

Clore, G. L. (1985, August). *The cognitive consequences of emotions and feelings.* Paper presented at the meeting of the American Psychological Association, Los Angeles.

Clore, G. L., & Byrne, D. (1974). A reinforcement affect model of attraction. In T. L. Huston (Ed.), *Foundations of interpersonal attraction* (pp. 143–170). New York: Academic Press.

Clore, G. L., Parrott, W. J., & Wilkin, N. (1989). *Does emotional bias occur during encoding or judgment?* Unpublished manuscript, University of Illinois.

Clore, G. L., Schwarz, N., & Kirsch, J. (1983, May). *Generalized mood effects on evaluative judgments.* Paper presented at the meeting of the Midwestern Psychological Association, Chicago.

Collins, J., & Clark, L. (1989). *Mechanisms of meaning.* Unpublished manuscript, University of Illinois.

Davitz, J. R. (1969). *The language of emotion.* New York: Academic Press.

Diener, E., Larson, R. J., & Emmons, R. A. (1984, August). *Bias in mood recall in happy and unhappy persons.* Paper presented at the meeting of the American Psychological Association, Toronto.

Dreben, E. K., Fiske, S. T., & Hastie, R. (1979). The independence of item and evaluative information: Impression and recall order effects in behavior-based impression formation. *Journal of Personality and Social Psychology, 37,* 1758–1768.

Easterbrook, J. A. (1959). The effect of emotion on cue utilization and the organization of behavior. *Psychological Review, 66,* 183–201.

Ekman, P. (1982). *Emotion in the human face.* New York: Cambridge University Press.

Ewert, O. (1983). Ergebnisse und Probleme der Emotionsforschung. In H. Thomas (Ed.), *Enzyklopädie der Psychologie: C, IV, Vol. 1. Theorien und Formen der Motivation* (pp. 398–452). Göttingen: Hogrefe.

Eysenck, M. W. (1976). Arousal, learning, and memory. *Psychological Bulletin, 83,* 389–404.

Fiedler, K. (1988). Emotional mood, cognitive style, and behavior regulation. In K. Fiedler & J. Forgas (Eds.), *Affect, cognition, and social behavior* (pp. 100–119). Toronto: Hogrefe International.

Fiedler, K., Pampe, H., & Scherf, U. (1986). Mood and memory for tightly organized social information. *European Journal of Social Psychology, 16,* 149–164.

Fiske, S. T. (1980). Attention and weight in person perception: The impact of negative and extreme behavior. *Journal of Personality and Social Psychology, 38,* 889–906.

Fiske, S. T., Kenny, D. A., & Taylor, S. E. (1982). Structural models for the mediation of salience effects on attribution. *Journal of Experimental Social Psychology, 18,* 105–127.

Forgas, J. P., & Moylan, S. (1987). After the movies: The effects of mood on social judgments. *Personality and Social Psychology Bulletin, 13,* 467–477.

Frijda, N. H. (1986). *The emotions.* Cambridge, England: Cambridge University Press.

Frijda, N. H. (1987). Emotions, cognitive structure, and action tendency. *Cognition and Emotion, 1,* 235–258.

Frijda, N. H. (1988). The laws of emotion. *American Psychologist, 43,* 349–358.

Fuhrman, R., & Ostrom, T. M. (1989). *Memory for AIDS information.* Manuscript submitted for publication.

Gallagher, D., & Clore, G. L. (1985, May). *Effects of fear and anger on judgments of risk and blame.* Paper presented at the meeting of the Midwestern Psychological Association, Chicago.

Hamilton, D. L., Katz, L. B., & Leirer, O. (1980). Cognitive representation of personality impressions: Organizational processes in first impression. *Journal of Personality and Social Psychology, 39,* 1050–1063.

Hasher, L., Rose, K. C., Zacks, R. T., Sanft, H., & Doren, B. (1985). Mood, recall, and selectivity in normal college students. *Journal of Experimental Psychology: General, 114,* 104–118.

Hastie, R. (1984). Causes and effects of causal attribution. *Journal of Personality and Social Psychology, 46,* 44–56.

Hastie, R., & Park, B. (1986). The relationship between memory and judgment depends on whether the judgment task is memory-based or on-line. *Psychological Review, 93,* 258–268.

Higgins, E. T. (1987). Self-discrepancy: A theory relating self and affect. *Psychological Review, 94,* 319–340.

Higgins, E. T. (1989). Knowledge accessibility and activation: Subjectivity and suffering from unconscious sources. In J. S. Uleman & J. A. Bargh (Eds.), *Unintended thought* (pp. 75–123). New York: Guilford Press.

Higgins, E. T., & King, G. (1981). Accessibility of social constructs: Information processing consequences of individual and contextual variability. In N. Cantor & J. F. Kihlstrom (Eds.), *Personality, cognition, and social interaction* (pp. 69–122). Hillsdale, NJ: Erlbaum.

Higgins, E. T., & Lurie, L. (1983). Context, categorization, and memory: The "change-of-standard" effect. *Cognitive Psychology, 15,* 525–547.

Higgins, E. T., Rhodewalt, F., & Zanna, M. P. (1979). Dissonance motivation: Its nature, persistence, and reinstatement. *Journal of Experimental Social Psychology, 15,* 16–34.

Higgins, E. T., Rholes, W. S., & Jones, C. R. (1977). Category accessibility and impression formation. *Journal of Experimental Social Psychology, 13,* 141–154.

Higgins, E. T., & Stangor, C. (1988). A "change-of-standard" perspective on the relations among context, judgment, and memory. *Journal of Personality and Social Psychology, 54,* 181–192.

Hildebrand-Saints, L., & Weary, G. (1989). Depression and social information gathering. *Personality and Social Psychology Bulletin, 15,* 150–160.

Holyoak, K. J., & Nisbett, R. E. (1988). Induction. In R. J. Sternberg & E. E. Smith (Eds.), *The psychology of human thought* (pp. 50–91). Cambridge, England: Cambridge University Press.

Isen, A. M. (1984a). The influence of positive affect on decision making and cognitive organization. In T. Kinnear (Ed.), *Advances in consumer research* (Vol. 11, pp. 530–533). Provo, UT: Association for Consumer Research.

Isen, A. M. (1984b). Toward understanding the role of affect in cognition. In R. S. Wyer, Jr., & T. K. Srull (Eds.), *Handbook of social cognition* (Vol. 3, pp. 179–236). Hillsdale, NJ: Erlbaum.

Isen, A. M. (1987). Positive affect, cognitive processes, and social behavior. In L. Berkowitz (Ed.), *Advances in experimental social psychology* (Vol. 20, pp. 203–253). New York: Academic Press.

Isen, A. M., & Daubman, K. A. (1984). The influence of affect on categorization. *Journal of Personality and Social Psychology, 47,* 1206–1217.

Isen, A. M., Daubman, K. A., & Gorgoglione, J. M. (1987). The influence of positive affect on cognitive organization. In R. E. Snow & M. J. Farr (Eds.), *Aptitude, learning, and instruction: Vol. 3. Conative and affective processes.* Hillsdale, NJ: Erlbaum.

Isen, A. M., Means, B., Patrick, R., & Nowicky, G. (1982). Some factors influencing decision making strategy and risk-taking. In M. S. Clark & S. T. Fiske (Eds.), *Affect and cognition: The 17th Annual Carnegie-Mellon Symposium on Cognition* (pp. 243–261). Hillsdale, NJ: Erlbaum.

Isen, A. M., Shalker, T. E., Clark, M. S., & Karp, L. (1978). Affect, accessibility of material in memory, and behavior: A cognitive loop? *Journal of Personality and Social Psychology, 36,* 1–12.

Izard, C. E. (1977). *Human emotions.* New York: Plenum.

James, W. (1950). *The principles of psychology* (Vol. 2). New York: Dover. (Original work published 1890)

Johnson, E., & Tversky, A. (1983). Affect, generalization, and the perception of risk. *Journal of Personality and Social Psychology, 45,* 20–31.

Kelley, H. H. (1972). *Causal schemata and the attribution process.* Morristown, NJ: General Learning Press.

Kelly, G. (1955). *The psychology of personal constructs.* New York: Norton.

Keltner, D., & Audrain, P. (1988). *Moods, emotions, and well-being judgments.* Unpublished manuscript, Stanford University.

Kruglanski, A. W. (1980). Lay epistemo-logic—process and contents: Another look at attribution theory. *Psychological Review, 87,* 70–87.

Kuhl, J. (1983). Emotion, Kognition and Motivation, II. *Sprache und Kognition, 4,* 228–253.

Lacey, J. I., & Lacey, B. C. (1970). Some autonomic nervous system relationships. In P. Black (Ed.), *Physiological correlates of emotion* (pp. 205–227). New York: Academic Press.

Laird, J., Wagener, J., Halal, M., & Szegda, M. (1982). Remembering what you feel: Effects of emotion on memory. *Journal of Personality and Social Psychology, 42,* 646–657.

Lazarus, R. (1966). *Psychological stress and the coping process.* New York: McGraw-Hill.

Lehmann, H. E. (1985). Affective disorders: Clinical features. In H. I. Kaplan & B. J. Sadock (Eds.), *Comprehensive textbook of psychiatry* (4th ed., pp. 786–811). Baltimore: Williams & Wilkins.

Leight, K., & Ellis, H. (1981). Emotional mood states, strategies, and state dependency in memory. *Journal of Verbal Learning and Verbal Behavior, 20,* 251–266.

Lewicka, M. (1986). *Decision making under approach and avoidance conditions.* Unpublished manuscript, University of Warsaw, Poland.

Leyens, J., Cisneros, T., & Hossey, J. (1976). Decentration as a means for reducing aggression after exposure to violent stimuli. *European Journal of Social Psychology, 6,* 459–473.

Lichtenstein, M., & Srull, T. K. (1985). Conceptual and methodological issues in examining the relationship between consumer memory and judgment. In L. F. Alwitt & A. A. Mitchel (Eds.), *Psychological processes and advertising effects: Theory, research, and applications* (pp. 113–128). Hillsdale, NJ: Erlbaum.

Lingle, J. H., & Ostrom, T. M. (1979). Retrieval selectivity in memory-based impression judgments. *Journal of Personality and Social Psychology, 37,* 180–194.

Manucia, G. K., Bauman, D. J., & Cialdini, R. B. (1984). Mood influences in helping: Direct effects or side-effects? *Journal of Personality and Social Psychology, 46,* 357–364.

Markus, H., & Zajonc, R. B. (1985). The cognitive perspective in social psychology. In G. Lindzey & E. Aronson (Eds.), *Handbook of social psychology* (3rd ed., Vol. 1, pp. 137–230). New York: Random House.

Marsh, K. L., & Weary, G. (1989). Depression and attributional complexity. *Personality and Social Psychology Bulletin, 15,* 325–336.

Martin, L. L., & Clark, L. F. (in press). Social cognition: Exploring the mental processes involved in human social interaction. In M. W. Eysenck (Ed.), *The international review of cognitive psychology.* Chichester, England: Wiley.

Martindale, C. (1981). *Cognition and consciousness.* Homewood, IL: Dorsey Press.

Masters, J. C., & Furman, W. (1976). Effects of affect states on noncontingent outcome expectancies and beliefs in internal or external control. *Developmental Psychology, 12,* 481–482.

Mecklenbräuker, S., & Hager, W. (1984). Effects of mood on memory: Experimental tests of a mood-state-dependent retrieval hypothesis and of a mood-congruity hypothesis. *Psychological Research, 46,* 335–376.

Mednick, S. A. (1962). The associative basis of the creative process. *Psychological Review, 69,* 220–232.

Nisbett, R. E., & Wilson, T. (1987). Telling more than we can know: Verbal reports on mental processes. *Psychological Review, 84,* 231–259.

Oatley, K., & Johnson-Laird, P. N. (1987). Towards a cognitive theory of emotions. *Cognition and Emotion, 1,* 29–50.

Obrist, P. A. (1981). *Cardiovascular psychophysiology.* New York: Plenum.

Ortony, A., Clore, G. L., & Collins, A. (1988). *The cognitive structure of emotions.* Cambridge, England: Cambridge University Press.

Ruehlman, L. S., West, S. G., & Pasahow, R. J. (1985). Depression and evaluative schemata. *Journal of Personality, 53,* 46–92.

Schachter, S., & Singer, J. E. (1962). Cognitive, social, and physiological determinants of emotional state. *Psychological Review, 69,* 379–399.

Scherer, K. R. (1984). Emotion as a multi-component process: A model and some cross-cultural data. In P. Shaver (Ed.), *Review of personality and social psychology: Vol. 5. Emotions, relationships, and health* (pp. 37–63). Beverly Hills, CA: Sage.

Schwarz, N. (1983). Stimmung als Information: Zum Einfluß von Stimmungen auf die Beurteilung des eigenen LLebens. In G. Luers (Ed.), *Bericht über den 33. Kongreß der Deutschen Gesellschaft für Psychologie in Mainz 1982.* Göttingen: Hogrefe.

Schwarz, N. (1987). *Stimmung als Information: Untersuchungen zum Einfluß von Stimmungen auf die Bewertung des eigenen Lebens.* Berlin: Springer-Verlag.

Schwarz, N. (1988). Stimmung als Information: Zum Einfluß von Stimmungen auf evaluative Urteile. *Psychologische Rundschau, 39,* 148–159.

Schwarz, N., & Clore, G. L. (1983). Mood, misattribution, and judgments of well-being: Informative and directive functions of affective states. *Journal of Personality and Social Psychology, 45,* 513–523.

Schwarz, N., & Clore, G. L. (1986, April). *Stimmungseinflüsse auf die Personenbeurteilung: Stimmungskongruente Enkodierung oder Stimmung als Information?* Paper presented at the 28th Tagung Experimentell Arbeitender Psychologen, Saarbruecken, Federal Republic of Germany.

Schwarz, N., & Clore, G. L. (1988). How do I feel about it? Informative functions of affective states. In K. Fiedler & J. Forgas (Eds.), *Affect, cognition, and social behavior* (pp. 44–62). Toronto: Hogrefe International.

Schwarz, N., Kommer, D., & Lessle, N. (1988). *Covariation perception as a function of mood states.* Unpublished manuscript.

Schwarz, N., Servay, W., & Kumpf, M. (1985). Attribution of arousal as a mediator of the effectiveness of fear-arousing communications. *Journal of Applied Social Psychology, 15,* 74–78.

Schwarz, N., & Strack, F. (in press). Evaluating one's life: A judgment model of subjective well-being.

In F. Strack, M. Argyle, & N. Schwarz (Eds.), *The social psychology of well-being*. Oxford: Pergamon Press.

Schwarz, N., Strack, F., Kommer, D., & Wagner, D. (1987). Soccer, rooms and the quality of your life: Mood effects on judgments of satisfaction with life in general and with specific life-domains. *European Journal of Social Psychology, 17*, 69–79.

Sherman, S. J., & Corty, E. (1984). Cognitive heuristics. In R. S. Wyer & T. K. Srull (Eds.), *Handbook of social cognition* (Vol. 1, pp. 189–286). Hillsdale, NJ: Erlbaum.

Sinclair, R. C. (1987). *Mood and impression formation*. Paper presented at the 58th annual meeting of the Eastern Psychological Association.

Sinclair, R. C. (1988). Mood, categorization breadth, and performance appraisal: The effects of order of information acquisition and affective state on halo, accuracy, information retrieval, and evaluations. *Organizational Behavior and Human Decision Processes, 42*, 22–46.

Spiesman, J., Lazarus, R. S., Mordkoff, A., & Davidson, L. (1964). Experimental reduction and stress based on ego defense theory. *Journal of Abnormal and Social Psychology, 68*, 367–380.

Srull, T. K. (1983). Affect and memory: The impact of affective reactions in advertising on the representation of product information in memory. In R. Bagozzi & A. Tybout (Eds.), *Advances in consumer research* (Vol. 10, pp. 324–328). Ann Arbor, MI: Association for Consumer Research.

Srull, T. K. (1984). The effects of subjective affective states on memory and judgment. In T. Kinnear (Ed.), *Advances in consumer research* (Vol. 11, pp. 530–533). Provo, UT: Association for Consumer Research.

Stein, N. L., & Levine, L. J. (1987). Thinking about feelings: The development and organization of emotional knowledge. In R. E. Snow & M. J. Farr (Eds.), *Aptitude, learning, and instruction: Vol. 3. Conative and affective processes* (pp. 165–197). Hillsdale, NJ: Erlbaum.

Strack, F., Schwarz, N., & Gschneidinger, E. (1985). Happiness and reminiscing: The role of time perspective, mood, and mode of thinking. *Journal of Personality and Social Psychology, 49*, 1460–1469.

Tölle, R. (1982). *Psychiatrie* (6th ed.). Berlin: Springer-Verlag.

Tversky, A., & Kahneman, D. (1974). Judgment under uncertainty: Heuristics and biases. *Science, 185*, 1124–1131.

Watkins, M. J. (1979). Engrams as cuegrams and forgetting as cue overload. A cueing approach to the structure of memory. In C. R. Puff (Ed.), *Memory organization and structure*. New York: Academic Press.

Wegner, D. M., & Vallacher, R. R. (1986). Action identification. In R. M. Sorrentino & E. T. Higgins (Eds.), *Handbook of motivation and cognition: Foundations of social behavior* (Vol. 1, pp. 550–582). New York: Guilford Press.

Weiner, B. (1985a). An attributional theory of achievement motivation and emotion. *Psychological Review, 92*, 548–573.

Weiner, B. (1985b). "Spontaneous" causal thinking. *Psychological Bulletin, 97*, 74–84.

Weyent, J. M. (1978). Effects of mood states, costs, and benefits of helping. *Journal of Personality and Social Psychology, 36*, 1169–1176.

Wong, P. T. B., & Weiner, B. (1980). When people ask "why" questions, and the heuristics of attributional search. *Journal of Personality and Social Psychology, 40*, 650–663.

Worth, L. T., & Mackie, D. M. (1987). Cognitive mediation of positive affect in persuasion. *Social Cognition, 5*, 76–94.

Wyer, R. S. (1980). The acquisition and use of social knowledge: Basic postulates and representative research. *Personality and Social Psychology Bulletin, 6*, 558–573.

Wyer, R. S., & Carlston, D. (1979). *Social cognition, inference, and attribution*. Hillsdale, NJ: Erlbaum.

Zajonc, R. B. (1980). Feeling and thinking: Preferences need no inferences. *American Psychologist, 35*, 151–175.

Zajonc, R. B. (1989, June). *Interaction of affect and cognition below the level of awareness*. Paper presented at the Conference on Evaluation and Emotion in Social Cognition, Sopot, Poland.

Zanna, M. P., & Cooper, J. (1974). Dissonance and the pill: An attribution approach to studying the arousal properties of dissonance. *Journal of Personality and Social Psychology, 29,* 703–709.

Zanna, M. P., & Cooper, J. (1976). Dissonance and the attribution process. In J. H. Harvey, W. J. Ickes, & R. F. Kidd (Eds.), *New directions in attribution research* (Vol. 1, pp. 199–217). Hillsdale, NJ: Erlbaum.

Zillman, D. (1978). Attribution and misattribution of excitatory reactions. In J. H. Harvey, W. I. Ickes, & R. F. Kidd (Eds.), *New directions in attribution research* (Vol. 2, pp. 335–368). Hillsdale, NJ: Erlbaum.

CHAPTER 16

Cognitive versus Traditional Motivational Models
Irreconcilable or Complementary?

JOEL WEINBERGER
Adelphi University
DAVID C. McCLELLAND
Boston University

Etymologically, "motivation" has its roots in the Latin word *movere*, which means "to move." In psychology, the study of motivation involves attempts to explain the psychological causes of action or behavior (movement). In accord with this, Heckhausen (1977) saw motivational models as attempts to explain the goal-directedness of behavior in general, as well as individual differences in choice of activity and in intensity and persistence of effort. Beyond this general definition, there exists no consensus on construing or explaining motivation. Kleinginna and Kleinginna (1981) unearthed 98 separate definitions of "motivation," embracing diverse phenomena and theoretical orientations.

This paper is concerned with contrasting and (we hope) reconciling two major approaches to motivation. The first stems from traditional motivation theory (McClelland, Atkinson, Clark, & Lowell, 1953) and sees motivation as primarily affective. The second is an offshoot of the so-called cognitive revolution launched by Miller, Galanter, and Pribram (1960) and Neisser (1967). It views motivation as a cognitive phenomenon.

We begin by reviewing McClelland's latest and most complete model of motivation (McClelland, 1985). We then briefly define cognitive science generally and cognitive psychology in particular. This is followed by a discussion of some influential cognitive conceptions of motivation (Cantor, Markus, Niedenthal, & Nurius, 1986; Carver & Scheier, 1981a, 1981b; Markus, 1977, 1983; Scheier & Carver, 1981; Trope, 1986a; Weiner, 1986a) that purport to offer an alternative to the traditional position.

Following the aforementioned reviews, we critically compare the cognitive and traditional approaches. We review some of the criticisms that have been leveled at the traditional model. We also examine what we perceive to be some of the inadequacies and gaps in cognitive conceptions.

Comparing the traditional and cognitive views shows that there is strong conflict between them; they seem, in fact, to be irreconcilable. We attempt to relieve this gloomy state of affairs by offering a theoretical resolution that, we believe, can account for both of the disparate viewpoints. We point out that, in effect, there are two kinds of motivation (cf. McClelland, Koestner, & Weinberger, 1989). One is affectively based and is better explained through the traditional (McClelland, 1985) model. The other is cognitively based and is more amenable to cognitive interpretions. These two types of motivation explain different phenomena and follow qualitatively different rules. They seem, for the most part, to work in parallel (i.e., they are orthogonal to each other). Hence, the apparently contrasting findings and conflicting theoretical interpretations of the cognitivists and the traditionalists are due to their study of disparate phenomena. Each view is correct within its purview, but inadequate when extended beyond its range. Both views are required for a complete understanding of motivated behavior. Data we have recently collected (Koestner, Weinberger, & McClelland, 1989; McClelland et al., 1989) are presented in support of our theoretical conceptions.

THE TRADITIONAL (McCLELLAND) MODEL OF MOTIVATION

In McClelland's (1985) model, the term "motive" is specific to times in which important learning takes place in connection with affect that is innately associated with what is called a "natural incentive." (These variables and terms are made clear below.) There are hypothesized to be a limited number of natural incentives and therefore a limited number of motives. Motivated activity can be said to be occurring when a person does something that will create a situation in which a natural incentive will be available. This behavior is usually something the person has learned to do. The incentive made available by the learned behavior then leads (automatically) to a pleasant affect. Experiencing this affect constitutes a "kick" or a "natural high" for the person and thereby reinforces the whole behavioral sequence. So a person learns to do things that will bring him or her into the presence of a natural incentive, which then allows him or her to experience the associated pleasant affect. The person also learns to recognize cues that signal the potential availability of a natural incentive, or the possibility of creating a situation that will contain such an incentive. To summarize: Through learning, certain cues lead the person to expect the availability of a natural incentive and its associated pleasant affect. Thus, these cues arouse an anticipatory goal state. This anticipatory goal state, this emotionally charged state of readiness or expectation, is the motive.

The reader will note that in this model, unlike many other major motivational models, the organism is generally not driven to end unpleasant states of affairs such as nervous system tension (e.g., Freud, 1915/1957), cognitive dissonance (Festinger, 1957), cognitive discrepancies (Higgins, 1987), or tissue deficits (Hull, 1943). To employ the old adage of the carrot and the stick, the traditional model tends to see motives as carrots drawing the organism into behavior rather than sticks driving the organism to action. One exception to this general rule is the need for affiliation (Atkinson, Heyns, & Veroff, 1954), which seems to have a large fear-of-rejection component (Boyatzis, 1972; McAdams, 1985). This anomaly has generated discomfort (stick motivation?) among traditional motivation researchers, with the result that recent work in the affiliative area has unearthed motives more in line with the appetitive model we have described (McAdams, 1985; Weinberger & McLeod, 1989). Of course, we do not deny that a great deal of motivated behavior is avoidance-oriented. Either these motives have yet to be discovered, or they constitute a different type of motive from those successfully described by the model and are therefore best explained via different (possibly cognitive) models of motivation (e.g., Higgins, 1987; Sorrentino & Short, 1986).

Derivation of the McClelland Model

The McClelland (1985) model just sketched draws on ethological understanding of motivated animal (see Hinde, 1970) and human (Eibl-Eibesfeldt, 1979) behavior. It also draws on Ekman's (1971, 1984) view of a limited number of innate emotional expressions and states.[1]

McClelland's (1985) notion of "natural incentive" is closely akin to what ethologists have termed a "sign stimulus." A sign stimulus is an aspect of the environment that automatically and innately releases an impulse to act in a specific manner (if the situation permits it). Such behavior usually enhances the likelihood of survival or procreation. Examples of this type of behavior abound in the animal kingdom. The pecking of gull chicks, for example, is released in part by a red dot on the bill of the parent gulls. Pecking at this dot gets the chicks fed and thereby helps them to survive (Tinbergen & Perdeck, 1950). The male stickleback fish is automatically stimulated to attack by the red belly of another male stickleback. This serves the function of protecting its mating territory (Tinbergen, 1951). Hinde (1970) provides many more such examples.

The ethological model has been productively applied to humans as well as animals. Thus Bowlby (1969, 1973, 1980) has developed a conception of infant attachment in humans based on the ethological imprinting work pioneered by Lorenz (1935). In Bowlby's model, separation from the primary caretaker (almost always the mother) automatically leads to proximity seeking (i.e., attempts to find and be in contact with the mother). When these attempts are successful, the infant experiences positive feelings of comfort. Such behavior helps to ensure the survival of the human infant in its "environment of evolutionary adaptedness." To be alone in such an environment could easily lead to death from predators or through exposure. In both the Bowlby (1969, 1973, 1980) and McClelland (1985) models, the human being's response to sign stimuli (natural incentives) is more flexible and less stereotyped than that of lower animals. Moreover, the behavior emitted in response to these natural incentives becomes more sophisticated with development. Finally because of his or her superior brain, the human being is better than are lower animals at learning how to create or seek out situations in which natural incentives will be available. Nevertheless, the basic principles are the same across species.

The McClelland (1985) model also parallels the ethological perspective in its emphasis on *neurohormones* as critical to motivated behavior (Hinde, 1970). In McClelland's model, specific neurohormones or patterns of neurohormones are tied to particular motive states.[2] McClelland (1989) has tentatively identified norepinephrine as related to the power motive and dopamine as connected to the affiliative motive.[3] The exact nature of this relationship is not yet clear. It may be that neurohormones function as both causes and effects of motivated states. This kind of interrelatedness is commonplace in the relationship between the endocrine system and behavior of lower animals (Wilson, 1975). Lehrman (1964, 1965), in his classic work on the courtship behavior of the ringdove, for example, demonstrated a complicated set of interconnections between hormone release and reception of external signals. Candland and Leshner (1971) found that hormones and dominance in male squirrel monkeys were also interrelated. Thus concentration of certain hormones predicted dominance order (hormone level as cause), but levels changed as ranks did (hormone level as effect). To return to the McClelland model, a person high in a motive may be characterized as having a chronically high level of the hormone pattern associated with that motive. He or she is therefore more likely to act in concert with that motive. In addition, behaving in a manner that brings about the natural incentive associated with the motive may result in an increase of that selfsame hormone pattern.

McClelland (1985) also posits an additional connection not explicitly discussed by ethologists. He suggests that each of the neurohormone patterns relates to a particular emotional experience. There are therefore a limited number of innate emotional experiences, each of which is tied to a specific motive state. Beginning with Darwin (1872), several theorists have presented evidence on facial expressions that supports the notion of a limited number of basic emotions (Boucher & Brandt, 1981; Eibl-Eibesfeldt, 1972; Ekman, 1972, 1984; Lorenz, 1965).

Schematic Representation of the McClelland Model

The McClelland (1985) model can be represented schematically in the following way:

> Cue (learned) → Emotionally charged anticipatory goal state (the motive) → Impulse to act → Learned behaviors → Natural incentive or sign stimulus → Consummatory response → Specific hormone pattern → Specific affect (indexed by expressive behaviors)

Affect appears at two points in this representation: first as the "emotionally charged anticipatory goal state (the motive)," and then as the "specific affect (indexed by expressive behaviors)." It is the latter, specific affect, that constitutes the core or goal of the motivated behavior. The emotionally charged anticipatory goal state (the motive) represents an anticipation of the specific affect. It keeps the organism on track so that it can come to experience the goal affect.

Learning enters the model in that the person knows how to come into contact with the incentive through learning (1) how to identify the cues that signal its appearance; (2) where such incentives or cues can be found; and/or (3) how to create a situation that will lead to the appropriate incentive. Individual differences are said to be due to (1) the inherent strength of the anticipatory goal state itself; (2) the variety of cues that trip off the anticipatory goal state; and/or (3) the extent to which cues trigger the anticipatory goal state. The first of these is probably related to degree of hormone release and heredity. The latter two are attributable to learning and refer to generality and strength of learning, respectively (cf. McClelland, 1985, 1989; McClelland & Pilon, 1983).

Assessment of Individual Differences in Motive Strength

Ideally, individual differences in the strength of the various motives would be assessed via physiochemical measurement, through analysis of specific hormone profiles. Although a start has been made in this direction (McClelland, 1989), as yet there are not enough data to enable us to identify the relevant profiles with complete confidence. Moreover, the extant technology is not yet sufficiently sophisticated (or easy to come by) to make this practical. The alternative has historically been to assess something closely akin to what Murray (1938) referred to as "needs," which he defined as

> a construct . . . which stands for a force (the physio-chemical nature of which is unknown) in the brain region, a force which organized perception, apperception, intellection, conation and action in such a way as to transform in a certain direction an existing, unsatisfying situation. (pp. 123–124)[4]

One of the main ways in which Murray (1938) studied needs was through the spontaneous fantasy elicited by his Thematic Apperception Test (TAT). The assumption underlying the use of this measure was that spontaneous fantasy reflects internally based motivational phenomena. That is, spontaneous fantasy is held to provide a relatively direct and accurate readout of motivational dynamics. Freud (e.g., 1933/1964) pioneered this idea in his work on dreams and free association. Murray (1936, 1938) substituted telling stories to a standardized set of ambiguous pictures for the less structured speech productions favored by Freud. Provision of such a set of stimuli to all subjects made these kinds of data more amenable to empirical analysis. The contribution of McClelland and Atkinson (1948; McClelland et al., 1953; McClelland, Clark, Roby, & Atkinson, 1949) to improving this technology was the empirical development of rigorous scoring systems to assess the strength of the motivated fantasies told in response to TAT cards. Thus individuals could now be assigned numbers corresponding to their levels of measured motivation. These TAT-based measures continue to be routinely employed in research based on McClelland's work (see, e.g., McAdams, 1985; Sorrentino & Short, 1986; Winter, 1973).

A concrete example may help make this conception clearer. We will illustrate with power motivation, but the same principles hold for other motivations (e.g., those for affiliation and achievement). Let us say that a person comes across an opportunity to have an impact (the basic natural incentive for power motivation). The person has learned that karate provides an opportunity to experience the "kick" or positive affective experience to be gained from hitting someone.[5] This knowledge arouses an emotionally charged anticipation (anticipatory goal state— the power motive) of being able to experience the emotion or affect (as reflected in epinephrine and norepinephrine release) associated with the impact incentive. In other words, power motivation is aroused. Depending on the strength of the association and various competing motives, this arousal will lead the person to seek opportunities to spar or possibly even get into fights. It also leads the person to acquire the skills needed to successfully experience the impact incentive. If he or she manages to strike an opponent, this functions as a natural incentive, which then results in the release of epinephrine and norepinephrine and the experience of a satisfying emotion. This emotional "kick" reinforces the sequence.

A person high in a motive is sensitive to and on the lookout for cues that signal the potential availability of the natural incentive related to that motive. His or her fantasy (assessed via a TAT-type measure) reflects this preoccupation. Such an individual comes to learn a variety of ways to recognize and take advantage of such cues. Also, as a person matures, he or she cognitively elaborates the natural incentive in a variety of ways. In the case of power motivation, the person high in this motive looks for and learns to identify ways of experiencing the impact incentive, and also gets attached to symbolic representations of simple physical impact. Thus he or she may collect prestige supplies (e.g., powerful cars, flashy jewelry, etc.), try to exercise control over others in politics or business, or even work to help powerless others (see Winter, 1973).

Support for the McClelland Model

Much of the model has been strongly supported. The ethological literature supporting the existence and importance of sign stimuli to motivated behavior is voluminous (Hinde, 1970; Hoyle, 1984). There are also a great many data, collected over 40 years, showing that certain stimuli arouse achievement, power, and affiliative behaviors. Such behaviors have been shown to vary across individuals in ways predictable from TAT-type measures (McClelland, 1985). Neurohormones associated with these behaviors and individual differences have been demonstrated for the power and affiliative motives (McClelland, 1989). Buck (1985) has related motivated affect and associated neurohormones to identifiable facial expressions.

Summary

For purposes of this chapter, the important points of the traditional (McClelland, 1985) model can be summarized as follows:

1. Motives are biologically based. Animals have the same sorts of motives as humans do. That is, they develop out of experience with the same type of natural

incentive (e.g., rats also get a positive emotional "kick" from the impact of attacking and biting; Panskepp, 1971). Humans, of course, have many more complex ways of symbolically representing the natural incentive and of finding means of experiencing the affect associated with them.

2. There are a limited number of basic motives.

3. Affect is at the core of a motive.

4. Each motive has a particular affect associated with it and possibly a unique hormone profile.

5. Motives have long-term effects on behavior.

6. Motives affect relatively unconstrained behavior more strongly than constrained behavior.

7. Motives are best assessed through indirect means such as spontaneous fantasy or expressive movements, rather than through conscious reports of goals and intentions.

COGNITION, COGNITIVE SCIENCE, AND COGNITIVE PSYCHOLOGY

Basics of Cognitive Science

The Latin root of "cognition" is *cognoscere*, which means "to know."[6] In accord with this, Stillings et al. (1987) have declared "perceiving and knowing" to be the domain of cognitive science. Cognitive science has generated great enthusiasm and has been hailed as the science of the mind (Gardner, 1987). In this conception, the "mind" is viewed as a complex system that receives, stores, retrieves, transforms, and transmits information. For this reason, cognitive science is also referred to as "information-processing theory."

Cognitive science is an interdisciplinary field that has had an impact on several areas of study. These include psychology, linguistics, philosophy, computer science, and neuroscience. Certain assumptions and standard terms are shared by all of these subdisciplines (cf. Stillings et al., 1987). The first concerns the nature of information and information processing. Information is seen as *patterned*, rather than as random. The processing of this information (the subject matter of cognitive science) is said to involve rule-driven manipulations of these patterns of information. The rules governing information processing are termed "algorithms." Algorithms (information-processing rules) are formal procedures or systems in the sense that they operate on the formal patterns of the information (or symbols representing the information) rather than on their meanings. Thus an algorithm is not restricted to a particular set of information, but can be applied to all structurally similar sets. Furthermore, no understanding of the meaning or underlying structure of the information is necessary for successful application of an algorithm. This means that a machine can carry out an algorithm as readily and as effectively as a human being, as long as the appropriate formal properties can be programmed into it. Cognitive scientists hold that an information-processing system is completely defined and can be understood in its entirety if the formal rules (algorithms) that it is applying can be specified.

A second assumption concerns the cognitive-science conception of "meaning." Meaning is understood to be a function of "symbols" and their significance. A symbol is said to "represent" what it stands for, so "representations" refer to symbiotically coded aspects of the world. An effective representation has a well-defined mapping to the object in the world that it represents. Algorithms then act on these representations. Thus, representations are the raw material upon which algorithms operate. Cognitive scientists believe that an organism (or a machine) produces meaningful behavior by performing formal operations (algorithms) on symbolic structures (representations) that bear a representational relationship to the world. This then produces meaningful results.

Cognitive science further holds that information processes can and should be studied independently of the physical systems (biological or physical, organism or machine) on which they operate. For this reason, an algorithm or representation is equally valid for a human being or a machine. The physics or biology of the information processor is studied elsewhere.

Cognitive Psychology

The brief exposition above relates to all of cognitive science. In this section, we explore the domain of cognitive psychology, which is concerned with human mental capabilities and functions. It is here that cognitive interpretations of human motivation have been offered.

The general model of cognitive psychology—what is frequently referred to as "cognitive architecture" or "the architecture of the mind" (Anderson, 1983)—is as follows. Psychological processes begin with stimulation of the sense receptors by external events. This supplies the information needed to interpret those events. So the senses pick up information; this is termed "perception." The world has structure (is patterned), and the information obtained via the sense receptors reflects this. So information enters in structured patterns.

Although the information obtained through the senses is patterned, it is not yet in a form that is comprehensible to or usable by the perceiver (receiver). The perceiver therefore operates on this information and transforms it into an interpretable (usable) representation. This representation preserves the formal structure of the original information. That is, the representation has an abstract structural similarity to the patterned information.[7] Such operations or information processing may be repeated several times, so that the original information may undergo several transformations. These transformations are accomplished through the operation of various algorithms. So information processing proceeds through a series of algorithms.

When all transformations of the information have been completed, the resulting representation is stored in the human neurophysical system. Such storage takes the form of an associative network with numerous connections, termed "nodes" by cognitive scientists.

Stored information can be retrieved to be used as is or to be further processed. Retrieval takes place through the activation of the appropriate associative network. Such activation spreads through the network along its links or nodes. This spreading occurs in many directions at once (i.e., in parallel, as opposed to serially). The part of the network with the most associative connections to whatever triggered the activation is most strongly activated. This part then becomes dominant and is retrieved.

The operation of the "cognitive architecture," as we have described it, can be summarized as proceeding through the following steps:

1. Information enters the sense organs in structured patterns.
2. This information is operated upon and transformed into representations that maintain the formal structure of the information.
3. The operations through which information is transformed follow rules termed "algorithms."
4. The transformed information is stored in associative networks.
5. Information is retrieved through activation of the appropriate associative network.

Most cognitive psychologists studying the aforementioned processes tend to focus on perception, learning, and memory (see, e.g., Solso, 1988). But cognitive notions have also been found to be relevant to the study of personality and motivation (see, e.g., Mook, 1987). A major concept utilized by these latter theorists is that of the "schema." Formally, a schema can be defined as a cluster of connected general propositions (i.e., a tightly linked associative network) that tends to be activated as a unit (Stillings et al., 1987). So simply put, a schema is an associative network that defines something. Let us elaborate on this. First, schemas are not logically or hierarchically organized; instead, they specify the general properties of events or objects in a "family resemblance" manner. That is, a schema is an associative network whose elements "go together" in a probabilistic, sometimes idiosyncratic manner. The organization of any of these associative networks is based on the unique experience of the individual. This means that the categories defined by schemas have "fuzzy" (as opposed to sharp) boundaries. Since schemas tend to be activated as a unit (Stillings et al., 1987), when one part of the associative network comprising the schema becomes activated, all of the schema is retrieved.

Schemas are said to exert a powerful influence on the way information is processed. They function like molds that are fit over incoming information and help the person to organize that information. They can also distort information so that it will more readily fit the mold. Schemas are therefore strongly assimilative in the Piagetian (Flavell, 1963) sense. There are several types of schemas, categorized according to the type of information they hold. They include object schemas (descriptions of external objects such as birds, trees, or buildings), frames (descriptions or complex visual scenes), personality schemas, the self-schema, scripts (schemas that code social situations such as going to a restaurant), and plans (schemas for behavior). Of all of these, it is the self-schema that has been most closely and frequently linked to motivational phenomena (e.g., Carver & Scheier, 1981a, 1981b; Cantor et al., 1986).

The self-schema is an extremely complicated and central cognitive structure. It refers to the cognitive model of the self and is composed of self-categorizations. Like all schemas, it exerts powerful effects on perception, memory, and thought. So information consistent with the self-schema is processed more efficiently and recalled better than information inconsistent with this schema. But because the self-schema is more central and complex than virtually any other schema, its influence is more far-ranging and pervasive. Much incoming information is evaluated relative to this schema and is then accepted or resisted on the basis of its fit. Other schemas are also strongly influenced by the self-schema. It is arguably the most important schema. Some cognitive views of motivation are overtly reliant on the self-schema as their central explanatory construct (e.g., Cantor et al., 1986; Carver & Scheier, 1981a, 1981b). Others do not always explicitly refer to the self-schema, but it plays a major role in their thinking nonetheless (e.g., Trope, 1983, 1986a, 1986b; Weiner, 1985, 1986a, 1987). We examine these models next.

COGNITIVE MODELS OF MOTIVATION BASED ON THE SELF-SCHEMA

Public and Private Selves: Carver and Scheier's Model

A view of motivation emphasizing the self that is very closely tied to the cognitive model described above is that of Carver and Scheier (1981a, 1981b; Scheier & Carver, 1981). In fact, their work can be seen as a direct outgrowth of the seminal information-processing conceptions of Miller et al. (1960). To Carver and Scheier, motivation can be completely understood through information-processing conceptions (also termed by them "cybernetics" or "control theory").

According to Carver and Scheier, the self-schema or self is the major information-processing or control system involved in motivational phenomena. (We use the terms "self" and "self-schema" interchangeably in this chapter.) The self, however, is not a unitary structure; it is multifaceted. That is, it consists of many semiautonomous, practically orthogonal aspects. (This parallels the Markus, 1977, and Cantor et al., 1986, notion of "multiple selves," to be discussed later.) Research conducted by these theorists has suggested to them that a particularly important distinction in the self is between what they term the "public" and "private" selves (cf. Buss, 1980; Fenigstein, Scheier, & Buss, 1975).

The public self is the aspect of the self exposed to public scrutiny through self-presentation or self-portrayal. This self is a social product that develops as the individual learns to take an outside perspective on himself or herself (i.e., becomes able to see himself or herself as others do).[8] The public self is typically activated in social situations. That is, to whatever extent this self guides behavior, it does so through consideration of how contemplated or planned behavior would be viewed and responded to by others. An individual motivated by this aspect of the self is socially aware.

The private self consists of aspects of the self that are internal rather than public. It includes personal concerns and private needs, as well as other aspects of the self often hidden from others. This aspect of the self manifests itself in self-consciousness or self-awareness.[9] To the extent that the private self influences behavior, an individual is aware of and likely to act on his or her thoughts, feelings, and attitudes. Such an individual is conscious of and responsive to transient affective states, bodily sensations, and behavioral dispositions.

Like any other schema, the self-schema must be accessed and activated before it can be expected to influence behavior. The particular aspect of the self that structures behavior, therefore, depends upon the aspect of the self that is most strongly activated. Carver and Scheier have focused on attention as a critical variable here. Attention to a specific self-aspect is held to be a necessary precondition for enabling that self-aspect (through activation) to have an impact on behavior. That is, a given aspect of the self will only influence behavior if it is taken as the object of the individual's attention (cf. Duval & Wicklund, 1972; Wicklund, 1979). Such attention can be characteristic of an individual, or it can be dictated by environmental exigencies. The former results in an almost continual and the latter in a temporary direction of attention.

Carver and Scheier have devised a self-report instrument to assess chronic tendencies to be attentive to either the public or private aspects of the self (i.e., the extent to which an individual habitually attends to his or her public vs. private self). They have also utilized experimental manipulations to alter momentary levels of public or private self-attention. An impressive body of evidence supports their conceptions (see Carver & Scheier, 1981b, and Scheier & Carver, 1981, for the relevant studies).

The use of self-report scales to measure the public and private selves suggests that the person is potentially aware of and able to report accurately on critical aspects of his or her self-concept. After all, a person cannot be expected to report on something he or she has no conscious knowledge of. The issue of awareness is a point to which we return when describing the other cognitive models of motivation. It becomes critical when we compare the cognitive and traditional models of motivation.

Possible Selves: The Model of Markus, Cantor, and Associates

The work of Markus (1977, 1983), Cantor (Cantor, Niedenthal, & Langston, 1987), and their associates (e.g., Cantor et al., 1986) focuses more on the self and its interactions with the environment than on information processing per se. Nonetheless, the model is clearly a cognitive one, relying as it does on self-schemas.[10] Motivation, according to these theorists, is largely manifested in the individual's understanding of himself or herself. In fact, these authors contend that motivation may not exist independently or outside of the self-concept.

Three constructs related to the self are most strongly implicated in motivational phenomena, according to this model. They are what Markus (1977) has termed "possible selves," what Cantor et al. (1987) have called "life tasks," and what Cantor et al. (1986) term the "working self-concept." "Possible selves" refer to all of the distinct notions the person has about what it is possible for him or her to become or be like. They include selves that the person could be, would like to be, feels he or she ought (or ought not) to be, and is afraid to be. Each self includes outcome expectations, feelings, and images associated with its attainment. Motivationally, they provide end states (i.e., incentives) to strive for or avoid.

"Life tasks" refer to issues the individual sees as important at a particular point in life. They provide the context in which behavior, particularly motivated behavior, occurs. Life tasks and possible selves are said to interact to produce motivated behavior. In pursuing particular life tasks, the individual is likely to be guided by relevant possible selves. The possible selves provide distinctive end states or goals for the person's predominant life tasks. Thus the goal of accomplishing a life task is the attainment or avoidance of a possible self. Life tasks, in turn, determine which of the possible selves will be salient and available to the person.

The particular possible self operating at any given time and thereby influencing information processing and behavior at that time is termed the "working self-concept" or "current self-concept." This current self-concept is a function of the current life task. That is, the current view of the self (i.e., the operative possible self) is selected from the collection of self-views (possible selves) made salient by the prevailing social context (life task). The activated subset of self-concepts (current self-concept) changes as the life tasks and salient features of the social environment change.

In the Cantor et al. (1986) model, no possible self is necessarily more important than any other. Thus there is nothing inherently special about achievement or affiliative motivation. They are attributable to the accessing of an achievement and an affiliative self-concept, respectively. These then interact with life tasks just as any other possible self does.

The Cantor et al. (1986) model has much in common with that of Carver and Scheier (1981a, 1981b; Scheier & Carver, 1981), beyond their common cognitive orientation. Both reject the idea of a single, monolithic self in favor of separate, even orthogonal selves. Carver and Scheier focus on the public and private selves. Markus (1977, 1983) and Cantor et al. do not emphasize any particular self-concept, but would seem to have no argument with the notions of public and private selves. Both models also stress the importance of the social context. In the Carver and Scheier model, the context directs attention to one of the selves. In the Cantor et al. model, context is provided by the relevant life task, which then recruits the appropriate possible self. Attention is implicit in this notion. Finally, the two conceptions agree on awareness. The individual is held to be at least potentially aware of and able to report accurately on his or her various selves, as well as on the life task he or she is involved in. Cantor et al. (1986) state this quite plainly: "Most people reveal an extensive understanding of themselves" (p. 97). Furthermore, they assert that "elements of self-knowledge are accessible, can be reported and reflected on by the individual, and are implicated in individuals' strategies of action" (p. 100).

The Achievement Motivation Models of Weiner and of Trope

The investigations of both Weiner (1985, 1986a) and Trope (1975, 1983, 1986a, 1986b) derive more directly from *attribution theory* than from cognitive science per se. But although cognitive science and attribution theory have relatively independent histories, they do converge, as we try to show. Moreover, Weiner and Trope are avowedly cognitive in their orientations, and their models are fully compatible with classical cognitive-science conceptions.

Attribution theory begins with the assumption that people always seek to explain their experiences. In order to do so, they attribute events to identifiable causes (Shaver, 1975); hence the name "attribution theory." The attempt to match an experience with its cause has been termed "causal search" (Forsyth, 1980; Kelley, 1971). The solutions people come up with for their causal searches and the strategies they use to come up with them constitute the subject matter of attribution theory (Jones & Davis, 1965; Kelley, 1967, 1971, 1973).

The attribution theory emphasis on the strategies people utilize for their causal searches is its point of convergence with standard cognitive-science conceptions. Causal search strategies can be identified with the cognitive-science notion of algorithms. And, as the reader will recall, the particular algorithm employed depends to a large degree on which schema is operating. A theorist seeking to bridge the fields of attribution theory and standard cognitive psychology would have to focus on causal search strategies (algorithms) in the context of an operative schema. This is just what Weiner and Trope have done. They have chosen to concentrate on the operation of the self-schema associated with achievement. Thus they have concerned themselves with the information-processing strategies (causal search strategies) or algorithms characteristic of the achieving self.

For both Weiner and Trope, the event of significance to the achieving self (i.e., the event to be explained) is success or failure at a task. Such events activate the self-schema termed the "achieving self." To explain this success or failure, a causal search is begun. The strategies used to explain success or failure vary as a function of the salience of the achieving self for a particular individual. Following traditional motivational nomenclature, Weiner and Trope refer to individual differences in the salience or centrality of the achievement self-concept as differences in "achievement motivation." They assess such individual differences through self-report measures such as the Mehrabian (1969) achievement scales.[11]

Weiner's (1979, 1986a) research has shown that people high in what he terms achievement motivation (people for whom the achieving self is particularly salient or central) show different information-processing strategies (attribute success and failure to different causes) than do people low in achievement motivation (people for whom the achieving self is not salient or central). Individuals high in achievement motivation tend to attribute success to high ability and effort. They tend to attribute failure to a lack of effort and possibly to bad luck. People low in achievement motivation, on the other hand, tend to attribute success to luck and task facility (easiness of task). Given failure, they tend to assume a lack of ability.

In Trope's (1983, 1986a, 1986b) model, the central purpose of causal search following success or failure is to obtain accurate information concerning ability.[12] Such information is termed "diagnostic." He found (Trope, 1975; Trope & Brickman, 1975) that individuals high in achievement motivation were more likely to seek out diagnostic information than were individuals low in achievement motivation. In these early studies, diagnosticity was confounded with high ability, so that it was not clear whether the key variable was veridical information or positive information about ability. This was corrected in later studies (e.g., Trope, 1980), which found that individuals high in achievement motivation were more interested in learning about both high and low ability levels than were those low in achievement motivation.[13]

Both Trope and Weiner assume awareness of and ability to accurately report on critical aspects of the self on the part of the actor. They employ self-report measures of achievement motivation, make success or failure on a task explicit to their subjects, and ask for reports of attributions. Weiner (1986b) has been quite explicit about this. He embraces the study of conscious processes and eschews formulations relying on unconscious processes: "considering how life is spent and what is reflected upon—direct access to the determinants of motivation and emotion is quite possible. For most of us at most times, a royal road to the unconscious is less valuable to the motivation researcher than the dirt road to consciousness" (p. 285).

The views of Weiner and of Trope are easily reconciled with and can be seen as complementary to those of Carver and Scheier (1981a, 1981b; Scheier & Carver, 1981) and Cantor et al. (1986). All are cognitive and all focus on the self as the central instigator of motivated behavior. Furthermore, all see awareness as central and therefore rely almost exclusively on self-report. Carver and Scheier and Cantor et al. have concentrated on the multifaceted nature of the self and on its general operation. Carver and Scheier have also focused on two important dimensions of the self—the public and private selves. Cantor et al. and Carver and Scheier can be said to have investigated the macrostructure of the self. Weiner and Trope have taken a more fine-grained approach. They have examined the operation of a particular aspect of the self, namely, the achieving self. Thus they can be said to have attended to the microstructure of the self.

Summary

For our purposes, the relevant points of the cognitive-based motivation theories we have covered are as follows:

1. Motivation is centered upon and flows from the self.
2. The self is multifaceted.
3. The particular aspect of the self that is operative depends on the social context and on attentional processes.
4. People are aware of and can accurately report on their motivations, attributions, and attentional processes.

In the next section, we compare the cognitive with the traditional view of motivation.

COMPARING THE TRADITIONAL AND COGNITIVE VIEWS OF MOTIVATION

The McClelland model is biological and emphasizes affect. It sees human motivation as continuous with animal motivation (albeit far more flexible and sophisticated). It draws on the field of ethology to connect human and animal motivation. There are hypothesized to be a limited number of motives, possessed by everyone to varying degrees. Neurohormone profiles may underlie the motives. Motives are held to affect long-term outcomes and relatively unconstrained behaviors. And, finally, people are said to be relatively unaware of and unable to directly report on their motives, which are therefore more clearly reflected in their recurrent fantasies than in their self-descriptive statements. As a consequence, motives are best measured indirectly through spontaneous stories told to ambiguous pictures.

The cognitive views of motivation are quite different. First, they emphasize information processing over biology. Instead of making analogies between humans and lower animals, cognitive psychologists tend to compare human functioning with information processing by computers. Instead of ethology, artificial intelligence is called upon. There is, in principle, no limit to the number of motives, and certainly nothing inherently unique about achievement, power, or affiliation. There are as many possible motivators of behavior as there are self-categorizations or possible selves. In principle, a motivation researcher could just as easily study the masculine or feminine self-categorization as the achievement self-categorization. For that matter, a chess player self-concept could be just as valid a motivator as an achievement or power self-concept. The differences among the various self-categorizations are in their specific content and possibly the extent of their associative networks. The number of self-categorizations should vary from individual to individual in an idiosyncratic manner. The structure of each self-concept should also vary idiosyncratically, so that one person's achieving self may be very different from another's. Finally, self-concepts are not innate but learned, and they are learned relatively late in development. A sense of self, the ability to take roles, and an understanding of the attributes of each potential self-concept must be present before a person can form a coherent self-schema.

Self-schemas are likely to have sporadic effects on behavior. Which one is activated and for how long depend on the environmental context and on attentional processes. As these shift, so does the operative self-concept. Thus short-term, within-situation behavior is more easily predicted than is long-term, cross-situation behavior. Finally, people can report accurately on their self-categorizations, which can therefore be measured through direct questioning and straightforward self-report measures.

It is clear that the two views of motivation differ on almost every important feature. There is apparently no point of connection between them. This is reflected in their motive measures, which tend to have a zero-order correlation (cf. McClelland et al., 1989). It is no wonder, then, that proponents of each model have attacked the other as inadequate. We briefly describe some critiques of each model, as well as some rejoinders, and then offer our resolution of this dilemma.

Criticisms of the Traditional Model

Critiques of McClelland's model tend to focus on either motive measurement (Entwisle, 1972), the model's alleged mechanistic orientation (Mancuso & Mascolo, 1987), or apparent inconsistencies in the predictive power of the motives (Cantor et al., 1986). We begin with criticisms of assessment.

Assessment
Entwisle (1972) estimated the test–retest reliability of the TAT measure used to assess need for achievement to be between .20 and .40. She also conducted item analysis (interitem reliability) and determined that a person's score on any particular TAT picture was not related to his or her score on any other TAT picture (*r*'s = .30–.40). She concluded that the TAT measure was not reliable and therefore could not be valid.

The so-called inadequacy of the TAT motive measure is more apparent than real. McClelland (1985) has discussed the criteria for good measurement as they relate to TAT assessment. He showed that this measure had adequate sensitivity, uniquely reflected changes in the variables of interest, and had validity and utility. As far as reliability was concerned, there was more than adequate interrater reliability (*r*'s ≥ .85). Interitem reliability, one of the areas cited by Entwisle as low, is not an appropriate criterion for this sort of measure. The different TAT pictures are not meant to be equivalent assessors of the motive. Instead, each picture represents an *independent estimate* of the true motive score. And independent measures contribute more to prediction if they are uncorrelated (cf. Lundy, 1985; McClelland, 1980).

This brings us to the issue of test–retest reliability, where Entwisle (1972) also reported a low coefficient. First, even if one were to accept Entwisle's reliability estimates, this would not necessarily mean that the measure was invalid. Even a test with such a high degree of error could be theoretically useful in group prediction (Brody, 1983). Next, it has been shown that conditions of test administration can affect scores (Lundy, 1985). Scores are most valid under relaxed conditions and least valid under ego-involving conditions. (This is an important point, and we come back to it later.) Finally, Winter and Stewart (1977) found that subjects were biased against reporting the same story themes on two separate occasions. But when they were explicitly told that they could repeat stories, test–retest reliability became quite respectable (r's of about .60).

Another argument concerning mode of measurement is based on the fact that self-report and TAT measures of motives do not correlate. This is patently true (see McClelland et al., 1989). Cognitivists have argued that this lack of correlation betokens the invalidity of the TAT. The so-called poor reliability of the TAT is then called in to buttress this argument. Traditional theorists have, of course, taken the opposite tack (as we explicate below)—namely, that the two measures do not correlate because self-report does not measure motives. There is a third alternative, however. This is that the two measures do not correlate because they measure different things, which are, in reality, orthogonal to each other (Biernat, 1989; Koestner et al., 1989; McClelland et al., 1989). We see this as the solution to the cognitive versus traditional dilemma, and we expand on it later.

"Mechanistic" Nature of the Model

It appears that criticisms leveled against the reliability of TAT measurement are without serious merit. What about the argument that the model is a holdover of anachronistic mechanistic views? Mancuso and Mascolo (1987) have charged the model with championing a conditioning theory of motivation. They argue that it employs the explanatory concepts of classical conditioning to explain the growth of and changes in motivated behaviors. In line with this, they identify natural incentives with unconditioned stimuli and consummatory responses with unconditioned responses. They then affirm that the model proposes that natural incentives (unconditioned stimuli) become associated with previously neutral stimuli through temporal contiguity. These previously neutral stimuli then come to function as conditioned stimuli and elicit the consummatory responses (unconditioned responses) originally evoked by the natural incentives (unconditioned stimuli). As a result of this classical conditioning, people come to respond to the conditioned stimulus as they previously responded to the unconditioned stimulus.

The Mancuso and Mascolo (1987) account is seriously flawed. First, their understanding of classical conditioning is inaccurate (see Rescorla, 1988). More importantly, they have misrepresented the McClelland (1985) model. It does not hold that control of motivated behavior passes from natural incentives (which Mancuso & Mascolo identify with unconditioned stimuli) to something else (which they identify with conditioned stimuli). Instead, motives lead people to find ways to seek out and/or create situations where natural incentives will be available. The natural incentive then functions as it always has.

Mancuso and Mascolo (1987) are also in error when they assert that the model explains the development of individual differences in motives through instrumental conditioning—in other words, that people differ in the strength of their motives because they have been differentially reinforced by socializing agents for expressing them. Mancuso and Mascolo argue that opportunities to obtain the natural incentives identified by McClelland (1985) are limitless. Given this, they cannot see how any socializing agent can set up a reinforcement schedule capable of controlling the frequency of motivated behavior. Thus, they conclude, there is no way for individual differences to arise. Once again, their reasoning is faulty. Socializing agents are not limited to simple rewards and punishments or to making incentives more or less available, as Mancuso and Mascolo's critique implies. The literature on intrinsic motivation has clearly shown that motivation can be powerfully altered without any change in the availability of incentives or in reinforcement contingencies (Deci & Ryan, 1985). The bulk of this work has demonstrated that it is all too easy to stunt the initiation and persistence of motivated behaviors through apparently innocuous feedback concerning past performance and expectations of future performance. Other work (e.g., Koestner, Ryan, Bernieri, & Holt, 1984) has shown that motivation can also be enhanced through variations in equally subtle feedback.

Mancuso and Mascolo's (1987) misunderstandings of the model are, we believe, due to a commonly held cognitive bias: That which does not fit into a cognitive framework must perforce be at least partly mechanistic and probably belongs to the behaviorist perspective. Weiner (1972) made a similar error when he placed traditional achievement motivation theory partway between the cognitive and mechanistic models of motivation. Again the reasoning seems to be that if something is not cognitive, it must be mechanistic. In fact, the McClelland model is neither.

Inconsistencies in Predictive Power

The final argument against the McClelland model has some merit. It is true, as Cantor et al. (1986) claim, that traditional (TAT) measures of motives are not always successful in predicting outcomes. It is also true, however (see below), that cognitive self-report measures have yielded mixed results. We believe that we can explain and tie together these inconsistencies in a theoretically meaningful way. We make this attempt later in the chapter.

Criticizing the Cognitive Viewpoint

We begin our critique of cognitive conceptions by pointing out some difficulties with cognitive science generally. These relate largely to its *almost total neglect of affect.* The tenuous connection between cognition and behavior is also briefly mentioned. Moving to the motivation models, we discuss some problems with the type of data collected and with some inconsistency of results. We also note some problems with self-report.

Cognition, Affect, and Motivation

That cognitive theorists give short shrift to affect and motivation has been pointed out by several reviewers. Both Kuhl (1986) and Hoffman (1986) have discussed this in Volume 1 of this handbook. Correcting this deficiency was, in fact, one of the reasons for starting this handbook (Sorrentino & Higgins, 1986). We would like to illustrate here the extent to which motivation and affect have been neglected by cognitivists. The terms "affect," "emotion," and "motivation" do not appear *at all* in an otherwise excellent introduction to cognitive science (Stillings et al., 1987). The same is true of a commonly used cognitive psychology text (Solso, 1988). Likewise, these terms do not appear in an authoritative edited book on cognitive science (Kintsch, Miller, & Polson, 1984). In 1980, the prestigious Nebraska Symposium on *Motivation* (italics ours) devoted 238 pages of its published proceedings to cognitive processes (Howe, 1981). "Affect" was never mentioned, the word "emotion" appeared on one page, and "motivation" appeared on nine pages, six of which referred to motivated retrieval and recall! Thus we are not just discussing insufficient attention to these areas, but rather an almost total dismissal of them. To the extent that cognitive models of motivation derive from cognitive science, they are relying on a data base and on conceptions that have virtually ignored affect and motivation. So extending cognitive theory to motivation may be stretching it beyond its range of convenience.

On those occasions when affect is considered by cognitivists, it is seen as a consequence of and secondary to cognition; it is quite literally an afterthought. But there is evidence that affect may precede cognition (Zajonc, 1980, 1984). Certainly lower animals, even quite primitive ones, evidence emotional, motivated behavior. Much of this behavior seems to be automatically elicited by hormonal and environmental stimuli rather than by complex cognitive processing, let alone attributions requiring awareness. If this occurs and is important in lower animals, it seems reasonable to assume that humans demonstrate similar functioning. To think otherwise is to argue for a radical discontinuity between humans and lower animals.

The Type of Data Collected and the Results Obtained in Cognitive Models of Motivation

As they themselves admit, cognitive researchers are often unable to bridge the gap between cognition and behavior (Nisbett & Ross, 1980). The data presented by cognitive motivational theorists are no exception. Much of this work does not deal with actual behavior; instead, it involves asking subjects what they would do in hypothetical or actual situations. Alternatively, subjects may be asked to role-play some scenario and then to report on their understanding of the situation and what they would do next in it (e.g., Brophy & Rohrkemper, 1981; Graham, Doubleday, & Guarino, 1984; Niedenthal, Cantor, & Kihlstrom, 1985; Nurius & Markus, 1984; Weiner, 1980a, 1980b; Weiner, Russell, & Lerman, 1979). Cognitive models explain the results of such studies very cleanly. But these investigations are asking for cognitive judgments. It is hardly surprising that cognitive conceptions predict cognitive judgments. The connections to actual behavior are assumed but often not tested.

The cognitivists' reliance on self-report can also be problematic. Nisbett and Wilson (1977) have shown that people's self-reports cannot always be trusted. People are often unaware of what they are like and why they do what they do. McClelland and his associates (McClelland, 1980, 1985; McClelland et al., 1953, 1989) have presented a large body of data showing that self-reports do not predict motivated behaviors. As a result, they concluded that self-reported motives are not true motives. There is, however, an equally large body of data relating cognitive assessments (self-reports) and cognitive manipulations (focusing of attention) to actual motivated behavior. Thus, as discussed earlier, Carver and Scheier (1981a) have shown that experimentally manipulating self-directed attention results in predictable changes in performance. Likewise, they have shown that self-reports of chronic or habitual self-attention can predict such performance. And Trope (1983, 1986a) summarized data demonstrating that achievement performance could be predicted via self-reported achievement motivation. So the assertions denying the relationship of self-report and cognitive variables to motivated behavior are clearly incorrect. And yet there exist the data showing no such relationship. We attempt to resolve these contradictions in the next section.

TWO KINDS OF MOTIVATION

We believe that cognitive and traditional models differ because they study qualitatively different types of motivation. One kind is tied to conceptions of the self, is almost wholly a product of relatively sophisticated learning occurring subsequent to language acquisition, and is activated by anything that makes a relevant aspect of the self salient (e.g., ego involvement, self-directed attention, powerful demand characteristics, etc.). Since this type of motivation requires a capacity to develop self-concepts, it is unique to humans. Because there are in principle an unlimited number of potential self-concepts, there are an almost unlimited number of potential motivators. Moreover, since the content of self-concepts depends entirely on learning, each can be organized in an almost unlimited number of ways. As a consequence, there are large differences in what motivates different individuals. People have access to their self-concepts and can report on them, probably because of their relatively late acquisition and ties to language. This type of motivation is best understood through cognitive principles, which emphasize information-processing notions such as schemas, the self, idiosyncratic organization, and attentional processes. It is best assessed via self-report.

The second kind of motivation is more primitive. It is based on a limited number of biologically based needs that exist in everyone. These needs are innate and continuous with those of animals, differing only in their flexibility. Individual differences in this type of motive are attributable to variation in genetic endowment and/or early (largely prelinguistic) learning. These motives are triggered by relevant environmental variables. They tend to have long-term effects and are most easily expressed in nondemanding, free-response situations. They are best measured in such a situation as well. For this reason, they have been assessed through projective (TAT-type) stories.

The two kinds of motivation outlined above are essentially orthogonal. That is, they operate independently of one another. Thus one or the other (or a combination thereof) may be operative at any particular time. Cognitively based motives are most likely to be active in well-defined social situations calling for specific kinds of behavior. Traditionally defined motives are most likely to evidence themselves in unstructured situations that allow for variability in responding.

One major reason for the confusion between cognitive and need-based motivation is that the constructs employed by the theorists of each school have often been given the same names. Thus Weiner (1972, 1985, 1986a) and Trope (1983, 1986a, 1986b) call behavior rooted in an achieving self-concept "achievement motivation." But the traditional view also has a construct termed "achievement motivation" (McClelland, 1985; McClelland et al., 1953). If, however, qualitatively different phenomena are being examined by these two models, the use of the same name by both is improper and misleading (cf. Kagan, 1988). An early study in the achievement literature (deCharms, Morrison, Reitman, & McClelland, 1955) suggested that the variable assessed via the TAT be referred to as "need for achievement" (*n* Achievement, or *n* Ach) and the variable assessed through self-report be termed "value of achievement" (*v* Ach). The "need" term has continued to be used to refer to the TAT-based variable, but the "value" term has come to take on a different meaning in psychology. It is now generally utilized to describe beliefs concerning the desirability of goals and ways of behaving (Chaiken & Stangor, 1987; Rokeach, 1973, 1979).

Value is therefore no longer an appropriate way to describe motives rooted in self-conceptions. As a consequence, we refer in the remainder of this chapter to these kinds of motives as "self-attributed motives" (cf. Koestner et al., 1989; McClelland et al., 1989). This reflects their relationship to the self and the fact that they are measured through self-report. We employ the prefix *san* to refer to self-attributed needs; this complements the traditional use of the prefix *n*, which has historically referred to the needs implicit in TAT stories. We use the term "implicit motives" to reflect their mode of measure (i.e., the fact that the person does not explicitly describe himself or herself as having the motive). Thus TAT-assessed motives are referred to as *n* Ach, *n* Power (*n* Pow), *n* Affiliation (*n* Aff), and so on, whereas self-reported motives are referred to as *san* Achievement (*san* Ach) and so on. The former are herewith termed "implicit motives" and the latter "self-attributed motives." It is our hope that this usage will be adopted by others in the field.

Below, we offer evidence to support our interpretation of self-attributed and implicit motives. This evidence bears on variables most likely to elicit each kind of motivation; some experiments explicitly designed to test our hypotheses concerning differences in the arousal and functioning of implicit and self-attributed motives; and some developmental and longitudinal data bearing on the different precursors of the two types of motives.

EVIDENCE FOR THE TWO KINDS OF MOTIVATION

The first piece of evidence suggesting that implicit and self-attributed motives are qualitatively different is a negative one. As we mentioned earlier, the two types of motives almost never correlate significantly with each other. McClelland et al.

(1953) were the first to report this, and it has been found repeatedly since then (e.g., Atkinson & Litwin, 1960; Biernat, 1989; Child, Frank, & Storm, 1956; de Charms et al., 1955; Halisch & Heckhausen, 1987; Heckhausen, 1980; Heckhausen & Halisch, 1986; Holmes & Tyler, 1968; Koestner et al., 1989; Korman, 1974; Kreitler & Kreitler, 1976; McClelland, 1958; Rokeach, 1973). This shows that whatever these two measures are looking at, they are not equivalent.

The next set of data shows that the lack of correlation does not bespeak the invalidity of one or the other measure. Instead, it reflects a theoretically meaningful qualitative difference in what the two types of measures are getting at— namely, self-attributed and implicit motives. Each type of motive predicts different classes of behavior. Implicit motives (measured through TATs) tend to be predictive of long-term, relatively unconstrained behavioral trends, whereas self-attributed motives (assessed via self-report) tend to predict short-term responses to more specific situations or choice behaviors. For example, *n* Ach has been shown to predict entrepreneurial activity over time in both the United States (McClelland, 1965) and India (McClelland, 1987). Similarly, the inhibited power motive (a subtype of *n* Pow) predicted managerial success in a major corporation over 16 years (McClelland & Boyatzis, 1982); it also predicted elevated blood pressure over 20 years following college graduation (McClelland, 1979). Likewise, intimacy motivation (a TAT construct developed by McAdams, 1985), evidenced at age 30, predicted marital happiness and psychosocial adjustment at age 47 (McAdams & Vaillant, 1982). Many of these studies also collected self-report motive measures; these, however, had no long-term predictive validity.[14]

In contrast to implicit motives, self-attributed motives seem better able to predict short-term behavior in highly structured situations. And they do best when the structure is ego-involving and/or directs attention to various aspects of the self. The work of Carver and Scheier (1981b) reviewed earlier demonstrates the importance of self-directed attention. Likewise, the investigations of Markus and Cantor and their associates (e.g., Cantor et al., 1986) show that the relevance of a situation to the individual's life task is critical to the predictive power of self-attributed needs. And Trope (1983, 1986a) has shown the importance of ego-involving aspects of the task, in that success and failure and their causes are made salient in his studies. An investigation by Patten and White (1977) illustrates the point neatly. Self-report measures of achievement (*san* Ach) predicted performance on a laboratory task only when there was an external goad for achieving (ego-arousing instructions). Under neutral conditions, *san* Ach did not relate to performance. Implicit motives do not fare well in situations conducive to the predictive power of self-attributed motives. Thus Clark and McClelland (1956), McClelland et al. (1953), and Wendt (1955) all failed to demonstrate any effect of *n* Ach on performance when external prompts and/or ego-involving instructions were utilized.

Several studies have focused on and provided evidence supportive of the existence of the two orthogonal types of motivation we have been discussing. The earliest was reported by deCharms et al. (1955). They showed that *san* Ach but not *n* Ach (which did not correlate) predicted susceptibility to expert opinion.

Heckhausen and Halisch (1986) conducted a more extensive study. First, they found the usual zero-order correlation between *san* Ach and *n* Ach. More critical was the different pattern of findings for each type of motive. Thus *n* Ach predicted the number of job-related activities spontaneously and successfully carried out, whereas *san* Ach predicted setting high levels of aspiration and reporting high levels of ability.

In a very recent study, Biernat (1989) also found the aforementioned types of differences in the predictive powers of *san* Ach and *n* Ach. After she had obtained the usual lack of correlation between the *san* Ach and *n* Ach measures, she found that they predicted different aspects of performance. The implicit motive (*n* Ach) predicted the solving of mental arithmetic problems (cf. Wendt, 1955), whereas the self-attributed motive (*san* Ach) predicted subjects' choice of whether or not they wanted to be a leader, as well as their choice of adjectives descriptive of a hypothetical person.

In the affiliative domain, Constantian (cited in McClelland, 1985) collected both self-report and TAT measures of affiliation (*san* Aff and *n* Aff, respectively). She found that *n* Aff predicted whether a person would be talking with someone, when beeped randomly throughout several days, more strongly than did *san* Aff. On the other hand, *san* Aff predicted subject reports of affiliative preferences (e.g., whether a person said he or she would rather go to a movie alone or with someone else) better than did *n* Aff.

In none of the studies described above did self-attributed motives predict implicit-motive-related behaviors or vice versa. Thus, they all support our argument that there is a qualitative difference between self-attributed and implicit motives. Moreover, evidence has been adduced in both the achievement and affiliative domains. So these findings are not restricted to achievement. None of these studies, however, were conducted with our theoretical formulations in mind. We turn next to some recent work explicitly designed to test our model.

We (Koestner et al., 1989) asked college students to associate and later recall picture–word pairs. In one condition, this was all they were told. In another condition, an achievement incentive was introduced by making repeated references to doing better at the task. Introducing the achievement incentive was generally effective in improving performance across all subjects. More theoretically relevant was the finding that this incentive was particularly effective for those high in *san* Ach. The incentive had no effect whatsoever on subjects high (or low, for that matter) in *n* Ach.

The same subjects discussed above were then asked to work on word-finding puzzles that varied in their level of difficulty or challenge (challenge or optimal uncertainty is the natural incentive for *n* Ach). No explicit ego-involving achievement incentive was given for this task. Here, the results showed that subjects high in *n* Ach performed relatively better on a challenging than on an easy puzzle, whereas subjects low in *n* Ach showed the reverse pattern. Performance was not predicted in any way by *san* Ach.

In another experiment, we (Koestner et al., 1989) generalized these findings to the power domain. Here, subjects were presented with pictures of two adults in an office or factory setting. The subject's task was to determine which one was the boss. (This is part of a social perception test designed by Sternberg, 1986.) One group was simply asked to perform the task; this was the no-incentive condition. The other group was told that a high score indicated superior ability to influence or manage others; this was the incentive condition. The implicit motive (*n* Pow) predicted overall performance on this task across the two groups. The self-attributed motive (*san* Pow) only predicted performance in the incentive condition.

The results of these experiments all support our distinction between implicit and self-attributed motives. Implicit motives were more likely to predict unconstrained behaviors, such as spontaneous job-related activities (Heckhausen & Halisch, 1986), mentally solving arithmetic problems (Biernat, 1989), frequency of affiliative activity (Constantian, cited in McClelland, 1985), and performance on challenging puzzles and ability to accurately recognize employer–employee relationships (Koestner et al., 1989). Self-attributed motives, on the other hand, were more predictive of choice behaviors, such as level of aspiration (Heckhausen & Halisch, 1986), wanting to be a leader and picking descriptive adjectives (Biernat, 1989), and stating preferences about being with others (Constantian, cited in McClelland, 1985). Self-attributed motives were also effective at predicting behaviors following ego-involving instructions (i.e., situations in which the self was explicitly brought into focus), such as telling subjects that a task was achievement-related (Patten & White, 1977) or that doing better was desirable or indicated superior ability (Koestner et al., 1989). Self-attributed motives were also shown to be sensitive to demand characteristics related to choice, such as susceptibility to expert opinion (deCharms et al., 1955).

Our model also holds that implicit and self-attributed motives should have different child-rearing antecedents. Implicit motives are said to be largely built on genetics and early affective learning, whereas self-attributed motives are more dependent upon later-developing symbolic representational capacities, most notably language-mediated cognitive structures.[15] We now present some preliminary evidence supporting this aspect of the model.

Data collected by Watson and Ramey (1972) support the notion that implicit motives begin very early in life. They reported that infants as young as 6 weeks of age learned to respond so as to cause changes in their environment (movement of a mobile). Changes not contingent on their behavior did not affect responding. Moreover, the mothers of these infants reported that the babies who controlled movement experienced more positive affect toward these changes than did the babies who had no such control. This type of behavior sounds very much like an early example of *n* Ach. The infant gains an affective kick from overcoming a challenge (learning to create movement). It would be difficult to posit *san* Ach at such an early age, since an achieving self-concept or the idea of success versus failure can hardly be assumed to have developed by 6 weeks.

There are also data showing that the child-rearing antecedents of the two types of motives differ. These data are from a follow-up study of 5-year-old children whose mothers were extensively questioned about their child-rearing practices (Sears, Maccoby, & Levin, 1957). At age 31, these same children (now obviously adults) were assessed for both implicit and self-attributed motives (see McClelland & Pilon, 1983; McClelland et al., 1989).

Table 16.1 shows the early child-rearing practices that were significantly correlated with adult implicit motives, as well as those child-rearing practices that correlated significantly with self-attributed motives. As the table illustrates, the two types of motives show different developmental antecedents. Moreover, the differences are in accord with our model. First, the predictors of the implicit motives generally occur earlier in a child's life than do the predictors of the self-attributed motives. Furthermore, the particular correlates make theoretical sense. Thus the predictors of *n* Ach involve mastery of internal bodily states (hunger and elimination). The predictor of *san* Ach involves explaining the nature of a task and the child's responsibilities toward it. This clearly involves more linguistically coded information than do the precursors of *n* Ach. Scheduled feeding involves no verbal communication. For this sample, toilet training also involved

TABLE 16.1   Correlations of Child-Rearing Variables with Implicit and Self-Attributed Motives in Adulthood (*n* = 76–78)

	Correlation with	
Child-rearing variable	n *Achievement*	san *Achievement*
Scheduling of feeding	.33*	.06
Severity of toilet training	.41***	−.10
Early tasks set for child	−.10	.31**
	n *Power*	san *Power*
Permissiveness for sex and aggression	.31**	.08
Punishes aggression to parents	−.17	.32**
Frequency mother spanks	−.07	.39**
	n *Affiliation*	san *Affiliation*
Mother unresponsive to infant crying	.27*	.02
Child told not to fight back	.11	.27*

Note. From "How Do Self-Attributed and Implicit Motives Differ?" by D. C. McClelland, R. Koestner, and J. Weinberger, 1989, *Psychological Review, 96*, 690–702. Copyright by the American Psychological Association. Reprinted by permission.

*p < .05.
**p < .01.
***p < .001.

little speech, as training was reported to be complete for the majority of these children by 19 months (Sears et al., 1957).

The power motives show a similar pattern. Implicit power (*n* Pow) is associated with permissiveness toward sex and aggression. This does not mean that parents verbally encourage such behavior, but rather that it is tolerated or ignored. Again, symbolic representational capacity and verbal mediation do not seem to be factors. In order for a mother's spanking (which predicts *san* Pow) to be effective, however, a child must possess sufficient symbolic representational capacities to understand the nature of the transgression for which he or she is being punished, as well as future consequences for repeated offenses. The parent usually accompanies the spanking with explicit verbal statements emphasizing just these factors.

The affiliative findings are not as reliable as the others, but they are consistent with them. Implicit affiliation (*n* Aff) is correlated with the nonverbal behavior of ignoring some of the infant's behavior (crying). When it is kept in mind that *n* Aff has a strong fear-of-rejection component (Boyatzis, 1972; McAdams, 1985), this association makes sense. Self-attributed affiliation (*san* Aff) is associated with maternal verbal instructions to be nice and not to fight back.

The pattern of findings is remarkably consistent, especially given the 25-year interval between assessments. Implicit motives are acquired earlier in life than are self-attributed motives. Implicit motives are built on largely nonverbal affective experiences, whereas self-attributed motives are built on more highly symbolic representational capacities, such as linguistically coded communications and instructions. Thus these findings complement the experimental results we have presented earlier. Self-attributed motives stem from (often linguistically based) self-concepts. They affect behavior when (and apparently only when) these self-concepts are activated. Implicit motives are affectively based and have no direct language referent; they are activated by cues intrinsic to a task.

CONCLUSIONS AND SPECULATIONS

In this chapter, we have presented overviews of a traditional model and some cognitive models of motivation. We have shown that conflicts between the two models arise because they are concerned with qualitatively different phenomena. We have presented some research data to support our argument. On the basis of these experimental, developmental, and longitudinal studies, we have concluded that the two types of motives are built on different bases, are acquired in different ways and at different stages in development, and are triggered by different variables.

It seems counterintuitive at first blush to have two orthogonal systems, within the same organism, subserving similar behavior. What can be the purposes of such a dual system? And if our conceptions are accurate, where would each system be housed? Our discussion of these issues is largely speculative but empirically testable.

Other Two-System Theories

First, it is not so unusual to posit two generally noninteracting parallel systems subserving similar areas of functioning. Paivio (1971, 1978a, 1978b, 1986) has offered a model similar to ours to account for visual information processing. According to this dual-coding model, visual experience is registered in two functionally independent systems, one verbal and the other nonverbal. The verbal system deals with linguistic information, whereas the nonverbal system processes perceptual–motor information. Even though the two representational systems are functionally independent, appropriate experiences can produce referential connections between them. So the two systems can interact.

Based on Paivio's conceptions and influenced by psychoanalytic theory, Bucci (1985, 1989) has developed yet another dual-coding model. She, like Paivio, posits independent verbal and nonverbal systems. The verbal system in her model, as in Paivio's, utilizes the abstract code of language and logic. This system generally encodes verbal information and stores it in linguistic form. The nonverbal system, on the other hand, is organized according to analogical principles. That is to say, categorization is based on experiences' looking or feeling similar, occurring together in time or place, and/or having similar structure or form. Affect is likely to be associated with this system. The range of contents of this system include sensory, motor, and visceral aspects of experience. Encoding such experiences creates knowledge, expectations, and beliefs that exist outside of language. This system may exist in other species and in children prior to language acquisition; it also continues to operate throughout life. The parallels between Bucci's model and ours are striking. Like implicit motives, the nonverbal system is analogically rather than linguistically organized. Affect is important to both, and both are said to be present in lower animals and preverbal children. Similarly, the verbal coding system can be identified with our notions of self-attributed motives. Both rely on logical and linguistic organization. Finally, both the dual-coding model and our motivational model posit a functional independence of their two major constituent systems.[16]

Psychoanalytic theory also bears a strong similarity to our motivational conceptions. Thus Freud (1923/1961) saw the id and the ego as functionally independent parts of the mind. According to Freud, the id is an irrational, affect-laden structure whose contents are continuous with those of lower animals. Its reasoning is analogical rather than logical, and its operation is typically not available to awareness. Freud believed id needs to have profound, lifelong effects, which are most strongly shaped by early preverbal experiences.

Freud's (1923/1961) description of the id coincides quite nicely with our understanding of implicit motives. The longitudinal findings we have discussed earlier enhance this convergence. Thus McClelland and Pilon (1983) found that implicit motives were predicted by such child-rearing variables as scheduled feeding, strictness of toilet training, and permissiveness toward sex and aggression. These empirical findings are remarkably similar to what classical Freudians have asserted (see, e.g., Fenichel, 1945).

The psychoanalytic view of the ego also ties in well with our model. It can be identified with self-attributed motives. The ego develops later than the id, is concerned with practical affairs, and is organized logically. Freud (1923/1961) did not grant the ego much power or independence in accounting for behavior. This parallels McClelland's initial position (McClelland et al., 1953) on self-attributed motives (then termed "values"). Later psychoanalysts, however (e.g., Hartmann, 1939/1958; White, 1960) saw this as a deficiency in psychoanalytic theory and reconceptualized the ego as having its own motives independent of the id. This development parallels our present understanding of self-attributed motives (McClelland et al., 1989).

Why Two Motive Systems?

Connecting our model with that of psychoanalysis enables us to speculate on the underlying reason for the existence of the two motive systems, on why they are independent, and on how they can be made more congruent. Simply put, implicit needs (id needs, in psychoanalytic jargon) are the more basic, primitive, animalistic needs. Animals act on these needs more or less automatically. The human cognitive system of self-attributed motives (the ego) provides the human being with an escape from the automatic processing characteristic of lower animals. That is, self-attributed motives are able to temporarily override implicit motives. Cognitive investigators have, in fact, found that intentions and current concerns can temporarily override more primitive automatic functioning (Bargh, 1984; Logan, 1980; Posner & Snyder, 1975). In the field of memory, this has been termed "suppression of prepotent responses" (Kinsbourne, 1987).

In evolutionary terms, a conscious, cognitive motivational system can be said to have been built "on top," so to speak, of a more primitive, animalistic motivational system. The evolutionary advantage of such an arrangement is enormous. It allows for much greater flexibility of behavior, thereby increasing the likelihood of survival. The automatic (implicit) motivational system is poorly equipped to make plans or set specific goals that can take contextual circumstances into account. The cognitive self-attributed motive system can do all of these things and is therefore adaptation-enhancing. It gives humans a tremendous advantage over lower animals.

Where Are the Systems Located?

Let us now speculate a bit on where the motivational systems may be located. Since the implicit motives are apparently built on direct experiences of affect that are also characteristic of animals, they must be controlled by parts of the brain common to both humans and animals. Midbrain structures may serve as a candidate here. If the midbrain is implicated in implicit motives, these motives may be tied to physiological systems known to be controlled by midbrain structures. And, as we have mentioned earlier, there are data suggesting such a connection. Thus implicit motives have been shown to be related to neurohormone release (McClelland, 1989). So it may be that implicit motives are mediated through midbrain structures governing the autonomic nervous system (cf. McClelland et al., 1989).

Self-attributed motives, on the other hand, require symbolic representational capacities such as language and are unique to humans. Therefore, they must be housed in an area of the brain that differentiates humans from animals. The highly developed cerebral cortex of humans, where language is processed, seems to fit the bill. Humans have, of course, a much more highly developed cerebral cortex than any other animal; moreover, language, which is apparently unique to humans, is controlled by cortical structures.

Congruence of the Systems

The final issue concerns the lack of association between the two motive systems. Why do the systems not become more congruent over time? All of us are familiar with the experience of wanting to act (or to refrain from acting) in a certain way but being unable to do so consistently. Self-attributed and implicit motives are often discordant. It was precisely symptomatology that was contrary to stated desires that led Freud (Breuer & Freud, 1893–1895/1955) to become interested in what we call implicit motives. He discovered that implicit motives are best identified by analyzing the affect-laden associative networks of fantasy (he used dreams and free association for this purpose). Our view is similar in that we too assess such motives through an analysis of fantasy (although TAT-based scoring systems are used in place of dreams and free association).

So it is not unusual for these two motive systems to be orthogonal. But Freud also believed that they could be made more congruent. Moreover, he argued that increasing their convergence would lead to improved psychological functioning. The techniques employed by psychoanalysis to this end focus on rigorous self-observation. Such observation can help bring implicit motives into awareness, where the more flexible cognitive systems can be brought to bear on them. And Bucci (1985, 1989) has argued that accurate labeling of the contents of the nonverbal system (which we here identify with implicit motives) by the verbal system (which we here identify with self-attributed motives) leads to an adaptation-enhancing reorganization of experience. Borrowing from Paivio (1971, 1986), she terms such verbal labeling of nonverbal referents "referential activity," and she has presented data that support her notions. This suggests that the two motivational systems can interact in special circumstances and that such interactions can potentially enhance adaptive functioning.

Summing Up

We have tried to cover a lot of ground in this chapter. We have discussed and compared traditional and cognitive models of motivation. We have tried to demonstrate, through presentation of empirical data and logical argument, that there are two functionally autonomous kinds of motivation. We have then tried to account for this dual motivational system. Finally, we have tried to draw some important practical implications from our model.

We believe that an understanding of how implicit and self-attributed motives function not only is theoretically important, but has important implications for psychological well-being. The model is still in its formative stages. Future research is needed to clarify it and apply it to some real-life situations.

Notes

1. The work of Eibl-Eibesfeldt (1972), of Lorenz (1965), of Plutchik (1980), and of Buck (1985) also supports the conception of a limited number of emotional states reflected in expressive behavior.

2. This parallels Murray's (1938) classic notion that what he termed "needs" had a physiochemical substrate in the brain.

3. As yet, no neurohormone has been tied to the achievement motive.

4. So, as we have mentioned before (see note 2), the view that motives have a neurohormone substrate (McClelland, 1985) was proposed early by Murray (1938). But although Murray's (1938) views are closely related to and strongly influenced the McClelland (1985) model, there are some important differences between them. Thus Murray, like other motivational theorists we have contrasted with McClelland (Festinger, 1957; Freud, 1915/1957; Higgins, 1987; Hull, 1943), saw his motivational construct (needs) as acting to alter unsatisfying situations, whereas McClelland, as we have described earlier, sees motivated behavior as being in the service of leading to a satisfying state of affairs.

5. The impact incentive of the power motive need not be physical aggression, as in this example. A person could have impact through a political movement or through writing a book as well. We have chosen a physical example because of its ease of exposition.

6. Although in its original usage "cognition" referred to overtly conscious knowledge about some aspect of the world, it has been broadened to include any knowledge structure, whether conscious or nonconscious (Kuhl, 1986).

7. This is similar to the classic gestalt concept of isomorphism (Kohler, 1930, 1969).

8. The public self parallels the self as it has been discussed in the classic symbolic interactionism works of Cooley (1902) and Mead (1934), as well as the more recent but equally influential writings of Goffman (1959, 1974) on self-presentation.

9. Personality theorists who have focused on the private self include Allport (1961), Lecky (1945), Maslow (1970), and Rogers (1947).

10. Markus (1977) defines a "self-schema" as a "cognitive generalization about the self, derived from past experience, that organizes and guides the processing of self-relevant information contained in the individual's social experiences" (p. 64). A series of such schemas comprises the "self-concept."

11. We adopt the term "achievement motivation" here because that is what Weiner (1972, 1985, 1986a) and Trope (1975, 1983, 1986a, 1986b) term the construct. We argue later in this chapter, however, that what Weiner and Trope call "achievement motivation" differs in theoretically important ways from the variable referred to by McClelland and his associates (McClelland, 1985; McClelland et al., 1953), and should therefore be called something else.

12. Sorrentino and Hewitt (1984), however, have presented evidence showing that this is only true for what they term "uncertainty-oriented" individuals. The type of person they term "certainty-oriented" seeks to avoid diagnostic information. (See also Sorrentino & Short, 1986.)

13. Trope (1986a) has offered an interesting integration of his early and late studies, wherein he hypothesizes that diagnostic information serves to increase self-esteem in the long run.

14. Bray, Campbell, and Grant (1974), in a study of managerial success, offer a particularly compelling example of the failure of a variety of self-report measures of motivation to predict long-term outcomes.

15. Although we attribute these later-developing motives to learning, they could have a genetic link as well (cf. Sorrentino & Short, 1986).

16. Raynor and McFarlin (1986) and Sorrentino and Short (1986) also posit two orthogonal motivational systems, although their conceptions differ considerably from ours.

References

Allport, G. W. (1961). *Pattern and growth in personality.* New York: Holt, Rinehart & Winston.

Anderson, J. R. (1983). *The architecture of cognition.* Cambridge, MA: Harvard University Press.

Atkinson, J. W., Heyns, R. W., & Veroff, J. (1954). The effect of experimental arousal of the affiliation motive on thematic apperception. *Journal of Abnormal and Social Psychology, 49,* 405–410.

Atkinson, J. W., & Litwin, G. H. (1960). Achievement motive and test anxiety conceived as motive to approach success and motive to avoid failure. *Journal of Abnormal and Social Psychology, 60,* 52–63.

Bargh, J. A. (1984). Automatic and conscious processing of social information. In R. W. Wyer, Jr., & T. K. Srull (Eds.), *Handbook of social cognition* (Vol. 3, pp. 1–44). Hillsdale, NJ: Erlbaum.

Biernat, M. (1989). Motives and values to achieve: Different constructs with different effects. *Journal of Personality, 57,* 69–95.

Boucher, J. D., & Brandt, M. E. (1981). Judgment of emotion from American and Malay antecedents. *Journal of Cross-Cultural Psychology, 12,* 272–283.

Bowlby, J. (1969). *Attachment and loss: Vol. 1. Attachment.* New York: Basic Books.

Bowlby, J. (1973). *Attachment and loss: Vol. 2. Separation.* New York: Basic Books.

Bowlby, J. (1980). *Attachment and loss: Vol. 3. Loss.* New York: Basic Books.

Boyatzis, R. E. (1972). A two factor theory of affiliation motivation. Unpublished doctoral dissertation. Harvard University.

Bray, D. W., Campbell, R. J., & Grant, D. L. (1974). *Formative years in business: A long term study of managerial lives.* New York: Wiley.

Breuer, J., & Freud, S. (1955). Studies on hysteria. In J. Strachey (Ed. and Trans.), *The standard edition of the complete psychological works of Sigmund Freud* (Vol. 2, pp. 1–307). London: Hogarth Press. (Original work published 1893–1895)

Brody, N. (1983). *Human motivation: Commentary on goal-directed action.* New York: Academic Press.

Brophy, J. E., & Rohrkemper, M. M. (1981). The influence of problem ownership on teachers' perceptions of and strategies for coping with problem students. *Journal of Educational Psychology, 73,* 295–311.

Bucci, W. (1985). Dual coding. A cognitive model for psychoanalytic research. *Journal of the American Psychoanalytic Association, 33,* 571–608.

Bucci, W. (1989). A reconstruction of Freud's tally argument: A program for psychoanalytic research. *Psychoanalytic Inquiry, 9,* 249–281.

Buck, R. (1985). Prime theory: An integrated view of motivation and emotion. *Psychological Review, 92,* 389–413.

Buss, A. H. (1980). *Self-consciousness and social anxiety.* San Francisco: W. H. Freeman.

Candland, D. K., & Leshner, A. I. (1971). Formation of squirrel monkey dominance order is correlated with endocrine output. *Bulletin of the Ecological Society of America, 52,* 54.

Cantor, N., Markus, H., Niedenthal, P., & Nurius, P. (1986). On motivation and the self-concept. In R. M. Sorrentino & E. T. Higgins (Eds.), *Handbook of motivation and cognition: Foundations of social behavior* (Vol. 1, pp. 96–121). New York: Guilford Press.

Cantor, N. J., Niedenthal, P., & Langston, C. (1987). Life-tasks, self-concept ideals, and cognitive strategies in a life transition. *Journal of Personality and Social Psychology, 53,* 1178–1191.

Carver, C. S., & Scheier, M. F. (1981a). *Attention and self-regulation: A control theory approach to human behavior.* New York: Springer.

Carver, C. S., & Scheier, M. F. (1981b). A control systems approach to behavioral self-regulation. In L. Wheeler (Ed.), *Review of personality and social psychology* (Vol. 2, pp. 107–140). Beverly Hills, CA: Sage.

Chaiken, S., & Stangor, C. (1987). Attitudes and attitude change. *Annual Review of Psychology, 38,* 575–630.

Child, I. L., Frank, K. F., & Storm, T. (1956). Self-ratings and the TAT: Their relations to each other and to adulthood background. *Journal of Personality, 25,* 96–114.

Clark, R. A., & McClelland, D. C. (1956). A factor analytic integration of imaginative and performance measures of the need for achievement. *Journal of General Psychology, 55,* 73–83.

Cooley, C. H. (1902). *Human nature and the social order.* New York: Scribner's.

Darwin, C. (1872). *The expression of the emotions in man and the animals.* London: John Murray.

deCharms, R., Morrison, H. W., Reitman, W. R., & McClelland, D. C. (1955). Behavioral correlates of directly and indirectly measured achievement motivation. In D. C. McClelland (Ed.), *Studies in motivation* (pp. 414–423). New York: Appleton-Century-Crofts.

Deci, E. L., & Ryan, R. M. (1985). *Intrinsic motivation and self-determination in human behavior.* New York: Plenum.

Duval, S., & Wicklund, R. A. (1972). *A theory of objective self-awareness.* New York: Academic Press.

Eibl-Eibesfeldt, I. (1972). Similarities and differences between cultures in expressive movements. In R. A. Hinde (Ed.), *Nonverbal communication.* Cambridge, England: Cambridge University Press.

Eibl-Eibesfeldt, I. (1979). *Ethology: The biology of behavior.* New York: Holt, Rinehart & Winston.

Ekman, P. (1971). Universal and cultural differences in facial expressions of emotion. In J. K. Cole (Ed.), *Nebraska Symposium on Motivation* (Vol. 19, pp. 207–283). Lincoln: University of Nebraska Press.

Ekman, P. (1984). Expression and the nature of emotion. In K. R. Scherer & P. Ekman (Eds.), *Approaches to emotion* (pp. 319–343). Hillsdale, NJ: Erlbaum.

Entwisle, D. R. (1972). To dispel fantasies about fantasy-based measures of achievement motivation. *Psychological Bulletin, 77,* 377–391.

Fenichel, O. (1945). *The psychoanalytic theory of neurosis.* New York: Norton.

Fenigstein, A., Scheier, M. F., & Buss, A. H. (1975). Public and private self-consciousness. *Journal of Consulting and Clinical Psychology, 37,* 75–86.

Festinger, L. (1957). *A theory of cognitive dissonance.* Evanston, IL: Row, Peterson.

Flavell, J. H. (1963). *The development psychology of Jean Piaget.* New York: Van Nostrand.

Forsyth, D. R. (1980). The function of attributions. *Social Psychology Quarterly, 43,* 184–189.

Freud, S. (1957). Instincts and their vicissitudes. In J. Strachey (Ed. and Trans.), *The standard edition of the complete psychological works of Sigmund Freud* (Vol. 14, pp. 111–140). London: Hogarth Press. (Original work published 1915)

Freud, S. (1961). The ego and the id. In J. Strachey (Ed. and Trans.), *The standard edition of the complete psychological works of Sigmund Freud* (Vol. 23, pp. 3–69). London: Hogarth Press. (Original work published 1923)

Freud, S. (1964). New introductory lectures on psycho-analysis. In J. Strachey (Ed. and Trans.), *The standard edition of the complete psychological works of Sigmund Freud* (Vol. 22, pp. 3–184). London: Hogarth Press. (Original work published 1933)

Gardner, H. (1987). *The mind's new science: A history of cognitive revolution.* New York: Basic Books.

Goffman, E. (1959). *The presentation of self in everyday life.* Garden City, NY: Doubleday.

Goffman, E. (1974). *Frame analysis: An essay on the organization of experience.* Cambridge, MA: Harvard University Press.

Graham, S., Doubleday, C., & Guarino, P. A. (1984). The development of relations between perceived controllability and the emotions of pity, anger, and guilt. *Child Development, 55,* 561–565.

Halisch, F., & Heckhausen, H. (1987). Motive-dependent vs. ability-dependent valence functions for success and failure. In F. Halisch & J. van den Bercken (Eds.), *International perspectives on achievement and task motivation.* Lisse, The Netherlands: Swets & Zeitlinger.

Hartmann, E. (1958). *Ego psychology and the problem of adaptation* (D. Rapaport, Trans.). New York: International Universities Press. (Original work published 1939)

Heckhausen, H. (1977). Achievement motivation and its constructs: A cognitive model. *Motivation and Emotion, 4*, 283–329.

Heckhausen, H. (1980). *Motivation und Handlung* [*Motivation and action*]. Berlin: Springer-Verlag.

Heckhausen, H., & Halisch, F. (1986). *"Operant" versus "respondent" motive measures: A problem of validity or of construct?* Münich: Max-Planck-Institut für Psychologische Forschung.

Higgins, E. T. (1987). Self-discrepancy: A theory relating self and affect. *Psychological Review, 94,* 319–340.

Hinde, R. A. (1970). *Animal behavior: A synthesis of ethology and comparative psychology.* New York: McGraw-Hill.

Hoffman, M. L. (1986). Affect, cognition, and motivation. In R. M. Sorrentino & E. T. Higgins (Eds.), *Handbook of motivation and cognition: Foundations of social behavior* (Vol. 1, pp. 244–280). New York: Guilford Press.

Holmes, D. S., & Tyler, J. D. (1968). Direct versus projective measures of achievement motivation. *Journal of Consulting and Clinical Psychology, 32,* 712–717.

Howe, H. E., Jr. (Ed.). (1981). *Nebraska Symposium on Motivation* (Vol. 29). Lincoln: University of Nebraska Press.

Hoyle, G. (1984). The scope of neuroethology. *Behavioral and Brain Sciences, 7,* 367–412.

Hull, C. L. (1943). *Principles of behavior.* New York: Appleton-Century-Crofts.

Jones, E. E., & Davis, K. E. (1965). From acts to dispositions: The attribution process in person perception. In L. Berkowitz (Ed.), *Advances in experimental social psychology* (Vol. 2, pp. 219–266). New York: Academic Press.

Kagan, J. (1988). The meanings of personality predicates. *American Psychologist, 43,* 614–620.

Kelley, H. H. (1967). Attribution theory in social psychology. In D. Levine (Ed.), *Nebraska Symposium on Motivation* (Vol. 15, pp. 192–238). Lincoln: University of Nebraska Press.

Kelley, H. H. (1971). *Attribution in social interaction.* Morristown, NJ: General Learning Press.

Kelley, H. H. (1973). The processes of causal attribution. *American Psychologist, 28,* 107–128.

Kinsbourne, M. (1987). Brain mechanisms and memory. *Human Neurobiology, 6,* 81–92.

Kintsch, W., Miller, J. R., & Polson, P. G. (Eds.). (1984). *Method and tactics in cognitive science.* Hillsdale, NJ: Erlbaum.

Kleinginna, P. R., Jr., & Kleinginna, A. M. (1981). A categorized list of emotion definitions, with suggestions for a consensual definition. *Motivation and Emotion, 5,* 345–379.

Koestner, R., Ryan, R. M., Bernieri, F., & Holt, K. (1984). Setting limits on children's behavior: The differential effects of controlling versus informational styles on intrinsic motivation and creativity. *Journal of Personality, 52,* 233–248.

Koestner, R., Weinberger, J., & McClelland, D. C. (1989). *How motives and values interact with task and social incentives to affect performance.* Unpublished manuscript, McGill University.

Kohler, W. (1930). The new psychology and physics. *Yale Review, 19,* 560–576.

Kohler, W. (1969). *The task of gestalt psychology.* Princeton, NJ: Princeton University Press.

Korman, A. (1974). *The psychology of motivation.* Englewood Cliffs, NJ: Prentice-Hall.

Kreitler, H., & Kreitler, S. (1976). *Cognitive orientation and behavior.* New York: Springer.

Kuhl, J. (1986). Motivation and information processing. In R. M. Sorrentino & E. T. Higgins (Eds.), *Handbook of motivation and cognition: Foundations of social behavior* (Vol. 1, pp. 404–434). New York: Guilford Press.

Lecky, P. (1945). *Self consistency: A theory of personality.* New York: Island Press.

Lehrman, D. S. (1964). The reproductive behavior of ringdoves. *Scientific American, 211,* 48–54.

Lehrman, D. S. (1965). Interaction between internal and external environments in the regulation of the reproductive cycle of the ringdove. In F. A. Beach (Ed.), *Sex and behavior* (pp. 355–380). New York: Wiley.

Logan, G. D. (1980). Attention and automaticity in Stroop and priming tasks: Theory and data. *Cognitive Psychology, 12,* 523–553.

Lorenz, K. Z. (1935). Der kumpan in der umvelt des vogels. *Zeitschrift für Ornithologie, 83,* 137–213, 289–413.

Lorenz, K. (1965). *Evolution and modification of behavior.* Chicago: University of Chicago Press.

Lundy, A. C. (1985). The reliability of the Thematic Apperception Test. *Journal of Personality Assessment, 49*, 141–145.

Mancuso, J. C., & Mascolo, M. F. (1987). Re-cognizing achievement motivation. *Motivation and Emotion, 11*, 323–330.

Markus, H. (1977). Self-schemata and processing information about the self. *Journal of Personality and Social Psychology, 35*, 63–78.

Markus, H. (1983). Self-knowledge: An expanded view. *Journal of Personality, 51*, 543–565.

Maslow, A. H. (1970). *Motivation and personality.* New York: Harper & Row.

McAdams, D. P. (1985). *Power, intimacy and the life story.* Homewood, IL: Dorsey Press.

McAdams, D. P., & Vaillant, G. E. (1982). Intimacy motivation and psychosocial adaptation: A longitudinal study. *Journal of Personality Assessment, 46*, 586–593.

McClelland, D. C. (1958). Methods of measuring human motivation. In J. W. Atkinson (Ed.), *Motives in fantasy, action and society* (pp. 7–42). Princeton, NJ: Van Nostrand.

McClelland, D. C. (1965). N Achievement and entrepreneurship: A longitudinal study. *Journal of Personality and Social Psychology, 1*, 389–392.

McClelland, D. C. (1979). Inhibited power motivation and high blood pressure in men. *Journal of Abnormal Psychology, 88*, 182–190.

McClelland, D. C. (1980). The merits of operant and respondent measures. In L. Wheeler (Ed.), *Review of personality and social psychology* (Vol. 1, pp. 10–41). Beverly Hills, CA: Sage.

McClelland, D. C. (1985). *Human motivation.* Glenview, IL: Scott, Foresman.

McClelland, D. C. (1987). Characteristics of successful entrepreneurs. *Journal of Creative Behavior, 3*, 219–233.

McClelland, D. C. (1989). Motivation factors in health and disease. *American Psychologist, 44*, 675–683.

McClelland, D. C., & Atkinson, J. W. (1948). The projective expression of needs: 1. The effect of different intensities of the hunger drive on perception. *Journal of Psychology, 25*, 205–222.

McClelland, D. C., Atkinson, J. W., Clark, R. A., & Lowell, E. L. (1953). *The achievement motive.* New York: Appleton-Century-Crofts.

McClelland, D. C., & Boyatzis, R. E. (1982). The leadership motive pattern and long-term success in management. *Journal of Applied Psychology, 67*, 737–743.

McClelland, D. C., Clark, R. A., Roby, T. B., & Atkinson, J. W. (1949). The projective expression of needs: IV. The effect of the need for achievement in thematic apperception. *Journal of Experimental Psychology, 39*, 242–255.

McClelland, D. C., Koestner, R., & Weinberger, J. (1989). How do self-attributed and implicit motives differ? *Psychological Review, 96*, 690–702.

McClelland, D. C., & Pilon, D. A. (1983). Sources of adult motives in patterns of parent behavior in early childhood. *Journal of Personality and Social Psychology, 44*, 564–574.

Mead, G. H. (1934). *Mind, self, and society.* Chicago: University of Chicago Press.

Mehrabian, A. (1969). Measures of achieving tendency. *Educational and Psychological Measurement, 29*, 445–451.

Miller, G. A., Galanter, E., & Pribram, K. H. (1960). *Plans and the structure of behavior.* New York: Holt, Rinehart & Winston.

Mook, D. G. (1987). *Motivation: The organization of action.* New York: Norton.

Murray, H. A. (1936). Techniques for a systematic investigation of fantasy. *Journal of Psychology, 3*, 115–143.

Murray, H. A. (1938). *Explorations in personality.* New York: Oxford University Press.

Neisser, U. (1967). *Cognitive psychology.* New York: Appleton-Century-Crofts.

Niedenthal, P. M., Cantor, N., & Kihlstrom, J. F. (1985). Prototype matching: A strategy for social decision-making. *Journal of Personality and Social Psychology, 48*, 575–584.

Nisbett, R., & Ross, L. (1980). *Human inferences: Strategies and shortcomings of social judgment.* Englewood Cliffs, NJ: Prentice-Hall.

Nisbett, R. E., & Wilson, T. D. (1977). Telling more than we can know: Verbal reports on mental processes. *Psychological Review, 84*, 231–259.

Nurius, P., & Markus, H. (1984). The mutable self-concept: *Social context as reflected in self-knowledge.* Unpublished manuscript, University of Michigan.

Paivio, A. (1971). *Imagery and verbal processes.* New York: Holt, Rinehart & Winston.

Paivio, A. (1978a). A dual coding approach to perception and cognition. In H. L. Pick & E. Saltzman (Eds.), *Modes of perceiving and processing information* (pp. 39–51). Hillsdale, NJ: Erlbaum.

Paivio, A. (1978b). The relationship between verbal and perceptual codes. In E. C. Carterette & M. P. Friedman (Eds.), *Handbook of perception: Perceptual coding* (pp. 375–397). New York: Academic Press.

Paivio, A. (1986). *Mental representations: A dual coding approach.* New York: Oxford University Press.

Panskepp, J. (1971). Aggression elicited by electrical stimulation of the hypothalamus in albino rats. *Physiology and Behavior, 6,* 321–329.

Patten, R. L., & White, L. A. (1977). Independent effects of achievement behavior. *Motivation and Emotion, 1,* 39–59.

Plutchik, R. (1980). *The emotions: A psycho-evolutionary synthesis.* New York: Harper & Row.

Posner, M. I., & Snyder, C. R. (1975). Attention and cognitive control. In R. L. Solso (Ed.), *Information processing and cognition: The Loyola Symposium.* Hillsdale, NJ: Erlbaum.

Raynor, J. O., & McFarlin, D. B. (1986). Motivation and self-system. In R. M. Sorrentino & E. T. Higgins (Eds.), *Handbook of motivation and cognition: Foundations of social behavior* (Vol. 1, pp. 315–349). New York: Guilford Press.

Rescorla, R. A. (1988). Pavlovian conditioning: It's not what you think it is. *American Psychologist, 43,* 151–160.

Rogers, C. R. (1947). Some observations on the organization of personality. *American Psychologist, 2,* 358–368.

Rokeach, M. (1973). *The nature of human values.* New York: Free Press.

Rokeach, M. (1979). *Understanding human values: Individual and societal.* New York: Free Press.

Scheier, M. F., & Carver, C. S. (1981). Public and private aspects of self. In L. Wheeler (Ed.), *Review of personality and social psychology* (Vol. 2, pp. 189–216). Beverly Hills, CA: Sage.

Sears, R. R., Maccoby, E. E., & Levin, H. (1957). *Patterns of child rearing.* Evanston, IL: Row, Peterson.

Shaver, K. S. (1975). *An introduction to attribution processes.* Cambridge, MA: Winthrop.

Solso, R. L. (1988). *Cognitive psychology* (2nd ed.). Newton, MA: Allyn & Bacon.

Sorrentino, R. M., & Hewitt, E. (1984). Uncertainty-related properties of achievement tasks as a function of uncertainty-orientation and achievement-related motives. *Journal of Personality and Social Psychology, 47,* 884–899.

Sorrentino, R. M., & Higgins, E. T. (1986). Motivation and cognition: Warming up to synergism. In R. M. Sorrentino & E. T. Higgins (Eds.), *Handbook of motivation and cognition: Foundations of social behavior* (Vol. 1, pp. 3–20). New York: Guilford Press.

Sorrentino, R. M., & Short, J. C. (1986). Uncertainty orientation, motivation, and cognition. In R. M. Sorrentino & E. T. Higgins (Eds.), *Handbook of motivation and cognition: Foundations of social behavior* (Vol. 1, pp. 379–403). New York: Guilford Press.

Sternberg, R. J. (1986). *Intelligence applied: Understanding and increasing your intellectual skills.* New York: Harcourt Brace Jovanovich.

Stillings, N. A., Feinstein, M. H., Garfield, J. L., Rissland, E. L., Rosenbaum, D. A., Weisler, S. E., & Baker-Ward, L. (1987). *Cognitive science: An introduction.* Cambridge, MA: MIT Press.

Tinbergen, N. (1951). *The study of instinct.* Oxford: Clarendon Press.

Tinbergen, N., & Perdeck, A. C. (1950). On the stimulus situation releasing the begging response in the newly hatched herring gull chick. *Behaviour, 3,* 1–39.

Trope, Y. (1975). Seeking information about one's own ability as a determinant of choice among tasks. *Journal of Personality and Social Psychology, 32,* 1004–1013.

Trope, Y. (1980). Self-assessment, self-enhancement and task preference. *Journal of Experimental Social Psychology, 16,* 116–129.

Trope, Y. (1983). Self-assessment in achievement behavior. In J. M. Suls & A. G. Greenwald (Eds.), *Psychological perspectives on the self* (Vol. 2, pp. 93–121). Hillsdale, NJ: Erlbaum.

Trope, Y. (1986a). Self-enhancement and self-assessment in achievement behavior. In R. M. Sorrentino & E. T. Higgins (Eds.), *Handbook of motivation and cognition: Foundations of social behavior* (Vol. 1, pp. 350–378). New York: Guilford Press.

Trope, Y. (1986b). Testing self-enhancement and self-assessment theories of achievement motivation: A reply to Sohn's critique. *Motivation and Emotion, 10,* 247–262.

Trope, Y., & Brickman, P. (1975). Difficulty and diagnosticity as determinants of choice among tasks. *Journal of Personality and Social Psychology, 31,* 918–925.

Watson, J. S., & Ramey, C. G. (1972). Reactions to response-contingent stimulation in early infancy. *Merrill-Palmer Quarterly, 18,* 219–228.

Weinberger, J., & McLeod, C. (1989). *The need to belong: A psychoanalytically-based affiliative motive in the McClelland-Atkinson tradition.* Paper presented at the meeting of the American Psychological Association, New Orleans.

Weiner, B. (1972). *Theories of motivation: From mechanism to cognition.* Chicago: Rand McNally.

Weiner, B. (1979). A theory of motivation for some classroom experiences. *Journal of Educational Psychology, 71,* 3–25.

Weiner, B. (1980a). A cognitive (attributional)–emotion–action model of motivated behavior: An analysis of judgments of help-giving. *Journal of Personality and Social Psychology, 39,* 186–200.

Weiner, B. (1980b). May I borrow your class notes? An attributional analysis of judgments of help-giving in an achievement-related context. *Journal of Educational Psychology, 72,* 676–681.

Weiner, B. (1985). An attributional theory of achievement motivation and emotion. *Psychological Review, 92,* 548–573.

Weiner, B. (1986a). *An attributional theory of motivation and emotion.* New York: Springer.

Weiner, B. (1986b). Attribution, emotion, and action. In R. M. Sorrentino & E. T. Higgins (Eds.), *Handbook of motivation and cognition: Foundations of social behavior* (Vol. 1, pp. 281–312). New York: Guilford Press.

Weiner, B. (1987). The role of emotions in a theory of motivation. In F. Halisch & J. Kuhl (Eds.), *Motivation, intention and volition* (pp. 22–30). New York: Springer.

Weiner, B., Russell, D., & Lerman, D. (1979). The cognition–emotion process in achievement-related contexts. *Journal of Personality and Social Psychology, 37,* 1211–1220.

Wendt, H. W. (1955). Motivation, effort and performance. In D. C. McClelland (Ed.), *Studies in motivation.* New York: Appleton-Century-Crofts.

White, R. W. (1960). Competence and the psychosexual states of development. In M. R. Jones (Ed.), *Nebraska Symposium on Motivation* (Vol. 8, pp. 97–141). Lincoln: University of Nebraska Press.

Wicklund, R. A. (1979). The influence of self on human behavior. *American Scientist, 67,* 187–193.

Wilson, E. O. (1975). *Sociobiology: The new synthesis.* Cambridge, MA: Harvard University Press.

Winter, D. G. (1973). *The power motive.* New York: Free Press.

Winter, D. G., & Stewart, A. J. (1977). Power motive reliability as a function of retest instructions. *Journal of Consulting and Clinical Psychology, 45* 436–440.

Zajonc, R. B. (1980). Feeling and thinking: Preferences need no inferences. *American Psychologist, 35,* 151–175.

Zajonc, R. B. (1984). The interaction of affect and cognition. In K. R. Scherer & P. Ekman (Eds.), *Approaches to emotion* (pp. 239–246). Hillsdale, NJ: Erlbaum.

Author Index

Abele, A., 545
Abeloff, M. D., 134
Abelson, R. P., 4, 15, 96, 98, 101, 111, 113–116, 118, 119, 408, 412, 453, 485
Ables, R. P., 408, 409
Aboud, F., 391
Abrahams, S., 231
Abramowitz, A. I., 304
Abramson, L. Y., 27, 73, 75–77, 269, 373, 410, 488, 492, 505, 547, 549
Ach, N., 54, 57, 58
Adams, G. R., 213
Adams, H. E., 528
Adams, J. A., 6
Adelmann, P. K., 134
Aderman, D., 286
Adler, T., 172, 388
Adorno, T. W., 112, 299, 337
Afton, A. D., 493
Agustsdottir, S., 97
Ahrens, A. H., 504, 505
Ajzen, I., 5, 165, 183, 334, 338, 339, 355, 358, 362, 363n, 364n, 501, 502
Alba, J. W., 485, 489, 494, 518
Allan, L. G., 474
Allen, B. P., 377
Allen, H. M., 304
Allen, J. L., 290, 377
Allen, S. W., 466
Alloy, L. B., 73, 75–77, 269, 284, 410, 488, 504, 505, 547, 549
Allport, F. H., 97
Allport, G. W., 113, 118, 182, 370, 408, 413, 591n
Alon, S., 231
Alstatt, L., 281
Alston, W. P., 370, 371, 381, 384
Altshuler, J., 377
Anderson, C. A., 488, 498, 500, 505
Anderson, J. R., 85, 109, 110, 569
Anderson, N. H., 540
Anderson, R. C., 97, 237, 485
Anderson, R. E., 487
Andrew, R. J., 140
Andrews, L., 283
Angell, M., 507
Antoni, M., 22
Appleman, A. J., 355
Apsler, R., 277
Apter, M. J., 223n
Arbuthnot, J., 209, 210
Arcelus, F., 304
Archer, R. L., 273
Arieti, S., 392

Arkes, H. R., 485, 488
Arkin, R. M., 334, 355, 356, 513
Arnold, M. B., 543
Aronson, E., 408, 409, 412, 413, 423
Asch, S. E., 344, 362
Athay, M., 415
Atkinson, J. W., 27, 44, 54, 55, 64, 105, 112, 118, 119, 152, 170, 177, 180, 181, 186, 187, 196, 199, 201, 206, 223n, 234, 251, 339, 562, 564, 566, 583
Atkinson, R. C., 473
Audrain, P., 536, 538, 542
Austin, G. A., 415
Averill, J. R., 272, 276

Backman, C. W., 408, 411, 413–415, 418, 428, 439
Baddeley, A. D., 430
Balaban, T., 387
Baldwin, M. W., 486
Balloun, J. L., 74
Bandura, A., 11, 27, 151, 153, 154, 156, 161, 162, 172, 177, 178, 187, 229–232, 235, 387
Bar-Hillel, M., 347, 502
Bar-Tal, D., 334, 339
Bar-Tal, Y., 334
Barbee, A. P., 267, 275
Barber, J. D., 299
Barclay, C. R., 495
Barclay, J., 205
Barenboim, C., 371
Bargh, J. A., 79, 81, 84, 93–96, 100, 106–109, 111–115, 117, 119–121, 312, 323, 335, 423, 440n, 454, 456, 485, 489, 511, 540, 589
Barker, R. G., 106
Barnett, L. W., 139
Baron, J., 78, 79, 504, 510
Baron, R., 123
Baron, R. A., 141
Baron, R. J., 12
Baron, R. M., 254, 275
Baron, R. S., 278
Barsalou, L. W., 459
Barta, S. G., 27
Barter, J., 38
Bartlett, F. C., 485
Batson, C. D., 273, 282, 287, 289, 290
Baumann, D. J., 265, 280, 282, 550
Baumeister, R. F., 410, 415, 431
Baumgardner, A. H., 334, 356, 415, 437, 513
Baumgardner, M. H., 469, 470, 489
Beattie, A. E., 116
Beattie, J., 510
Beck, A., 492

Beck, A. T., 78
Beck, P., 319
Beckmann, J., 62, 74, 102
Bee, H., 204
Bem, D. J., 240, 333, 409, 414, 486
Bem, S. L., 397
Bemporad, J., 392
Ben-Yair, E., 234, 251
Ben Zur, H., 430
Benenson, J., 388, 433
Bensley, L. S., 139
Benson, D. F., 12
Beourne, E., 215
Berg, J. H., 273
Berglas, S., 97, 334, 356, 513
Berkowitz, L., 270, 275, 277, 409
Berlyne, D., 440*n*
Berlyne, D. E., 230, 339
Berndt, T. J., 377, 378, 379
Bernieri, F., 579
Berridge, K. C., 460
Berscheid, E., 43, 334, 354, 361, 364*n*, 385
Berzonsky, M. D., 207
Beyth, R., 490
Biernat, M., 578, 583-585
Bigner, J. J., 371
Bilsky, W., 157
Birch, D., 55, 118, 119, 170, 177, 199, 201, 223*n*, 339
Birnbaum, M. H., 78
Bjork, R. A., 452, 455, 464, 468
Black, J. B., 485
Blackwell, J., 389
Blake, F., 311
Blaney, P. H., 24, 268, 490, 527, 529
Blank, A., 116, 123, 278
Blankenship, V., 109, 186
Blascovitch, J., 428, 437
Blasi, A., 153
Blatt, M. M., 210
Blaxton, T. A., 464
Bless, E., 277
Bless, H., 279, 287, 546, 550
Bloom, H. S., 304
Blumer, C., 488
Boag, L. C., 392
Bobko, P., 177
Bobocel, R., 200, 300, 349
Bobrow, D. G., 72, 109, 431
Bodenhausen, G. V., 528
Boehm, L., 488
Boggiano, A. K., 231, 251, 394
Bohner, G., 279, 546, 550
Boissevain, J., 426
Boland, F., 138
Bolen, D., 392
Bolland, J. M., 310
Bollnow, O. F., 536, 537
Bond, R. N., 94, 106, 277
Bonoma, T. V., 409
Borgida, E., 98
Boring, E. G., 63, 96, 108
Borman, C., 85
Boucher, J. D., 565
Bourne, L. E., 72
Bower, G. H., 44, 267-269, 284, 485, 491, 528-531, 534, 540, 541

Bowers, K. S., 454
Bowlby, J., 285, 564
Bowman, C., 274
Boyatzis, R. E., 564, 583, 587
Boyd, R. W., 302
Boyer, J. L., 281
Bradley, G. W., 410
Branch, L. G., 139
Brand, J. F., 97
Brandt, M. E., 565
Branscombe, N. R., 85, 466
Bransford, D. E., 462
Bransford, J. D., 485
Braun, O. L., 463
Bray, D. W., 591*n*
Brehm, J. W., 27, 39, 58, 62, 75, 116, 210, 412
Brent, E., 301, 316
Breuer, J., 131, 590
Brewer, M. B., 94, 458
Brewer, W. F., 105, 494, 495
Breznitz, S. J., 430
Brickman, P., 26, 86, 390, 392, 506, 575
Broadbent, D. E., 12, 456, 545
Broadbent, K., 491, 492
Brock, T. C., 74, 83, 277
Brockner, J., 27, 62
Brody, N., 474, 577
Brody, R., 321, 322
Bromley, D. B., 369, 371-373, 376, 382, 383, 385, 394
Brooks, L. R., 457, 458, 466, 474
Brophy, J. E., 580
Brown, A. S., 487
Brown, D. R., 151, 152
Brown, J., 469, 471, 472, 489
Brown, J. D., 20, 410, 434, 437, 483, 488, 505, 507
Brown, R., 109, 153
Brown, R. W., 235, 236
Brown, S. A., 45
Brown, S. R., 310, 324
Brown, T. A., 302, 305
Brownbridge, G., 38
Brownlee, E. A., 415
Broxton, J. A., 418
Bruner, J. S., 84, 97, 111, 112, 182, 299, 335, 415, 455, 460, 485, 489, 545
Brunson, B. I., 24
Bryan, J. W., 396, 397
Bucci, W., 588, 590
Buchanan, B., 62
Buchanan, W., 281
Buck, R., 284, 288, 428, 433, 567, 591*n*
Bulman, R. J., 390, 513
Burger, J. M., 28, 355
Burgio, K. L., 27
Busemeyer, J. R., 11, 12
Bush, R., 425
Buss, A. H., 112, 386, 455, 571
Buss, D. M., 105, 110, 115, 370, 381
Bussey, K., 387
Bycio, P., 142
Byrne, D., 197, 538

Cacioppo, J. T., 97, 112
Calveric, B. R., 375
Camhy, M., 394, 400

Campbell, A., 300, 301, 320
Campbell, D. T., 335
Campbell, J., 20, 437, 513
Campbell, J. D., 371, 410
Campbell, J. E., 304
Campbell, R. J., 591*n*
Candee, D., 152, 153, 177, 186
Candland, D. K., 565
Cantor, N., 4, 6, 44, 98, 106, 111, 112, 114, 115,
    118, 423, 453, 472, 487, 562, 571-573, 575,
    577, 579, 580, 583
Cantor, N. J., 572, 573
Capitman, J. A., 5
Carlsmith, J. M., 270, 277, 285, 412, 423
Carlson, M., 265, 281, 287
Carlston, D., 529
Carlston, D. E., 114, 540, 541
Carmichael, L., 488
Carpenter, K. M., 499
Carroll, J. S., 498
Carson, R. C., 415
Carson, T. P., 528
Carter, D. B., 396
Carter, S. R., III, 131
Carver, C. S., 3, 5, 8, 11, 17, 22-24, 26, 27, 29,
    31, 34, 39, 40, 42, 44, 45, 60, 111, 274,
    427, 562, 571-573, 575, 581, 583
Case, R., 80, 193, 383
Casey, E. S., 495
Caspi, A., 385
Cataldo, E. F., 304
Cauble, M., 218
Cervone, D., 177
Chabassol, D. J., 204
Chaiken, S., 94, 97, 349, 361, 435, 486, 518, 582
Chambers, W., 5
Chambliss, C. A., 28
Chanowitz, B., 116, 123, 278
Chapanis, A., 409
Chapanis, N. P., 409
Chaplin, R., 74
Chaplin, W. F., 370
Chapman, D. W., 63
Chard, F., 273
Charlin, V., 265
Chase, W. G., 308, 485
Chatman, J., 62
Cheesman, J., 469
Cheng, P. W., 79
Chew, C. H., 134
Chi, M. T. H., 80, 308
Chidester, T., 416
Chiesi, H. L., 485
Chilamkurti, C., 375
Child, J. L., 583
Christiansen, B. A., 45
Christie, R., 299
Chrosniak, L. D., 487
Chwalisz, K., 43
Cialdini, R., 375
Cialdini, R. B., 265, 271, 276, 277, 278, 280-
    282, 284, 287, 290, 437, 499, 547, 550
Cisneros, T., 552
Citrin, J., 305
Citron, C. C., 387
Clark, D. M., 528, 531
Clark, L., 539, 542

Clark, L. F., 541
Clark, M., 269, 271
Clark, M. S., 265, 268, 270, 278, 281, 284, 528,
    540
Clark, R. A., 105, 562, 566, 583
Clark, R. D., III, 276
Clarke, G. L., 418
Clayton, J. P., 224*n*
Clayton, V., 205, 207
Clore, G. L., 29, 279, 527-529, 531, 532, 534-
    538, 541, 542, 545
Cofer, C. N., 133
Cohen, A. R., 62, 83, 412
Cohen, C. E., 97
Cohen, J. D., 10
Cohen, N. J., 451
Cohen, O., 237
Cohen, P. R., 268
Coke, J. S., 273
Colby, A., 223*n*
Collins, A., 29, 537
Collins, J., 457, 539, 542
Collins, J. C., 474
Collins, R. L., 410
Condry, J., 258
Connell, J. P., 230
Conner, J. M., 387
Conover, P. J., 310, 313-317, 323
Contrada, R. J., 179
Converse, P. E., 302, 314, 320, 323
Converse, P. S., 300
Conway, M., 486
Cook, T. D., 469
Cooley, C. H., 591*n*
Cooley, C. S., 414
Cooper, E. E., 231
Cooper, J., 333, 387, 398, 412, 529, 542
Corbit, J. D., 136
Corkin, S., 451
Corty, E., 540
Cowan, C. L., 275
Cowan, W. B., 108, 119
Cox, M. G., 370
Coyne, J. C., 421
Craik, F. I. M., 465
Craik, K. H., 370, 381
Crandall, J. E., 273
Crary, W. G., 424
Creighton, J., 507
Crocker, J., 308, 370, 485, 504
Crockett, W. H., 371
Crosniak, L. D., 492
Cross, H. J., 210
Cross, S., 507
Croyle, R. T., 398
Csikszentmihalyi, M., 66, 232
Cunniff, C., 94
Cunningham, J. D., 355
Cunningham, M. R., 267, 271-273, 275, 282,
    283, 285
Curtis, R. C., 421, 437

Dafoe, J. L., 231
D'Agostino, P. R., 112, 116, 334, 357, 359-361
Dallas, M., 465, 468, 469, 473
Damon, W., 402*n*
Daniels, D., 380

Daniels, D. H., 433
Daniels, L., 270
Darby, B., 271
Darley, J. M., 12, 414, 415, 421, 499
Darlington, R. B., 277
Darwin, C., 140, 565
Daubman, K. A., 279, 548
Davidson, J. R., 74
Davidson, L., 552
Davis, K. E., 334, 355, 356, 503, 574
Davis, O., 303
Davitz, J. R., 544
Dawkins, R., 12
DeAngelis, D. L., 42
deCharms, R., 230, 582, 583, 585
Deci, E. L., 229–233, 235, 240, 252, 579
DeCooke, P. A., 495
DeCotis, K. M., 391
DeCourville, N., 486
Dellarosa, D., 72
Dembo, T., 53, 180
Dempster, F. N., 80
De Nicholas, M. E., 278
Dennett, D. C., 93, 99, 106, 120, 121
Derlega, V., 122
Dermer, M., 334, 385
Derogatis, L. R., 134
Devine, P. G., 94, 95, 98, 409
Diener, C. I., 24
Diener, E., 9, 38, 43, 531
Dignan, M. H., 221
Dipboye, R. L., 413
DiVitto, B., 374
Dix, T., 375
Dixon, N. F., 469, 470, 472
Dizadji, D., 19
Dodson, J. D., 54
Dooling, D. J., 485
Doren, B., 491, 529
Dornbusch, S. A., 425
Doubleday, C., 580
Dovidio, J. F., 276, 277, 290
Downs, A., 303
Draft, D., 438
Dreben, E. K., 540
Dritschel, B. H., 491, 492, 505
Dull, V., 458
Dunbar, K., 10
Dunn, D. S., 438
Dunning, D., 502
Dupree, D. A., 105
Durso, F. T., 487, 488
Duval, S., 10, 265, 274, 275, 572
Duval, V. H., 274
Dweck, C., 388, 433
Dweck, C. S., 6, 24, 32, 391
Dywan, J., 462, 464, 466, 472, 473

Eagly, A., 97
Eagly, A. H., 518
Easterbrook, J. A., 278, 432, 545, 551
Eastman, C., 151, 162
Eaton, W. O., 397
Ebbesen, E., 453
Ebbesen, E. B., 97, 495
Eccles, J., 172, 173
Eccles, J. E., 388

Eccles-Parsons, J., 194
Edwards, C. P., 209
Edwards, W., 343
Efran, J. S., 131, 140–142
Eibl-Eibesfeldt, I., 564, 565, 591n
Eich, E., 490
Eisenberg, N., 275, 276, 375, 393, 398, 399
Ekman, P., 140, 544, 564, 565
Ellenberger, M. F., 472
Elliott, E. S., 6, 32
Ellis, H., 548
Ellsworth, P., 140
Ely, R. J., 416, 422, 435, 437
Emler, N., 156
Emmons, R. A., 6, 17, 37, 38, 62, 111–114, 118, 531
Entin, E. E., 196
Entwisle, D. R., 577
Eppler, M., 432
Epstein, S., 377, 414–416, 428, 432
Erber, R., 98, 278, 309, 324, 334, 354, 361
Erffmeyer, E. S., 500
Ericsson, K. A., 68, 107
Eriksen, C. W., 467, 475
Erikson, E. H., 201, 202, 213, 215, 299
Eshel, Y., 433
Evans, M., 485
Ewen, R. B., 213
Ewert, O., 536
Eysenck, M. W., 545

Fabes, R. A., 276
Fair, P. L., 276
Farrell, D., 62
Fazio, R., 5
Fazio, R. H., 12, 94, 95, 111, 112, 182, 183, 185, 412, 427, 435, 456, 499
Feather, N. T., 27, 44, 55, 112, 118, 151, 152, 154–160, 162–171, 173–177, 179–182, 184, 185, 187, 196, 234, 251, 269, 506
Feigenbaum, R., 355
Feldman, N. S., 98, 378, 379, 381, 385, 395
Feldman, S., 310, 313–317, 323
Felson, R. B., 425
Feltz, D. L., 500
Fenichel, O., 588
Fenigstein, A., 112, 571
Ferguson, T. J., 374, 376, 379
Fernald, A., 432
Festinger, L., 180, 230, 333, 363, 392, 398, 408, 411, 414, 563, 591n
Festinger, L. A., 53, 54, 74
Fetzer, B. K., 504
Fiedler, K., 529, 544, 548–550, 554
Finke, R. A., 488, 499
Finn, S. E., 386
Fiorina, M., 320
Fischer, L. W., 193, 201
Fischhoff, B., 78, 438, 489, 490, 502, 506, 513
Fishbein, M., 5, 165, 183, 334, 355, 358, 501, 502
Fisk, A. D., 117
Fiske, S. T., 95, 96, 98, 106, 115, 119, 120, 179, 270, 271, 307–309, 324, 334, 354, 361, 362, 370, 396, 533, 540, 545
Flavell, J. H., 383, 570
Flay, B. R., 469

Fletcher, G. J. O., 371, 486
Flett, G. L., 375, 389
Fogarty, J. J., 491
Fogarty, S. J., 268
Foley, H. J., 488
Foley, M. A., 487, 488, 492
Folger, R., 75
Follansbee, D. J., 24
Fondacaro, R., 83
Fong, G. T., 79
Ford, D. H., 4, 42
Forest, D., 269, 283
Foreyt, J. P., 139
Forgas, J. P., 269, 284, 547
Forsyth, D. R., 574
Fowles, D. C., 133
Frank, K. F., 583
Frank, M. G., 493, 494
Frankel, G., 265
Frankiewicz, R. G., 218
Franks, J. J., 462
Fraser, S. C., 121
Freedman, I., 230
Freedman, J. L., 121, 277
Freedman, M. R., 485
Freeman, S. J., 211
Fremouw, W. J., 138
Frenkel-Brunswik, E., 112, 299, 337
Frese, M., 60
Freud, S., 3, 21, 131, 299, 563, 566, 588, 589,
    591n
Freund, T., 112, 337-339, 345-348, 357, 363n,
    364n
Frey, D., 75, 362
Frey, K. S., 387, 389, 397, 399
Friedman, A., 106
Friedman, M. L., 216, 220, 221
Friedman, S., 94
Friesen, W. V., 140
Frijda, N. H., 30, 32, 33, 36, 41, 527, 543, 544,
    554, 555
Froming, W. J., 5
Fromkin, H. L., 83
Fromm, E., 299
Frost, R. O., 283
Fuhrman, R., 545
Fuhrman, R. W., 98
Fulero, S., 485
Fultz, J., 276, 290
Furman, W., 269, 270, 284, 547

Gaa, J. P., 218
Gaertner, S. L., 276, 277
Gaines, B., 410
Galanter, E., 7, 96, 453, 562
Gale, R. M., 517
Gallagher, D., 43, 537, 542
Gallistel, C. R., 60
Ganellen, R. J., 5, 40
Gardner, B. T., 9
Gardner, H., 568
Gardner, R. A., 9
Garfinkel, P. E., 135, 139
Garner, D. M., 135, 139
Garrett, J. B., 167
Gaschke, Y. N., 284
Gatlin, D. S., 304

Gavanski, I., 509, 510, 512
Gazzaniga, M. S., 432, 455
Gelman, R., 459
Genung, V., 385
George, A. L., 299
George, J. L., 299
Gerard, H. B., 62, 74, 75
Geva, N., 269
Ghiselin, B., 109
Gibbons, F. X., 24, 274, 427
Gibson, J. J., 63, 123, 254
Giebink, J. W., 211
Gilbert, D. T., 94, 429, 431
Giles, M. W., 304
Gilligan, C., 155, 208
Gilovich, T., 493, 494, 512
Gitta, M. Z., 200, 212, 223n, 300, 349
Giuliano, T., 423, 427
Glasberg, R., 391
Gleicher, F. H., 509
Gnepp, J., 375
Goethals, G. R., 414, 486
Goffman, E., 106, 415, 421, 426, 591n
Goldberg, J., 80
Goldberg, L. R., 370
Goldman, M. S., 45
Goldman, R., 97
Goldstein, D., 488
Goldstein, K., 411
Gollin, E. S., 371
Gollwitzer, P. M., 18, 55, 61-63, 67, 69-71, 73-
    77, 80, 81, 83, 96, 102, 108, 110, 111, 114,
    186, 544
Gomes, M., 105
Goodman, C. C., 84
Goodman, J., 499
Goodman, S., 304
Goodnow, J. J., 415
Gordon, J., 136, 139
Gordon, S. E., 97, 370
Gorgoglione, J. M., 548
Gorkin, L., 435
Gottman, J. M., 387
Gouaux, C., 269
Govender, R., 94
Graf, P., 96
Graham, S., 580
Granberg, D., 301, 316
Grant, D. L., 591n
Gray, G., 5
Gray, J., 133
Gray, J. A., 41
Graziano, W., 334, 385
Graziano, W. G., 283
Green, M. L., 283
Greenberg, J., 39, 40, 58, 273, 355, 424, 483
Greene, D., 230, 231, 251
Greenwald, A. G., 410, 412, 432, 469, 470, 489,
    497, 500
Gregory, W. L., 499
Grev, R., 267
Griffin, D. W., 502, 503, 505
Griffin, J. J., 410
Griffin, M., 495
Griffitt, W., 269
Griffitt, W. B., 269
Grill, H. J., 460

Gross, A., 277
Gruder, C. L., 469
Grusec, J. E., 375, 392, 393, 398, 399
Gschneidinger, E., 491, 539
Guarino, P. A., 580
Gurin, G., 301
Gutkin, D. S., 208, 209

Ha, Y.-W., 415, 510
Haan, N., 218
Hacker, W., 60
Hafer, C. L., 221
Hagen, J. W., 81
Hager, W., 529
Hagerman, S., 27
Haith, M., 432
Halal, M., 268, 529
Hale, G. A., 81
Halisch, F., 583-585
Hall, C. S., 411
Hall, E. G., 500
Hamel, J. A., 359
Hamill, R., 311, 312, 317
Hamilton, D. L., 97, 548
Hamilton, J. C., 415
Hancock, R. D., 435
Handley, R., 134
Hanges, P. J., 45
Hanna, S. E., 197
Hannah, D. B., 370
Hanson, C., 517
Harackiewicz, J., 231, 258
Harbluk, J. L., 489
Hargis, K., 265, 275, 289
Harlow, H. F., 230
Harrison, A. A., 415
Hart, D., 402n
Hartmann, E., 589
Hartwick, J., 97
Harvey, J. H., 334, 355
Hasher, L., 452, 485, 488, 489, 491, 494, 495, 518, 529
Hashtroudi, S., 487, 492
Hastie, R., 319, 440n, 455, 471, 475, 533, 540, 546
Hatfield, E., 122, 204
Havemann, E., 204, 218
Hay, J., 122
Hayden, T., 370
Hayward, S., 193
Heatherton, T. F., 138
Heckhausen, H., 24, 55-58, 60, 63, 67, 69, 70, 73, 74, 80, 81, 102, 110, 152, 161, 162, 170, 179, 180, 186, 187, 562, 583-585
Heider, F., 230, 249, 333, 355, 369, 392, 398, 408, 409, 411, 503
Helle, P., 40
Heller, J. F., 229-232, 251, 252, 334, 433
Heller, K. A., 377, 378, 379
Hemsley, G. D., 440n
Hendersen, R. W., 170
Hendrick, C., 204, 210
Hennigan, K. M., 469
Hensler, C. P., 304
Herman, C. P., 135, 136, 138
Herr, P. M., 95
Herren, L. T., 269

Herrnstein, R. J., 153
Hersh, R. H., 208, 209
Hershey, J. C., 504, 510
Herstein, J. A., 318, 319, 322
Hervitz, E. F., 499
Hewitt, E., 337
Hewitt, E. C., 197-200, 223, 300, 349
Heyns, R. W., 564
Hibscher, J., 135
Higgins, D. S., 105
Higgins, E. T., 6, 17, 38, 41, 42, 79, 83, 84, 94, 95, 97, 100, 102, 105-107, 109, 111-114, 116, 143, 170, 171, 180, 183, 194, 198, 200, 203, 206, 229, 232, 234-237, 243, 249, 271, 274, 276, 277, 312, 323, 335, 360-362, 379, 383, 385, 386, 389, 399, 423, 427, 436, 440n, 456, 459, 465, 485, 488, 489, 507, 511, 528, 534, 541-543, 547, 551, 553-555, 563, 564, 579, 591n
Higgins, R. L., 20, 410
Hildebrand-Saints, L., 547
Hill, C. A., 421, 426, 427, 437
Hillgruber, A., 58
Hilton, D. J., 106
Hilton, J. L., 421
Hinde, R. A., 564, 565, 567
Hinich, M., 303
Hintzman, D. L., 457, 458
Hirst, W., 517
Hirt, E. R., 498
Hirtle, S. C., 308
Hitch, G., 430
Hixon, J. G., 429, 432
Hoch, S. J., 78
Hoffman, J., 388
Hoffman, M. L., 29, 142, 179, 392, 433, 579
Hofstadter, D. R., 509
Hofstede, G., 338
Hogan, H. P., 488
Hogan, R., 209
Holender, D., 455, 468
Holmes, D. S., 583
Holstein, C. B., 209, 210
Holt, K., 579
Holtz, R., 274
Holyoak, K. J., 546
Homer, P. M., 185
Hooley, J. M., 134
Hormuth, S. E., 273
Hornstein, H. A., 265
Hossey, J., 552
Houston, J. P., 204, 207
Hovland, C. I., 469
Howard, K. I., 143
Howard-Pitney, B., 98
Howe, H. E., Jr., 580
Hoyle, G., 567
Hubbard, M., 362, 505
Hubert, S., 540
Hull, C. L., 3, 132, 278, 410, 563, 591n
Hull, J. G., 9
Hult, R. E., 218, 219
Humphrey, G., 63
Hunt, J. M., 230
Hunt, W. A., 139
Huntley, C. W., 433
Hurst, P., 194

Huston, T. L., 439
Hyland, M., 32, 39

Ickes, W. J., 83
Inhelder, B., 203, 309
Insko, C. A., 75
Iran-Nejad, A., 38
Isen, A. M., 265, 267–271, 277, 279, 281, 283, 284, 287, 490, 527, 528, 540, 547, 548, 550, 554
Izard, C. E., 232, 544

Jackson, D. N., 375
Jacoby, L. L., 96, 451, 452, 457, 462–466, 468–473, 489
Jaffe, J. H., 136
Jahoda, M., 299
James, W., 93, 99, 107, 108, 436, 552
Janis, I. L., 74, 438
Janoff-Bulman, R., 26, 512
Jarvik, M. E., 136
Jasechko, J., 469, 471, 472, 489
Jecker, J. D., 74
Jensen, A. M., 392
John, O. P., 95, 370
Johnson, D. E., 377
Johnson, E., 269, 533, 542, 547
Johnson, J. T., 510
Johnson, M. K., 452, 462, 471, 482, 485, 487–489, 492, 494–496, 498, 499, 514, 518
Johnson, T. J., 355
Johnson, V., 218
Johnson-Laird, P. N., 140, 363n, 415, 453, 518, 543, 555
Jones, C. R., 84, 335, 456, 528
Jones, E. E., 62, 75, 97, 113, 117, 118, 123, 334, 355, 356, 410, 431, 440n, 493, 503, 513, 574
Jones, M., 372, 376
Jones, S. C., 410
Jordan, C., 389
Josephson, J., 375, 377
Judd, C. M., 4
Juola, J. F., 473

Kagan, J., 204, 218
Kahan, T. L., 494
Kahle, L. R., 185
Kahneman, D., 78, 103, 346, 415, 427, 431, 432, 457, 461, 462, 473, 489, 499, 501, 502, 508, 509, 512, 528
Kahneman, E., 187
Kanfer, F. H., 11, 12, 27
Kanter, R. M., 62
Kardes, F. R., 94
Karlovac, M., 380
Karniol, R., 230
Karp, L., 265, 528
Karylowski, J., 265
Kassin, S. M., 382
Katz, D., 182
Katz, L. B., 97, 548
Kauff, D. M., 474
Kaufman, C. M., 437
Kay, B. A., 44
Kayne, N. T., 504
Keasey, C. B., 210

Keats, J. G., 397
Keel, R., 385
Kelley, C. M., 96, 451, 462–464, 466, 468–473, 489
Kelley, D. J., 267, 275
Kelley, H. H., 62, 122, 242, 256, 333, 334, 343, 354–356, 385, 360, 363, 369, 370, 374, 532, 537, 574
Kelly, G., 544
Kelly, G. A., 39, 115, 415
Kelman, H. C., 205
Kelso, J. A. S., 6, 44
Keltner, D., 536, 538, 542
Kenny, D. A., 275, 533
Kenrick, D. T., 265, 271, 272, 281
Kernell, S., 304, 320
Kerr, K. L., 500
Key, V. O., Jr., 302
Kidd, R. F., 277
Kiersted, G., 19
Kiesler, L. A., 62
Kiesler, S. B., 74
Kiewiet, D. R., 305
Kihlstrom, J. F., 4, 6, 44, 98, 111, 114, 118, 423, 580
Kim, H., 278
Kim, J. I., 361, 362
Kim, J. K., 452
Kimble, G. A., 21, 99
Kinder, D. R., 301, 304, 305, 308, 316
King, G., 84, 95, 107, 111, 135, 427, 551
King, G. A., 312, 335, 360
Kinney, R. F., 75–77
Kinsbourne, M., 589
Kintsch, W., 518, 580
Kirsch, J., 528
Klahr, D., 27
Klar, Y., 334, 339
Klayman, J., 415, 510, 511
Kleck, R. E., 134
Klein, D. C., 277
Klein, R., 106, 143, 198, 232, 277
Klein, S. B., 132
Klein, Z., 433
Kleinginna, A. M., 562
Kleinginna, P. R., Jr., 562
Klerman, J. L., 276
Klinger, C. A., 394
Klinger, E., 6, 17, 27, 39, 40, 55, 109, 119
Klinger, M. R., 500
Klopfer, W. G., 425
Knight, L., 138
Koenigsberg, H. W., 134
Koeske, R., 308
Koestner, R., 563, 578, 579, 582–586
Kohlberg, L., 152–155, 158, 177, 186, 201, 202, 208, 209, 211, 218, 219, 223n, 370, 387, 393, 394, 396, 398, 400
Kohler, W., 591
Kolers, P. A., 457
Kolodner, J. L., 457
Kommer, D., 539, 549
Konecni, V. J., 277
Koriat, A., 438
Korman, A., 583
Korman, A. K., 424
Kornadt, H. J., 64

Kozlowski, L. T., 136
Kramer, D. A., 209
Kramer, G., 303
Kramer, G. H., 304
Krames, L., 142
Krantz, S. E., 269
Kreitler, H., 583
Kreitler, S., 583
Kruglanski, A. W., 112, 161, 230-232, 234, 235,
    240, 252, 333, 334, 337-339, 342-349,
    351-353, 357, 359, 363n, 364n, 540
Krull, D. S., 94, 416, 417
Kuczynski, L., 392
Kuhl, J., 4, 40, 55, 60, 83, 109, 110, 112, 118,
    119, 151, 152, 171, 177, 180-182, 186, 453,
    461, 554, 579, 591n
Kuiper, N. A., 504
Kukla, A., 22, 39, 58
Kuman, P., 440
Kumpf, M., 531
Kuna, P. H., 139
Kunda, Z., 97, 339, 487, 494, 495, 512, 513
Kunst-Wilson, W. R., 415
Kupfersmid, J. H., 211
Kurland, D. M., 80
Kutkus, A., 75

Lacey, B. C., 543
Lacey, J. I., 543
Laird, J., 529
Laird, J. D., 268
LaKind, E., 265
Lamberth, J., 197
Landau, M. O., 282
Landauer, T., 270
Landers, D. M., 500
Landman, J., 509
Lane, R. E., 299, 322
Langer, E. J., 77, 93, 94, 116, 123, 278, 438
Langston, C., 572
Langston, C. A., 112
Lank, C., 138
Lanzetta, J. T., 134
Larish, D. D., 10
Larkin, J. H., 308
Larson, R. J., 531
Larter, W. M., 308
LaRue, A., 456, 459
Larwill, L. K., 474
Lasswell, H. D., 299
Latham, G. P., 8
Lau, B., 224n
Lau, R. R., 297, 304, 305, 307, 309, 312, 317,
    321, 323, 324
Lauterbach, K., 105
La Voie, L., 40
Lazarus, R., 551
Lazarus, R. S., 34, 428, 432, 552
Leach, K., 487
Leary, M. R., 27
Lecky, P., 408, 411, 414-416, 428, 439, 591n
Leggett, E. L., 32, 391
Lehman, D. R., 79
Lehmann, H. E., 552
Lehrman, D. S., 565
Leight, K., 548
Leippe, M. R., 469, 470, 489

Leirer, O., 548
Leirer, V. O., 97
Lepper, M. R., 230-233, 236, 238, 240, 242,
    244-247, 251, 256, 270, 361, 362, 392, 498,
    505
Lerman, D., 580
Lerner, M., 85
Leshner, A. J., 565
Lessle, N., 549
Leventhal, H., 83
Levi, A., 333, 334, 360
Levin, H., 586
Levine, L. J., 553, 555
Levinger, G., 439
Levinson, D. J., 112, 299, 337
Levitt, K., 96, 432
Levy, G. D., 396
Levy, P. E., 437
Lewicka, M., 554
Lewin, K., 24, 53, 54, 97, 102, 109, 110, 115,
    118, 123, 160, 177, 180, 301, 340
Lewis, M., 193, 432
Lewis, T., 231
Lewis-Beck, M. S., 304, 305
Leyens, J., 552
Liberman, A., 97, 518
Liberman, D., 218
Libet, B., 108, 120
Lichtenstein, E. H., 105
Lichtenstein, M., 540
Lichtenstein, S., 78, 438, 502
Lichtman, R. R., 34
Lightner, J. M., 334
Lin, S., 502
Lindsay, D. S., 487, 489, 495, 499
Lindskold, S., 410, 431
Lindzey, G., 113, 411
Lingle, J. H., 540, 541
Linville, P. W., 436
Lisle, D. J., 438
Litman-Adizes, T., 27
Litt, J., 94
Little, B. R., 6
Litwin, G. H., 583
Liu, J., 489
Liu, T. J., 493
Livesley, W. J., 369, 371-373, 376, 382, 383,
    385, 394
Lobel, M., 410, 414, 437
Locke, D., 153, 155
Locke, E. A., 8, 177
Lockhart, R. S., 465
Lodge, M., 311, 318, 319, 322
Loevinger, J., 220
Loftus, E. F., 489, 495
Logan, G. D., 95, 96, 108, 119, 454, 458, 589
Lombardi, W., 109, 114, 335
Lombardi, W. J., 94
Lombardo, J. P., 281
Lord, C. G., 361, 362
Lord, R. G., 45
Lorenz, K. Z., 564, 565, 591n
Lowell, E. L., 105, 562
Luchins, A. A., 84
Ludwig, A. M., 136
Lui, L., 458
Luiten, A., 376

Lumsdaine, A. A., 469
Lund, A., 424
Lund, M., 62
Lundy, A. C., 577
Luria, Z., 396, 397
Lurie, L., 243, 541

Maccoby, E. E., 392, 586
MacFarlane, S., 272
MacIver, D., 390
Mackay, D. M., 7
Macker, C. E., 277
Mackie, D. M., 277, 279, 550
MacLennan, R. N., 375
Maddux, J. E., 178
Mahoney, H. J., 453
Maides, S. A., 359
Main, D. S., 394
Malanchuk, O., 310
Malone, B., 156
Maltese, J., 136
Mamberg, M. H., 269
Mancuso, J. C., 577-579
Mandel, M. R., 276
Mandler, G., 42, 109, 474
Mann, L., 74, 438
Manne, S., 265
Manning, M. M., 178
Manucia, G. K., 280, 282, 283, 550
Maoz, I., 237
Maracek, J., 416, 423, 435
Marcel, A. J., 107, 467-469
Marcia, J. E., 213, 215-218, 220, 221
Marcus, D. E., 387, 396
Marken, R. S., 14
Markus, H., 6, 36, 424, 427, 453, 483, 485, 495, 506, 507, 543, 562, 571-573, 580, 591n
Marlatt, G. A., 136, 139, 499
Marmurek, H. C., 440n
Marriott, M., 457
Marsh, K. L., 548
Martin, D. J., 77, 492
Martin, L., 39
Martin, L. L., 109, 114, 118, 119, 541
Martindale, C., 550
Maruyama, M., 42
Marziali, E., 143
Marzillier, J. S., 151, 162
Mascolo, M. F., 577-579
Maslow, A. H., 20, 284, 285, 299, 591n
Masters, J. C., 269, 270, 284, 547
Matarazzo, J. D., 139
Matter, J., 545
Matteson, R., 215, 216
Matthews, K. A., 24
Matthews, L. L., 290
Matthews-Simonton, S., 507
Mavin, G. H., 95, 312, 535
Maxeiner, M. E., 27
Mayer, F. S., 265
Mayer, J. D., 269, 274, 275, 277, 284, 491, 529
Mayseless, O., 342-345, 357, 359, 362
Mazlish, B., 299
McAdams, D. P., 564, 566, 583, 587
McArthur, L. Z., 94, 106, 123, 254, 355, 374
McBride, L., 216
McCall, G. J., 418

McCall, R. J., 285
McCann, C. D., 83, 97, 112, 113, 237
McCarrel, N. S., 462
McCauley, R. N., 495
McClelland, D., 105
McClelland, D. C., 56, 159, 160, 177, 206, 285, 562-567, 577, 578, 580, 582-586, 588-591
McClelland, J. L., 10, 457
McConahay, J. B., 304
McConnell, H. K., 486
McConville, B. J., 392
McCreath, H., 375
McDermott, H., 308
McDougall, W., 131, 132
McFarland, C., 486, 487, 494, 495, 508, 509
McFarlin, D. B., 182, 193, 194, 196, 197, 214, 428, 429, 437, 592n
McGinnies, E., 112
McGlynn, R. P., 5
McGraw, K., 311
McGuire, W. J., 408, 409
McKeithen, K. B., 308
McLachlan, D. R., 489, 514
McLeod, C., 564
McMillen, D. L., 274, 277
McNeill, D., 109
Mead, G. H., 414, 415, 416, 591n
Means, B., 269, 277, 547
Mecklenbräuker, S., 529
Medin, D. L., 457, 458
Mednick, S. A., 550
Meece, J. L., 172
Mehrabian, A., 574
Meichenbaum, D. H., 499
Meilman, P. W., 217
Melisaratos, N., 134
Mellers, B. A., 78
Meltzer, A. H., 304
Merikle, P. M., 469
Merluzzi, T. V., 27
Metcalfe, J., 490
Mettee, D. R., 416, 423, 435
Meyer, D. E., 109
Meyer, W. U., 58
Michela, J. L., 355
Michotte, A. E., 57
Midgley, C., 388
Milberg, S., 278
Milberg, S. J., 116
Millar, K. U., 39, 40, 42
Millar, M. G., 39
Miller, A. H., 302, 310, 311, 313, 319
Miller, A. T., 383, 389, 390
Miller, D. T., 334, 355, 358, 359, 457, 493, 508, 509, 512
Miller, F., 334
Miller, F. D., 94
Miller, G. A., 7, 96, 98-100, 102, 103, 107, 108, 110, 111, 114, 118, 453, 562, 571
Miller, I. H., 27
Miller, J. G., 209, 384, 386
Miller, J. R., 580
Miller, K., 421, 437
Miller, L. C., 105, 111, 113, 114, 117
Miller, N., 265, 281
Miller, P. A., 275
Miller, P. H., 81

Miller, R. L., 392
Miller, W., 277
Miller, W. E., 302
Miller, W. S., 300, 301
Millon, T., 216
Mills, C. J., 94
Mills, J., 269
Milojkovic, J. H., 502
Mineka, S., 170
Minsky, M., 106, 485
Mirels, H. I., 167
Mischel, H. N., 153-156
Mischel, W., 27, 83, 106, 153-156, 370, 385, 453
Mitchell, T. R., 161, 179
Miyamoto, S. F., 425
Mohr, D. M., 372
Monroe, K. R., 298, 304
Monson, T., 334, 385
Monson, T. C., 385
Montello, D. R., 272
Mook, D. G., 284, 570
Moore, B., 275
Moore, B. S., 271, 493
Moore, S. G., 392
Moran, G., 216
Mordkoff, A., 552
Moreland, R. L., 428
Morelli, G., 209
Morgan, M., 231
Mori, D., 432
Morrison, H. W., 582
Morton, J., 456, 465
Moscovitch, M., 514
Moskowitz, G. B., 95
Motowildo, S. J., 177
Mowday, R. T., 62
Moylan, S., 269, 547
Munic, D., 135
Munro, G., 213
Murgatroyd, S., 223*n*
Murphy, D. R., 487
Murray, E. J., 28
Murray, H., 113
Murray, H. A., 3, 566, 591*n*

Nakamura, Y., 474
Neely, J. H., 95, 96
Neely, R., 274
Neisser, U., 96, 98, 99, 103, 485, 493, 517, 562
Neuberg, S. L., 98, 115-117, 361, 362
Newcomb, T. M., 408, 409, 418
Newell, A., 15, 44, 98, 107, 119
Newman, L. S., 377, 378, 386, 394
Newton, J. W., 163-166, 175, 185
Newtson, D., 235
Ney, L. G., 487
Nicholls, J. G., 230, 382-384, 390, 391, 433
Nichols, M. P., 131, 140-142
Nie, N. H., 302
Niedenthal, P., 453, 562, 572
Niedenthal, P. M., 580
Nigro, G., 493
Nisbett, R., 78, 187
Nisbett, R. E., 79, 107, 230, 361, 377, 454, 455, 463, 493, 539, 546, 580
Nitsch, K. E., 462

Norman, D. A., 7, 17, 72, 96, 103, 107-111, 118, 120, 431
Norman, W. H., 27
Norton, L. W., 178
Nowicky, G., 269, 547
Nurius, P., 6, 36, 427, 453, 506, 562, 580

Oatley, K., 140, 543, 555
O'Brien, G. E., 167-170, 175
Obrist, P. A., 543
Odbert, H. S., 370
Odum, E. P., 418
Ogilvie, D. M., 42
O'Heeron, R. C., 134
Olejnik, A. B., 456, 459
Olinger, L. J., 504
Olson, J. M., 83, 200, 300, 349
Olthof, T., 376
O'Malley, M. N., 283
Ordeshook, P., 303
Ordeshook, P. C., 303
O'Reilly, C. O., III, 62
Orpen, C., 425
Ortony, A., 29, 37, 308, 537, 553, 555
Orvis, B. R., 355
Osgood, E. E., 408, 409, 411
Oster, H., 140
Ostrom, T. M., 319, 540, 541, 545
Overton, W. F., 205, 207, 387, 396
Oyserman, D., 507

Paivio, A., 588, 590
Palys, T. S., 6
Pampe, H., 529
Panskepp, J., 568
Papanek, M. L., 545
Park, B., 4, 319, 475, 533, 540
Parrott, W. J., 535
Parsons, J. E., 385, 386, 388, 391
Pasahow, R. J., 549
Patane, M. J., 179
Patrick, R., 269, 547
Patten, R. L., 583, 585
Patterson, J. R., 156
Paulhus, D. L., 96, 432
Pavelchak, M. A., 179, 334
Pavlov, L. P., 416
Peevers, B. H., 371, 382, 383
Pelham, B. W., 94, 416, 417, 419, 420, 429, 434, 436, 437, 439, 440*n*
Pennebaker, J. W., 131, 133, 134, 137, 141
Perdeck, A. C., 564
Peri, N., 349, 351, 352, 354
Perlmuter, L. C., 21, 99
Perloff, L. S., 504
Pervin, L., 6
Pervin, L. A., 86, 112, 120, 418
Peterson, C., 493
Peterson, L. M., 24, 27, 34
Petrocik, J. R., 302
Petty, R. E., 97, 112
Phillips, L. D., 502
Piaget, J., 120, 201-203, 205, 206, 210, 309
Pichert, J. W., 97, 237, 485
Pietromonaco, P., 83, 94, 115, 456
Piliavin, J. A., 276
Pilon, D. A., 566, 586, 588

Pittman, N. L., 116
Pittman, T. S., 112, 116, 229–232, 251, 252, 258, 334, 356, 357, 359–361, 410, 426, 431, 433
Pliner, P., 135, 435
Plutchik, R., 591
Podd, M. H., 211, 215, 218
Polanyi, M., 461
Polivy, J., 131, 135, 138, 142–144
Polson, P. G., 580
Pomper, G. M., 302
Porter, C. A., 493
Porter, L. W., 62
Posner, M. I., 84, 95, 96, 100, 117, 119, 453, 589
Post, R. M., 491
Post, T. A., 487
Post, W. M., 42
Postman, L., 112
Powell, M. C., 94, 95
Powers, W. T., 7, 12–16, 18, 19, 44
Pratkanis, A. R., 469, 470, 489
Pratto, F., 94, 95, 111–113, 115, 312
Predmore, S., 410, 426
Prentice-Dunn, S., 9
Press, A. N., 371
Preston, E., 361
Pretty, G. H., 232
Pribram, K. H., 7, 96, 453, 562
Price, H. D., 304
Prinz, W., 4
Prior, J. B., 319
Prüm, E., 57
Pryor, J. B., 27
Purohit, A. P., 392
Pyszczynski, T., 39, 40, 273, 483
Pyszczynski, T. A., 355, 424

Quanty, M. B., 141
Quattrone, G. A., 463, 511

Rabkin, E. S., 71
Raine, A. S., 302
Ramey, C. G., 585
Raphael, D., 207
Rapkin, D., 136
Ratajczak, H., 69
Ray, C., 223*n*
Raye, C. L., 471, 487–489, 492, 494–496, 518
Raynor, J. O., 27, 55, 158, 182, 193, 194, 196, 197, 206, 214, 377, 428, 429, 592*n*
Read, D., 509
Read, L., 136
Read, S. J., 105, 111, 113, 114, 117, 399, 415–417, 421, 422, 424–427, 435, 437
Reckman, R. F., 486
Redler, E., 392, 393, 398, 399
Reeder, G. D., 371
Regan, D. T., 277
Regan, J. W., 277
Reich, W., 299
Reis, H., 432
Reiss, S., 235, 240, 256
Reitman, J. S., 308
Reitman, W. R., 54, 582
Rempel, J. K., 474
Renwick, S., 156

Rescorla, R. A., 578
Rest, J. R., 152–154, 156, 158, 177, 186
Reus, V. I., 491
Revelle, W., 177
Reynolds, K. D., 499
Rhodebeck, L. A., 304
Rhodewalt, F., 97, 542
Rholes, 84, 97, 335, 369–377, 379, 380, 382, 383, 389–391, 394, 456, 488, 528
Rice, T. W., 304
Rich, A. R., 27
Richards, B. S., 218
Richardson, K. D., 437
Richardson-Klavehn, A., 452, 455, 464, 468
Ridgeway, D., 276
Riegel, K. F., 212
Riker, W., 303
Rimm, C., 204
Rips, L. J., 473
Risse, G., 452
Roby, T. B., 566
Rodin, J., 138, 289
Roediger, H. L., 464
Rogers, C. R., 20, 134, 135, 432, 591*n*
Rogers, M., 265, 273, 275, 286
Rogers, R. W., 9
Rogoff, B., 209
Rohrkemper, M. M., 580
Rokeach, M., 154, 156, 157, 159, 160, 163, 173, 182, 184, 185, 198, 204, 216, 337, 582, 583
Roney, C. J. R., 193, 197–200, 204, 206, 211, 214, 216, 221
Ronnis, D. L., 412
Rook, K., 83
Rosch, E., 236
Rose, K. C., 491, 529
Rosenbaum, D. A., 6, 14, 16
Rosenberg, M. J., 408, 411
Rosenblatt, P. C., 62
Rosenbloom, P. S., 107, 119
Rosenhan, D. L., 265, 271, 275, 289
Ross, J., 391
Ross, L., 78, 187, 362, 367, 376, 384, 498, 502, 503, 505, 580
Ross, M., 230, 232, 242, 334, 355, 358, 359, 486, 487, 494, 495, 497
Rotenberg, K. J., 371, 375, 376, 379, 383
Roth, S., 27
Rothbart, M., 116, 485
Rothenberg, A., 139
Rothstein, M., 230
Rotter, J. B., 27, 179, 230
Rowe, I., 218, 220
Rubin, D. B., 418
Rubin, J. Z., 62
Ruble, D. N., 79, 98, 231, 251, 369, 371, 373–383, 385–389, 391, 393–395, 397–400
Ruehlman, L. S., 549, 552
Rueter, H. H., 308
Rule, B. G., 374, 376
Rumelhart, D. E., 71, 308, 457
Rusbult, C. E., 62
Rushton, C., 223*n*
Rushton, J. P., 392
Russell, D., 580
Russell, J. A., 276
Rutter, M., 392

Ruvolo, A., 506
Ryan, R. M., 229-233, 240, 252, 579

Saari, L. M., 8
Sagotsky, G., 231
Salancik, G. R., 62, 486, 487
Salmoni, A. W., 6
Salovey, P., 265, 268, 271, 273, 275, 286, 289
Salt, P. S., 276
Sanbonmatsu, D. M., 94
Sanders, D. Y., 274
Sanford, N., 299
Sanford, R. N., 112, 299, 337
Sanft, H., 491, 529
Sanitioso, B., 512
Sanitioso, R., 97
Sanitioso, R. S., 487
Sansone, C., 258
Scarlett, H. H., 371
Schachter, S., 42, 131, 138, 276, 460, 542
Schacter, D. L., 468, 489, 514
Schaffer, M. M., 457, 458
Schaller, G. B., 272
Schaller, M., 265, 276, 282, 287, 290, 547, 550
Schaller, S., 276
Schank, R. C., 4, 15, 98, 101, 104-106, 110, 111,
    113-116, 118, 119, 453, 457
Scheff, T. J., 141
Scheier, M. F., 3, 8, 11, 17, 22-24, 26, 27, 29,
    31, 39, 42, 44, 45, 60, 111, 112, 562, 571-
    573, 575, 581, 583
Schemrer, F. W., 334
Schenkel, S., 216
Scherer, K. R., 555
Scherf, U., 529
Schiffenbaur, A., 269
Schlenker, B. R., 27, 117, 409, 410, 413, 421,
    428, 431, 439
Schlosberg, H., 80
Schmale, A. H., 272
Schmalt, H. D., 170
Schmidt, G. W., 410
Schmidt, R. A., 6, 16
Schneider, D. J., 131
Schneider, K., 170
Schneider, S. K., 510
Schneider, W., 10, 117, 453, 454, 455
Schoeneman, T. J., 414
Schooler, J. W., 488
Schpitzajzen, A., 338
Schroeder, D. A., 290, 377
Schwartz, B., 76
Schwartz, G. E., 276
Schwartz, J., 106
Schwartz, J. M., 359
Schwartz, M. F., 271
Schwartz, S. H., 157
Schwartz, P., 278, 289
Schwartzman, D. F., 499
Schwarz, N., 279, 491, 527-529, 531, 532, 535-
    537, 539-542, 545, 546, 549, 550, 552
Scott, J., 492
Seamon, J. G., 474
Sears, D. O., 304-307, 321, 323, 408, 409
Sears, P. S., 53, 180
Sears, R. R., 586, 587
Sechenov, I. M., 99

Sechler, E. S., 498, 505
Secord, P. F., 371, 382, 383, 408, 411, 414, 415,
    418
Sedikides, C., 98
Segal, J. A., 304
Seligman, C., 232
Seligman, M. E. P., 27, 277, 373
Selz, O., 54
Semmer, N., 60
Serbin, L. A., 387
Servay, W., 531
Shaffer, D. R., 204, 210, 217, 265, 267, 283, 284
Shaklee, H., 489, 506
Shalker, T. E., 265, 269, 528
Shallice, T., 17, 96, 103, 107-111, 118, 120, 239,
    453, 454
Shantz, C. U., 382
Shapiro, B., 432
Shapiro, M. J., 302
Sharp, C., 311
Shaver, K. S., 574
Shaw, K. N., 8
Sheffield, F. D., 469
Shell, R., 375
Shepsle, K., 323
Sherk, L., 270
Sherman, R. T., 500
Sherman, S. J., 4, 435, 482, 498-500, 507, 510,
    511, 540
Sherrod, D. R., 493
Sherwood, J. J., 425
Shiffman, S., 136, 139
Shiffrin, R. M., 10, 117, 453, 454, 455
Shoben, E. J., 473
Short, J. C., 83, 158, 182, 193, 197, 210, 214,
    217, 223n, 234, 337, 338, 377, 429, 440n,
    458, 564, 566, 591n, 592n
Showers, C., 4
Shrauger, J. S., 410, 414, 424, 428, 431, 439
Shu-Fang Dien, D., 219
Shulman, R. F., 486
Shyi, G. C.-W., 488
Sibicky, M. E., 290
Sicoly, F., 359, 487
Sigwart, C., 60
Silka, L., 58
Silver, R. C., 38, 40, 109, 119
Silverman, I., 424
Silvern, L., 193, 201
Simmonds, S. F., 283, 287
Simmons, J. L., 418
Simon, D. P., 308
Simon, H. A., 15, 22, 68, 98, 104, 107, 108, 308,
    320, 485
Simonton, O. C., 507
Simpson, D. D., 319
Simpson, E. L., 219
Simutis, Z., 392
Sinclair, R. C., 548, 549
Singer, J. A., 268, 276
Singer, J. E., 42, 131, 542
Singer, J. L., 276
Skelton, J. A., 97
Skinner, B. F., 3
Skov, R. B., 499, 510, 511
Skowronski, J., 540
Slaby, R. G., 387, 397

Slovic, P., 78, 79, 187
Slowiaczek, L. M., 511
Slugoski, B. R., 106
Slusher, M. P., 488
Smetana, J. G., 377, 378
Smith, D., 273
Smith, E. E., 457, 473
Smith, E. R., 44, 85, 94, 98, 100, 110, 334, 457, 458, 466
Smith, G. F., 377
Smith, M. B., 182, 299, 409
Smith, R. A., 309, 324
Smith, T. W., 231
Smythe, W. E., 457
Snell, J., 501
Sniderman, P., 321, 322
Snyder, C. R., 20, 410, 435, 589
Snyder, C. R. R., 95, 96, 453
Snyder, M., 415, 423, 427, 485, 487, 510
Snyder, M. L., 334, 338, 357, 360
Solomon, G. S., 274
Solomon, R. L., 136, 137
Solomon, S., 58
Solomon, S. K., 485
Solso, R. L., 570, 580
Sorrentino, R. M., 83, 105, 113, 137, 158, 182, 193, 197-200, 204, 206, 210-212, 214, 216, 217, 221, 223n, 234, 300, 337, 338, 349, 361, 379, 429, 435, 440n, 458, 463, 470, 564, 566, 579, 591n, 592n
Sparling, S., 277
Speer, L. K., 304
Spence, K. W., 278, 460
Spencer, J. A., 138
Spielman, L. A., 94
Spiesman, J., 552
Spilich, G. J., 485
Spiro, R. J., 485
Spores, J. M., 371
Sprecher, S., 122
Sproule, C. F., 27
Squire, L. R., 451
Srull, T. K., 4, 29, 32, 81, 84, 97, 98, 112-114, 236, 453, 456, 466, 529, 539, 540, 542
Stangor, C., 79, 235-237, 243, 361, 387, 397, 398, 489, 541, 582
Stark, H. A., 468
Stark, L. H., 136
Staub, E., 270
Steele, C. M., 139, 410, 413, 428, 439, 489
Steers, R. M., 62
Stein, N. L., 553, 555
Stein-Seroussi, A., 429
Steinberg, J., 267
Steinmetz, J. L., 498
Steller, B., 70
Stelmach, G. E., 10
Stephens, D., 385
Stephenson, B., 426
Sterling, B., 277
Sternberg, R. J., 585
Stewart, A. J., 577
Stigler, G., 304
Stillings, N. A., 568, 570, 580
Stipek, D. J., 380, 388-390, 433
Stitch, M. H., 281
Stock, C. B., 499

Stokes, D. E., 300
Stoltenberg, C. D., 178
Storm, T., 583
Stotland, E., 26
Strack, F., 279, 491, 498, 531, 539, 540, 542, 545, 550, 552
Strauman, T., 143, 198, 232, 277
Strauman, T. J., 106, 271, 276, 277
Stroh, P., 311
Stucky, R. J., 20
Stunkard, A. J., 139
Stuss, D. T., 12
Suengas, A. G., 491, 492, 494
Suinn, R., 500
Sulin, R. A., 485
Sullivan, E. V., 220
Suls, J., 208, 209
Sumner, W. G., 411
Sushinsky, L. W., 235, 240, 256
Swann, W. B., Jr., 12, 399, 408, 410, 411, 413-419, 421-429, 431, 432, 434-439, 440n, 510
Sweeney, P. D., 428
Switzer, G. E., 280, 282, 283
Szegda, M., 268, 529

Tait, R., 109, 119
Taliaferro, A., 273
Tannatt, L., 433
Tannenbaum, P. H., 408, 409, 411
Taylor, B. R., 509
Taylor, R., 491
Taylor, S. E., 20, 34, 98, 106, 270, 271, 307, 308, 396, 410, 414, 434, 437, 483, 485, 488, 505, 507, 510, 533
Taylor, T. H., 487, 495
Teasdale, J., 373
Teasdale, J. D., 27, 178, 268, 491, 528, 531
Tedeschi, J. T., 409, 410, 431
Tellegen, A., 38
Teraspulsky, L., 377
Tesser, A., 20, 39, 109, 114, 118, 119, 410, 414, 436, 437, 440n, 513
Tetlock, P. E., 98, 300, 333, 334, 355, 360, 361, 362
Thein, R. D., 81, 94, 95, 111, 115, 312, 440n, 540
Thibaut, J. W., 97, 113, 117, 118, 123, 363
Thomas, D., 204
Thompson, W. C., 275
Thoresen, C. E., 453
Threlkeld, J., 135
Tice, D. M., 415
Tinbergen, N., 564
Toda, M., 82
Tölle, R., 552
Tolman, E. C., 27
Tomkins, S. S., 140, 271, 432
Tomlinson-Keasey, C., 205
Toppino, T., 488
Tota, M. E., 94, 96, 114
Town, J. P., 334
Tracy, J. J., 210
Traupmann, J., 122
Travis, C. C., 42
Trope, Y., 197, 229, 234, 235, 237, 241-243, 251, 256, 402n, 416, 428, 562, 571, 574, 575, 581-583, 591

Trzebinski, J., 5, 105
Tubbs, D., 5
Tufte, E. R., 304
Tulving, E., 468, 484, 514
Turiel, E., 209, 210
Turnbull, W., 508
Turner, T. J., 485
Turtle, J. W., 509
Tversky, A., 78, 187, 269, 346, 415, 427, 431, 461, 462, 473, 489, 499, 502, 509, 511, 528, 533, 542, 547
Tykocinski, O., 170, 399
Tyler, J. D., 583
Tyler, T. R., 114, 118, 304, 305
Tyrrell, D. J., 94

Uleman, J. S., 93-96, 99, 106, 120, 370
Underwood, B., 271, 275, 493
Uranowitz, S. W., 485
Utne, M., 122

Vaillant, G. E., 583
Vallacher, R. R., 6, 12, 16-19, 21, 59, 108, 235, 236, 244, 454, 545
Vallone, R. P., 502
Van de Kamp, M. E., 500
van Dijk, T. A., 518
Van Hook, E., 17, 38
van Roozendaal, J., 374
Van Selst, M., 96
Van Zandt, B. J. S., 474
Vazquez, C. V., 77
Veitch, R., 269
Velten, E., 271, 276
Verba, S., 302
Vernon, P., 113
Veroff, J., 151, 152, 159, 177, 564
Vesonder, G. T., 487
Vincent, J., 271
Viscusi, D., 269, 547
Volanth, A. J., 269
Von Bargen, D., 397
von Cranach, M., 60
Vookles, J., 170, 399
Voss, J. F., 485, 487
Vroom, V. H., 161, 179

Wachtel, P. L., 418
Waddell, B. A., 270, 284
Wadden, T. A., 139
Wade, C., 372, 376, 390
Wadell, B., 528
Wageman, R., 231
Wagener, J., 529
Wagener, J. J., 268
Wagner, D., 539
Wagner, J. A., 218
Wahler, R. G., 493
Walhood, D. S., 425
Walker, L. D., 377
Walker, L. J., 218
Wallace, J., 277
Wallington, S. A., 277
Walster, E., 74
Walter, A. A., 488
Walter, C. B., 6
Walters, C., 389

Walters, J., 370
Wang, A. Y., 487
Warr, P., 38
Warren, R. E., 84
Warrington, E. K., 451
Warsh, S., 135
Wason, P. C., 363n, 415
Waterman, A. S., 214-216
Waterman, C. K., 214-216
Waters, E., 276
Watkins, M. J., 529
Watson, D., 38
Watson, D. L., 42
Watson, J. S., 585
Watt, H. J., 63
Wattenberg, M. P., 310, 319
Weary, G., 20, 355, 547, 548
Weatherford, M. S., 303
Weber, M., 167
Weber, R., 370
Wegner, D. M., 6, 12, 16-19, 21, 59, 108, 131, 137, 138, 235, 236, 244, 427, 454, 545
Weiby, M., 355
Weimer, W. B., 335
Weinberg, R. A., 224n
Weinberger, D. A., 276
Weinberger, J., 562-564, 586
Weiner, A. S., 207
Weiner, B., 27-29, 55, 118, 132, 162, 171, 177-179, 181, 197, 284, 285, 334, 355, 359, 360, 373, 471, 545, 562, 571, 574, 575, 579, 580, 582, 591
Weingartner, H., 491
Weinstein, N. D., 410, 504
Weiskrantz, L., 451
Weiss, M. G., 81
Weiss, R., 218
Weiss, R. F., 281
Wellborn, J. G., 230
Wells, G. L., 509, 510, 512
Wells, R. S., 203
Wendt, H. W., 583
Wenzlaff, R. M., 416
Wessler, R., 220
West, S. G., 549
Weyent, J. M., 271, 280, 283, 550
White, L. A., 583, 585
White, R. W., 182, 230, 285, 299, 589
White, T. L., 131
White, W., 440n
Whitehouse, K., 473
Wicklund, R. A., 10, 18, 62, 66, 75, 83, 210, 274, 275, 334, 338, 357, 360, 412, 461, 463, 488, 572
Wilensky, R., 98, 100, 104, 105, 110, 111, 114, 115, 118, 119
Wilkin, N., 535
Williams, J. M. G., 491-493, 505
Williams, M., 277
Wills, T. A., 34, 410, 437
Wilson, E. O., 3, 418, 565
Wilson, G. D., 156
Wilson, T., 539
Wilson, T. D., 5, 107, 432, 438, 454, 455, 463, 580
Wimer, S., 370
Winograd, T., 72

Winter, D. G., 566, 567, 577
Winter, L., 94, 95
Witherspoon, D., 452, 465, 466, 474
Wolff, P. L., 267, 275
Wolff, W., 433
Woloshyn, V., 468, 470, 471
Wonderly, D. M., 211
Wong, P. T. P., 27, 545
Wood, J. V., 34
Wood, M. E., 371
Woodworth, R. S., 80
Woolever, D. K., 27
Wooley, O. W., 135
Wooley, S. C., 135
Worchel, S., 75
Worth, L. T., 277, 279, 287, 550
Wortman, C. B., 27, 38-40, 513
Wright, H. F., 106
Wright, J. B., 334
Wright, J. C., 385
Wright, R. A., 58, 179
Wright, T. L., 178
Wundt, W., 268
Wurf, E., 507
Wyer, R. S., Jr., 4, 29, 32, 84, 97, 98, 112-114,
    236, 370, 453, 456, 466, 528, 529

Yaniv, I., 109
Yarkin, K. L., 334
Yarrow, M. R., 371
Yerkes, R. M., 54
Yinon, Y., 282
Yoken, C., 143

Zacker, J., 216
Zacks, R. T., 491, 529
Zajonc, R. B., 83, 96, 134, 415, 428, 431,
    432, 483, 485, 495, 506, 538, 539, 543,
    580
Zakai, D., 349, 351, 352
Zangwill, O. L., 494
Zanna, M. P., 83, 333, 474, 486, 529,
    542
Zax, M., 141
Zbrodoff, N. J., 96
Zeevi, G., 230
Zehner, K. S., 498
Zeiss, A. R., 453
Zevon, M. A., 38
Zillman, D., 107, 529, 542
Zubek, J. M., 158, 193, 377
Zuckerman, M., 334, 355, 358, 410
Zukier, H., 84

Subject Index

Ability perceptions, 388–392
Abstinence violation effect, 136
Abstract representations, 107
Accessibility, 236, 243, 244, 248
  definition, 335
  memory biases, 488, 489
  and predicting the future, 499
  and self-verification, 435
Accountability
  and closure, 362, 363
  and social judgment, 98
Achievement
  expectancies and valences, 181, 182
  motivation model, 574, 575, 582, 591n
  resultant values, 196, 197
  and self-evaluation, children, 388–392
  self-verification role, 423
ACT* model, 109, 110
Action, 3–45
  mind-set role, 63–67
  phase model, 53–62
  role of emotions, monitoring, 29–43
  Rubicon model, 55–62
Action identification, 6
Action orientation, 461, 463
Action-oriented representations, 105
Active processes (see Effortful processes)
Activity engagement
  affective responses, 239, 240
  determinants, 236, 237
  inferences, 240–243
  and intrinsic-extrinsic motivation, 252–259
  stability and change, 243–247
  theory of, 229–264
Activity level, and mood, 276–278
Actual-ideal self discrepancy, 41, 42
Adjustment heuristic, 502
Affective states
  cognition interaction, theory, 142–144
  and disengagement, 39, 40
  and expectancies, 26, 28
  generalization, 533, 539
  informative function, 527–555
  judgment basis, 538–541
  mental processing effects, 543–555
  metamonitoring role, 30–43
  and mixed feelings, 37–39
  and self-enhancement, 428–434, 436–439
  valences interface, 179
Affective value, 194–201
Affiliative need, 564
Affordances, 123n
Aggression, 385, 386

Agitated negative emotions, 553, 554
Alcohol
  rebound effects, 136, 139
  and self-regulation, 9
Algorithms, 568–570, 574
Allocation of attention, 81, 82
Altruistic behavior (see also Helping behavior)
  and dispositional constructs, 392–394
  and happiness motivation, 287
Ambiguity tolerance
  certainty orientation, 216
  nonspecific closure need, 337
American Voter, The (Campbell), 300–302
Amnesia, 451, 452
Analytic memory processing, 474
Analytic reasoning, 549, 550
Anchoring effects
  and closure need, 346, 347
  probability judgments, 502
Androgyny, 224n
Anger, and helping behavior, 278
Anorexia nervosa, 135, 139
Anti-plans, 116
Anxiety, interruption role, 42, 43
Apperception, 491, 492
Appetitive behavior, 135, 136
Approach situations, 553, 554
Arousal
  helping behavior role, 277, 278, 284
  in inhibitors, 134
  and mood, 276–278
  perception of, 342, 343
Artificial intelligence models, 98, 99
Associative network model
  and awareness, 109, 110
  cognitive psychology, 569, 570
Atkinson's risk-taking model, 54, 55
Attention (see also Self-attention)
  and mind-sets, 81, 82
  mood effects, 271–276, 288, 545, 548
Attitudes
  activation of, 182–186
  behavior link, 183
  influence on memory, 486
Attribute ambiguity, 357
Attribution theory, 574
Attributions (see also Causal attributions)
  cognitive science relationship, 574
  debiasing of, 361, 362
  epistemic motivation, 357–360
  and expectancies, affect, 26, 28, 29
  and focus, 493, 494
  and need for closure, 354–360

Attributions (*continued*)
   temporal factors, 493, 494
   unconscious memory influence, 472–475
Authoritarian Personality, The (Adorno), 299
Authoritarianism
   dispositional judgments, 377
   nonspecific closure need, 337
   uncertainty orientation, 205, 206, 216
Autobiographical memory
   biases, 488, 489
   in depression, 505
   mood effects, 491
   truncated searchers, 489
Automaticity, 93–103
   versus conscious processing, 117–122
   and determinism, 120–122
   feedforward control, 9, 10
   goal activation, 96, 100, 111
   hierarchical feedback, 16
   individual variability, 115, 116
   and mind-sets, 84
   motivation, 100–112
   in social interaction, 93–130
   versus unconscious memory theory, 454, 455
Auto-motives, 93–130
Availability
   and accessibility, 335
   in predicting the future, 499
   and unconscious memory, 473
Avoidance situations, 553, 554
Awareness, 106–109

Bandura's theory, 11, 28
Behavior intentions
   versus goal intentions, 57, 61
   and predictability of behavior, 501, 502
Berscheid's theory, 43
Bias
   closure need effect, 335, 356, 361, 362
   and mind-sets, 73–79
   and preconceptions, 485–487
Binge behavior, 135, 136
Bowlby's model, 564
Bucci's model, 588, 590
Bulimia nervosa, 139

"Can" self, 508
Cantor's model, 572–574, 583
Capture error, 103
Carver and Scheier's model, 571, 572, 583
Category accessibility
   versus mind-set theory, 84
   motivation as, 455–459
   versus unconscious memory theory, 455–459
Catharsis of emotion, 141, 142
Causal attributions, 333–364
   and algorithms, 574
   and closure need, 354–360
   developmental trends, 376, 377
   epistemic motivation, 359, 360
   motivation and information role, 333–364
Causal reasoning
   cognitive science explanation, 574
   negative affect relationship, 545, 546, 549
Central-incidental learning task, 81
Certainty orientation
   cognitive level, 204–207

ego identity, 216, 217
individual differences, 197, 198
moral thinking, 158, 210
nonspecific closure need, 338
personality functioning, 197–201
self-verification, 435
Change decision experiment, 69, 70
Choice motivation, 55
Chronically accessible goals, 111–119
Chronically accessible political constructs, 312, 313, 317
Chunking
   affective state effect, 548
   political cognition, 308, 309
Closed-mindedness, 204, 210
Closure need
   attributions role, 354–360
   in epistemic motivation, 335–342
   experimental studies, 342–354
   and personality, 337, 338
   social interaction implications, 363
Cognition
   emotion interaction, theory, 142–144
   interactions across time, 482–484
   and mind-sets, 67–82
   political motivation, 306–323
Cognitive architecture, 570
Cognitive capacity, 551, 552
Cognitive consistency (*see* Consistency motive)
Cognitive constructs, 312, 313
Cognitive development
   and dispositional constructs, 383, 384
   stage theory, 203–207
   and uncertainty orientation, 203–207, 218, 219
Cognitive dissonance (*see* Dissonance models)
Cognitive models, 562–592
   criticisms, 579–581
   theoretical basis, 562–576
Cognitive psychology, 569–571, 579–581
Cognitive science, 568, 569, 579, 580
Cognitive structures
   and goals, 4–6
   political cognition, 312, 313
Cognitive tuning, 67–73
Commitment, 62
Comparator, 7
Compensatory self-enhancement, 410
Competence, 233, 234
Concrete thought, 204–207
Confabulation, 488
Confidence
   and closure need, 349–354
   and predicting the future, 502–506
Conflict
   and goal hierarchies, 17
   mixed emotions, 37–39
Congruence bias, 510
Congruous information, 71–73
Conscious processing (*see* Effortful processes)
Consciousness
   "edit" function, 454
   goal formulation, 453–455
   and self-enhancement, 433
Conservatism Scale, 156
Conservative politics, 313, 314, 323*n*

Consistency motive (*see also* Self-verification)
  and behavior, children, 398, 399
  development of, 393
  historical perspective, 411–413
  and self-enhancement theory, 410, 411
  source of, 399
  and theoretical trends, 408, 409
Construction, 483
Context-specificity, 461
Control concept
  connotations, 27–29
  and determinism, 120–122
  job-seeking behavior study, 167–171
  nonspecific closure need, 357, 359
  self-verification role, 415, 416
Control motive, 116, 415, 416
Counterexplanation task, 505
Counterfactuals, 508–510
Creativity, 550, 551
Cued recall experiment, 71–73
Cultural factors
  dispositional constructs, 384, 385
  and stage theory, 219, 220
Current concerns theory, 55, 109
Current processing goal, 98, 99
Current self-concept, 573

Debiasing, 361, 362
Decision making, 278–280, 288
Declarative knowledge, 44*n*
Defining Issues Test, 156
Deindividuation, 9
Dejected negative emotions, 553, 554
Deliberative mind-sets, 64–75
  illusion of control study, 75–78
  and open-mindedness, 79–82
  probability judgments, 78, 79
Delinquent adolescents, 507
Delusional syndromes, 488
Denial, 134, 135
Depressed children, 392
Depression
  analytical reasoning, 549, 552
  autobiographical memory, 505
  biased imagination, 504, 505
  disengagement theory, 39, 40
  helping behavior, 550
  information seeking, 547, 548
  overgeneral encoding, 492, 493
  social interaction choices, 418
Depressive realism
  analytic reasoning, 549, 552
  illusion of control study, 78
  and imagination, 504, 505
Determinism, 120–122
Dialectical theory, 212
Dichotic listening study, 95
Dieters, 135, 136, 138, 139
Directed recollection, 471, 472
Discounting, 358
Discrepancy concept (*see* Self-discrepancy)
Disengagement
  behavioral consequences, 24, 25
  and negative affect, 39, 40
  override function, 40
  and self-regulation, 22–29, 39, 40
Disequilibrium, 210, 211

Dispositional constructs, 369–402
  changes in, 382–386
  cognitive factors, 383, 384
  concept, 370–386
  cultural factors, 384, 385
  in depressed children, 392
  developmental aspects, 369–402
  interpersonal perceptions, children, 394–396
  invariance perception, 388–394
  matching rule, 379–382
  motivational factors, 384–386
  prediction studies, 373–378, 503, 504
  rules for, 379–382
  in self-evaluation, 388–392
  versus situational factors, 493, 494
  temporal perspective, 493, 494
  and valences, 380, 381
Dispositionalism, 503
Dissonance models (*see also* Consistency
    motive)
  helping behavior, 277
  versus Rubicon model, 62
  theoretical trends, 408–410
Divided attention, 471, 472
Dopamine, 565
Drives
  motivational underpinning, 132, 133
  unconscious memory influences, 459–461
Drug addiction, 139
Drug withdrawal, 136, 137, 139
Dual-coding model, 588
Dynamic orientation, 461, 463

Eastern value system, 219
  dispositional constructs, 384, 385
  uncertainty orientation, 224*n*
Eating behavior, 135, 136, 138, 139
Ecological perception, 122*n*, 123*n*
Economics, 302–304, 320
Efficacy expectations, 27–29, 161, 162
Effortful processes
  versus automatic processes, 117–122
  and determinism, 120–122
  feedback control, 7–10
  and goal precedence, 118, 119
  and mind-sets, 84
  response to environment role, 94–96, 120–122
  social interactions, 94–97
Ego functioning, 21, 22, 589
Ego identity
  moral development relationship, 218, 219
  uncertainty-orientation role, 213–219
"Elan to maximize," 284–286
Elation (*see* Happiness)
Elderly
  formal thought potential, 207
  moral reasoning, 211
Electroencephalography, 108
Emotion
  behavioral cue role, 140–142
  catharsis role, 141, 142
  cognition interactions, theory, 142–144
  informative function, 536–538
  metamonitoring function, 29–43
  in self-evaluation, children, 391, 392
Empathy (*see* Helping behavior)

Employment, 166–171
Encoding
    influence of preconceptions, 485–487
    mood effects, 534, 535, 548, 549
    and type of focus, 492, 493
Environmental control, 120–122
Episodic memory
    attributions influence, 472–475
    automaticity theory comparison, 454, 455
    motivation influence, 451–481
    versus priming theory, 457–459
Epistemic motivation
    attribution theory implications, 357–360
    dimensions, 334–352
    experimental studies, 342–354
    and social interaction, 363
Erikson's ego identity stages, 213–219
Ethological model, 564, 565
Evaluative judgments (see Judgment)
Evaluative mind-sets, 66, 67
Executive process, 99
Expectancy
    and action, values, 151–192
    and affect, 26, 28
    conceptual analysis, 27–29, 159–163, 178–180
    in goal attainment, 22–26
    influence on recall, 485
    and self-regulation, 22–24
    thought processes, 34, 35
    types of, 161, 162
    and valences, 180–182
Expectancy–value model, 151–192
    comparative analysis, 177, 178
    unconscious memory comparison, 461
Expressed emotion, 134
Expressive behavior, inhibition, 137
Externality, 138
Extrinsic motivation, 229–264
    and activity engagement, 252–259
    versus intrinsic motivation, 229–235
Eyewitness testimony, 489

Facial expression, 134
Failure expectancy, 24
Failure feedback, 389, 390
Fairy tale experiment, 70, 71
Fame judgment task, 469, 470
Familiarity
    and moral level, 211
    unconscious memory role, 473
Fantasy, 566
Fear
    and expectancies, 24
    misattribution, 537
Feedback control
    effortful action, 7–9
    hierarchical organization, 12–22
    role of emotions, 29–43
    self-regulation, 4–12
    self-verification role, 424–427
Feedforward control, 9, 10
Feelings-as-information, 527–555
Festinger's theory, 409, 411
Field theory
    goal activation, 102
    political motivation applications, 301
Flow experience, 66

Fluency heuristic, 473
Focus phenomenon, 491–494
"Foot-in-the-door" effect, 393
Foreclosed identity status, 216, 217, 220, 221
Formal thought, 204–207
Frames, and recall, 485–487
Free will, 120
"Freezing" effects
    and closure need, 338, 339
    debiasing, 361, 362
    impression formation, 345
Freudian theory
    id energy, 132
    and McClelland's model, 588, 589
    personality, 21, 22
    political motivation application, 299
Friendship
    negative self-view factor, 434
    self-verification influence, 417–420, 434
Fundamental attribution error
    overconfidence factor, 503
    overriding influences, 98
Future self, 506–508

Gamblers, biased beliefs, 512
Gender constancy, 387, 396, 397, 400, 401
General encoding, 492, 493
Generalization
    and affective states, 533, 534
    uncertainty-oriented, 205
Generosity-stinginess dimension, 378
Gestalt theory, 411
Goal detector, 104
Goal intention
    action phase, 57–62
    automatic activation, 100, 111
    versus behavioral intention, 57, 61
    social judgment influence, 96, 97
Goal-oriented persons, 223n
Goals
    and affect, 39
    automatic activation, 96, 99–119
    cognitive models, problem, 98, 99
    disengagement, 22–29, 39
    hierarchy of, 12–22
    phase model, 53–55
    precedence relationships, 118, 119
    in self-regulation, 4–12
    unconscious memory influences, 453–455
Group performance, 437
Guilt, 227

Habit, 459–461, 476
Happiness, 265–296
    decision-making influence, 278–280
    ethological perspective, 272, 273
    and helping behavior, 265–296
    (mis)attribution studies, 531–533
    mood management hypothesis, 282–284
    and motivation, 280–286
    theoretical framework, 266–268
Health beliefs, 512
Hedonic relevance, 355, 356
Helping behavior, 265–296
    and arousal, 276–278
    attention effects, 271–276
    decision making, 280

depression effect, 550
ethological perspective, 272
mood effect, 265-296, 550
mood management hypothesis, 281-284
motivation, 280-286
self-enrichment theory, 284-286
self-focus role, 273-276
Hierarchical model, 12-22
Higgins's model, 41, 42
Hindsight bias, 490, 511, 513
Homeostasis, 282-286
"Homunculus" problem, 99
Hormones, 565
"How Shall a Thing Be Called?" (Brown), 235
Hunger, 135, 136
Hypothesis generation
  bias, 510
  and closure need, 343, 344
Hypothesis-testing activities, 415
Hysteria, 139

Ideal self
  discrepancy effects, 41, 42
  feedback control systems, 14, 15
  future self predictions, 507, 508
  hierarchical model, 20, 21
  and self-enhancement, 436
Identity development
  and performance, 217
  self-esteem, 220, 221
  uncertainty-orientation role, 213-217
Illusion of control, 75-78
Illusion of invulnerability, 504, 505
Imagination tasks, 499, 500, 504, 505, 507
Impartiality, 74, 75
Implemental mind-sets, 65-73
  illusion of control, 75-78
  and open-mindedness, 79-82
  probability judgments, 78, 79
Implicit motives, 582-591
Important self-views, 436
Impression formation
  motivational influences, 97, 98
  primacy effects, closure, 344, 346
Individual variability
  chronic social constructs, 115-117
  motive strength, 566, 567
Information function, feelings, 527-555
Information-gathering strategies, 510-513
Information processing
  in political cognition, 322, 323
  theory of, 568-571
Information seeking, 547, 548
Information value, 194-201
Inhibitory processes, 131-147
  costs of, 133-137
  and emotion, 140-142
  physiology, 133, 134
Instinct, 132, 133
Intentional processes (see Effortful processes)
Intentions
  action phase, 57, 61
  and behavior, 501, 502
  behavioral prediction comparison, 501
  unconscious memory influence, 453, 454
Internal cues, 131-147
Internalization, children, 392-394, 399

Interpersonal interactions
  children's dispositional constructs, 394-396
  self-verification motive, 417-423
Interruption
  and anxiety, 42, 43
  in self-regulation, 22-29
Intrinsic motivation, 229-264
  and activity engagement, 252-259
  versus extrinsic motivation, 229-235
Invariant dispositions, 388-394
Invulnerability illusion, 504, 505

James, William, 108
Job-seeking behavior, 166-171
Judgment
  and affective state, 538-541
  debiasing of, 362
  epistemic model, 361
  information-functions hypothesis, 528-530
  motivations, 333-364
  recall relationship, 540, 541
  unconscious memory influence, 473, 474

Kohlberg's stage theory, 202, 208-212, 218-221
Külpe, Oskar, 63

Labeling, 392, 393
Lay epistemics (see Epistemic motivation)
Legal precedent example, 457, 458
Lewin, Kurt
  and automatic processes theory, 102, 106
  goal theory, 53, 54, 102
  political motivation application, 301
Liberal politics, 313, 314, 323*n*
Life satisfaction, 531
Life tasks, 573
Logogen model, 456-459

Mandler's theory, 42, 43
Markus's model, 572-574, 583
Maslow's theory, 20, 21
Matching rule, 379-382
McClelland's model, 563-568, 576-579
Means-end analysis, 15, 16
Memory (see also Episodic memory;
    Unconscious memory)
  attributions, 472-475
  mood effects, 268, 269, 491, 492
  self-verification, 424
  temporal factors in bias, 484-517
  unconscious influences, 451-481
  veridicality, 494-497
Mental processes, 543-555
Metamonitoring, 29-43
Meta-script, 15
Michigan approach, 297, 298, 300-302, 319, 320
Mindlessness
  versus auto-motive model, 123*n*
  and mood, 278-280
Mind-sets, 53-92
  and action phase, 63-67
  affective state effects, 544, 545
  and biased interferences, 73-79
  cognitive functioning role, 67-82
  correlates, 82-85
  historical background, 63

Mind-sets (*continued*)
  mechanisms, 82–85
  and open-mindedness, 79–82
(Mis)attribution studies, 531–533
Misprediction, 518*n*
Mixed feelings, 37–39
Mobile allocation of attention, 81, 82
Models, 562–592
Mood
  autobiographical memory effect, 491
  decision-making role, 278–280
  and helping behavior, 265–296
  informative function, 527–555
  memory effects, 268, 269
  and motivation, helping, 280–286
  orientation to environment, 274–276
  remembering bias role, 490, 491
Mood-congruent recall, 268, 269
  autobiographical memory, 491
  and helping behavior, 270
  versus information-functions hypothesis,
    528–530
Mood dependence, 490, 491
Mood-incongruent recall, 529
Mood management hypothesis, 281–284
Moral development
  cultural perspective, 219–221
  and dispositional constructs, 392–394
  and ego identity, 218, 219
  stage theory, 202, 208–212, 219–221
  uncertainty orientation effect, 208–212, 218–
    221
Moral judgment
  components, 152, 153
  individual differences variables, 158
  motivational versus developmental analysis, 177
  reasoning in, 152–155
  stages in, 155–159
  theories of, 152–155
  uncertainty-orientation effect, 208–212
  value preference role, 155–159
  and volition, 186
Moratorium effects, 211, 214, 215
Motivation
  and attributions, closure, 354–363
  automatic activation, 100–112
  development of, 111, 112
  dispositional constructs, 304–306
  helping behavior, 265–296
  interactions across time, 484
  McClelland's model, 562–592
  and mood, 280–286
  social cognition influence, 97, 98
  unconscious influences, memory, 451–481

Natural incentive, 564, 578
Need for achievement, 582
Negative affect (*see also* Sadness)
  attention effect, 271–276, 545, 548, 549
  causal reasoning, 545, 546, 549, 550
  decision-making influence, 278–280
  and disengagement, 39, 40
  helping behavior effect, 265–296, 549
  information-processing effect, 544–555
  and positive affect, 37, 38
Negative self-concept
  affect regulation, 437

cognitive consistency experiment, 412, 413
compensatory self-enhancement, 410
  salience factor, 435
  self-enhancement theory, 434–436
  self-verification theory, 417–423, 427–429,
    434–436
  social interaction choices, 417–423, 437
Neurohormones, 565, 591*n*
"New Look" research, 97, 455, 459, 475
Nodes, 569, 570
Noise judgment task, 474, 475
Nonanalytic memory processes, 474
Nonspecific closure need, 337–342
  attributions effect, 354–360
  epistemic motivation, 337–342
  experimental studies, 342–354
  and personality type, 337, 338
  social interactions implication, 363
Nonverbal system, 588
Norepinephrine, 565
Normal-vote theory, 301
Noticer, 104
Noun span, 80, 81

Obesity, 138, 139
Obsessive–compulsive disorder, 139
On-line judgments, 541
Open-loop control, 10
Open-mindedness, 79–82
Opponent process theory, 136
Orientation, 461–463
Ought self, 41, 507
Outcome expectancy
  conceptual connotations, 27–29, 161, 163,
    187*n*
  in expectancy-value approach, 187*n*
  monitoring of, 34, 35
Overconfidence, and predictions, 502–506
Overmotivation, 54

Paivio's model, 588
Patterned information, 568
Perception, and unconscious memory, 464–467
Perseveration, 40
Person perception (*see also* Dispositional
    constructs)
  unconscious memory influence, 465, 466
Personal efficacy, 28
Personal strivings, 6
Personality, 193–228
  change, 194–201
  chronic motivations, 113
  hierarchical model, 20, 21
  uncertainty orientation influence, 197–221
Personality Research Form, 375
Persuasion
  depression effects, 549, 550
  and mood, 279
Physical activity, 276–278
Physical appearance, 420
Piaget's stage theory
  dispositional constructs, 383
  and uncertainty orientation, 203–207, 218, 219
Political chronicities, 312, 313, 317
Political motivation, 297–329
  cognitive approaches, 306–323
  cost orientation, 321

economic basis, 302–304, 320
impression-based strategy, 318, 319
information-processing theories, 322, 323
memory-based strategy, 318, 319
Michigan approach, 300–302, 319, 320
psychodynamic theory, 299, 300
rational-choice theory, 302–304, 320
self-interest, 302–304, 321, 322
symbolic politics theory, 304–306
Positive affect (*see also* Happiness)
attention effect, 271–276, 548
creativity, 550, 551
and decision making, 278–280
helping behavior effect, 265–296
information-processing effect, 544–555
mood management hypothesis, 282–284
and negative affect, 37, 38
Positive self-concept, 434, 435
Possible selves, 506–508, 572–574
Power motive, 566, 567, 587
Powers's model, 12–15, 44*n*
Preconceptions, 485–487
Preconscious (*see also* Automaticity)
and social interaction, 93–130
Predictability need, 416
Predicting the future, 500–505
Prejudice, 206
Preservation goals, 116
Primacy effects, 344–346
Priming
versus unconscious memory, 456–459, 464–467
word identification, 464–467
Principle control, 14, 18–22
Private self, 571, 572, 591*n*
Proactive goals, 118, 119
Probability judgments, 78, 79
Procedural knowledge, 44*n*, 547
Process-oriented persons, 223*n*
Program control, 15–19
Projection
in political choice, 315, 316
and unconscious memory, 463
Projective techniques
chronic motive activation, 105
and unconscious memory studies, 475
Prosocial behavior (*see also* Helping behavior)
consistency motive, 398
and dispositional constructs, 392–394
Protestant Ethic Scale, 167
Psychodynamic theory
and McClelland's model, 588, 589
personality, 21
political motivation, 299, 300
versus unconscious memory theory, 451
Psychological career, 195, 215, 216
Psychological situation, 106
Public self, 571, 572
Purposive goals, 120

Q-sort, 310

Rational choice, 302–304, 306, 307, 320
Reactive goals
definition, 101, 102
in social interaction, 104–106, 115–117
Readiness potential, 108
Reading a word, 465

Reality monitoring, 487–490
Rebound effects, 138, 139
Recall (*see also* Mood-congruent recall)
influence of preconceptions, 485–487
judgment relationship, 540, 541
mood effect, 268, 269
in self-verification, 424
Recognition memory, 474
Reconstruction, 483
Reference values
emotions role, monitoring, 32
in metamonitoring, 36, 37
in self-regulation, 8, 9, 14, 15
time dependence, 37
Repressors, 134
Restrained eaters, 135, 136, 138
Resultant value, 196
Retrieval-based judgments, 541
Risk-taking model, 54, 55
Rokeach Value Survey, 156
Rubicon model
action phases, 55–62
versus hierarchical models, 60

Sadness, 265–296
ethological perspective, 272, 273
and helping behavior, 265–296
mood management hypothesis, 281, 282
and motivation, 280–286
theoretical framework, 266–268
Schemas
in cognitive psychology, 570, 571
in goal specification, 4–6
influence on recall, 485–487
motivation model, 571–576
political cognition, 307–323
unconscious memory comparison, 455–459
Scripts, 15
Selective attention, 423–426
Self-actualization, 20, 21
Self-attention
feedback process, 8, 9
and helping behavior, 274–276
mood effects, 273, 274
and self-regulation, 8–12
Self-attributed motives, 582–591
Self-awareness, 9–12
Self-blame, 513
Self-certainty, 422, 423
Self-concept (*see also* Negative self-concept)
social interaction choices, 417–423
verification motive, 414–420, 434–436
Self-consistency (*see* Consistency motive)
Self-determination, 233, 234
Self-discrepancy
and affect, 180
and expectancy–value theory, 183, 184
feedback, 426, 427, 435
future self application, 507, 508
uncertainty orientation, 198
Self-efficacy
versus expectancy–value theory, 177, 178
and expectation, 162
job-seeking behavior study, 167–171
Self-enhancement, 408–441
affective aspects, 428–434, 436–439
and cognitive-consistency theory, 409–411

Self-enhancement (*continued*)
  compensatory version, 410
  developmental aspects, 432, 433
  historical influences, 410, 411
  mental processes, 429–434, 438, 439
  versus self-verification theory, 427–441
Self-esteem, 20 (*see also* Self-enhancement)
Self-evaluation
  and achievement, children, 388–392
  dispositional construct development, 388–392
  intrinsic-extrinsic motivation, 232
  role of emotions, 391, 392
Self-fulfilling prophecy effects, 499
Self-guide, 6
Self-handicapping, 513
Self-image, 214–217
Self-interest, 302–304, 320
Self-regulation, 3–52
  and disengagement, 22–29, 40
  emotions, metamonitoring, 29–43
  feedback control, 4–12
  feedforward process, 9, 10
  hierarchical model, 12–22
  principles of, 3–52
Self-reported motivation, 580–587
Self-schema, 571–576 (*see also* Schemas)
  cognitive structure, 571
  definition, 591*n*
Self-serving biases, 355, 356, 512
Self-verification, 408–441
  and affect, 436–439
  cognitive aspects, 428–434
  developmental perspective, 432, 433
  friendship choices, 417–420
  identity cues, 420, 421
  mental processes, 429–434, 438, 439
  origins, 414–417
  pragmatics, 436–439
  selective attention, 423–426
  self-discrepant feedback effect, 426, 427
  versus self-enhancement theory, 427–441
  social interaction role, 415, 417–423
  strategies, 417–426
  theory of, 414
Semantic-dispositional category, 381
Sequence control, 15, 19
Sex roles
  consistency motive, 398, 399
  invariant perception of, 387, 396, 397
  uncertainty orientation, 224*n*
Sign stimulus, 564
Simulation heuristic, 499
Situation-specific goals, 114, 115
Situational norms, 106
Skin conductance, 134
"Sleeper" effect, 469
Smoking behavior, 136, 139
Social approval, 356
Social comparison
  self-evaluation development, 388
  and self-verification, 437
Social environment, 417–423
Social interaction
  auto-motive model, 111–122
  children's constructs, 394–396
  and closure need, 363

conscious versus automatic processing, 117–122
  and epistemic motivation, 363
  negative self-concept influence, 417–420
  preconscious determinants, 93–130
  self-verification function, 415, 417–420
Social judgment, 93, 94
Social perception
  automatic influences, 93, 94
  mood effects, 269
Social traits (*see* Trait constructs)
Social withdrawal, 385, 386
Socialization, 393
Source goal, 103
Source monitoring, 487–490
Specific closure need
  attributions effect, 355, 356
  in epistemic motivation, 335–342
  experimental studies, 342–354
Spontaneous recollection, 471, 472
Stage theory, 201–221
State orientation, 461, 463
Static orientation, 461, 463
Stereotypes
  automatic processes, 95
  and closure need, 347–349
  debiasing, 361, 362
  influence of expectancies, 485, 488
  motivational influences, 97, 98
Strategic self-presentation, 429–439
Stroop paradigm, 95, 96
Subjective confidence, 342, 343
Subjective well-being, 531
Suicide, 492, 493
Supervisory attentional system, 103
Symbolic politics theory, 304–306
Synchronization, 212

Task complexity, 540
Telic Dominance Scale, 223*n*
"Test-operate-test-exit" model, 102
Thematic Apperception Test, 463, 566, 567, 577, 578
  reliability, 577, 578
Thought sampling experiment, 67–69, 75
Thought suppression, 137, 138
Thresholds, 489
Time dependence of reference values, 37
"Tip-of-the-tongue" phenomenon, 109
Tool versus object metaphor, 461–463, 471, 472
TOTE model, 102, 103, 453
Traditional motivation models, 562–592
Trait constructs (*see also* Dispositional constructs)
  and automatic processing, 95
  chronic accessibility, 113
Trauma, 137
Trope's model, 574, 575, 583
Truncated searches, 489
Type-of-inference approach, 231–234
Type-of-motivating property, 249–252
Type-of-need approach, 231–233

Uncertainty orientation, 193–228
  cognitive development interpretation, 203–207, 218, 219
  cultural perspective, 219–221

dialectical theory, 212
ego identity development, 213-219
individual differences, 197, 198
moral development, 208-212, 218, 219
moral thinking, 158
and nonspecific closure need, 337, 338
personality functioning, 194-201
self-discrepancy, 198
self-verification, 435
Unconscious, political motivation, 299, 300
Unconscious memory
automaticity comparison, 454, 455
versus conscious influences, 453-455
controversy, 467, 468
empirical issues, 464
and habit, 476
motivational influences, 451-481
opposition studies, 467-472
and orientation, 461-463
Unemployment, 166-171

Valences
conceptual analysis, 178-180
dispositional construct formation, 380, 381
and expectations, 180-182
and values, 159-178
Value-expressive sets, 113, 114, 118

Value of achievement, 582
Values
and actions, model, 151-192, 196
activation of, 182-186
affect role, 184, 185
influence on moral reasoning, 155-159
motivational versus developmental analysis, 177
versus motives, 159
personality influence, 174-201
socialization effect, 156, 157
volition role, 186
Velocity analogy, 30, 33
Velton Mood Induction Procedure, 271, 276
Volition, and values, 186
Volitional strength, 57, 58
Volutionale Objektion, 102
Voter Decides, The (Campbell), 301

Weiner's model, 574, 575
Western value systems, 219, 224*n*, 384, 385
Will psychology, 54, 58, 60, 102
Word identification, 464-467
Working self-concept, 573
Würzburg school, 63, 96

Yerkes-Dodson law, 54